Drug-Induced Neurological Disorders

Drug-Induced Neurological Disorders

K. K. Jain

MD, FRCS(C), FRACS, MFPM, FFPM
Consultant in Pharmaceutical Medicine
Basel, Switzerland

2nd completely revised edition

Hogrefe & Huber Publishers
Seattle · Toronto · Bern · Göttingen

This book is dedicated to my wife Verena and my children Eric, Adrian and Vivien Jain for their patience and understanding during its preparation.

Library of Congress Cataloging-in-Publication Data

Jain, K.K. (Kewal K.)
Drug-induced neurological disorders. 2nd ed.
Includes bibliographical references and index.

1. Nervous system – Diseases – Etiology. 2. Neuropharmacology. 3. Drugs – Side effects. I. Title.
RC 346J35   2001   616.8'0471   C99-932047-5

Canadian Cataloguing in Publication Data

Jain, K.K. (Kewal K.)
Drug-induced neurological disorders / K.K. Jain. – 2nd ed.
  p.; cm.
Includes bibliographical references and index.

1. Neurotoxicology. 2. Drugs – Side effects. 3. Neuropharmacology. I. Title.
[DNLM: 1. Nervous System Diseases – chemically induced. WL 140 J25d 1999]
RC347.5.J35   2001   616.8'0471 – dc21   99-042853

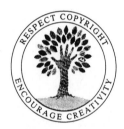

ISBN 0-88937-219-5
Hogrefe & Huber Publishers, Seattle • Toronto • Bern • Göttingen

© 2001 by Hogrefe & Huber Publishers

USA: P.O. Box 2487, Kirkland, WA 98083-2487
                        Phone (425) 820-1500, Fax (425) 823-8324
CANADA: 12 Bruce Park Avenue, Toronto, Ontario M4P 2S3
                        Phone (416) 482-6339
SWITZERLAND: Länggass-Strasse 76, CH-3000 Bern 9
                        Phone (031) 300-4500, Fax (031) 300-4590
GERMANY: Rohnsweg 25, D-37085 Göttingen
                        Phone (0551) 49609-0, Fax (0551) 49609-88

Printed in Germany

Foreword

When a new drug first enters preclinical studies, these are directed to determine the mechanism of primary action, pharmacokinetics, and in vivo toxicity. Though screening tests are undertaken, very little information is usually obtained on secondary activities of the drug and on its interaction with other drugs.

When a potential pharmaceutical compound moves from the preclinical to the clinical phase of study, this introduces another order of complexity, mainly the difference between human metabolism and that of animals. Moreover, the complexity of the human nervous system and human awareness provides the basis for a whole new series of effects and side effects. Some of these become obvious in Phase I trials in humans, but the number of subjects is always small at this stage. As the drug moves into Phase II and Phase III studies, less frequent toxicity reactions begin to be experienced. These include the development of antibodies with a host of immunologically mediated side effects. Additionally, in the human population, there are some individuals with unusual metabolisms who produce abnormal pharmacokinetics, and hence high blood levels of the drugs. Phase III and IV studies that are used to assess efficacy and the risk-benefit ratio of a medication often involve 500 to 5000 patients. With this number, it might be expected that most of the potential side effects of a drug would have been discovered by the end of this stage of pharmaceutical development.

Unfortunately, this is not so. Some idiosyncratic reactions have an incidence of only 1 in 10,000 or 1 in 100,000 patients. If the idiosyncratic reaction is fatal, even reactions with this rarity may lead to withdrawal of the trial medication. Additionally, many of the uncommon adverse drug reactions (ADRs) go unrecognized for a considerable period after the drug is released. Reasons include that the ADR is very different in type from the primary effect of the drug, that the ADR is very similar to a spontaneous human disease, or that the ADR only results from drug interaction with other drugs or metabolic disorders. It is not until a pattern of such disorders is recognized in a cohort of patients taking a certain drug that it comes under suspicion for being responsible for an ADR.

Post-marketing surveillance by pharmaceutical companies is especially important for recognition of these ADRs. Companies are generally effective in collecting and cataloging such reports. The World Health Organization maintains a registry of adverse drug reactions. The medical/scientific literature is also an important vehicle for reports of potential ADRs, for this is often the mechanism by which clinicians raise the first suspicions that an unusual medical complication might be an ADR. When a very unusual medical condition is first seen, it is never certain whether it is due to a drug or not. When it is seen a second and a third time in relation to treatment with a certain drug, than the association becomes more likely. It is essential that physicians have a high index of suspicion. Undoubtedly, a very large number of such ADRs are missed, either because the physician was suspicious but never saw a second instance of the disorder, or was too busy to report it. The rate of reporting of ADRs is undoubtedly quite low throughout the world.

However, to be set against this low rate of recognition of ADRs is the fact that the literature and pharmaceutical industry data banks are full of single case reports of potential complications of every drug. A glance at the Physicians' Desk Reference reveals the enormous range of complications of each drug that the practicing physician is warned about. One of the problems of such product information is that ADRs recognized early in the development of a drug, even though they may be extremely rare, tend to get fossilized in this information. No attempt is ever made to eliminate reference to such side effects that turn out to have extremely low frequencies. It is likely that many such reports of apparent ADRs are not due to the drug in question, or are rare idiosyncratic reactions. From a scientific point of view, one would like some index of the frequency of each suggested ADR. Unfortunately, not only is the frequency of reporting low, but certainty of the causality is often absent, and the denominator of drug dose times patient years is unknown. We might hope that patient data banks in this computer age would help. Record linkage studies such as those by Mayo Clinic or in Oxford may help, but rarely are pharmaceutical agents sufficiently clearly targeted for these studies to produce information on more than the common ADRs and common drugs.

Turning to the nervous system, we are all aware that over the last 15 years there has been an enormous explosion in knowledge of basic neurosciences. In particular, enormous strides have been made in the understanding of basic neurochemical mechanisms of the action of the nervous system, and the discovery of new classes of receptors, neurotransmitters, second messengers, and fields of neuronal functions. Each discovery has opened the way for the development of new, highly directed, and potent pharmaceutical agents. As the range in potency of these has increased, the potential for drug interaction has also increased exponentially. Such interactions can include the development of excessive therapeutic action, the blocking or abnormal increase in a normal neurological function, or frank neurotoxicity. Again, such changes will not be recognized as a specific ADR without the presence of a very observant neurologist with a high index of suspicion. The complexity of the nervous system and the rapid advance in the development of neuroactive substances explains why neurology is the major discipline experiencing this exponential rise in drug-induced disorders.

How can we improve the dissemination of information about neurological ADRs? One source of information is the Physicians' Desk Reference. For each drug, there are a reported series of complications divided under region of the body. Under the central nervous system, almost all drugs are reported to cause nausea, drowsiness, dizziness, and tremor. It is interesting that these are also the most frequent side effects experienced by subjects taking placebo medication in double-blind controlled trials. Hence, they may not be due to the specific effect of the drug in question. Another source of information is to review textbooks of disease. In the field of neurology, each chapter or monograph includes some description of drug toxicity affecting this system. Textbooks of neuropharmacology and therapeutics of neurological disease often have important information, but are never comprehensive. They only deal with the most common complications that are well recognized. The data banks of ADRs, such as those of the WHO and individual pharmaceutic firms, can be helpful. However, for the practicing clinician, one has to have developed a suspicion that the unusual neurological reaction is due to a certain drug before one can approach any of these data banks. Access to pharmaceutical company reports may be difficult, for these companies are often unwilling to provide full information, and the rate at which ADRs are reported and their statistical reliability has already been discussed.

Often the neurologist comes at the situation from a different direction. The patient is exhibiting an unusual neurological syndrome, and the suspicion arises whether this could be due to an ADR. It must be remembered that polypharmacy is the order of the day, particularly in the elderly, where, if there are not five different diseases each receiving three different medications, the individual is quite unusual!

Hence, there is a great need for a monograph such as that of Dr. Jain. This attempts to collate the frequency of the rare drug-induced neurological disorders affecting each area of the nervous system and each of the many neurological functions within each area. Dr. Jain brings an unusual experience to this task. He is a neurosurgeon and neurologist who, for many years, has been a medical advisor to the pharmaceutical industry. He has an understanding of the records of ADRs in the pharmaceutical firms, and hence has access to many that are normally not surveyed in producing a compilation of drug-induced neurological disorders. He has also undertaken a very exhaustive review of the clinical literature dealing with neurological ADRs. The reader is provided with a very succinct collection of this information arranged in the clinically relevant format of individual regions of the nervous system and neurological functions.

Dr. Jain well recognizes the limitations and drawbacks of the data sources concerning ADRs that I have highlighted above. His first chapter on epidemiology and clinical significance is an excellent critical review of this field. The reader will do well to come back again and again to these points in reading the remainder of the book. In summary, there is an enormous amount of information in this book that will be of great use to the practicing neurologist.

Walter G. Bradley, D.M., F.R.C.P.
Professor and Chairman
Department of Neurology
University of Miami School of Medicine
Miami, Florida, USA

Preface to the Second Edition

A considerable amount of new information on adverse reactions to drugs has been published during the four years since the publication of the first edition. The information could fit into the chapters as organized for the first edition and no change was made in the number of chapters. Several new drugs, including some biotechnology preparations, have been introduced in medical practice and their adverse effects have been included in this edition. Considerable new information about older drugs and the pathomechanism of drug-induced neurological disorders is now available. A symptom index has been added to lead the reader to the appropriate table in the text which lists the drugs associated with that symptom or disease. A description of the role of individual drugs can be found in the following text in the same chapter. The bibliography has now been enlarged to include 3,835 citations. There were many more that could not be included due to limitation of space.

The author gratefully acknowledges the useful suggestions provided by the readers of the first edition and these were taken into consideration during the preparation of the second edition. I would like to thank Mr. Robert Dimbleby, Editor, International Division of Hogrefe & Huber for his personal attention to this project.

K. K. Jain

Preface to the First Edition

The purpose of this book is to present an account of drug-induced neurological disorders (DIND) which should be considered in the differential diagnosis of various neurological conditions. Although adverse drug reactions are under-reported, there is a vast literature on this subject but hitherto no book has been available on this subject. Publications on this subject are scattered in various journals and monographs, covering several medical subspecialties, and are not easily accessible to a practicing physician.

Using my background knowledge of neurology and of monitoring the safety of pharmaceutical products, I have critically evaluated over 5000 publications on this topic. About 3000 of these have been selected as references and information has been organized into tables and a readable text. Each disorder is discussed with listing of responsible drugs rather than description of all neurological adverse effects of individual drugs. Some drugs appear in more than one chapter. A physician investigating drug-induced peripheral neuropathy needs only to refer to the relevant chapter which contains cross references to other neurological effects of some of these drugs.

Pathomechanisms of various types of DIND has been discussed as these are important for the understanding, prevention, and treatment. This subject will also be of interest to neurologists as well as health professionals working in the area of drug safety for the pharmaceutical industry and the health authorities.

I would like to acknowledge the useful advice and help of Prof. P. Krupp, Head International Pharmacovigilance, Sandoz Ltd., Basel, during preparation of this book. Finally, I would like to thank both directors of Hogrefe & Huber Publishers, Dr. Christine Hogrefe and Dr. Thomas Tabasz, as well as the editor Mr. Robert Dimbleby for their personal attention to this project.

K. K. Jain

Table of Contents

Chapter 1
Epidemiology and Clinical Significance

Introduction and Terminology

The term "drug-induced neurological disorders (DIND)" as used here refers to unintended or undesirable effects on the nervous system caused by drugs or associated with drug use. Such disorders are classified as iatrogenic disorders, a term which also covers other illnesses such as ones caused by other therapies, e.g., surgical procedures, or even neglect in carrying out treatment which results in harm or injury to the patient. The use of the word "induced" within the term DIND does not necessarily imply a proven causal relationship of the drug to the disorder. The drug may affect the nervous system directly (primary neurotoxicity) or indirectly by other systemic disturbances caused by the drug (secondary neurotoxicity). DIND includes disorders caused by inappropriate use or overdose of a drug or interaction with other drugs but environmental and industrial toxins are excluded.

Terms that are used commonly in reference to adverse effects of drugs are defined by the World Health Organization (WHO) as follows:

Adverse Event/Adverse Experience (AE). This is any untoward medical occurrence that may present during treatment with a pharmaceutical product but which does not necessarily have a causal relationship with this treatment.

Adverse Drug Reaction (ADR). This is an event which is related or suspected to be related to the trial medicine. An ADR is a response to a drug which is noxious and unintended, and which occurs at doses normally used in man for prophylaxis, diagnosis, or therapy of disease, or for modification of physiological function.

Side Effect. This is any unintended effect of a pharmaceutical occurring at doses normally used in humans which is related to the pharmacological properties of the drug.

Historical Aspects

The concept of harm resulting from medical treatment is more than 3,500 years old. The Code of Hammurabi in the seventh century BC prescribed penalties for physician errors that resulted in harm. Similarly, the Roman law in the first century AD included penalties for such harms. Complications of medical treatment have been described all the great medical writers throughout the past centuries. Around the middle of twentieth century, with the development of pharmacotherapy, increasing attention was given to adverse drug reactions. They were not viewed merely as iatrogenic phenomena but rather inevitable consequences of medical progress and introduction of new drugs. Among the earliest adverse effects of therapies to be recognized were those of the nervous system. Polyneuropathies as complications of vaccinations were recognized in 1934 (Cathala 1934) and encephalopathies in 1949 (Globus and Kohn 1949). Payk (1974) was the first to separate complications resulting from treatment of neurological disorders from neurological complications resulting from treatment of other systems. Around the same time pathogenesis of iatrogenic neurologic disorders was discussed under a dozen categories, nine of which concerned adverse drug effects (Yajnik and Solanski 1972). Most of the complications related to antibiotic and hormone therapy. The first work to focus on iatrogenic pathology in neurology was published in 1975 (Arnott and Caron 1975). There was, however, a concern regarding the increasing number of adverse effects and surveillance systems were developed during the past 20 years for collection and analysis of adverse drug reactions.

Epidemiology of DIND

The exact incidence of DIND is unknown. Reported adverse effects of drugs on the nervous system form only a small proportion of all neurological disorders but they are under-recognized and under-reported. ADRs, both from clinical trials and postmarketing surveillance, are usually reported to the manufacturers of the product involved. The manufacturers make the initial assessment of these reports and file the ADRs with the health authorities of the countries involved according to the regulatory requirements. The World Health Organization also maintains a data base for ADRs. The reporting rate of ADRs is low and even in countries with well organized safety surveillance systems such as Sweden and the United Kingdom, all the ADRs are not reported.

The incidence of ADRs in hospitalized patients has been determined by meta-analysis of 39 prospective studies from US hospitals (Lazarou et al 1998). The overall incidence of serious ADRs was 6.7% and of fatal ADRs was 0.32% of hospitalized patients making these the fourth leading cause of death in the US after heart disease, cancer and stroke. The incidence is much higher than that assumed from the spontaneous reporting system which identifies only about 1 in 20 ADRs.

Only a small fraction of the ADRs are published as case reports or as a part of the results of clinical trials of new drugs. Most of the information received by the pharmaceutical companies is inadequate for establishing the diagnosis of drug-induced neurological disorders but it is used for answering questions from physicians and for making decisions for inclusions of adverse reactions in basic drug information and package insert.

Most of the products listed in the Physicians' Desk Reference include a mention of at least one untoward effect which relates to the nervous system. Entries in the list of adverse reactions is not always based on medical judgment but may be a measure to protect the manufacturer against legal liability by having declared that such an adverse reaction has been reported. The ADR may not be causally related to the drug and this information is not of significant practical value for a neurologist.

The frequency of occurrence of adverse events (AE) in clinical trials can be calculated and compared with that in the placebo group. An AE is considered to be an ADR only if the relation to the drug is proven or suspected. Because the size of the clinical trials is limited and seldom involves more than 500 patients, rare ADRs cannot be expected to show up in these trials. Postmarketing surveillance continues for the lifetime of a drug to detect such ADRs. The frequency of occurrence of ADRs in this phase is difficult to determine because of poor reporting rate and lack of knowledge of the denominator. The number of patients exposed to the drug is sometimes estimated from the quantity of the drug sold and the standard dose for a patient. These figures are not reliable because the amount of drug used by individual patients varies a great deal and all the drugs sold are not administered to the patients.

Another way to estimate the frequency of drug-induced neurological disorders is to review the case records from hospitals. Of 1500 neurological consultations at John Hopkins Hospital, 14% of the conditions were iatrogenic but only 1% of these were drug-related (Moses and Kaden 1986). In UK, 2% of the neurological admissions to a general hospital were drug-induced (Morrow and Patterson 1987).

Assessment of Adverse Drug Reactions

Causality Assessment. Several methods of causality assessment of adverse drug reactions (ADRs) are in use which include questionnaires, algorithms, and computerized Bayesian approach. None of these methods have found universal application because they are tedious, time consuming, and expensive. Stephens (1987) reviewed 22 methods of causality assessment and concluded that Bayesian approach (Naranjo et al 1992) was the only reliable method. In practice causality is usually assessed by global judgment, i. e., opinion of the causal relation of the drug to the event after taking into consideration the available relevant information such as the temporal relationship, results of dechallenge (discontinuation of the medication) and rechallenge (re-exposure to the medication), etc. The importance attached to each of these factors varies among the assessors and often no reason is given why a particular causality rating was assigned to an AE. In order to standardize the assessment of AEs, Jain (1995) has devised a method of triage of the AEs using a questionnaire with the following seven questions:

1. Is there a biological explanation (pathomechanism) for the AE?
2. Is the AE temporally related to the drug AE ?
3. Is dechallenge positive?
4. Is rechallenge positive?
5. Is the event already known and documented?
6. Is the AE known to occur during the course of the natural disease?
7. Is the AE known with the concomitant drug?

The answers are weighted and scored to allocate the ADRs to the following categories: A (Probable); B (Possible); O (Unlikely or insufficient information for assessment). These are approximate terms because of soft nature of the data available. The term definite is used rarely. Possible means that such a reaction can take place with the drug and sometimes this term is used simply because the possibility cannot be excluded.

Diagnostic Assessment. ADRs are often reported as symptoms and these should be linked to a provisional neurologic diagnosis. There are two limitations to this assessment:

1. The assessor does not have access to the patient and further information is usually difficult to obtain.
2. Drug safety specialists are rarely neurologists and the average medical assessor does not the have adequate neurological knowledge to carry out this step.

Evaluation of Literature. Publications showing the association of various drugs with DINDs fall into the following categories:

– *Single case reports.* This is the weakest evidence particularly if the case is not well documented. Unfortunately this constitutes the bulk of the literature on adverse reactions to drugs. Such case reports are usually not peer-reviewed. Reputable journals insist on minimum essential information before publishing these reports but many inadequately documented reports also get published in obscure journals. Whether the causal relationship is proven or not, such reports cannot be ignored. Some of these reports may encourage other physicians to submit similar unreported cases for publication.

– *Multiple case reports.* This is a stronger evidence than that provided by single case reports.

– *Reports of clinical trials of new drugs.* These provide a useful source of adverse events for assessment.

– *Drug safety reviews.* These serve a useful purpose of analyzing the cumulative evidence in literature. A good review should provide a critical analysis of the information, comments on pathomechanisms of DIND, and possibly suggestion for prevention and treatment.

– *Toxicology studies.* Animal experimental studies provide toxicological information which may or may not be relevant to humans DINDs but may provide an insight into pathomechanisms.

– *Epidemiological studies.* These are the most useful source of information, particularly if they are properly designed prospective studies.

– *Textbooks on adverse drug reactions.* Some well known DINDs are listed in recognized textbooks of adverse drug reactions and can be quoted even though reference to the original source is not always provided.

Some authors have attempted to stratify the information on ADRs according to the strength of evidence into various levels. The major drawback is that a rigid system of evaluation cannot be applied to "soft" data that is available from drug safety literature. The quality of information available varies from one drug to another and application of strict criteria of evaluation might exclude information which may useful even though it is anecdotal. Evidence is presented as available and pathomechanisms are described where possible. Drugs frequently mentioned and reported in relation to certain disorders are marked with asterisks in various tables and the readers are left to make their own judgment.

Clinical Significance

Drug-induced neurological disorders (DIND) can mimic neurological disorders due to other causes. However, when there is a reasonable suspicion of association with a drug or a known or plausible pathomechanism for DIND, the drug should be considered in the differential diagnosis. For practical purposes ADRs in the categories A (probable) and B (possible) are taken into consideration.

DINDs are presented according to various neurological systems. It has the advantage that a physician or a neurologist who is investigating a patient with a neurological problem has access to information about drugs which can cause that problem. One drawback is that ADRs seldom involve only one neurological system. There may be involvement of other systems of the body or involvement of another neurological system.

Assessment of a DIND in a patient receiving a multimodal treatment is difficult. Patients undergoing organ transplants are liable to neurological complications of the primary disease, the procedure and the drugs which include immunosuppressants and antibiotics which are liable to induce neurological disorders. Critical decisions need to be made in case of liver and heart transplants. For this an understanding of the pathomechanism of neurological disorders and their natural history is important. An immunosuppressant may not need to be discontinued if the evidence for causal relationship is weak and the neurological complications are transient. In a study on liver transplant, the time of occurrence of CNS complications and the risk factors identified suggest that the pre-transplant condition and the surgical phase are the two most critical periods for developing CNS complications. Patients undergoing liver transplant with a severe pre-transplant medical disorders are at higher risk of experiencing CNS complications (Guarino et al 1999).

Neurologic Symptoms as ADRs

ADRs can present with a neurologic symptom which may be an entity in itself with several mechanisms and a number of widely differing pharmaceutical agents may be the causative agents. An example is headache which is discussed in Chapter 6. The following are some of the symptoms and their causes which can be ADRs of drugs:

Drop Attacks and Falls. The following can be considered in the investigation of a patient with drop attacks and falls:
– Behavioral toxicity
– Dementia
– Movement disorders, e. g., parkinsonism
– Loss of consciousness due to syncope or seizures
– Transient ischemic attacks
– Neuromuscular disorders: neuropathy and myopathy
– Myelopathy
– Cerebellar disorders
– Vestibular disorders

Neurogenic Bladder. A patient who presents with neurogenic bladder dysfunction can have any of the following drug-induced causes:
– Encephalopathy
– Myelopathy
– Autonomic neuropathy

Ataxia. A patient presenting with ataxia may have the following drug-induced causes affecting different parts of the CNS:
– Cerebellar: degeneration or hemorrhage.
– Cerebral: encephalopathy
– Spinal cord: myelopathy with posterior column involvement.
– Brainstem: transient ischemic attacks
– Frontal lobe lesions in encephalomyelitis

Vertigo and Dizziness. Different drugs may produce these symptoms by a number of neurological as well as systemic disturbances such as the following:
Neurological:
– Vestibulotoxicity, e. g., aminoglycoside antibiotics
– Cerebellar dysfunction, e. g., anticonvulsants

– Depression of central integrative centers, e. g., hypnotics

Systemic:
– Hypotension
– Vasculitis
– Hematological disorders.

Dysarthria. This is disturbance of normal speech articulation and can be affected by drugs acting at different levels of the nervous system:
– *Cerebral cortex.* Slurring of speech can be due to effect of sedative-hypnotic drugs on the cerebral control of speech.
– *Central anticholinergic effect* of some drugs such as tricyclic antidepressants can lead to speech block, i. e., halt in normal speech patterns.
– *Cerebellum.* Scanning speech can result from drugs such as lithium and phenytoin which have a toxic effect on the cerebellum.
– *Neuromuscular blockade,* an adverse effect of drugs such as aminoglycoside antibiotics, can produce a myasthenic syndrome and cause fatigability of speech.
– *Oro-facial movement disorder* in tardive dyskinesia due to neuroleptic therapy can make articulation difficult.

Vomiting. Nausea and vomiting are prominent symptoms of a variety of neurological disorders. No clear protective role, such as that of vomiting associated with gastric irritants, can be defined for this. The pathomechanism of vomiting is neurological: stimulation of the vomiting center in the brainstem. Vomiting is associated with the following neurological disorders which can be drug-induced:
– Raised intracranial pressure: benign intracranial hypertension
– Encephalopathy
– Aseptic meningitis
– Headache

Some drug-induced disorders are distinct neurological syndromes such as tardive dyskinesia, serotonin syndrome, and eosinophilia myalgia syndrome. However, they need to be differentiated from naturally occurring neurological disorders.

Concluding Remarks

Drug-induced neurological disorders may be more frequent that they have hitherto considered to be. They can mimic naturally occurring neurological disorders or induce drug-specific syndromes. Further studies are required to determine the pathomechanisms and the incidence of these disorders. The current methods of data collection for adverse effects of drugs are inadequate. In order to improve the current situation, it would be important to establish registries for drug-induced neurological disorders.

References

Arnott G, Caron JC: Iatrogenic pathology in neurology. Lille Med 1975; 20 (special number): 294–298.

Cathala JU: La paralysie post-sérothérapie. Presse Méd 1934; 42: 65–67.

Globus JH, Kohn JL: Encephalopathy following pertussis vaccine prophylaxis. JAMA 1949; 141: 507–509.

Guarino M, Stracciari A, D'Alessandro R, et al: Risk factors for central nervous system complications after liver transplantation. Presented at the American Academy of Neurology Meeting, Toronto, Canada, 20 April, 1999.

Jain KK: A short practical method for triage of adverse drug reactions. Drug Information Journal 1995; 29: 339–342.

Lazarou J, Pomeranz BH, Corey PN: Incidence of adverse drug reaction in hospitalized patients. JAMA 1998; 279: 1200–1205.

Morrow JI, Patterson VH: The neurological practice of a general hospital. JNNP 1987; 50: 1397–1401.

Moses H, Kaden I: Neurologic consultations in a general hospital: spectrum of iatrogenic disease. Am J Med 1986; 81: 955–958.

Naranjo CA, Shear NH, Lanctot KL: Advances in the diagnosis of adverse drug reactions. J Clin Pharmacol 1992; 32: 897–904.

Payk TR: Iatrogenic injuries in neurology. Fortschr Neurol Psychiatr Grenzgeb 1974; 42: 97–111.

Stephens MDB: The diagnosis of adverse medical events associated with drug treatment. Adv Drug React Ac Poison Rev 1987; 1: 1–35.

Yajnik HV, Solanski SV: Iatrogenic neurological disorders. Ind J Med Sci 1972; 26: 419–427.

Chapter 2
Pathomechanisms of Drug-Induced Neurological Disorders

Introduction

Pathomechanisms of drug-induced neurological disorders (DIND) vary considerably and most of them remain unexplored. It is sometimes difficult to draw a line between desirable and undesirable effect of a drug for neurological disorder. For example, intravenous diazepam may control status epilepticus but will make the patient drowsy for a while. Such transient neurological disturbances are considered a minor inconvenience, leave no permanent sequelae, and are overweighed by the therapeutic benefits of the drug. On the other hand, central nervous system (CNS) may be affected by drug for disorders of other systems. Various pathomechanisms of DIND will be discussed under the following three categories:
- Direct mechanisms or primary neurotoxicity
- Indirect mechanisms, i. e., neurotoxicity is due to drug- induced disturbances of other organs
- Predisposing or risk factors for DIND:
  · related to the patient
  · related to the drug.

These mechanisms are discussed briefly in this chapter and further details are given in chapters dealing with individual disorders.

Direct Neurotoxicity

Role of the Blood-Brain-Barrier (BBB). This barrier usually prevents the access of drugs to the fluid spaces of the brain. For direct neurotoxic effects the drugs usually have to cross the BBB. Despite this barrier, lipid-soluble molecules as benzodiazepines readily enter the brain. A drug has to have the property of crossing the BBB to have therapeutic effect on the CNS.

Damage to the BBB facilitates the passage of drugs which normally do not cross the BBB. Diseases in which BBB is damaged such as multiple sclerosis, malignant brain tumors and meningitis would facilitate the direct neurotoxic effect of drugs. This point is discussed in further detail under the factors related to the patient.

Damage to BBB. The access is facilitated if the BBB is damaged and the effect of drugs is seen in areas which lack BBB. Drugs may bypass the BBB by retrograde intra-axonal transport. In case of peripheral nerves, BBB may be deficient in posterior root ganglia and perineurium making them susceptible to peripheral neuritis. Damage to the BBB can occur in a number of diseases which can predispose the patient to DIND when a neurotoxic drug is administered. Adriamycin, when injected into the cerebral ventricles of mice, passes into the surrounding parenchyma and is detected in the nuclei of both neurons and neuroglia (Bigotte and Olsson 1984). Therefore, it can be assumed that when adriamycin is given to patients with disturbance of BBB, the drug may spread to the brain in the same way.

Retrograde Axonal Transport. It is a well established fact that neurons have the capacity to incorporate substances at the periphery of the axons and that material can be transported within the axons to the perikaryon by means of retrograde axonal transport. When toxic substances are picked up by axons and transported to perikaryon, death or degeneration of the neuron results, a phenomenon called "suicidal axonal transport". Selective nerve cell degeneration has been induced in the trigeminal ganglion of the mouse by injecting adriamycin around the intact sensory nerve terminals (Bigotte and Olsson 1987).

Direct Mechanisms of Neurotoxicity

These mechanisms are listed in Table 2.1.

Table 2.1. Direct mechanisms of neurotoxicity

Disturbances of brain energy metabolism
 – ATP synthetase inhibition
 – Uncoupling
 – Disturbances of oxygen consumption
 – Enzymatic dysfunction
 – Selective vulnerability of the central nervous
   system
Sequelae of disturbances of brain energy metabolism
 – Ca^{2+}ion entry in the cell
 – Oxygen free radical formation
 – Excitatory amino acids
Ion channel disturbances
Mitochondrial dysfunction
Neurotransmitter disturbances
Metabolite-mediated toxins
Astrogliosis
Drug-induced selective cell death
Unknown mechanisms

Disturbances of Brain Energy Metabolism

These play an important role in drug-induced neurotoxicity. Various disturbances of brain energy metabolism are:

ATP Synthetase Inhibition. Adenosine triphosphate (ATP) plays an important role in the brain. Under normoxic conditions ATP is synthesized almost exclusively by oxidative phosphorylation in the mitochondria and only a small portion comes from glycolysis. The rate of ATP production varies with rapid synthesis in areas of higher functional activity. ATP level is a reliable indicator of pathological events such as hypoxia, ischemia, hypoglycemia, seizures, and toxic effects of drugs which may disrupt the homeostasis of brain metabolism by hindering energy production or enhancing energy consumption. Oligomycin is an example of a drug which inhibits ATP synthetase (Jung and Brierly 1983).

Uncoupling. There must be an adequate rate of electron flow and oxygen delivery as well as efficient coupling between electron transport and oxidative phosphorylation to maintain a balance between energy production and utilization. Uncoupling is dissociation of oxidative phosphorylation following its inhibition, for example, by barbiturates (Brody and Bain 1954).

Disturbance of Oxygen Consumption. Oxygen deficiency whether due to hypoxia, ischemia or drug effects, leads to depletion of glycogen stores and impaired mitochondrial respiration. ATP production is decreased. The resulting neuronal damage may be transient, reversible, or irreversible depending on the duration and extent of hypoxia. Oxygen transport from the blood to the tissues becomes impaired after chronic exposure to ethanol resulting in oxygen deficiency which restricts the synthesis of ATP.

Enzymatic Disturbances. Adenosine which is formed by enzymatic dephosphorylation of adenosine monophosphate (AMP) has an inhibitory effect on the central nervous system. The action of this enzyme is inhibited by theophylline intoxication leading to convulsions (Jensen et al 1984).

Selective Vulnerability of the Central Nervous System. Brain cells are selectively vulnerable because they express specifications which mediate essential functions, for example, neurotransmitter uptake. Neurons at specific sites are more vulnerable than those in other areas (Baumgarten and Zimmerman 1992).

Sequelae of Disturbances of Brain Energy Metabolism

Sequelae of metabolic disturbances of the brain are: Ca^{2+} entry into neurons, free radical formation, and excitatory amino acids.

Ca^{2+} Entry in Neurons. Ca^{2+} normally acts as a second messenger and plays an important role in membrane stabilization and regulation as well as neurotransmitter release. However, it can also cause cell death under certain circumstances. Ca^{2+} enters the postsynaptic neurons mostly through receptor operated calcium channels which lie on dendrites. The most important transmitters are glutamate and related amino acids. The best known is N-methyl-D-aspartate (NMDA) receptor linked to calcium channels. Stimulation of this receptor allows mainly Ca^{2+} and some Na^+ to enter the cell. Inside the neuron Ca^{2+} is a signal which is changed into various cell responses. During energy deficit Ca^{2+} may rise manifold and set off metabolic reactions with formation of free fatty acids (FFA) and cell destruction. Increased level of Ca^{2+} in mitochondria activates various dehydrogenases and alters the metabolic flux into the citric acid cycle. Cell viability is threatened when calcium homeostasis fails and calcium-activated reactions run out of control. There is considerable evidence for a link between Ca^2 influx and neuronal necrosis.

Free Radicals. A free radical is an agent with an unpaired electron in its orbit. Oxygen radicals are produced by normal cellular metabolism but are usually kept under control by several defense mechanisms. Such defense mechanisms may be overwhelmed when there is increased production of oxygen free radicals by hypoxia and disturbance of cellular metabolism. Central nervous system is particularly vulnerable to free radical damage because of its high lipid content.

Superoxide radical is water soluble but it can cross membranes through the anion channels and enter the extracellular space. Seizures are one manifestation of the attack of free radicals on neuronal membranes. Drug-induced seizures lead to increase of brain levels of FFA. Superoxide may arise from further metabolism of FFA. Oxygen radicals may also increase the permeability of BBB. Free radical mechanisms may contribute significantly to the expression of harmful properties of diverse, unrelated neurotoxic agents (Bondy 1992).

Excitatory Amino Acids. Current evidence suggests that poorly controlled release of these amino acids, their insufficient clearance from the extracellular space and breakdown of surrounding GABA-ergic inhibition transform the excitatory transmitters into potential toxins (Olney 1990). Pathogenesis of excitotoxic cell damage is shown in Figure 2.1.

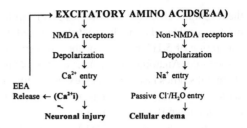

Figure 2.1. Pathogenesis of excitotoxic cell damage (modified from McDonald and Johnson 1990).

Mitochondrial Dysfunction

Mitochondrial DNA is susceptible to mutations by endogenous as well as exogenous factors. Increased sensitivity to mutagenic factors may account for the mitochondrial DNA polymorphism within ethnic groups and mitochondrial disease associated with all mitochondrial DNA mutations, including DNA depletion (Tritschler and Medori 1993). Mitochondrial damage is known to be caused by classic poisons such as cyanide and carbon monoxide. Some drugs such as zidovudine used for treatment of AIDS can also impair the mitochondrial function. Patients on prolonged zidovudine therapy develop a mitochondrial myopathy with ragged red fibers, the pathologic hallmark of mitochondrial disorders (Dalakas and Pezeshkpour 1990).

Neurotransmitter Disturbances

Neurotransmitter disturbances are an important pathomechanism of adverse reactions of several drugs such as antidepressants which are aimed at manipulating this system for therapy. Some neurotransmitters involved in DIND are: serotonin (5-HT), norepinephrine (NE), dopamine (DA), and acetylcholine (ACh).

Serotonin (5-HT). Both excess and depletion of this neurotransmitter can produce neurological disorders. Examples of drugs which produce depletion of serotonin are substituted amphetamine derivatives: 3,4-methylenedioxyamphetamine (MDMA, ecstasy), p-chloramphetamine (PCA), and fenfluramine.

All of these drugs release serotonin and cause depletion of 5-HT from most axon terminals in

the forebrain. Decrease in brain levels of serotonin are considered to be due to drug-induced degeneration of 5-HT neurons or their projections
to the brain. Anatomical and neuroimmunocyto-
chemical studies have provided evidence for the
axonal degeneration as well as reinnervation but
it is not known if a normal pattern is established
(Molliver et al 1990). MDMA use has been
shown to produce depletion of dopamine and
produce parkinsonism.

There is controversy regarding the effect of fenfluramine. Low doses of this drug which are effective in suppressing food intake in rats do not have
effect on the integrity of the 5-HT terminals in spite
of increase in brain levels of 5-HT. Higher doses,
however, deplete brain 5-HT and produce toxic effects (Zaczek et al 1990). Dexfenfluramine, a drug
used as an appetite suppressant has been withdrawn from the market as an antiobesity drug.
Studies in monkeys indicate that dexfenfluramine
can produce serotonergic deficits as long as 12 to
17 months after treatment (McCann et al 1994).
The drug is said to "prune" neurons and result in
depletion of serotonin in the brain. This study can
be criticized because serotonin depletion is hardly
an indicator of neurotoxicity. Moreover, it may
take high decreases in serotonin, perhaps 80% to
90%, before functional problems appear. In another study on mice it was shown that dexfenfluramine produces hypothermia which protects the
animals against neurotoxicity (Miller and O'Callaghan, 1994). Antidepressants which block serotonin uptake increase brain levels of serotonin and
may produce serotonin syndrome.

Pathogenesis of serotonin syndrome by drug-induced excess of serotonin is described in Chapter
21.

Norepinephrine. Blockage of NE uptake by antidepressants can cause tremor (Richelson 1990).

Dopamine. Blockage of dopamine uptake by antidepressants can lead to psychomotor activation
and aggravation of psychoses. Dopamine depletion may result from enhanced metabolism of
dopamine via MAO activity. This may explain
why neurotoxicity of levodopa can be reduced
by MAO-B inhibitor deprenyl (Mena et al 1992).

Acetylcholine. ACh binding sites on cholinergic
nerve terminals or sites postsynaptic to choliner-

gic neurons (nicotine receptors) are well known
targets of neurotoxins. Atropine is an example of
such a drug which can produce memory impairment by reducing ACh in the brain.

Metabolite-Mediated Neurotoxicity

The best example of metabolite mediated neurotoxicity is the use of designer drugs containing
the contaminant MPTP (1-methyl-4-phenyl-
1,2,5,6-tetrahydropyridine). Their use results in
severe Parkinsonian syndrome. MPTP leads to
selective destruction of dopamine cell bodies in
the substantia nigra and the loss of the striatonigral pathways. MPTP is not a neurotoxin itself;
it is converted in the glia to 1-methyl-4-phenyl-
pyridinium ion (MPP$^+$) by monoamine oxidase B
(MAO B) via the intermediate MPDP. MPP$^+$ is a

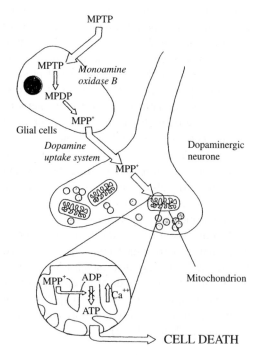

Abbreviations: ADP/ATP = adenosine di/triphosphate;
MPDP = 1-methyl-4-phenyl-1,2,5,6,-dihydropyridine;
MPP$^+$ = 1-methyl-4-phenylpyridinium ion

Figure 2.2. Mechanism of neurotoxicity caused by 1-
methyl-4-phenyl-1,2,5,6-tetrahydropyridine   (MPTP).
Reproduced from Pirmohamed M & Park K: The role of
active metabolites in drug toxicity. Drug Safety 1994; 11:
114–144 (by permission).

substrate for the dopamine reuptake systems and accumulates within dopaminergic neurons, where it binds to neuromelanin, a black pigment found in the nigral nerve cells of primates. MPP^+ is then concentrated in the mitochondria where it is thought to inhibit oxidative phosphorylation, leading to ATP depletion and changes in intracellular calcium concentration with subsequent cell death. This mechanism is illustrated in Figure 2.2.

Astrogliosis

Traditionally the induction of gliosis has been regarded as relatively late step in the cascade of events that follow neural cell damage. Gliosis as measured by an increase in glial fibrillary acidic protein, can coincide with the earliest evidence of cell damage, often within hours of toxin exposure. Perhaps a signal common to a variety of toxicants initiates this response and further investigations are worthwhile for determining the common mediators of neurotoxicity.

Drug-Induced Selective Cell Death

Drugs may induce death of a selective population of neurons. Cyclosporine-induced selective cell death of oligodendrocytes has been shown in cortical cultures (McDonald et al 1996). This may help to explain the involvement of brain white matter in cyclosporine toxicity in humans. Pharmacological strategies such as the use of neurotrophic factors may prove useful in enhancing the benefit-risk ratio of using this drug.

Unknown Mechanisms

Some drugs such as fluorinated quinolone antibiotics are associated with neurotoxicity but PET scanning shows no abnormality of cerebral blood flow and metabolism (Bednarczyk et al 1992). The mechanism of several other DINDs remains unknown.

Methods of Assessing Neurotoxicity

Study of adverse effects of chemical, physical, or biological factors on the function and/or structure of the nervous system is called neurotoxicology and is a branch of toxicology. Most of the studies on neurotoxicology have taken place within the last ten years. A comprehensive but handy review of this topic is to be found in a volume edited by Tilson and Mitchell (1992). Most of the studies in neurotoxicology concern exposure to environmental and industrial chemicals and measurement of effect in experimental animals. The information accumulated in this fashion is not nec-

Table 2.2. Methods for assessing neurotoxicity.

Animals studies
 – The neurotoxicology of cognition: attention, learning, and memory
 – Behavioral changes
 – Effect on motor function
 – Electrophysiological studies: EEG and evoked potentials
 – Effect of neurotoxicants on brain chemistry: neurotransmitter changes
 – Metabolic mapping with deoxyglucose auto-radiography
 – Morphological changes in the nervous system
  • Axonal degeneration detected by silver stains
  • Increase in glial fibrillary acidic protein (GFAP). Used as a marker
 – Developmental neurotoxicology: effect on neurodevelopment
Cell cultures as alternatives to conventional animal toxicity. In vitro models
Molecular biological approaches
 – Genetic and molecular analysis of proteins using DNA technology
 – In situ hybridization
 – Ion channel neurotoxicity: receptor and ligand binding neuronal injury
 – Study of myelin injury
 – Immunological methods
  • immunohistochemistry
  • study of cell adhesion and proliferation
Human studies
 – Clinical neurological examination
 – Neuropsychological tests
 – Behavioral test batteries
 – EEG and action potentials
 – NMR imaging to evaluate drug concentration and metabolism
 – Positron emission tomography (PET)
 – Brain imaging studies for detection of lesions: CT and MRI scans

essarily relevant to the study of neurological adverse effects resulting from the use of therapeutic substances in human patients. Never-the-less, the methods used are important for the investigation of the potential neurotoxicity of a drug. Some of these methods are used for testing neurotoxicity in the preclinical stage of drug development. These methods are listed in Table 2.2.

A discussion of these methods of assessing neurotoxicity is beyond the scope of this work. Some of the newer approaches will be mentioned briefly here.

Glial Fibrillary Acidic Protein (GFAP) Assay. GFAP levels increase in the areas of the brain damaged by neurotoxic chemicals. GFAP assay can detect nervous system damage missed by standard histological screens. An example of this is the damage to the rat olfactory bulb caused by the chemical β,β-iminodiproprionitrile (IDPN) detected by GFAP assay whereas a variety of standard assays could find no damage (Lorens et al 1993). Neurotoxicologists now hope that the GFAP results can help them find a similar human biomarker that would reveal exposure to neurotoxicants. Whereas increase in GFAP result from cellular damage caused by chemical exposures, drugs administered at therapeutic doses do not cause the same response.

GFAPβ mRNA is an alternative transcript of the GFAP gene. Northern blot assay enabled further studies on the regulation of GFAPβ expression in vivo. Since it is well-known that neuronal brain injury is one of the most powerful inducers of GFAP, Condorelli et al (1999) examined the expression of GFAPα and β after a neurotoxic lesion in the rat hippocampus. Results obtained show a parallel increase in both GFAP transcripts with an identical time-course, suggesting that regulatory regions of the gene influence in similar way the rate of transcription at the two different start sites (alpha and beta) or that a similar post-transcriptional mechanism is involved in regulating both mRNA isoforms.

Immunohistochemistry. This is a powerful tool for evaluating neurotoxic effect of drugs. It allows one to demonstrate neurotoxic effects of a substance through altered morphology or loss of stained structure as in the classical methods of histochemistry. In addition it can reveal the neurochemical identity of the affected structures. This technique has been used for demonstrating neurotoxicity of fenfluramine. It is a versatile and sensitive technique for localizing antigens of interest in the central nervous system with a high degree of resolution. Depletion of antibodies may not necessarily indicate neurotoxicity and this is a limitation of this technique. Immunohistochemistry is also being used to examine functional neuroanatomy by elucidating changes in the expression of proteins which appear to relate to drug treatment or neuronal injury.

In situ Hybridization Histochemistry. This methods utilizes standard physicochemical rules for DNA and RNA duplex formation, allowing one to form hybrids between mRNA molecules and labelled probes with complementary nucleotide sequences within the tissues. This technique is reviewed in more detail by Jain (1999b). This technique provides a new window into the brain and a view of protein synthetic machinery of individual brain cells. The practical utility of this method in elucidating the drug action in the brain is still limited till the techniques are refined.

Secondary Drug-Induced Neurological Disorders

Central nervous system is affected by changes in other organs. Many of the neurological disorders are secondary to diseases of other organs. Similarly, CNS is affected by ADRs affecting other body systems. Such DINDs are referred to as secondary to distinguish them from primary DINDs for discussion of pathomechanisms. Examples of secondary DINDs according to the primary system involved are listed below.

Drug-Induced Cardiovascular Disorders. Several such ADRs can affect the brain by affecting the CBF and cerebrovascular system. Some examples are:

– Drug-induced cardiac arrhythmias can lead to dizziness, syncope, and cerebral ischemia.
– Severe drug-induced hypotension, particularly in the elderly hypertensives with athero-

sclerosis may lead to cerebral ischemia and possible cerebral infarction.

– Drug-induced hypertension may lead to hypertensive encephalopathy or cerebral hemorrhage.

Drug-Induced Hematological Disorders. The most important of these are coagulation disorders which can lead to cerebral hemorrhage or thrombosis. Leukocytosis produced by granulocyte colony stimulating factor may produce cerebral microcirculatory disturbances.

Drug-Induced Respiratory Disorders. These can lead to decreased ventilation and cerebral hypoxia.

Drug-Induced Renal Disorders. Renal failure can lead to uremia and uremic encephalopathy.

Drug-Induced Hepatic Disorders. These can lead to hepatic encephalopathy. Increased activity of GABA-ergic system is considered to play a role in the pathogenesis of hepatic encephalopathy in patients with acetaminophen-induced hepatic failure. Benzodiazepines can augment the GABA-ergic tone through a receptor-mediated mechanism and there is a rational basis for the use of benzodiazepine-receptor antagonists such as flumazenil for the treatment of hepatic encephalopathy (Basile et al 1991).

Drug-Induced Electrolyte and Metabolic Disorders. An example of this is convulsions resulting from drug-induced hyponatremia, hypoglycemia, and hypomagnesemia. Hyponatremia can produce cerebral edema and rapid correction of hyponatremia can produce central pontine myelinolysis.

Drug-Induced Vitamin Deficiency. Drugs may increase the need of vitamins and may produce relative deficiency of vitamins particularly during illness which may increase the requirement of vitamins (Roe 1992). Drug-induced vitamin deficiency is well known and this may involve vitamins of the B group such as B_1, B_6, and B_{12}. Peripheral neuropathy associated with isoniazid has been attributed to B_6 deficiency (Ochoa 1970). Histamine H_2-receptor antagonists can cause vitamin B_{12} deficiency and these patients may present with ataxia, dementia, and impaired

position or vibration sense in addition to megaloblastic anemia (Force and Nahata 1992).

Drug-Induced Endocrine Disorders. Hypothyroidism due to sulfonamides, lithium, and para-aminosalicylic acid can lead to psychoses, depression, decline of mental function, carpal tunnel syndrome, ataxia, and seizures. Hyperthyroidism can produce tremor and myopathy.

Risk Factors Related to the Patient

Risk factors which predispose a patient to the development of DIND are shown in Table 2.3.

Table 2.3. Conditions which predispose a patient to DIND.

Genetic predisposition: pharmacogenetic factors
Old age
Patients with history of neurological disorders
Use by normal subjects of drugs indicated for neurological disorders
Compromised brain function
– degenerative brain disease
– intracranial space occupying lesions
– brain damage, e. g., stroke or head injury
Conditions increasing permeability of BBB, e. g., meningitis
Systemic diseases, for example, those involving the kidneys and the liver, AIDS
Non-compliance

Pharmacogenetics

Pharmacogenetics is term is applied to the influence of genetic factors on the action of drugs. It is the study of the linkage between the individual's genotype and the individual's ability to metabolize a foreign compound. It focuses on genetic contribution to drug action as opposed to genetic causes of disease. Genetic factors represent an important source of interindividual variations in drug response and has led to the recognition of the discipline of pharmacogenetics.

An increasing number of monogenic traits have been reported that give rise to altered drug pharmacodynamics or pharmacokinetics. Examples of single-gene phenomena are seen both in drug metabolism and pharmacologic effects. P (pigment)-450 enzymes are controlled by genes called CYP (cytochrome P). There are 27 families of CYP450 and many of the enzymes are polymorphic. For practical purposes these enzymes in the human liver can be divided into two phases (West et al 1997; Linder et al 1997):

1. Phase I enzymes. These are predominantly oxidative. Principle ones are:
   - Cytochromes P-450 (CYP) with subtypes CYP1A2, CYP2A6, CYP2B, CYP2C19, CYP2D6, CYP2E1, CYP3A.
   - NADPH-quinone
   - Oxidoreductase
2. Phase II enzymes. These are conjugative and often couple with the byproducts of phase I. Principle ones are:
   - Glutathione-S-transferase
   - Sulfotransferase
   - N-acetyl transferase
   - UDP-glucuronosyltransferase

Overall, in poor metabolizers, whether phase I or phase II, there is limited metabolism in most patients unless another major metabolic pathway involving other enzymes exists. Drug metabolism also depends on whether the parent compound is a prodrug that forms an active metabolite, and poor metabolizers under this condition will form only trace amounts of an active compound.

Inter- and intra-individual variability in pharmacokinetics of most drugs is largely determined by variable liver function as described by parameters of hepatic blood flow and metabolic capacity. Among the factors affecting these parameters are genetic differences in metabolizing enzymes. Clinically relevant genetic polymorphisms have been found in cytochrome P450-mediated oxidation of debrisoquine and sparteine (CYP2D6) which represents 25% of the major isoforms of P450 responsible for drug metabolism.

Genetic aberrations associated with adverse reactions are of two types. The vast majority arise from classical polymorphism in which the abnormal gene has a prevalence of more than 1% in the general population. Toxicity is likely to be related to blood drug concentration and, by implication, to target organ concentration as a result of impaired metabolism. The other type is rare and only in 10,000 to 1 in 100,000 persons may be affected.

Most idiosyncratic drug reactions fall into the latter category. Examples of adverse reactions with a pharmacogenetic basis are malignant hyperthermia and extrapyramidal movement disorders in psychiatric patients on neuroleptic therapy.

Genotyping may be able to identify individuals at risk of reactions to certain drugs (Jain 1999a) but multiple genes involved in drug reactions may be difficult to detect and a patient may have a life-threatening reactions due to other factors which influence the onset of drug reactions such as drug-disease interaction and drug-drug interaction.

Old Age

The elderly are frequently on multi-drug therapy and are two to three times more likely than young persons to experience adverse reactions to drugs. Some of the changes with aging which predispose the aged to adverse effects of drugs are:

– Reduction in lean body mass
– Albumin decreases by about 25% in the elderly, making more free drug available in the serum.
– Decreases in liver blood flow and hepatic cell and enzyme function result in decreased drug metabolism.
– Decreases in the blood flow to the kidneys and in the number of functional glomeruli result in decreased creatinine clearance.
– Age-related changed in the brain. These include the loss of neurons, decreased dendritic connections between neurons, decreased cerebral blood flow, and decreased number of neurotransmitters. To some extent these changes offer additional explanation why the elderly are more sensitive to psychotropic drugs.

Elderly patients are particularly prone to adverse effects of psychotropic agents, including benzodiazepines because of the altered pharmacokinetics (Jenike 1988). Memory and psychomotor impairment are more pronounced in the elderly on benzodiazepine treatment as compared with younger controls (Pomara et al 1991). The elderly are more sensitive to the central effects of drugs.

It is known that geriatric patients are at greater risk of neurological complications during surgical procedures, due in part to altered response to anesthetic drugs. The aged are sensitive to and require smaller doses of anesthetics to produce anesthesia. Experiments in rats have shown that aging potentiates the cerebral metabolic depression produced by midazolam (Baughman et al 1987). In a study by Greenblatt et al (1991), triazolam was shown to cause a greater degree of sedation and psychomotor impairment in healthy elderly persons than in younger persons who received the same dose. These results were considered to be due to reduced clearance and higher plasma concentration of triazolam rather than due to increased intrinsic sensitivity to the drug.

The elderly are frequent users of antirheumatic agents and also are more prone to show CNS toxicity of these agents. Tinnitus is a well known reversible ADR of salicylates. Because the early symptoms may be overlooked, an elderly patient with salicylate intoxication may present with encephalopathy: confusion, agitation, slurred speech, hallucinations, seizures and coma (Iobst et al 1989).

The incidence of tardive dyskinesia is higher among the elderly patients than in young patients on neuroleptic therapy (Waddington and Youssef 1985) and this complication is more likely to be irreversible in older patients (Smith and Baldessarini 1980). Parkinsonian side effects are more common in the younger patients than in the older ones but choreiform side effects increase with age (Moleman et al 1986).

Pregnancy and Prenatal Exposure to Drugs

Exposure of the fetus to certain drugs in the earlier phases of pregnancy may produce congenital malformations of the nervous system. This topic is not included in this book. Prenatal exposure to drugs, both therapeutic and recreational, has been documented to produce cognitive disturbances in early childhood. These may be subtle developmental abnormalities that may not be detected at birth but manifest later on in childhood.

Some tests such as Fagan's Test of Infant Intelligence which evaluates visual recognition memory, can detect abnormalities in infants between the ages of 6 and 12 months who have a history of in utero exposure to drugs (Struthers and Hansen 1992). These abnormalities are predictive of neuropsychological deficits that manifest later in childhood and enables their identification before the children reach school age. Cognitive performance in adult age has been documented to impaired as a result of in utero exposure to phenobarbital given for the treatment of epilepsy (Reinisch et al 1995).

Patients with History of Neurological Disorders

Patients who have had neurological signs and symptoms in the past are more likely to have a recurrence of these as adverse drug reactions. History of headaches, seizures, and movement disorders should be taken into consideration when prescribing drugs which are known to produce these ADRs. Patients with underlying movement disorders such as Tourette's syndrome and tardive dyskinesia are more liable to develop carbamazepine-induced tics (Kurlan et al 1989).

Use by Normal Subjects of Drugs Indicated for Neurological Disorders. Drugs given to modulate CNS function counteract an abnormal function and aim to achieve a balanced neurological status. Use of such drugs by volunteers in studies and misuse by persons without neurological disease may produce disturbances of neurological function. Neurological patients who have been taking certain medications for long periods usually develop tolerance to minor adverse reactions seen at the start of the therapy. Another mechanism, for example in epileptic patients on antiepileptic drugs, is enhanced metabolism by hepatic p450 enzyme. Non-epileptic patients taking these drugs for the first time may show adverse effects after doses which are well tolerated by patients on chronic AED therapy.

Patients with Compromised Brain Function

The human brain has a considerable reserve capacity and plasticity which enables it to function without obvious deficits even after parts of it are rendered inactive. However, any further insult such as drug toxicity may lead to decompensation and manifestations of neurological disorders. Some examples are:

Degenerative Brain Diseases. Patients with Alzheimer's disease show an exaggerated response to sedative and hypnotic drugs. Patients with underlying organic brain disease are more prone to CNS depressant effects of benzodiazepines. Severe neuroleptic sensitivity has been described in patients with senile dementia of the Lewy body type: 54% of these patients showed this reaction as compared to 7% of the patients with Alzheimer's disease.

Intracranial Space Occupying Lesions. Patients with a unilateral large chronic subdural hematoma may not show any hemiplegia but on intravenous injection of valium, such patients have been observed to manifest hemiplegia from which they recover after the effect of valium wears off. This unmasking of occult neurological deficit was made during cerebral angiography under local anesthesia in the pre-CT era (Jain 1974). A more recent study has shown that sedatives can unmask focal neurological deficits (Thal et al 1996). Preoperative midazolam or fentanyl in patients with brain tumor or stroke exacerbation of pre-existing neurological deficit. The sedative-induced changes ranged from unilateral mild weakness to complete hemiplegia but were transient in nature.

Brain Damage. Adolescents with brain damage are more prone to develop carbamazepine neurotoxicity (Parmalee and O'Shanik 1988). Patients with stroke are subject to increased lithium neurotoxicity (Moskowitz and Altschuler 1991).

Disturbances of Blood Brain Barrier (BBB)

Conditions which disrupt BBB such as head injury, infections, and cerebrovascular accidents may allow systemic drugs, that normally do not cross BBB, to reach the brain tissues and produce toxic effects. Patients with meningitis are more liable to develop neurotoxicity of antibiotics due to penetration of BBB.

Systemic Diseases

Patients suffering from systemic diseases are more prone to develop adverse reactions to drugs. DINDs are more likely to develop in patients with diseases of the kidneys and liver. Patients with AIDS have multiple diseases and impairment of immune system. They have a disproportionate share of adverse drug reactions including those involving the nervous system. These patients do not tolerate tricyclic antidepressant well because of the anticholinergic effects of these drugs. They are more prone to develop drug-induced peripheral neuropathy with zidovudine (see Chapter 11).

Non-Compliance

Neurological patients may not be able to comply with the proper drug use. An epileptic patient may forget to take medications and have breakthrough seizures.

Risk Factors Related to Drugs

Factors related to the drugs which influence neurotoxicity are:
- *Dose*. Some of the neurotoxic effects are dose-related and some occur only as an overdose effect. Management of non-neurotoxic side effects of drugs enable higher doses of these drugs to be given leading to neurotoxicity. An example of this high-dose chemotherapy enabled by the addition of granulocyte colony stimulating factor (filgrastim) which counteracts neutropenia. Eventually neurotoxicity becomes the limiting factor with this approach (Leyvraz et al 1993).
- *Rate of drug delivery*. Faster rates of intravenous delivery of some drugs may produce

transient neurological disturbances. Some novel controlled release preparations have less tendency to produce adverse reactions (Florence and Jani 1994). Examples of this are controlled release preparations of levodopa and theophylline which have lowered the CNS adverse reactions.

– *Route of administration*. Some drugs, which usually do not cross the BBB, have neurotoxic effects only when applied directly to the CNS such as by intrathecal or intraventricular routes. Intravenous administration has usually more pronounced effects than oral ingestion. Some of these routes of drug delivery have their own complications. Intrathecal baclofen pump infections can produce meningitis. A case has been reported with such a pump infection where the presenting manifestation was tetraparesis (Samuel et al 1994). The patient required with the use of local irrigation of the pump system with antibiotics.

– *Impurities in drug*. Drug impurities may be responsible for the neurotoxicity, e. g., tryptophan and eosinophilia-myalgia-syndrome (see Chapter 20).

– *Drug interactions*. Interactions may occur with concomitant medications

– *Drug-disease interaction*. Drug may have an unfavorable influence the course of the neurological condition being treated.

– *Drug withdrawal*. Withdrawal of drugs after prolonged use may produce neurological disorders.

Drug Interactions

A drug-drug interaction occurs when pharmacologic action of a drug is altered by coadministration of second drug. This may result in an increase or decrease of the known effect of either drug or a new effect which is seen with neither of the drugs. Drug-drug interactions are classified on the basis of mechanism that is involved primarily. These are as follows:

– *Pharmacokinetic* interactions occur as the drug is transported to and from its site of action, and the result is a change in plasma level or tissue distribution of the drug.

– *Pharmacodynamic* interactions occur at biologically active (receptor) sites and result in a change in the pharmacologic effect of a given plasma level of the drug.

– *Idiosyncratic* interactions occur unpredictably in a small number of patients and are unexpected from known pharmacologic actions of individual drugs. Their mechanisms are generally unclear but may be based on genetic susceptibility.

Factors which increase the likelihood of clinically significant interactions with psychotropic drugs are:
– Use of drugs that induce or inhibit hepatic microsomal enzymes
– Drugs that have a low therapeutic index
– Drugs that have multiple pharmacologic actions
– High risk patients (elderly, medically ill, etc)

Interactions leading to DIND usually occur under the following circumstances:
– Enhancement of neurotoxicity of drug for CNS disorders interacting with another CNS drug or a non-CNS drug which affects its metabolism.
– Enhancement of potential neurotoxicity by interaction between drugs for non-CNS disorders.

Drugs for CNS Disorders. The concentration of drugs for CNS disorders may rise to toxic levels because of concomitant drugs which interference with drug metabolism and clearance. One of the common mechanisms is that plasma levels of a CNS drug is raised by other drugs which inhibit the hepatic microsomal p450 metabolism. Drug interactions in psychopharmacology have been reviewed by Callahan et al (1993). Some of the important drug interactions are shown in Table 2.4. These are only some examples and further interactions are mentioned in various other chapters.

The use of two CNS drugs can have adverse interactions. Such an interaction can take place if one drug is substituted for the other after an inadequate washout period. Hypertension with stupor has been reported after a switch of two Monoamine oxidase (MAO) inhibitors isocarboxacid and phenelzine (Safferman and Masiar 1992).

Table 2.4. Neurological disorders due to drug interactions of psychopharmaceuticals.

Drug	Interaction with	Neurological ADRs	Mechanism	Reference
Antipsychotic 1/clo-zapine	Antipsychotic 2/lithi-um	Disorientation, trem-or, ataxia, seizures	Combined neurotoxicity of two antipsychotics	Meyer et al (1996); Blake et al (1992)
Benzodiazepines (BZD)	Omeprazole	Ataxia	Increase of plasma levels of BZD by p450 inhibition	Marti-Mosso (1992)
Carbamazepine (CBZ)	Erythromycin	Neurotoxicity of car-bamazepine	Increase of plasma levels of CBZ by p450 inhibition	Wroblewski et al (1986)
Clozapine	Benzodiaze-pines/Lorazepam	Excessive sedation, ataxia	Pharmacodynamic	Cobb et al (1991)
Ergotamine	Sumatriptan	Increased peripheral vasospasm in mi-graine	Pharmacodynamic interaction at 5-HT postsynaptic level between an agonist and an antagonist	Schorderet and Ferrero (1996)
Lithium	Diuretic	Lithium neurotoxici-ty	Decreased renal clearance of lithium	Schwarcz (1982)
MAO inhibitor: mo-clobemide	Fluoxetine (SSRI, a selective serotonin reuptake inhibitor)	Serotonin syndrome	Accumulation of serotonin due to in-hibition of degrad-ing action of MAO	See Chapter 21
Phenytoin (PHT)	Fluoxetine	Neurotoxicity of phenytoin	Increase of plasma levels of PHT by p450 inhibition	Jalil (1992)
Selective mono-amine oxidase inhib-itor/selegiline	Pethidine	Restlessness, irrita-bility, delirium	Dopamine was im-plicated	
Tricyclic anti-depres-sants (TCA)/ imipra-mine	Selective serotonin reuptake inhibitor/ fluoxetine	Accentuation of anti-depressant effect	Increase of plasma levels of TCA by p450 inhibition	Aranow et al (1989); Leroi and Walentynowicz (1996)

Drug-Disease Interaction. The drug may have an unfavorable effect on the course of the neu-rological disease. There are several such happen-ings particularly in degenerative disorders. It is difficult to determine whether the adverse effect is the natural course of the disease or if the drug induces neurological deterioration. One example would be an epileptic patient with an organic brain lesion whose seizures continue to deterio-rate with antiepileptic therapy. Optimal doses of the drug may not be able to control seizure ac-tivity due to progression of the underlying le-sion. Interferon-beta has been approved as a therapy for multiple sclerosis but a recent study

reported development of active lesions during the first three months in treated patients whereas none of the control patients had a relapse during that period (Rudge et al 1995). The rate of ap-pearance of new lesions declined after active treatment was stopped indicating that interferon-beta causes activation of the disease process. Long-term interferon-beta therapy, however, downregulates interferon gamma production and decrease clinical activity.

Drugs for Non-CNS Indications. Interaction of two such drugs can raise the plasma levels of one of these which is known to cause DIND. In one report addition of a quinolone raised theophylline serum levels by more than 100% and led to seizures in one-third of the patients (Grasela and Dreis 1992).

Neurological disorders have been reported in an elderly patients where chloroquine was used concomitantly with NSAIDs (Rollof and Vinge 1993). Although each of these drugs can cause neurologic adverse effects, a pharmacodynamic and/or pharmacokinetic interaction was considered to have contributed in this case.

Drug Withdrawal

Discontinuation of several drugs after prolonged therapeutic use may produce a withdrawal reaction with neuropsychiatric symptoms. This is to be distinguished from withdrawal syndromes seen in drug dependence. Manifestations of withdrawal of several drugs will be mentioned in various chapters of this book. Withdrawal phenomena are particularly associated with antidepressants and antipsychotics.

Antidepressants. Withdrawal phenomena following abrupt or progressive cessation of antidepressant medications are well recognized. These occur after all types of antidepressants including tricyclics, monoamine oxidase inhibitors and selective serotonin reuptake inhibitors. Mood changes resulting from withdrawal are difficult to distinguish from the symptoms of depression but other symptoms such as sleep disturbances, delirium and movement disorders may also occur (Lejoyeux et al 1996).

Incidence of antidepressant withdrawal syndrome varies from 16% to 80% in various studies. Risk factors for the development of this syndrome include long term use of the drug and concomitant discontinuation of a centrally acting comedication such as anticonvulsant carbamazepine. Pathophysiology of this syndrome is varies according to the type of antidepressant.

– *Tricyclic antidepressants (TCAs).* The most well documented hypothesis of pathophysiology is the effect on cholinergic system. Most of the symptoms are explained as a cholinergic rebound because TCAs produce muscarinic cholinergic receptor blockade resulting in development of tolerance and increase in postsynaptic density of muscarinic receptors. Movement disorders may be due to disturbance of cholinergic-dopaminergic balance in the nigrostriatal and mesocortical systems respectively. Parkinsonism may be associated with dopamine receptor blockade. Because TCAs also affect the noradrenergic system, abrupt withdrawal increases noradrenaline turnover which explains anxiety and agitation.

– *Monoamine oxidase inhibitors (MAOIs).* These drugs can exert an amphetamine-like effect and explains the similarity of MAOI withdrawal to amphetamine overdose. MAOIs downregulate and subsensitize α_2 adrenergic receptors in animals and humans (Cohen et al 1982). These effects provide a theoretical basis for MAOI withdrawal-induced psychosis.

– *Selective serotonin reuptake inhibitors (SSRIs).* CNS withdrawal symptoms of SSRIs are usually seen with paroxetine which as a short half-life and rarely with fluoxetine and sertraline (Stahl et al 1998). CNS withdrawal symptoms include dizziness, headache, seizures, paresthesias, vertigo and tremor. Psychiatric withdrawal symptoms more likely to be seen with fluoxetine include nervousness, anxiety, depression, suicide attempt, psychotic depression aggression and agitation. Because the psychiatric symptoms of antidepressant discontinuation include changes in mood, affect, appetite, and sleep, they are sometimes mistaken for signs of a relapse into depression. The mechanism of withdrawal reactions is not well understood but it is postulated that discontinuation events result from a sudden decrease in the availability of synaptic serotonin in the face of down-regulated serotonin receptors. In addition, other neurotransmitters, such as dopamine, norepinephrine, or gamma-aminobutyric acid (GABA), may also be involved. Individual patient sensitivity may also be a factor in SSRI discontinuation phenomena.

Antipsychotics. A variety of symptoms follow the discontinuation of phenothiazines, thioxanthenes and butyrophenones. The most common are nausea, vomiting, anorexia, paresthesias, anxiety, agitation, restless and insomnia. Patients may experience vertigo, paresthesias, myalgia and tremor. Symptoms usually appear a few days after discontinuation of the drug and resolve in 1–2 weeks.

The pathophysiology of antipsychotic withdrawal may involve drug-induced supersensitivity of muscarinic cholinergic and dopaminergic systems because antipsychotics bind to dopaminergic, muscarinic and adrenergic receptors. Long-term treatment with antipsychotic agents may result in dopaminergic rebound in the chemoreceptor trigger zone which may account for withdrawal-associated nausea and vomiting.

Management of antipsychotic agent withdrawal phenomena is symptomatic. Anxiety and agitation should be watched carefully as this may progress to psychosis and require increase in the dose of antipsychotic.

Discontinuation syndromes. The existence of discontinuation syndromes following treatment with neuroleptic (antipsychotic) drugs was first outlined in the mid-1960s but the effects of such syndromes have been neglected since then. Tranter and Healy (1998) have reviewed evidence for the existence and nature of discontinuation syndromes following neuroleptics through reports of difficulties following the use of dopamine blocking antiemetics, the use of chlorpromazine to treat tuberculosis, the use of antidepressant-neuroleptic combinations in affective disorders, the occurrence of tardive syndromes and studies designed to establish the existence of discontinuation syndromes in schizophrenia. Combined these bodies of data point strongly to the existence of discontinuation syndromes after cessation of treatment with neuroleptics which may involve features other than motor dyskinesias.

Concluding Remarks

Knowledge of the pathomechanism of drug-induced neurological disorders (DIND) is helpful in their assessment. More is known about this subject than is generally assumed. Several hypotheses still need further investigation. Better understanding of the pathomechanisms of DIND will improve their management.

References

Aranow RB, Hudson JI, Pope HG, et al: Elevated antidepressant plasma levels after addition of fluoxetine. Am J Psychiatry 1989; 146: 911–913.

Basile AS, Hughes RD, Harrison PM, et al: Elevated brain concentrations of 1,4-benzodiazepines in fulminant hepatic failure. NEJM 1991; 325: 473–478.

Baughman VL, Hoffman WE, Anderson S, et al: Cerebral vascular and metabolic effects of fentanyl and midazolam in young and aged rats. Anesthesiology 1987; 67: 314–319.

Baumgarten HG, Zimmerman B: Cellular and subcellular targets of neurotoxins: the concept of selective vulnerability. In Herken H, Hucho F (Eds.): Selective neurotoxicity, Berlin, Springer-Verlag, 1992, pp 1–27.

Bednarczyk EM, Green JA, Nelson AD, et al: Comparative assessment of the effect of lomofloxacin, ciprofloxacin, and placebo on cerebral blood flow, and glucose and oxygen metabolism in healthy subjects by positron emission tomography. Pharmacotherapy 1992; 12: 369–375.

Bigotte L, Olsson Y: Cytotoxic effects of adriamycin on the central nervous system of the mouse—cytofluorescence and electronmicroscopic observations after various modes of administration. Acta Neurol Scand 1984; 70(suppl 100): 55–67.

Bigotte L, Olsson Y: Degeneration of trigeminal ganglion neurons caused by retrograde axonal transport of doxorubicin. Neurology 1987; 37: 985–992.

Blake LM, Marks RC, Luchins DJ: Reversible neurological symptoms with clozapine and lithium. J Clin Psychopharmacology 1992; 12: 97–99.

Bondy SC: Reactive oxygen species: relation to aging and neurotoxic damage. Neurotoxicology 1992; 13: 87–100.

Brody TM, Bain JA: Barbiturates and oxidative phosphorylation. J Pharmacol 1954; 110: 148–156.

Callahan AM, Fava M, Rosenbaum JF: Drug interactions in psychopharmacology. Psychiatric Clinics of North America 1993; 16: 647–671.

Cobb CD, Anderson CB, Seidel DR: Possible interaction between clozapine and lorazepam. Am J Psychiatry 1991; 148: 1606–1607.

Cohen RM, Campbell IC, Dauophin M, et al: Changes in alpha and beta receptor densities in rat brain as a result of treatment with monoamine oxidase inhibitor antidepressants. Neuropharmacology 1982; 21: 293–298.

Condorelli DF, Nicoletti VG, Dell'Albani P, et al: GFAPβ mRNA expression in the normal rat brain and after neuronal injury. Neurochem Res 1999; 24: 709–714.

Dalakas MC, Pezeshkpour GH: Mitochondrial myopathy caused by long-term zidovudine therapy. NEJM 1990; 322: 1098–1105.

Florence AT, Jani PU: Novel oral drug formulations: their potential in modulating adverse drug effects. Drug Safety 1994; 10: 233–266.

Force RW, Nahata MC: Effect of histamine H_2-receptor antagonists on vitamin B_{12} absorption. Ann Pharmacother 1992; 26: 1283–1286.

Gordon M, Preiksaitis HG: Drugs and aging brain. Geriatrics 1988; 43: 69–78.

Grasela TH, Dreis MW: An evaluation of qulinolone-theophylline interaction using food and drug administration spontaneous reporting system. Arch Int Med 1992; 152 :617–621.

Greenblatt DJ, Harmatz JS, Shapiro L, et al: Sensitivity to triazolam in the elderly. NEJM 1991; 324: 1691–1698.

Iobst WF, Bridges CR, Regan-Smith MG: Antirheumatic agents: CNS toxicity and its avoidance. Geriatrics 1989; 44: 95–102.

Jain KK: Genomics. Waltham, Massachusetts, Decision Resources Inc, 1999a.

Jain KK: Molecular Diagnostics. Waltham, Massachusetts, Decision Resources Inc, 1999b.

Jain KK: Use of diazepam in carotid angiography. Canad J Neurosc 1974; 1: 141–142.

Jalil P: Toxic reaction following the combined administration of fluoxetine and phenytoin: two case reports. JNNP 1992; 55: 412–413.

Jenike MA: Psychoactive drugs in the elderly: antipsychotics and anxiolytics. Geriatrics 1988; 43: 53–65.

Jensen MH, Jorgensen S, Nielsen H, et al: Is theophylline-induced seizures in man caused by inhibition of cerebral 5'-nucleotidase activity. Acta Pharmacol Toxicol 1984; 55: 331–334.

Kriegelstein J, Nuglisch J: Metabolic disorders as consequences of drug-induced energy deficits. In Herken H, Hucho F (Eds.): Selective neurotoxicity, Berlin, Springer-Verlag, 1992, pp 11–139.

Kurlan R, Kersun J, Behr J, et al: Carbamazepine-induced tics. Clin Neuropharmacol 1989; 12: 293–302.

Lejoyeux M, Ades J, Mourad I, et al: Antidepressant withdrawal syndrome. CNS Drugs 1996; 5: 278–292.

Leroi I, Walentynowicz MA: Fluoxetine-imipramine interaction. Cand J Psychiatry 1996; 41: 318–319.

Leyvraz S, Ketterer N, Vuichard P, et al: Sequential high-dose combination chemotherapy with granulocyte colony-stimulating factor and peripheral blood progenitor cells in patients with solid tumors: intensification limited by non-hematologic toxic effects. JNCI 1993; 85: 1962–1964.

Linder MW, Prough RA, Valder R: Pharmacogenetics: a laboratory tool for optimizing therapeutic efficacy. Clin Chem 1997; 43: 254–266.

Lorens J, Crofton KM, O'Callaghan JP: Administration of 3,3'-iminodiprioprionitrile to the rat results in region-dependent damage to the central nervous system at levels above the brain stem. J Pharmacol Exp Ther 1993; 265: 1492–1498.

Machover Reinisch J, Sanders SA, Lykke Mortensen E, et al: In utero exposure to phenobarbital and intelligence deficits in adult men. JAMA 1995; 274: 1518–1525.

Marti-Mosso JF: Ataxia following gastric bleeding due to omeprazole-benzodiazepine interaction. Ann Pharmacother 1992; 26: 429–430.

McCann U, Hatzidimitriou G, Ridenour A, et al: Dexfenfluramine and serotonin neurotoxicity: further preclinical evidence that clinical caution is indicated. J Pharmacol Exp Ther 1994; 269: 792.

McDonald JW, Goldberg MP, Gwag BJ, et al: Cyclosporine induces neuronal apoptosis and selective oligodendrocyte death in cortical cultures. Ann Neurol 1996; 40: 750–758.

McDonald JW, Johnston MV: Physiological and pathological roles of excitatory amino acids during central nervous system development. Brain Res Rev 1990; 41: 41–70.

McKeith I, Fairbairn A, Perry R, et al: Neuroleptic sensitivity in patients with senile dementia of Lewy body type. BMJ 1992; 305: 673–678.

Mena MA, Pardo B, Casarejos MJ, et al: Neurotoxicity of levodopa on catecholamine-rich neurons. Movement Disorders 1992; 7: 23–31

Meyer M, Baldessarini RJ, Goff DC, et al: Clinically significant interactions of psychotropic agents with antipsychotic drugs. Drug Safety 1996; 15: 333–346.

Miller DB, O'Callaghan JP: Environment-, drug- and stress-induced alterations in body temperature affect the neurotoxicity of substituted amphetamines in the C57BL/6J mouse. J Pharmacol Exp Ther 1994; 270: 752–760.

Moleman P, Janzen G, von Bargen BA, et al: Relationship between age and incidence of parkinsonism in psychiatric patients treated with haloperidol. Am J Psychiatry 1986; 143: 232–234.

Molliver ME, Berger UV, Mamounas MA, et al: Neurotoxicity of MDMA and related compounds: anatomic studies. Ann NY Acad Sc 1990; 600: 640–663.

Moskowitz AS, Altschuler L: Increased sensitivity to lithium-induced neurotoxicity after stroke. J Clin Psychopharmacol 1991; 11: 272–273.

Negrotti A, Calzetti S, Sasso E: Calcium-entry blockers-induced parkinsonism: possible role of inherited susceptibility. Neurotoxicology 1992; 13: 261–264.

Ochoa J: Isoniazid neuropathy in man: quantitative electronmicroscopic study. Brain 1970; 93: 831–850.

Olney JW: Excitotoxic amino acids and neuropsychiatric disorders. Ann Rev Pharmacol Toxicol 1990; 30: 47–71.

Parmalee DX, O'Shanick GJ: Carbamazepine-lithium toxicity in brain-damaged adolescents. Brain Injury 1988; 2: 305–308.

Pomara N, Deptula D, Singh R, et al: Cognitive toxicity of benzodiazepines in the elderly. In Salzman C, Lebowitz BL (Eds.): Anxiety in the elderly, New York, Springer-Verlag, 1991, pp 175–190.

Richelson E: Antidepressants and brain neurochemistry. Mayo Clin Proc 1990; 65: 1227–1236.

Roe DA: Effect of drugs on vitamin needs. Ann NY Acad Sc 1992; 669: 156–164.

Rollof J, Vinge E: Neurologic adverse effects during concomitant treatment with ciprofloxacin, NSAIDS, and choloroquine: possible drug interactions. Ann Pharmacother 1993; 27: 1058–1059.

Rudge P, Miller D, Crimlisk H, et al: Does interferon-beta cause initial exacerbation of multiple sclerosis. Lancet 1995; 345: 580.

Safferman AZ, Masiar SJ: Central nervous system toxicity after monoamine oxidase inhibitor switch: a case report. Ann Pharmacother 1992; 26: 337–338.

Samuel M, Finnerty GT, Rudge P: Intrathecal baclofen

pump infection treated by adjunct intrareservoir antibiotic instillation. JNNP 1994; 57: 1146–1147.

Schorderet M, Ferrero JD: Drug-drug interactions at receptors and other active sites. In D'Arcy PF, McElnay JC, Welling PG (Eds.): Mechanism of drug interactions, New York, Springer-Verlag, 1996, pp 215–233.

Schwarcz G: The problem of antihypertensive treatment in lithium patients. Compr Psychiatry 1982; 23: 50–54.

Smith JM, Baldessarini RJ: Changes in prevalence, severity, and recovery in tardive dyskinesia with age. Arch Gen Psychiatry 1980; 37: 1368–1373.

Stahl SM: Basic psychopharmacology of antidepressants, part I: antidepressants have seven distinct mechanisms of action. J Clin Psychiatry 1998; 59(suppl 4): 5–14.

Struthers JM, Hansen RL: Visual recognition memory in drug-exposed infants. Developmental and Behavioral Pediatrics 1992; 13: 108–111.

Thal GD, Szabo MD, Lopez-Bresnahan M, et al: Exacerbation or unmasking of focal neurologic deficits by sedatives. Anesthesiology 1996; 85: 21–25.

Tilson HA, Mitchell CL: Neurotoxicology. New York, Raven Press, 1992.

Tranter R, Healy D: Neuroleptic discontinuation syndromes. J Psychopharmacol 1998; 12: 401–406.

Tritschler H-J, Medori R: Mitochondrial DNA alterations as a source of human disorders. Neurology 1993; 43: 280–288.

Waddington JL, Youssef HA: Late onset voluntary movements in chronic schizophrenia: age-related vulnerability to "tardive" dyskinesia independent of extent of neuroleptic medication. Ir Med J 1985; 78: 143–146.

West WL, Knight EM, Pradhan S, et al: Interpatient variability: genetic predisposition and other genetic factors. J Clin Pharmacol 1997; 37: 635–648.

Wroblewski BA, Singer WD, Whyte J: Carbamazepine-erythromycin interaction. JAMA 1986; 255: 1165–1167.

Zaczek R, Battaglia G, Culp S, et al: Effects of repeated fenfluramine administration on indices of monoamine function in rat brain: pharmacokinetic, dose response, regional specificity and time course data. J Pharmacol Exp Ther 1990; 253: 104–112.

Zornberg GL, Bodkin JA, Cohen NM: Severe adverse interaction between pethidine and selegiline. Lancet 1991; 337: 246.

Chapter 3
Drug-Induced Encephalopathies

Introduction

The term "encephalopathy" has been used in the literature to characterize a constellation of symptoms and signs reflecting a generalized disturbance of brain function. Here the term is restricted to non-inflammatory organic disturbances of the brain. Encephalopathy may be acute or chronic. Encephalopathy and seizures may occur either together or separately but seizures are usually an acute manifestation. The manifestations vary according to the involvement of brain structures. Paralysis and coma may occur in severe cases. The causes are varied and may be toxic, metabolic, degenerative, vascular or posttraumatic, etc. Toxic and metabolic encephalopathies are usually reversible. Periodic triphasic waves are seen on EEG examination in patients with metabolic and some drug-induced encephalopathies. EEG may be normal or show only non-specific disturbances. A classification of drug-induced encephalopathies is shown in Table 3.1.

The term "leukoencephalopathy" is a special type of encephalopathy which indicates lesions of the white matter which may be viral or toxic or ischemic or immunologic in origin. The evidence for this pathology should ideally be based on brain imaging (ideally MRI) or neuropathological examination. The former is not always carried out in practice and the latter is usually limited to brain biopsy or autopsy. In case of uncertainty or lack of evidence, it may be preferable to refer to leave these cases under the broader category of encephalopathy. Leukoencephalopathy may be reversible or irreversible depending upon the nature of brain lesions and progression of the disease. The disease process may be localized as in the case of posterior leukoencephalo-

Table 3.1. Classification of drug-induced encephalopathies

Encephalopathy: non-specific drug-induced disturbance of brain function
Encephalopathies secondary to drug-induced metabolic disorders:
– Hepatic encephalopathy and hyperammonemia
– Hypoglycemic encephalopathy
– Hyponatremic encephalopathy
– Uremic encephalopathy
– Wernicke's encephalopathy
Leukoencephalopathy: encephalopathy with white matter lesions
– Secondary leukoencephalopathy: drug-induced hypertension
Syndromes associated with drug-induced encephalopathy:
– Reye's syndrome
– Toxic encephalopathy of the newborn
Encephalitis or encephalomyelitis: inflammatory or infectious lesions of the CNS

pathy with involvement of the parieto-occipital region.

The terms "encephalitis" or "encephalomyelitis" indicate widespread inflammatory disease of the CNS. Among therapeutic substances, only vaccines for viral diseases can be linked to encephalomyelitis.

Some of the clinical manifestations of encephalopathies are covered in other chapters; disturbances of consciousness (Chapter 4), neuropsychiatric disorders (Chapter 5), seizures (Chapter 7), movement disorders (Chapter 8), and cerebellar disorders (Chapter 15). This chapter is an overview of CNS adverse effects referred to as encephalopathies and which involve disturbance of more than one CNS function.

Encephalopathies are common with overdosage of drugs and environmental toxins. The coverage in this chapters is restricted mainly to encephalopathies associated with the therapeutic use of drugs. Encephalopathy may be secondary to other drug-induced disorders such as hepatic encephalopathy, hypertensive encephalopathy, uremic encephalopathy, hyponatremia and hypoglycemia. In Reye's syndrome there is multiorgan involvement including the brain.

Drugs Associated with Encephalopathy

Drugs which have been reported to be associated with encephalopathy are shown in Table 3.2.

Table 3.2. Drugs reported to be associated with encephalopathy

Acyclovir
*Alum
Antiepileptic drugs
Antineoplastic drugs
Baclofen
*Bismuth
*Bromides
Cephalosporins
Digoxin
DMSO
Fat emulsion therapy
Filgrastim
H_2-receptor antagonists
HOPA
Intrathecal contrast agents. methotrexate, iohexol
Intravenous immunoglobulin
Isoniazid
Levodopa
*Lithium
Mefloquine
OKT3
Penicillin
Podophyllin
PSC833
Stem cell transplantation
Sulfonamides
Theophylline

*Frequently reported.

Acyclovir

Acyclovir is used for the treatment of herpes simplex virus encephalitis. Rashiq et al (1993) have reviewed 35 patients reported to have developed neuropsychiatric symptoms during acyclovir therapy in an attempt to define acyclovir neurotoxicity and distinguish it from viral encephalitis. Acyclovir encephalopathy was distinguishable from viral encephalitis by sudden onset, absence of fever or headache, lack of focal neurologic findings and normal CSF findings. Symptoms appeared within two days of start of acyclovir and resolved within several days after discontinuation of the drug. The most common risk factors were the concomitant use of other potentially neurotoxic medications and chronic renal failure. Acyclovir has also been known to induce renal failure (Hernandez et al 1991).

Encephalopathy with coma has been reported in patients with renal disease and herpes simplex or zoster after treatment with oral aciclovir. These patient recovered after discontinuation of aciclovir and hemodialysis (Gil-Paraiso et al 1994; Mataix et al 1994). Encephalopathy has also been reported as an idiosyncratic reaction with normal blood levels of aciclovir in patients with renal disease. It has been reported in patients with renal disease on dialysis (MacDiarmaid-Gordon et al 1992; Peces et al 1996; Kitching et al 1997; Gomez Campdera et al 1998). It occurs in patients on peritoneal dialysis for renal disease after start of acyclovir therapy because acyclovir peritoneal clearance is negligible (Guilhem et al 1991).

Management. Dose of acyclovir should be lowered in patients with risk factors such as renal disease. A loading dose of 400 mg and a maintenance dose of 200 mg is recommended. Hemodialysis has been recommended as a diagnostic as well as therapeutic measures in such patients if aciclovir assay is not easily available (Beales et al 1994). Due to its slow protein binding, low steady state volume of distribution and high water solubility, acyclovir is an ideal drug for hemodialysis to enhance its elimination (Leikin et al 1995).

Alum

Aluminum encephalopathy associated with hemodialysis, also called dialysis encephalopathy, is well known. Its manifestations include dysarthria, myoclonus, dementia and seizures. Aluminum toxicity has been described in infants and children with abnormal renal function who are treated with oral or intravenous solutions containing aluminum. Alum bladder irrigation (Aluminum ammonium sulfate or aluminum potassium sulfate) is used for hematuria and several cases of acute encephalopathy have been reported following this procedure (Perazella and Brown 1993; Murphy et al 1992). The risk factors for this complication are renal failure and concomitant high-dose chemotherapy.

Normally alum is an astringent and when applied locally, it prevents its own absorption. However, in patients with damage to bladder epithelium resulting from chemotherapy, alum cannot serve the astringent function and may be absorbed. Several cases of aluminum encephalopathy have been reported following use of bone cement ionocem (IONOS, D-8031 Seefeld/Obb, Germany), a biomaterial that is widely used in Europe (Renard et al 1994; Hanston et al 1994). This finding has been contested by Reusche et al (1995) who have used this material for skull reconstruction inhuman patients and have not observed any substantial increase of aluminum in the CSF/cerebral tissue or any detrimental clinical sequences.

Management. Dialysis-associated encephalopathy must be taken into account as a possible cause of etiologically uncertain neuropsychiatric symptoms in patients on chronic hemodialysis. The diagnosis of aluminum-induced neurotoxicity is established by observing characteristic EEG changes which may precede clinical abnormalities by several months. Aluminum concentration in the plasma gives a reasonably accurate measure of the aluminum burden of the body. Values above 100 mg/L indicate that neurotoxicity can occur and 200 mg/L is associated with overt signs of neurotoxicity. Preventive measures include avoidance of excessive use of aluminum containing drugs and monitoring of serum aluminum levels in patients undergoing dialysis. Aluminum toxicity can actually be treated and reversed by using the chelator desferrioxamine as a therapeutic agent (Alfrey and Froment 1990).

Neuropathology. Experimental aluminum en-

cephalopathy has been produced in the rabbit as an evidence for aluminum-induced neurodegeneration (Rao et al 1998) and unless definitive evidence is available, aluminum remains a strong suspect in neurotoxicology. Examination of brain of an elderly patient who died as a sequel of aluminum encephalopathy showed characteristic argyrophilic, aluminum-induced lysosomal intracytoplasmic inclusions in the choroid plexus epithelium, cortical glia and numerous neuron populations. Laser microprobe mass analysis (LAMMA) confirmed manifold increase in subcellular aluminum content, especially in the neuronal cytoplasm, also demonstrated by atom absorption spectrometry (Reusche et al 1999).

Antiepileptic Drugs (AEDs)

Valproic acid, vigabatrin, lamotrigine, phenytoin, and carbamazepine have been reported to be associated with encephalopathy.

Valproic Acid (VPA). VPA-induced encephalopathy is characterized by somnolence, reduced motor activity and severe deterioration of cognitive and behavioral abilities. It should be distinguished from VPA intoxication, which is associated with increased VPA blood levels. Most reports of VPA-associated encephalopathy are about children where VPA was used in combination with other AEDs and serum ammonia concentration was elevated. Other cases have been described in adults (Visticot and Montreul 1994; Bauer and Elger 1993; Jones et al 1990; Gobel et al 1999) where encephalopathy occurred after the initiation of VPA therapy and resolved after discontinuation of therapy.

Pathomechanism. Mechanisms of encephalopathy may include interactions of the hepatic enzymes, a direct toxic effect on the cerebral receptors, as well as drug interactions. Possible explanations of VPA-associated encephalopathy are:
– Toxic effect of VPA on the brain, particularly, interaction with GABA receptors.
– VPA-induced hepatic failure leading to hepatic encephalopathy (Donat et al 1979).
– VPA-induced hyperammonemia. Various causes of hyperammonemia during treatment

with VPA are not clear but it may be due to depletion of mitochondrial acetyl CoA. VPA or its metabolites may act by inhibiting the activity of ornithine transcarbamylase (OTC) and carbonyl-phosphate synthetase (CPS). Patients with partial deficiency of OTC (Leào 1995) and CPS appear to be more susceptible to VPA-induced hyperammonemia. Hyperammonemia during VPA treatment may be asymptomatic and is not an indication for reducing or eliminating VPA therapy (Murphy and Marquart 1982).

– Lam et al (1997) report a patient who developed MELAS (mitochondrial myopathy, encephalopathy, lactic acidosis and stroke-like episodes) after start of VPA therapy. A nucleotide 3243 A→G mutation, which predisposes the patient to the detrimental effects of valproate on oxidative phosphorylation, was detected in the mitochondrial DNA.

– Mechanism of anticonvulsant effect of VPA is believed to involve elevation of GABA by inhibition of degradation enzymes of GABA Shunt. Experiments on mice have shown that higher doses of VPA significantly increase the brain levels of glutamate which opposes the action of GABA (Miyazaki et al 1988). This may be an explanation of VPA-associated encephalopathy.

– VPA encephalopathy may be a manifestation of VPA-induced aggravation of epileptic activity which may cause progression of focal epilepsy to grand mal seizures (Pakalnis et al 1989; Rangel et al 1988; Tartara and Manni 1985).

Management. Diagnostic tests for the detection of ornithine transcarbamylase deficiency must be performed before prescribing valproate for patients with a history of encephalopathy (Oechsner et al 1998). VPA should not be given to patients suspected of having mitochondrial diseases. VPA-induced encephalopathy is usually reversible after discontinuation of VPA. General management requires correction of hyperammonemia if present. L-carnitine or citrullin supplementation has been used but the rationale is unclear.

Phenytoin. Most of the reports of neurotoxicity

of phenytoin concern cerebellar disorders (see Chapter 15). Encephalopathy has been reported as a toxic effect of chronic use of phenytoin (Engel et al 1971; Ricart et al 1991; Nunez et al 1992; Lewin et al 1993).

Carbamazepine (CBZ). Encephalopathy with brainstem dysfunction has been reported as an effect of CBZ overdose (Salcman et al 1975; Donnet et al 1991; Kalaawi et al 1991). Encephalopathy has also been reported as an idiosyncratic reaction to CBZ (Smith 1991).

Vigabatrin. Two patients have been reported to have developed acute encephalopathy after starting vigabatrin therapy as an add-on to carbamazepine (Sälke-Kellermann et al 1993). Other cases have been reported of encephalopathy in patients on vigabatrin monotherapy (Ifergane et al 1998; Sharief et al 1993).

In animal toxicity studies, a consistent abnormal finding has been microvacuolation of the white matter of the brain but neuropathologic studies of the hippocampus excised at surgery in epileptic patients with long term treatment with vigabatrin have not shown any microvacuoles (Agosti et al 1990). A report of neuropathological examination in 5 patients on long-term vigabatrin therapy confirmed that no white matter vacuolation was seen (Sivenius et al 1993). MRI studies on a series of patients on vigabatrin therapy also did not reveal any evidence of white matter lesions (Cocito and Maffini 1995).

Lamotrigine. This new anticonvulsant is well tolerated and relatively free of CNS toxicity. A case is reported in which encephalopathy developed in a patient treated with lamotrigine following left frontal lobectomy for a low grade astrocytoma (Hennessy and Wiles 1996). The patient had high lamotrigine blood levels and recovery followed reduction of dose. The patient had been treated concomitantly by valproic acid as well and the serum levels were within normal limits.

Baclofen

This is a GABA derivative and is used for the treatment of spasticity. Spinal effects predominate when it is given within the therapeutic range but acute encephalopathy, manifested by impairment of consciousness, seizures, respiratory depression and hypotonia, has been reported with increasing toxic doses (Lee et al 1992). In the review by these authors, patients with chronic baclofen intoxication presented with hallucinations, impairment of memory, catatonia or acute mania. Periodic bursts of triphasic waves are seen on EEG of patients with baclofen intoxication and these changes resolve on discontinuation of baclofen and clinical recovery (Hormes et al 1988; Phillipi et al 1990). Lazzarino et al (1991) have reported a case of acute transient encephalopathy with confusion, drowsiness, myoclonic jerks, periodic triphasic sharp wave EEG patterns induced by low doses of baclofen. Baclofen encephalopathy is likely to develop in patients in renal failure particularly in presence of pre-existing cerebral damage (Himmelsbach et al 1992).

Intrathecal use of baclofen for spasticity is expanding now and overdosage by this route leads to coma and respiratory depression and is treated by physostigmine even though it is not a specific antidote (Muller-Schwefe and Penn 1989). Delhaas and Brouwers (1991) have reported 5 patients with similar problem and did not find physostigmine to be safe and effective in all the cases. Encephalopathy due to accidental overdose of baclofen has been reported in 6 children aged 2 to 6 years (Cooke and Glasstone 1994). Neurologic manifestations were impaired consciousness, convulsions, ataxia, and dilated pupils. They were managed with supportive treatment (gastric lavage and activated charcoal) and recovered.

Antineoplastic Drugs

Antineoplastic drugs are known to produce a non-specific encephalopathy. They are also known to produce leukoencephalopathy but the evidence for this is not always provided in the adverse drug reaction reports. Most of CNS effects are described in a subsequent section on leukoencephalopathy.

Bismuth

Bismuth subsalicylate is a component of widely used over-the-counter remedies. Reversible myoclonic encephalopathy due to intoxication by bismuth salts was first described by Burns et al (1974). Since then over 1000 cases have been reported in France (Martin-Bouyer et al 1980) and isolated cases have been reported from other countries. Encephalopathy has been reported to result from abuse of Peptobismol (Jungreis and Schaumburg 1993; Mendelowitz et al 1990). Bismuth-induced encephalopathy has also been reported following use of tri-potassium-dicitrato bismuthate in a patient with chronic renal failure (Playford et al 1990). A case of encephalopathy has also been reported following long-term extradural application of bismuth iodoform paraffin paste (Sharma et al 1994). Special presentation of encephalopathy include the following case reports:

– Encephalopathy with dementia (Kendel and Schäffer 1993).
– Encephalopathy resembling Creutzfeldt-Jacob disease (Von Bose and Zaudig 1991).
– Encephalopathy with myoclonus (Gordon et al 1995).

Slikkerveer and De Wolff (1994) have identified three facets of bismuth encephalopathy:
1. A prodromal phase lasting last from two to six weeks and characterized by gait disturbances and cognitive decline.
2. Clinical phase characterized by myoclonus, confusion, and dysarthria.
3. Recovery phase lasting four to six weeks. Symptoms usually clear spontaneously in the reverse order of their appearance after discontinuation of bismuth therapy.

A murine model for human bismuth encephalopathy has been reported where neurological signs (myoclonus, ataxia, tremor, and convulsions) have been produced by intraperitoneal injection of bismuth subnitrate (Ross et al 1988).

Diagnosis. The diagnosis of bismuth poisoning is supported by increased concentration of bismuth in the blood. Frontotemporal 4–6 Hz activity is seen in the frontotemporal region on EEG and increased density of the cerebral cortex has been noted on CT scanning. A radio-opaque substance can be seen on abdominal films in the large intestine of patients with barium intoxication.

Management. The following therapeutic measures should be considered in bismuth encephalopathy:
- Recovery usually occurs after discontinuation of bismuth intake.
- Evacuation of the bismuth from the intestine by gastrointestinal lavage.
- Dimercaprol has been found to be effective in treatment of bismuth encephalopathy (Molina et al 1989).

Bromides

Bromism is known as an effect of chronic ingestion of bromide salts which are often used as hypnotics (Michon et al 1989). The clinical picture is variable; confusion, drowsiness, hallucinations, extrapyramidal signs, etc.

Cephalosporins

Cephalosporins, like penicillin, can produce encephalopathy and seizures (see Chapter 7). Cefazolin encephalopathy has been reported mainly in patients with renal failure. Ortiz et al (1991) hypothesized that neurotoxicity of cephalosporins is due low serum protein concentration in renal failure patients. Cefazolin is highly protein-bound and decreased protein binding in renal failure may be responsible for neurotoxicity. A case of cephaloridine encephalopathy in a patient with renal failure has been reported by Taylor et al (1981).

Ceftazidime, a third generation cephalosporin, is structurally similar to penicillin. Absence status and toxic hallucinations have been reported following its use (Jackson and Berkovic 1992; Douglas et al 1988). Most of the neurotoxicity has been reported after intravenous use of this drug. Intraperitoneal ceftazidine is the recommended drug for treatment of peritonitis in general. Encephalopathy has been reported in an elderly patient after resolution of peritonitis by intraperitoneal ceftazidine (Lye and Leong 1994). The manifestations were impaired consciousness, bilateral slow waves on EEG, and myoclonus. The patient recurrent but had a recurrence of encephalopathy after repetition of ceftazidine for recurrence of peritonitis. Four patients were reported to develop encephalopathy with another third generation cephalosporin—cefuroxime (Herishanu et al 1998). All of these recovered within 48 hours after discontinuation of the drug.

Quinolone antibiotics are usually not associated with encephalopathy. There is one case report of a 4-year old girl with chronic renal insufficiency who developed encephalopathy after receiving two intravenous doses of ciprofloxacin to treat an infection (Rfidah et al 1995). An EEG showed a moderate excess of slow wave activity indicating a non-specific encephalopathy. Ciprofloxacin was discontinued and replaced by cefotaxime and the symptoms resolved within four days.

Digoxin

Extreme fatigue or drowsiness is common in patients receiving digitalis and may be attributed to cardiac failure. Two case reports in the literature suggest that such a manifestation may be due to digitalis encephalopathy. In both of the patients serum digoxin concentrations were over $4 \mu g/L$ and both recovered after discontinuation of digitalis with fall of digoxin levels to $0.3 \mu g/L$ in one patient and $0.7 \mu g/L$ in the other (Greenway et al 1996). Other causes of cerebral dysfunction were ruled out in these patients. It is recommended that serum digoxin levels should be checked in patients who present with abnormal cerebral dysfunction.

DMSO (Dimethylsulfoxide)

DMSO is approved for use as a bladder irrigant for interstitial cystitis. Its unapproved use extends to other indications. Transient encephalopathy was described in an elderly women on intravenous DMSO (Yellowlees et al 1980). Bond and Curry (1989) described an acute reversible encephalopathy in a patient with metastatic prostatic carcinoma who received several courses of intravenous DMSO in a "cancer clinic". Dhodapkar et al (1994) reported two patients who experienced severe reversible encephalopathy following infusion of peripheral blood stem cells cryopreserved in 10% DMSO. In one patient, reduction of DMSO level with plasmapheresis resulted in marked improvement in encephalopathy.

Fat Emulsion Therapy (FET)

This is used for parenterally administering calories and essential amino acids. Multi-organ failure in association with FET is known as "fat overload syndrome" (FOS). Schulz et al (1994) have described an encephalopathy with seizures as an initial manifestation of FOS and lipid deposits were demonstrated in area of cerebral infarction at autopsy.

Filgrastim

Filgrastim (granulocyte colony stimulating factor) is used for treating the neutropenia associated with cancer chemotherapy. A number of neurological adverse events have been reported in patients receiving this therapy in clinical trials but it is difficult to evaluate these because of advanced malignancy and multiple medications that these patients receive. The first published case of encephalopathy associated with filgrastim presented with cortical blindness and seizures in patient with ovarian cancer who had antineoplastic therapy with cyclophosphamide and cisplatin (Kastrup and Diener 1997). She had similar adverse events on a previous treatment with molgramostin, another colony stimulating factor used for the same indication. This resolved after discontinuation of molgramostin. EEG showed a left occipitotemporal focus with continuous spike-wave complexes. Filgrastim was discontinued and the patient was treated with phenytoin and valproic acid. Her symptoms resolved and there was no recurrence of seizures.

Histamine-2 (H₂)-Receptor Antagonists

H_2-receptor antagonists, particularly, cimetidine, are known to cause CNS toxicity manifested by confusion, agitation, hallucinations and seizures (Lipsy et al 1990; Cantu and Korek 1991). The underlying mechanism is blockage of CNS H_2-receptors. Ancillary mechanisms are cimetidine-induced release of norepinephrine in the hypothalamus, blocking of cholinergic receptors, inhibition of mitochondrial respiration and interaction with GABA receptors. Mental confusion and seizures have been observed in neurosurgical patients treated with intravenous famotidine and this was associated with renal failure and raised CSF concentrations of famotidine (Yoshimoto et al 1994).

HOPA (Calcium Hopantenate)

It is a complex of GABA and pantoic acid used in Japan for the treatment of mental retardation in children and dementia in the elderly. Several Japanese authors have reported encephalopathy with acidosis during HOPA treatment (Nakanishi et al 1990; Sasaki et al 1991; Kajita et al 1990).

It has been presumed that HOPA induces defects of coenzyme A because of its structure is common between HOPA and pantothenic acid. Dogs given increasing doses of HOPA over 8 weeks become comatose (Noda et al 1991). One group of dogs who received concomitant pantothenic acid did not develop any significant abnormality. The authors concluded that HOPA produces an acute encephalopathy in dogs by inducing a deficiency of pantothenic acid.

Intrathecal Contrast Agents

Methotrexate and iohexol, contrast materials used for lumbar myelography, have been reported to be associated with encephalopathy.

Metrizamide

– Metrizamide myelography can be associated with encephalopathy. Usui et al (1988) reported the case of a child with hydrocephalus in whom metrizamide shunt-gram was followed by disturbance of consciousness and extrapyramidal symptoms. There was periventricular penetration of contrast material into the medial part of thalamus and caudate nucleus, with resulting deficiency of the ascending noradrenergic reticular activating system and the nigrostriatal dopaminergic system.

Iohexol

– This is considered to have less neurotoxicity than metrizamide. However, three cases of encephalopathy have been reported following its use (Ceylan et 1993; Soriano-Soriano et al 1992; Donaghy et al 1985). Usual manifestations are coma and generalized slowing of EEG activity. Recovery is mostly spontaneous and dexamethasone has been considered to be beneficial.

Intravenous Immune Globulin (IVIG)

IVIG is being used for the treatment of immune thrombocytopenic purpura and Guillain-Barré syndrome. There are several spontaneous reports of this adverse reaction but only a few cases have been published. One patient experienced visual loss, confusion and seizures while receiving IVIG for Guillain-Barré syndrome (Harkness et al 1996). EEG showed widespread symmetric slow wave activity and MRI showed a small area of increased signal in the occipital area of the left occipital lobe. The patient recovered after discontinuation of IVIG. Another case is reported of a child treated with IVIG for immune thrombocytopenic purpura and developed hemiplegia and dysarthria following the infusion (Tsiouris and Tsiouris 1998). IVIG therapy was discontinued and the patient recovered. Mathy et al (1998) reported a patient who developed an acute encephalopathy during IVIG therapy. The signs and symptoms of the encephalopathy completely resolved after discontinuation of the treatment. There is a clinical similarity between these IVIG-related encephalopathy and the "reversible posterior leukoencephalopathy syndrome", described in the section on hypertensive encephalopathy.

The pathomechanism is not known but one possible explanation is transient hyperviscosity syndrome associated with rapid infusion of large doses of IVIG. Vasospasm is another explanation. Encephalopathy may be an immunoallergic reaction, caused by the entry of the exogenous IgG into the CSF compartment. CSF examinations usually show a neutrophilic or a mixed pleocytosis and aseptic meningitis has also been reported with IVIG (see Chapter 16).

Isoniazid

There is a case report of a girl who developed toxic encephalopathy 1 week after starting isoniazid 300 mg/day for a positive tuberculin test (Lopez Gaston and Carod Artal 1994). The symptoms included somnolence, disorientation, headache, nystagmus, and ataxia. EEG showed bilateral frontal slowing. Encephalopathy resolved 2 days after discontinuation of isoniazid. Encephalopathy recurred after resumption of isoniazid. Isoniazid-induced encephalopathy is rare with the use of therapeutic doses. .

Levodopa

Neufeld (1992) described four patients with idiopathic Parkinson's disease who developed a subacute encephalopathy and periodic triphasic EEG activity following an increase in dose of levodopa. These changes reverse following levodopa reduction or discontinuation.

Lithium

Toxic neuropathy has been described in patients receiving a combination of lithium and neuroleptics (Cohen and Cohen 1974; Biarez et al 1989; Schou 1990). Miller and Meninger (1987) reported that 27% of the patients on a combination of lithium and neuroleptics(developed neurotoxicity. Various clinical features reported include delirium, cerebellar dysfunction, and extrapyramidal signs. Lithium neurotoxicity syndrome is poorly defined, lacks diagnostic criteria, and is based mostly on anecdotal reports. El-Mallakh (1986) reviewed 213 published case reports of acute lithium toxicity occurring between 1948 to 1984. Although 95% of these patients had neurological signs, no factors that could have caused or contributed to lithium toxicity could be identified. However they graded acute lithium toxicity as follows:

– Grade I. Drowsiness, hypertonia, and muscle rigidity
– Grade II. Impaired consciousness progressing to lethargy
– Grade III. Seizures, stupor, and coma.

Kessel et al (1992) found no cases of neurotoxicity as defined in the earlier reports and it was considered to be an idiosyncratic reaction. A reversible Creutzfeldt-Jakob like syndrome with triphasic EEG waves has been described following use of lithium (Broussolle et al 1989; Smith and Kocen 1988).

Interactions with other drugs results in a higher incidence of lithium encephalopathy. Some drugs decrease the renal clearance of lithium and lead to toxic lithium blood levels. Lithium may have additive effects with psychopharmacologically active drugs. Some of the important interactions are with the following drugs:

– antipsychotics such as haloperidol
– antidepressants
– carbamazepine
– diuretics

There is no specific antidote for lithium toxicity. Long-term neurotoxic effects can be prevented in most of the cases. Even though high serum lithium levels are neurotoxic, a rapid decrease in high serum lithium concentrations may be even more toxic. Swartz and Dolinar (1995) have described such a case of a young woman with high serum lithium who developed encephalopathy after withdrawal of lithium and suggested that a 2 mEq/L/day decrease in lithium levels can be neurotoxic.

Mefloquine

Mefloquine is an effective prophylaxis and therapy for falciparum malaria. Neuropsychiatric

adverse reactions are well documented (see Chapter 5). An acute brain syndrome (encephalopathy) has been reported as an adverse effect of the therapy (Rouveix et al 1989; Bem et al 1992).

OKT3 (Muromonab CD3)

OKT3, a monoclonal antibody, is used as an immunosuppressive agent in patients receiving organ transplantation. Aseptic meningitis as a complication of this drug has been described in Chapter 16. Encephalopathy associated with OKT3 has also been reported (Coleman and Norman 1990; Min and Fallo 1993). Various clinical manifestations apart from aseptic meningitis are: convulsions, hallucinations, deterioration of mental function, and motor incoordination). A case of hemiparesis associated with OKT3 has also been reported (Osterman et al 1993).

The pathomechanism of encephalopathy is not known. It is believed that OKT3 induces a release of cytokines from lymphocytes or monocytes and these may mediate these symptoms. This has been described as "the cytokine release syndrome" or cytokine encephalopathy. Shihab et al (1993) consider delayed graft function as a significant risk factor for cytokine encephalopathy especially in diabetics. Delayed graft function might allow the retention of uremic toxins, which, in combination with cytokines, might mediate cytokine syndrome or it might cause the retention of released cytokines which, by themselves, mediate the syndrome. Brain swelling may be due to leakage from abnormal capillaries as an effect of cytokines.

Penicillin

Intravenous penicillin G has been reported to produce encephalopathy. The manifestations are progressive restlessness, mental confusion, hallucinations, and multifocal clonus. Penicillin encephalopathy has been produced experimentally and can be reversed by use of intravenous penicillamine (Raichle et al 1971).

Podophyllin

Podophyllin poisoning is uncommon and most reported cases result from accidental ingestion of podophyllin resin. Neurological manifestations of poisoning include encephalopathy, autonomic peripheral neuropathy, and cerebral involvement resulting in acute alterations of sensorium varying from mental confusion to coma. Podophyllin is a constituent of Chinese medicines and two cases of encephalopathy with peripheral neuropathy have been described after ingestion of such a substance. These patients developed cerebral atrophy documented by CT scan (Ng et al 1991).

The toxic agent responsible for podophyllin poisoning is considered to be podophyllotoxin (Filley et al 1982), a lipid-soluble compound that crosses cell membrane with ease. Neurotoxicity may be related to its in vitro ability to bind microtubular protein and inhibit axoplasmic flow. Colchicine and podophyllin toxins are structurally related and have similar clinical effects.

PSC833

PSC833 (Amdray, Novartis), a non-immunosuppressive cyclosporin analogue, is a P-glycoprotein (P-GP) inhibitor which is administered as an adjunct to chemotherapy. It overcomes the multidrug resistance (MDR) of P-GP-expressing tumors to chemotherapy by suppressing the activation of the MDR1 gene. PSC833 may affect the functional integrity of the BBB allowing increased penetration of certain chemotherapeutic drugs into the brain which may produce neurotoxicity (Schinkel et al 1996). It thus enhances, not only the therapeutic effect, but also the toxicity of chemotherapeutic agents as well other potentially neurotoxic drugs administered concomitantly. It is in phase III for treatment of ovarian cancer and acute myeloid leukemia. Cases of encephalopathy have been reported in clinical trials.

Stem Cell Transplantation

Autologous bone marrow transplantation (BMT) and peripheral blood stem cell transplantation (PBSCT) is increasingly used to treat hematological malignancies and solid tumors. The incidence of encephalopathy is 3.2% which is lower than in case of allogeneic BMT where there are added complications due to immunosuppressive therapy (Guerrero et al 1999). The higher reported incidence in some of the earlier studies (10% to 40%) is likely due to inclusion of cases which has suffered only confusion or somnolence or decrease in alertness. Some of the complications can also be attributed to the primary disease (malignancy) and other medications used.

Sulfonamides

Sulfonamide-induced toxic encephalopathy is considered to be rare. Patients with AIDS are more susceptible to adverse drug reactions including sulfonamides. Cases of encephalopathy associated with sulfadiazine therapy in AIDS patients have been reported (Reboli and Mandler 1992; Young 1989).

Trimethoprim-sulfamethoxazole is associated with aseptic meningitis (see Chapter 16). A case of encephalopathy as a part of general hypersensitivity reaction to trimethoprim-sulfamethoxazole has been reported (Theodorou et al 1995).

Sulfasalazine can produce encephalopathy by a hypersensitivity reaction causing cerebral microangiitis (Schoonjans et al 1993).

Theophylline

Seizures due to theophylline are well known (see Chapter 7). Maegaki et al (1993) have described two asthmatic children who developed semicoma following status epilepticus. CT scan showed long-lasting severe cortical edema which the authors considered to be characteristic of theophylline encephalopathy.

Encephalopathies Secondary to Drug-Induced Metabolic Disorders

Several encephalopathies are secondary to metabolic disorders associated drug-induced hepatic encephalopathy, hyperammonemia, Wernicke's encephalopathy, hypoglycemia and hyponatremia.

Hepatic Encephalopathy

Hepatic encephalopathy is characterized by disturbances of consciousness, personality changes, fluctuating neurological signs, asterixis (flapping tremor) and distinctive electroencephalographic changes. It may be acute and reversible or chronic and progressive. Coma and death may occur. A number of drugs associated with hepatic encephalopathy are shown in Table 3.3. There is a long list of other drugs which are hepatotoxic or produce fulminating hepatic failure which may be accompanied by hepatic encephalopathy.

Pathogenesis. The most important factor in the pathogenesis is severe hepatocellular function. Pathomechanism of drug-induced hepatic encephalopathy is not clear but various hypotheses are:

- Ammonia neurotoxicity. However, hyperammonemia may or may not be related to hepatotoxicity.
- Action of multiple neurotoxins

Table 3.3. Drugs which are associated with hepatic encephalopathy.

Acetaminophen overdose
Acetylsalicylic acid – high dose (DeLeeuw et al 1992)
Antineoplastic agents
Benzodiazepines
COX2 inhibitor (McCormick et al 1999)
Diuretics
Lanreotide, a somatostatin analog (Robin et al 1996)
Narcotics
Omeprazole (del Rio Fernandez et al 1997)
Propranolol, in patients with liver cirrhosis (Cales 1989)
Propylthiouracil (Kirkland 1990)
Terbinafine (Agarwal et al 1999)
Tuberculostatic agents (Moitinho et al 1996)
Valproic acid

- Imbalance of excitatory and inhibitory amino acids
- GABA hypothesis. Activation of brain receptors for benzodiazepines which is closely related to GABA receptor (Basile et al 1991). This may facilitate GABA neurotransmission (inhibitory). The role is uncertain because of the inconsistent effect of flumazenil in hepatic encephalopathy.
- Modestly elevated concentrations of ammonia, that commonly occur in liver failure, may contribute to the manifestations of hepatic encephalopathy by enhancing GABAergic inhibitory neurotransmission. This concept appears to unify the ammonia and GABAergic neurotransmission hypotheses (Jones and Basile 1998).

Hyperammonemia can occur as an adverse reaction to drugs without clinical evidence of liver disease. Examples of this are valproic acid (see under antiepileptic medications), cimetidine (Duval et al 1999) and antineoplastic therapy. High-dose 5-fluorouracil infusion therapy is associated with hyperammonaemia, lactic acidosis and encephalopathy (Yeh and Cheng 1997). Liaw et al (1999) identified 29 cancer patients who had 32 episodes of transient hyperammonemic encephalopathy related to continuous infusion of 5-fluorouracil. None of the patients had decompensated liver disease.

Management. Early recognition of hyperammonemia (before the ammonia level reaches 350 mmol/L) and institution of ammonia lowering agents is important to avoid further complications. Specific measures for treatment of hepatic encephalopathy are:

- Discontinuation of the offending drug
- Lowering of blood ammonia. Sodium benzoate and sodium phenylacetate have been used for antineoplastic-induced hyperammonemia (del Rosario et al 1997).
- Exclusion of protein from diet and of amino acids from parenteral nutrition
- Hemodialysis to remove toxic substances
- Chronic encephalopathy is effectively controlled by administration of lactulose.

Hypoglycemic Encephalopathy

Hypoglycemia induced or exacerbated by medications can result in convulsions, coma, and brain damage. Some of the drugs and the situations in which they produce hypoglycemia have been described in the literature (Seltzer 1979; Pandit et al 1993) and are listed in Table 3.4.

Table 3.4. Drugs and circumstances producing hypoglycemia.

Beta-blockers, by enhancing the action of insulin in
   diabetics
Captopril, in diabetic patients
Disopyramide, in patients with hepatic and renal disease
Ethanol, by potentiating hyoglycemia by other drugs
Insulin overdose
Lithium, long-term treatment in diabetics
Pentamidine, by inducing hemorrhagic pancreatitis
Quinine, during treatment of severe falciparum malaria
Salicylate poisoning
Streptozotocin, by cytolytic effect on beta cells of
   the pancreas
Sulfamethoxazole, in patients with renal failure
Temafloxacillin (a quinolone antibiotic withdrawn
   from market)

Hyponatremic Encephalopathy

Hyponatremia occurs in several systemic disease states and is also frequently drug-induced. Various pharmaceutical agents include those that interfere with the ability of the kidneys to excrete free water. They include sedatives, antidepressants, antiepileptics, analgesics, oral hypoglycemic agents, tranquilizers, narcotics, antineoplastic agents, and diuretics (Arieff 1993). Symptomatic hyponatremia leads to brain swelling, seizures and rise of intracranial pressure. Hypoxia is the major factor contributing to brain damage in patients with hyponatremia. Hypoxia leads to a failure of homeostatic brain ion transport, which allows the brain to adapt to increases in cell water.

In some drug-induced encephalopathies it is important to differentiate between direct neurotoxicity and that via hyponatremia as the management depends on the mechanism involved. A case of reversible encephalopathy due to hyponatremia resulting from ifosfamide infusion (also known to be directly neurotoxic) has been described (Cantwell

et al 1990). Correction of hyponatremia reversed the symptoms in this case. Encephalopathy with hyponatremia has been described with the antiepileptic drug oxcarbazepine (Rosendahl and Friis 1991). The importance of this observation is that seizures occurring in an epileptic patient on this drug may be due to hyponatremia rather than lack of efficacy of the drug. Water intoxication and hyponatremia have also been reported following use of an oxytocin nasal spray (Seifer et al 1985) and thiazide reserpine combinations (Yap and Lau 1992).

Management. This is determined largely by symptomatology. If the patient is asymptomatic, hyponatremia can be corrected by discontinuation of the drug and water restriction. If the patient is symptomatic, active therapy to increase the plasma sodium with hypertonic saline is indicated (Fraser and Arieff 1997). This should be done carefully as rapid correction may rarely lead to central pontine mylenosis.

Wernicke's Encephalopathy

This is also referred to as Wernicke's syndrome or Wernicke's disease or cerebral beri-beri and is an encephalopathy resulting from thiamine deficiency. It is usually associated with alcoholism is by no means confined to alcoholics. It occurs in anorexia nervosa, gastric plication, hyperemesis gravidarum, and prolonged fasting—conditions that are all associated with poor intake of vitamins. The clinical features are memory impairment, dysarthria, ataxia and ophthalmoplegia. The neuropathological lesions in fatal Wernicke's cases are in the paraventricular region of the thalamus and hypothalamus, mammillary bodies, the periaqueductal region, and the floor of the fourth

Table 3.5. Drug-induced Wernicke's encephalopathy.

5-fluorouracil with intravenous hyperalimentation
   (see text)
Amiloride-furosemide (see text)
Erbulazole, an experimental antineoplastic drug (De
Klippel et al 1991).
Glucose intravenous infusions in "at risk" patients
High-dose nitroglycerin (Nadel 1985)
Lithium-induced diarrhoea (Epstein 1989)
Tolazamide (Kwee and Nakada 1983)

ventricle. Causes of drug-induced Wernicke's encephalopathy are shown in Table 3.5.

Wernicke's encephalopathy and acute metabolic acidosis has been reported in a patient with gastric carcinoma who was given continuous infusion of 5-fluorouracil while receiving intravenous hyperalimentation (Kondo et al 1996). It manifested by confusion, diplopia, deafness and ataxia. The patient recovered after hemodialysis and intravenous thiamine. McLean and Manchip (1999) have described a case where this syndrome developed after long-term treatment with amiloride-furosemide for congestive heart failure. Furosemide is known to impede magnesium absorption in the kidneys by as much as 400%. Since magnesium is an essential factor in the conversion of thiamine into its active diphosphate and triphosphate esters, magnesium depletion may aggravate thiamine deficiency.

Intravenous infusions of glucose without thiamine supplementation should be avoided in patients at risk of developing Wernicke's encephalopathy. Treatment is discontinuation of the offending medication and administration of intravenous thiamine. Recovery takes place and severe neurological disability can be avoided if treatment is instituted early.

Drug-Induced Leukoencephalopathy

Drugs have been reported to be associated with leukoencephalopathy are shown in Table 3.6.

Amphotericin B

Intravenous amphotericin B (AmpB) is the drug of choice in the treatment of severe fungal infections although its systemic and renal toxicity is well known. Neurotoxicity, however, is less well-recognized. Ellis et al (1982) described the syndrome of progressive dementia, akinesia, mutism, and sphincter dysfunction complicating the treatment of a variety of mycoses with intravenous amphotericin B-methyl ester. Devinsky et al (1987) described a similar case associated with AmpB. Walker and Rosenblum (1992) have

Table 3.6. Drugs associated with leukoencephalopathy.

Amphotericin B
Antineoplastics*
cisplatin*
cytosine arabinoside
5-fluouracil
fludarabine
ifosfamide/mesna *
levamisole
methotrexate*
Arsenicals
Corticosteroids
Heroin
Immunosuppressive therapy with organ transplantation
Cyclosporine*
Tacrolismus* (FK506)
Interferons
Interleukin-2*
*Intravenous immunoglobulin

*Frequently reported.

reported two further cases of fatal leukoencephalopathy associated with intravenous administration of AmpB and reviewed the literature on this subject. Leukoencephalopathy with parkinsonian features has been described in children following bone marrow transplantation and high dose AmpB (Mott et al 1995). Although the course has been progressive and fatal in more than half of the reported cases, some recovered with residual neurological deficits. In other cases, it was shown to be reversible in early stages (Antonini et al 1996) with description of onset of hemiplegia after intravenous infusion of AmpB in one case on two occasions where recovery followed on both occasions within half an hour after discontinuation of the infusion (Devuyst et al 1995). The following clinical and pathological features were most commonly observed in the cases reported in the literature:
– The pathology and clinical course is less severe in patients with infections alone as compared to those with malignant disease where there is concomitant CNS adverse effect of chemotherapy.
– Most patients with malignant disease were immunosuppressed and received standard intravenous doses of AmpB for pulmonary aspergillosis, a complication of chemotherapy. None of the patients had clinical evidence of infection or a neoplastic process involving the CNS.

- Most patients with malignant disease had cranial radiation as well and treatment with a variety of antineoplastic and antimicrobial agents.
- Onset is either acute or a subacutely evolving neurologic disorder. It is characterized by a progressive dose-dependent course and is reversible if AmpB is discontinued early.
- Brain imaging studies showed abnormal findings. CT demonstrated hypodensity of white matter of the cerebral hemispheres, particularly in the frontal regions. MRI showed increased signals from cerebral white matter on T_2-weighted images from the frontal regions and basal ganglia.
- Neuropathologic findings are a diffuse non-inflammatory leukoencephalopathy characterized by florid astrogliosis, myelin loss, and infiltration of rarefied white matter by a large number of macrophages containing phagocytized myelin debris.

Pathomechanism. Normally AmpB does not penetrate the BBB but in some of the case described in literature, BBB may have been damaged by cranial radiation. There may also be an element of an idiosyncratic reaction in the development of this syndrome. The biologic effects of polyene macrolide antibiotics such as AmpB are chiefly mediated through their binding to cell membrane sterols including cholesterol. This results in a structural alteration which increases membrane permeability and permits leakage of intracellular constituents from susceptible cells. Cholesterol-rich myelin may be a target for binding of AmpB. AmpB-associated leukoencephalopathy has been reproduced in dogs (Ellis et al 1988).

Management. Patients receiving amphotericin should be monitored carefully for early signs of neurotoxicity. Early discontinuation of amphotericin may lead to recovery before irreversible lesions develop.

Antineoplastics

Neurotoxicity of antineoplastic agents is well known and this topic has been reviewed in an excellent monograph edited by Hildebrand (1990). Mechanisms of neurotoxicity of various compounds has been postulated but they do not necessarily correlate with the antineoplastic effect. Some of the explanations for the variations in neurotoxicity of various antineoplastic agents are:
- Individual characteristics and metabolites. Interactions with various enzymes.
- Dose
- Ability of various agents to cross the blood brain barrier which normally has a protective function against neurotoxicity
- Adjuvants used to increase penetration of blood brain barrier
- Combination with radiotherapy

Factors related to the patients which influence neurotoxicity include the following:
- Type of malignancy
- Presence of other systemic diseases
- Cerebral involvement with malignancies of other organs
  · metastases
  · paraneoplastic syndromes
- Patients with brain tumors have damage to the blood brain barrier with increased permeability

Cisplatin. Cisplatin is a metal coordination compound that was approved for use in 1979 for management of testicular cancer. The "cis" form exerts its biological effect by binding directly to DNA and formation of inter- and intra-strand links. Its effect is enhanced by other antineoplastic drugs and radiotherapy (Rosenberg 1984). Cisplatin is ototoxic (see Chapter 10) and induces peripheral neuropathy (see Chapter 11). Encephalopathy has been reported due to cerebral edema which may be secondary to hypo-osmolality induced by the drug. It is the most emetogenic of chemotherapeutic agents and this is the most obvious manifestation of neurotoxicity (Allen 1991). The emetic effects are most probably related to stimulation of the chemoreceptor trigger zones in the area postrema of the medulla.

A case of multifocal necrotizing leukoencephalopathy has been reported after cisplatin treatment (Bruck et al 1989). Another case of encephalopathy (manifested by mental confusion, drowsiness, seizures and visual disturbances) has been reported following cisplatin-based chemotherapy with bleomycin and vinblastine (Hitchins and Thomson 1988; Cohen and Cuneo 1983). A case of confusional state, without seizures but an epileptic EEG focus, has also been reported (Lyass et al 1998). There is unusual accumulation of cisplatin in the brains of patients who manifest encephalopathy perhaps via an altered BBB.

Cytosine Arabinoside (ARA-C). Neurologic toxicity of intravenous ARA-C is usually dose-related and predominantly cerebellar (see Chapter 15). Cerebral toxicity is reported to be less severe and may manifest as somnolence and confusion. A case has been reported of encephalopathy with hemiparesis and optic neuropathy (Hoffmann et al 1993). Subacute encephalopathy with prominent cerebellar dysfunction was reported in 8 of the 49 patients treated with high dose ARA-C (Lazarus et al 1981). The clinical features of intrathecal ARA-C include meningeal irritation, arachnoiditis, myelopathy and encephalopathy, manifested by seizures (Resar et al 1993; Phillips and Reinhardt 1991; Crawford et al 1986). Encephalopathy has also been reported following chemotherapy with a combination of ARA-C and flurabine both of which are structurally similar (Kornblau et al 1993).

The pathomechanism of ARA-C neurotoxicity is not known but the current concepts have been summarized by Resar et al (1993) as follows. CNS injury may be the result of ARA-C triphosphate (ARA-CTP), a cytotoxic substance or a metabolite such as uracil arabinoside. The primary determinants of cytotoxicity by ARA-CTP include the competitive inhibition of DNA polymerase alfa and direct incorporation into DNA. The concentration of ARA-CTP in the brain after intrathecal administration is sufficient to inhibit DNA synthesis and this may interfere with repair process in the CNS and replication of glial cells. Other mechanisms such as formation of arabinosylcytidine-choline may inhibit the synthesis of membrane glycolipids and glycoproteins in the CNS and contribute to neurotoxicity. However, it is difficult to establish a correlation between ARA-C metabolites in the CSF and clinical neurotoxicity in order to design a schedule of intrathecal ARA-C which may be effective but minimally neurotoxic. An interval of 2–3 days between intrathecal ARA-C treatments may reduce the risk of neurotoxicity.

5-Fluorouracil (5-FU). 5-FU is a derivative of the pyrimidine base uracil in which fluorine is substituted for the 5-position hydrogen. Manifestations of neurotoxicity are cerebellar disorders (see Chapter 15) and leukoencephalopathy. Several cases of multifocal inflammatory leukoencephalopathy have been reported with combined use of 5-FU and levamisole for adenocarcinoma of colon (Hook et al 1992; Neu and Ober 1992; Kimmel and Schutt 1993; Fassas et al 1994; Savarese et al 1996; Galassi et al 1996). Clinical manifestations varied from decline of mental function, ataxia, diplopia, and dysarthria to loss of consciousness. MRI showed multifocal periventricular enhancing white matter lesions. Cerebral biopsy in some cases showed active demyelinating disease. Most of the patients improved after cessation of therapy and treatment with corticosteroids although there were some residual neurological deficits.

Leukoencephalopathy in these cases is considered to be a toxic effect of 5-FU but a direct relationship has not been proven. Patients with decreased dihydropyrimidine dehydrogenase activity are at increased risk for experiencing leukoencephalopathy following 5-fluorouracil (Takimoto et al 1996). The comedication levamisole has also been reported to be associated with encephalopathy. Bilateral necrotizing leukoencephalopathy has been reported in a patient with combined chemotherapy including 5-FU, cyclophosphamide, and methotrexate (Gütling et al 1992).

A rare tumor lysis syndrome may occur along with fluorouracil-induced leukoencephalopathy. A fatal case due to this combination of adverse effects has been reported after fluorouracil monotherapy for colorectal cancer with hepatic metastases (Stephan et al 1995). The patient developed a generalized seizure, coma and uric acid nephropathy. This patient was considered to have experienced a chemotherapy-induced tumor lysis (confirmed by hepatic CT scan) rather than spontaneous tumor necrosis.

A similar case of leukoencephalopathy has been reported in a patient treated with 5-FU derivative hexylcarbonyl-5-FU (HCFU) mono-therapy (Aoki et al 1986). A case of leukoen-cephalopathy with loss of consciousness and CT appearance of low density lesions has been reported (Kamata et al 1988). HCFU passes readily through the BBB to provide 5-FU and its derivatives of which alpha-fluoro-beta-ala-nine is thought to be the culprit which produces leukoencephalopathy. Yamada et al (1989) have reviewed 24 cases of leukoencephalopathy re-sulting from use of HCFU (Carmofur) and re-ported in the Japanese literature. Another 5-FU derivative Tegafur which is used in Japan has also been reported to produce leukoencephalo-pathy (Dobashi et al 1994; Hata et al 1992; Hayashi et al 1992; Kawada et al 1991; Na-ganuma et al 1988).

Fludarabine. High doses of fludarabine are used for treatment of acute leukemia and have been reported to induce leukoencephalopathy (Cheson et al 1994). Lower doses are used in the treatment of chronic lymphocytic leukemia (CLL) and are generally considered to be safe. A case of fatal progressive multifocal leukoen-cephalopathy (confirmed by brain biopsy and neuroimaging) has been reported to develop 6 months after completion of a course with low dose (25 mg/m^2/day) fluarabine monotherapy for B-CLL (Zabernigg et al 1994). Lymphoma involving the brain was excluded at autopsy.

Ifosfamide/Mesna. Ifosemide (IFX), a structur-al isomer of cyclophosphamide, is active against several tumors. Unlike cyclophosphamide it has significant neurotoxicity. Combination with mesna (sodium 2-mercapto-ethane sulfonate) permits higher doses of ifosemide by detoxifying its urotoxic metabolite.

IFX encephalopathy is characterized by con-fusion, stupor and mutism. Several cases of ifosemide encephalopathy have been reported (Meanwell et al 1985; Beuzeboc et al 1988; Ghosn et al 1988; Danesh et al 1989; Miller and Eaton 1992). Incidence of encephalopathy is re-ported to vary from 11% to 18% (Merimsky et al 1992). Risk factors identified were low serum albumin indicative of hepatic dysfunction, high serum creatinine suggesting renal compromise, and presence of neoplastic disease in the pelvis.

Other risk factors are previous exposure to cis-platin and radiotherapy. Neurotoxic effects may range from subclinical EEG changes to severe irreversible encephalopathy and death. One rec-ommendation to prevent neurotoxicity is that ifosemide/mesna should not be given to patients with less than 20% probability of remaining free of CNS toxicity according to the nomogram pro-posed by Meanwell et al (1986).

Pathomechanism. Ifosemide is a prodrug which requires biotransformation to become cytotoxic. Neurotoxicity of ifosemide may be related to the high serum concentrations of chloracetaldehyde which is one of its major metabolites (Schoenide and Dana 1990). Chloracetaldehyde depletes in-tracellular glutathione concentration (Wagner 1994) Cerny and Küpfer (1992) have observed that a patient who developed encephalopathy on ifosemide therapy was a poor metabolizer of phenotype of carbocysteine, a situation in which endogenous cysteine is not available in sufficient amounts to produce the carbocysteine metabolite which is carboxymethyl thiocysteine. This pre-disposes to toxic effects of aldehydes. High se-rum creatinine concentration, presence of pelvic disease, fast infusion of IFX, and low serum al-bumin concentration are risk factors for IFX encephalopathy (Seddigh et al 1993). Stereose-lective study of urinary excretion of ifosfamide metabolites show that high R-3 dechloroacetal-dehyde concentration is linked with neurotoxici-ty in a subset of patients with overexpression of enzyme P450 (Wainer et al 1994).

Management. IFX neurotoxicity is dose-depend-ent and has been reported to be reversed in two patients by methylene blue as an antidote (Küp-fer et al 1994; Zulian et al 1995). These authors reported that prophylactic use in another patient prevented the onset of IFX neurotoxicity. Simo-nian et al (1993) reported that intravenous dia-zepam improved mental function and EEG in two patients with IFX encephalopathy.

Levamisole. This was originally used as an an-thelminthic agent but is now used as a chemo-therapeutic agent. Neurotoxic symptoms associ-ated with its use include confusion. tremor, and myalgia and a delayed encephalopathy has been reported (Zheng et al 1994). Leukoencephalopathy has been described in patients who received levamisole in combination with 5-fluorouracil. Chen et al (1994) described a case of multifocal leukoencephalopathy (confirmed by brain biopsy and MRI) in a patient who received a combination of 5-FU and levamisole. Despite continuation of 5-FU, resolution of contrast-enhancing lesions on MRI without further neurologic sequelae occurred when levamisole was stopped.

One case has been reported of multifocal leukoencephalopathy developing in a patient on levamisole monotherapy for malignant melanoma (Kimmel et al 1995). Another case was reported of multifocal leukoencephalopathy in a patient with hepatitis C who did not receive any other comedication (Lucia et al 1996). Clinical manifestations included lethargy, confusion, memory loss, dysphasia, weakness and ataxia. MRI showed multiple white matter lesions scattered throughout the cerebral hemispheres. The patient recovered completely after discontinuation of levamisole and corticosteroid therapy but the resolution of MRI lesions was incomplete.

Methotrexate (MTX). MTX is a structural analog of folic acid and is widely used as an antimetabolite in cancer chemotherapy. Its primary mechanism of action is inhibition of dihydrofolate with consequent depletion of intracellular folate pool. MTX also inhibits RNA, protein synthesis, glucose transport, and metabolism. Clinical expression of neurotoxicity of MTX depends on the route of administration, and the combined effect of drug concentration and dose.

Neurological complications of intrathecal MTX include arachnoiditis, myelopathy, and encephalopathy. The major risk factors are cumulative MTX dose and prior cranial radiation. CT scan as well as MRI are used for detection of leukoencephalopathy. Serial EEG may also be used for this purpose (Fuji et al 1988). MRI is considered to be more sensitive than CT scan. Early recognition is important as discontinuation of therapy leads to reversal of leukoencephalopathy (Gay et al 1989). Leukoencephalopathy was detected in 8 of 20 patients with acute lymphatic leukemia in early stages of treatment with intrathecal MTX and in 6 of these the lesions resolved after temporary or permanent interruption of therapy (Asato et al 1992).

High dose intravenous MTX has been reported to be associated with transient subacute leukoencephalopathy in 4 of the 83 patients with acute lymphatic leukemia (Sasazaki et al 1992). This complication usually appears after repeated courses of MTX treatment but a case of transient leukoencephalopathy has been reported following single high dose of intravenous MTX (Kubo et al 1992). Even low dose intravenous MTX has been reported to produce a delayed leukoencephalopathy (Boogerd et al 1988). Low dose oral methotrexate has also been reported to induce progressive multifocal leukoencephalopathy in a patient with rheumatoid arthritis (Worthley and McNeil 1995). One patient on alternating intrathecal MTX and ARA-C combined with radiotherapy, developed dementia and akinetic mutism and cerebral atrophy was shown on CT Jacobs et al (1991). In spite of discontinuation of treatment, the patient died of disseminated necrotizing encephalopathy.

Pathomechanism. Pathomechanism of MTX-induced leukoencephalopathy is not well understood but the following hypotheses have been considered (Phillips 1991):
– Cytotoxic effect on glial elements (Gregorios and Soucy 1990)
– Depletion of reduced folate in the brain
– Inhibition of cerebral protein and glucose metabolism
– Injury to cerebral vascular endothelium resulting in increased BBB permeability.
– Reduction of catecholamine neurotransmitter synthesis through direction inhibition of synthesis of tetrahydrobiopterin. This hypothesis is supported by the observation of increase of CSF biopterins in patients with MTX-induced encephalopathy (Netter et al 1991; Millot et al 1992).
– Release of adenine due to inhibition of purine synthesis (responsible for anti-inflammatory effect in patients with arthritis). This has been implicated in CNS neurotoxicity as increased concentrations of adenosine have been demonstrated in patients on MTX therapy (Bernini et al 1995).

Treatment. In the absence of a clear cut pathophysiological basis for MTX neurotoxicity, there is no definite treatment but the following drugs have been used:

- Intravenous leucovorine has been reported to reverse MTX-leukoencephalopathy (Cohen et al 1990).
- Intravenous aminophylline has been used to reverse MTX neurotoxicity as it displaces adenosine (implicated in neurotoxicity) from its receptor (Bernini et al 1995).

Vincristine. Hurwitz et al (1988) reported the case of a 8-year old child who developed a reversible encephalopathy as a result of conventional vincristine administration and bilateral radiolucencies were seen on CT scan. Cortical blindness has also been reported as an adverse reaction to vincristine (Merimsky et al 1992).

Miscellaneous Antineoplastic Drugs. A case of multifocal leukoencephalopathy has been reported in a patient with Wegner's granulomatosis treated with cyclophosphamide and corticosteroids (Choy et al 1992). A reversible encephalopathy (cortical blindness, seizures, paralysis, altered mental status) has been reported with fludarabine therapy (Cohen et al 1993). One case has been reported of leukoencephalopathy with enocitabine (behenoyl cytarabine) used for the treatment of acute myelogenous leukemia (Cho et al 1999). The patient has generalized seizures and MRI showed cortical and subcortical edema in posterior parietal region, temporal lobes and cerebellum. The patient recovered after discontinuation of enocitabine and treatment with anticonvulsants.

A fatal case of leukoencephalopathy has been described in a patient with non-Hodgkin's lymphoma treated with CHOP (cyclophosphamide, doxorubicin, vincristine and prednisone) followed by a stress dose of hydrocortisone (Cain et al 1998). Postmortem examination showed diffuse white matter edema with small areas of perivascular hemorrhages which were more marked in the left hemispheres. The etiology of leukoencephalopathy in this case was multifactorial.

Arsenicals

For thousands of years, arsenic and its compounds have been used for therapeutic purposes although the substance acquired its bad reputation due to its use for homicidal purposes. Neurological symptoms of acute arsenic poisoning include seizures and peripheral neuropathy is a more common sequel of chronic poisoning (see Chapter 11).

Organic arsenicals such as melarsoprol, which are used for the treatment of trypanosomiasis, can cause severe encephalopathy (Pialoux et al 1988; Arroz 1987). Convulsions and coma are frequent manifestations. It occurs in 7–13% of all cases treated with various schedules of this drug and may be fatal in up to 10% of cases. At autopsy the brain appears to be congested and swollen. Histological examination shows petechial hemorrhages and perivascular cuffing comprised of lymphocytes and macrophages. The pathologic changes in the brain are those of acute hemorrhagic leukoencephalopathy (Adams et al 1986). Hurst (1959) studied the lesions produced in the brains of monkeys by certain arsenical compounds. A single toxic dose of phenylarsine oxide as well as its triazine analog produces hemorrhagic and at times non-hemorrhagic necrosis at a number of sites in the brain. Neoarsphenamine did not produce any significant lesions. Some animals developed white matter gliosis. The authors concluded that none of the lesions of CNS were characteristic of arsenicals.

Melarsoprol-induced encephalopathy is probably an immune phenomenon rather than the result of dose-related arsenical toxicity. Trypanosomal antigens released after exposure to melarsoprol, presumably from the trypanosomes present in the brain (rather than the blood stream), bind to brain cells which eventually become the targets of antibodies and/or T-lymphocytes (Pepin and Milford 1991). Sub-curative chemotherapy may underlie the fatal post-treatment reactions seen in humans (Hunter et al 1992a). Oral prednisolone has been shown to reduce the incidence of encephalopathy induced by melarsoprol treatment of T. gambiense sleeping sickness (Pepin et al 1989). Hunter et al

(1992b) showed that, in the murine trypanoso-miasis model, azathioprine, a NSAID immuno-suppressant, ameliorated the post-treatment en-cephalopathy.

Corticosteroids

Glucocorticoids are frequently employed as im-munosuppressive agents and there are reports of occurrence and exacerbation of neurological im-mune-mediated conditions in patients receiving steroids. In a placebo-controlled trial, three of the five infants treated with dexamethasone for chronic lung disease, developed perivascular ab-normalities shown on cranial ultrasound exami-nation. One of these developed periventricular encephalomalacia subsequently (Noble-Jamie-son et al 1989). A case is reported of progressive multifocal leukoencephalopathy in a patient with multiple connective tissue disease who was treated with immunosuppressive therapy with low-dose corticosteroids for 12 years and azathioprine for 4 years (Schneider 1991).

Methylprednisolone is also used for the treat-ment of leukoencephalopathies. Steiner et al (1991) have studied the course of experimental allergic encephalitis (EAE) in rats and noted that methylprednisolone given prior to and during EAE significantly increased disease duration. In contrast, treatment with methylprednisolone af-ter onset of the disease was markedly beneficial.

Heroin

Spongiform leukoencephalopathy is a complica-tion of heroin addiction. Wolters et al (1982) re-ported 47 cases from Netherlands and the cause was known to be an unknown toxic factor. One case was reported from Germany (Haan et al 1983) and one case from Spain presented with both cerebral and cerebellar manifestations and died (Sempere et al 1991). Autopsy showed brain swelling and herniation. Extensive white matter spongiosis and vacuolization affecting the cerebrum and the cerebellum were seen mi-croscopically. Two similar cases have been re-ported in the United States following inhalation of heroin vapor (Kriegelstein et al 1997). MRI findings in these cases were symmetric lesions of high signal intensity in the occipital white matter, the posterior limb of the internal capsule and the splenium of the corpus callosum. These are considered to be characteristic of heroin-in-duced leukoencephalopathy. Both these patients survived with neurological deficits. The patho-mechanism remains unknown. None of the con-taminants found in the heroin sample are known to produce leukoencephalopathy.

Immunosuppressive Therapy with Organ Transplantation

Cyclosporin (CSP). CSP is the most widely used immunosuppressant to reduce the severity of graft versus host disease (GVHD) in organ transplantation. It is known to have toxic effects of the nervous system manifested by psychiatric disturbances, lethargy, tremor, visual disturb-ances, cerebellar ataxia and seizures. A rare com-plication is cortical blindness (Ghalie et al 1990). Some of these have been discussed individually in other chapters. Altogether, these manifesta-tions are, sometimes, referred to as encephalopa-thy (Truwit et al 1991). However, because of the white matter changes shown on MRI scan, the more appropriate term is leukoencephalopathy. CSP-leukoencephalopathy has been reported with the following organ transplantations:

– *Liver*. Neurological complications occur fre-quently in recipients of orthotopic liver trans-plantation. These complications include changes in mental status, seizures, severe headache and peripheral neuropathy. Neuro-logical complications can occur from a multi-plicity of factors which include the following:
  · Cerebrovascular accidents
  · CNS infections
  · Drug toxicity
  · Electrolyte disturbances
  · Metabolic factors
  · Preoperative hepatic encephalopathy
The role of drugs is difficult to determine be-cause there are no controls in the studies of liver transplantation where no immunosup-pressant is used. In one study encephalopathy

occurred in 46.1% of the patients but the percentage of those who developed leukoencephalopathy is not given (Menegaux et al 1994). In 27 of the 47 patients who developed neurological complications in this study, drug toxicity was the primary cause and the symptoms reversed with reduction of dosage or discontinuation of the drug. Cyclosporin and FK506, primarily during intravenous administration for the induction of immunosuppression accounted for 25 of the 27 neurological complications. In a comparison of CSP and FK506, the incidence of neurotoxicity was higher among patients treated with FK506 (21.3% vs 11.7%) than those treated with CSP (Mueller et al 1994). In another study 25% of patients developed CSP leukoencephalopathy after liver transplantation (de Groen et al 1987). In a study of 340 liver transplants, neurotoxicity was reported in only 12% of the cases and it was reverse in some of these by replacement of CSP by FK506 (Wijdicks et al 1995).

- *Kidney* (Berden et al 1985).
- *Bone marrow* (Reece et al 1991). One death occurred as a result of CSP-induced neurotoxicity during treatment with this agent following allogenic bone marrow transplantation for chronic myeloid leukemia (Gopal et al 1999). The patient had blurred vision, confusion and seizures. MRI showed diffuse white matter signal abnormality in the occipital regions, brainstem and thalamus. In spite of discontinuation of CSP and supportive treatment, the patient died. Autopsy showed edematous white matter with evidence of astrocyte injury and loss of cell processes between myelinated fibers and foot processes.
- *Heart* (McManus et al 1992).

Non-organ Transplant Indications for CSP. CSP neurotoxicity can occur unrelated to organ transplantation. Ettinger et al (1989) reported a patient with Wegner's granulomatosis who developed progressive multifocal leukoencephalopathy (PML) during CSP therapy. The patient died and the postmortem diagnosis was PML due to popova virus which may likely have been activated by CSP therapy. Monteiro et al (1993) described the case of a 16-year old girl who pre-sented with acute encephalopathy manifested by seizures two weeks after CSP and methylprednisolone treatment for idiopathic uveitis. MRI showed white matter changes. SCP was discontinued and intravenous phenytoin and diazepam were used for treatment. The patient recovered and was maintained on phenytoin and prednisolone therapy. Two months later, MRI changes resolved and the patient remained well. A case of acute leukoencephalopathy has been reported during CSP treatment in a patient with nephrotic syndrome (Shimizu et al 1994). The patient recovered after discontinuation of CSP and subcortical lesions shown on MRI resolved. Neurotoxicity has been reported after 4-month treatment with CSP treatment for rheumatoid arthritis (Kutlay et al 1997). The patient had multiple neurological symptoms including confusion, reduced visual acuity and ataxia. Recovery occurred after discontinuation of CSP. MRI was not done and it is not certain if there was any white matter abnormality.

Risk Factors. The following risk factors for CSP-leukoencephalopathy have been identified:

- Low serum cholesterol levels after liver transplantation (de Groen et al 1987). Possible explanations are:
  - CSP may interfere with the transport of cholesterol and other lipids into the brain and low cholesterol levels may magnify this effect.
  - Low concentration of LDL cholesterol may also lead to increased CSP delivery to astrocytes and thus increase neurotoxicity (de Groen et al 1988).
  - If total serum cholesterol is low, more CSP than usual may remain unbound and be able to pass the BBB and attach to its binding protein cycliphilin in the brain.
- Intravenous lipid solutions of CSP cause earlier and more severe symptoms than oral CSP (De Klippel et al 1992). Fat embolism leading to encephalopathy has also been reported to be induced by the drug's solvent.
- Children are more susceptible to neurotoxicity of CSP (Joss et al 1982).
- Impaired renal function. Nephrotoxicity may be due to CSP.

- Impaired liver function. Hepatoxicity may be due to CSP.
- Hypomagnesemia has been reported in recipients of allogenic bone marrow transplants who experience neurotoxicity of CSP (Thompson et al 1984). Hypomagnesemia is known to lower seizure threshold.
- Concomitant use of doxorubicin. Leukoencephalopathy has been reported after addition of doxorubicin to CSP therapy in a patient (Barbui et al 1992). One explanation is that BBB changes induced by CSP therapy may allow diffusion of doxorubicin (also a neurotoxin) into the brain. High brain levels of doxorubicin in the brain can inhibit P-glycoprotein in the brain capillary endothelial cells (Beck and Kuttesch 1992).
- Methylprednisone combined with CSP for prophylaxis of GVHD in bone marrow transplant patients (Reece et al 1991).
- Etoposide administration as a part of conditioning the patients for bone marrow transplantation (Reece et al 1991).
- Microangiopathy developing as a part of GVHD.
- Aluminum overload.
- Hypertension (Joss et al 1982).

Pathomechanism. The risk factors are well recognized but the mechanism of neurotoxicity of CSP is unknown. Concentration of CSP in the plasma of patients who develop leukoencephalopathy is usually within the therapeutic range. However, concentration of metabolites of CSP has been reported to be increased in these patients (Cilio et al 1993). These metabolites may accumulate in more vulnerable regions of the brain, particularly in the white matter, which has a high lipid content.

Endothelin (ET), a vasoconstrictor neuropeptide that has been implicated in cerebral vasospasm, may potentiate CSP-induced damage to the endothelium and promote CSP neurotoxicity (Truwit et al 1991). Normally the integrity of BBB restricts the movements of both CSP and ET. However, in many patients on CSP, conditions exist that disrupt the BBB and permit access of both ET and CSP to otherwise protected areas of the brain.

Management. CSP leukoencephalopathy is reversible after discontinuation of the drug and later institution of the drug at a lower dose appears to be a safe approach. However, a case of late onset of leukoencephalopathy after 3 years of use of CSP, and documented by CT scan showing hypodensity of white matter of the cerebellum has been reported by Welge-Lüsson and Gerhartz 1994). The patient improved after discontinuation of CSP but symptoms recurred after rechallenge. Withdrawal of the drug was followed by recovery and return of CT findings to normal. In patients undergoing treatment with CSP, risk factors for leukoencephalopathy should be corrected if possible, e. g., magnesium supplementation for hypomagnesemia.

Tacrolismus (FK506). FK506 is a biologically active macrolide antibiotic that was found to have a powerful immunosuppressant action. It is now approved for use in liver transplantation. Since its initial application to orthotopic liver transplantation, the use of FK506 has been associated with the development of a variety of major neurological complications including progressive multifocal leukoencephalopathy (Wothman et al 1994). Burkhalter et al (1994) reviewed the neurological complications seen in 100 consecutive orthotopic liver transplant recipients who received FK506 as the primary immunosuppressant agent. Major neurological complications occurred in 34% of the patients but no specific mention was made of leukoencephalopathy. Three patients in this series were diagnosed to have central pontine myelinolysis where the findings were confirmed by MRI. Central pontine myelinolysis after liver transplantation has been attributed to electrolyte disturbances (Estol et al 1989a) and seizures are explained by metabolic disturbances as well (Estol et al 1989b). It was concluded that major neurological complications after orthotopic liver transplantation are multifactorial and cannot be ascribed solely to FK506 toxicity.

Small et al (1996) described a tacrolismus-related syndrome in three patients that has similar radiographic and pathologic appearances and the analogous syndrome that occurs in patients taking cyclosporin. Other cases were reported with similar features (Nakamura et al 1998; Idilman et al 1998). Tacrolismus (like cyclosporin) binds to specific intracellular protein protein ligands which play a vital role in maintaining the stability of intracellular structures. The exact mechanism of demyelination has not been determined but it involves particularly the parietio-occipital region and the centrum semiovale. Although the syndrome is not associated with any particular (absolute) serum level of tacrolismus, it resolves spontaneously after decreasing the dose or discontinuing tacrolismus.

Interferons (IFNs)

Body's interferon system is well known as an antiviral and antitumor mechanism. Various interferons (α, β, γ) have been undergoing clinical trials in the treatment of viral and malignant diseases. It has even been used in the treatment of AIDS-related progressive multifocal leukoencephalopathy (Berger et al 1992). Although there was no improvement, it was not reported to cause any deterioration of the neurological status. Toxicity of IFN on various systems of the body is also well known and has been reviewed by Vial and Descotes (1994).

Interferon Syndrome. Manifestations of neurotoxicity can be termed as an "interferon syndrome". Disorders of cerebral function associated with interferons are:
– Neuropsychiatric:
  · confusion
  · thought blockage
  · memory disturbance
  · hallucinations
  · visuospatial disorientation.
– Leukoencephalopathy
– EEG changes
Psychiatric manifestations are prominent and are described in Chapter 5. Encephalopathy associated with IFN use and manifested by lethargy, anorexia, somnolence and confusion has been reported (Suter et al 1984). Signs of upper motor neuron lesion have also been reported (Smedley et al 1983; Vesikari et al 1988).

EEG from patients showing neurotoxic effects have revealed a diffuse slowing of the α rhythm and appearance of theta and delta waves, prominent in the frontal lobes and consistent with a diffuse encephalopathy (Quesada 1992).

Merimsky et al (1991) reported a patient with metastatic renal cell carcinoma treated with recombinant IFN-α-C who developed dementia, ataxia, confusion and cortical blindness. CT scan findings were compatible with leukoencephalopathy. It was considered to be a toxic effect rather than an allergic reaction (no antibodies to IFN in patient's serum) or the result of a viral infection as IFN acts as an inhibitor of viral replication. Mitsuyama et al (1992) reported a 78-year old patient with renal carcinoma treated with high dose infusion of IFN-α who developed an organic brain syndrome and MRI showed diffuse white matter lesions. Postmortem examination of the brain revealed changes compatible with those of Alzheimer's disease. This patient had cerebral atrophy prior to start of treatment and the authors considered the possibility that this may have predisposed the patient to neurotoxic effects of IFN. Seven of the nine patients with leptomeningeal disease given intraventricular IFN-α developed a progressive vegetative state but improved on discontinuation of the drug (Meyers et al 1991). Periventricular white matter changes were seen in three of the six patients on whom a CT scan was done. These patients had cranial radiotherapy prior to interferon treatment which might have predisposed them to this complication. An increased frequency of leukoencephalopathy was reported among 6 of 39 patients receiving prophylactic IFN-α after bone marrow transplantation following cranial irradiation and intrathecal methotrexate (Meyers et al 1987).

Headache and blurred vision has been reported in a patient after use of IFN-α2B for hepatitis C. MRI showed multiple small periventicular defects possibly of ischemic origin (Ene et al 1994). The patient recovered from the adverse effects after discontinuation of the drug but had a recurrence of these after restart of therapy 6 months later.

Pathomechanism of IFN Neurotoxicity. This is not well understood. Factors which predispose to IFN neurotoxicity are shown in Table 3.7.

Table 3.7. Factors predisposing to interferon neurotoxicity.

High dose
Route of administration with slow absorption
Intrathecal use of IFN
Elderly patients with cerebral atrophy
HIV positive patients
Acute viral infection with increased production of
   endogenous IFN. Therapeutic use of IFN in such
   patients may trigger coma (Russo et al 1989)

Characteristics of interferon neurotoxicity are:
– Usually there are no structural alterations in
   the brain.
– It is reversible.
– Areas of the brain with opiate receptors most
   susceptible.

Neurotoxicity is considered to be dose-related
and not due to any impurities in IFN-α (Rohatiner and Färkkila 1988). Bocci (1988) has reviewed the pathomechanisms of CNS toxicity of
IFN and other cytokines and concluded that direct interaction of these proteins may be possible

at level of circumventricular organs (area postrema, hypothalmic neurosecretory centers, vascular organ of the lamina terminalis) but appears
unlikely to be on cortical neurons and BBB. IFN-
γ has been shown to potentiate demyelination in
experimental allergic encephalomyelitis in addition to its effect on antigen presentation (Vass et
al 1992).

Acute and slowly reversible extrapyramidal disorder resembling Parkinson's disease and akathesia have been reported in patients receiving IFN-γ.
These symptoms resolved promptly following
benzatropine (an antimuscarinic agent) suggesting
that IFN may be a dopamine antagonist.

Integration of concepts of interaction between
the brain, the endocrine, and the immune systems in pathogenesis of neurotoxicity of IFN is
shown in Figure 3.1.

IFN-induced encephalopathy is usually reversible if IFN is discontinued. Symptoms may
regress partially when treatment is maintained
with the same dose or disappear with reduction
in dose. There is no antidote for IFN toxicity.

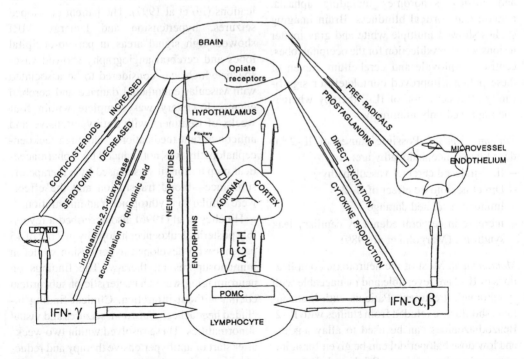

Figure 3.1. Pathomechanism of adverse effects of interferons on CNS interaction between brain, endocrine, and immune systems. POMC = Propriomelanocortin gene, IFN = Interferon

Interleukin-2 (IL-2)

Recombinant human interleukin-2 (IL-2) has been used in the treatment of solid tumors and appears to confer its antineoplastic effect via the activation of lymphoid precursor cells to lymphokine-activated killer (LAK) cells. It has also been used against HIV-1 infection. Neuropsychiatric complications occur in a third of the patients and 5% develop coma (Rosenberg et al 1989). Transient focal neurological deficits such as recurrent monocular blindness and quadrantanopia have been reported (Bernard et al 1990). A case of acute fatal leukoencephalopathy was reported after IL-2 therapy in a patient with normal neurological examination and it was considered to be possibly due to triggering of an immunologic reaction involving activated T lymphocytes directed against myelin (Vecht et al 1990).

Karp et al (1996) have reviewed the records of eight patients who developed focal neurological abnormalities out of a total of 1500 receiving IL-2 therapy for malignancy or HIV-1 infection. Initial confusion and delirium in these patients evolved into coma, ataxia, hemiparesis, seizures and cortical syndromes including aphasia, apraxia and cortical blindness. Brain imaging studies showed multiple white and gray matter lesions with a predilection for the occipital lobes, centrum semiovale and cerebellum. Seven of these patients improved completely or significantly after cessation of IL-2 therapy whereas one improved only minimally.

Pathomechanism. Possible causes of IL-2-induced leukoencephalopathy are:
- IL-2-induced cerebral vasculopathy
- Direct neurotoxic effect of IL-2
- Immune-mediated damage
- Increase in cerebral edema by capillary leak syndrome (Margolin et al 1989)

Management. Most of the neurotoxic complications of IL-2 are reversible and manageable with symptomatic treatment. Patients with brain tumors should be excluded from studies with IL-2. Benzodiazepines can be used to allay anxiety and low dose haloperidol can be given for agitation and hallucinations (Vial and Descotes 1992).

Hypertensive Leukoencephalopathy

Drug-induced hypertension may produce hypertensive encephalopathy which is a well known acute syndrome precipitated by sudden, severe hypertension. There is a disturbance of autoregulation that leads to severe vasospasm, petechial hemorrhages, microinfarcts and cerebral edema. Several drugs can induce hypertension (for references see Chapter 9). Hypertension may be also be associated with white matter changes and hypertensive encephalopathy could be termed leukoencephalopathy.

Delanty et al (1997) have described six dialysis-dependent chronic renal failure patients who developed hypertension, headache and seizures while on erythropoietin therapy. Four of these showed posterior white matter changes on neuroimaging. The patients recovered after discontinuation of erythropoietin and management with antihypertensives and anticonvulsants. A similar reversible posterior leukoencephalopathy has been described following blood transfusion in a patient who was not receiving any medications (Ito et al 1997). The patient developed seizures, hypertension and lethargy. MRI showed high signal areas in parieto-occipital lobes and cerebral angiography showed vasospasm which was considered to be associated with vascular endothelial damage and cerebral edema. Recovery was complete within four weeks of treatment with antihypertensive and anticonvulsant medications. Although leukoencephalopathy was not induced by a pharmaceutical preparation, it was caused by a therapeutic substance—blood transfusion and the effects were similar to erythropoietin administration.

Hinchey et al (1996) also described a reversible posterior leukoencephalopathy in 7 out of 15 patients who developed hypertension while on immunosuppressant therapy. The findings on neuroimaging were characteristic of subcortical edema without infarction. Clinical finding included headaches, confusion, seizures and visual abnormalities. These resolved within two weeks after start of antihypertensive therapy and reduction or withdrawal of immunosuppressants. The mechanism was considered to be a brain capillary leak syndrome related to hypertension, fluid retention and cytotoxic effect of immunosuppressant agents on the vascular endothelium.

Encephalomyelitis

Acute disseminated encephalomyelitis (ADEM) is a syndrome characterized by rapid development of multifocal neurological dysfunction. It occurrence is associated with immunization or vaccination (post-vaccinial encephalomyelitis) or systemic viral infections. Neurological sequelae of small pox vaccination marked the first time that complications following prophylactic immunization were recognized. The histological changes of post-vaccinial encephalomyelitis were recognized for the first time by Turnbull in 1912 (McAlpine 1931). These complications were not considered to be due to the direct cytopathologic effect of the virus but rather due to immune-mediated mechanisms directed against specific components of the CNS. Pathologically there is perivascular inflammation, edema and demyelination in the CNS.

The following vaccines have been reported to be associated with ADEM:
– Rabies
– DPT: diphtheria, pertussis, tetanus toxoid
– Rubella
– Measles
– Influenza
– Hepatitis B vaccine
– Japanese B encephalitis vaccine

Rabies. The incidence of encephalitis with original Pasteur vaccine, prepared in rabbit brain, was estimated to be 1:3000 to 1:35000 vaccinations. Various other preparations involving neural tissues continue to be associated with encephalomyelitis. Introduction of non-neural tissue vaccines, particularly human diploid cell vaccine, have markedly reduced but not eliminated the neurological complications.

Iizuka et al (1993) described a patient diagnosed as rabies vaccine encephalomyelitis in 1950 and died 37 years later. Post-mortem examination revealed extensive ischemic lesions in cerebral cortex and white matter with inflammatory lymphocytic infiltration.

Diphtheria Pertussis and Tetanus Toxoid (DPT). Most of the controversy regarding neurological complications surrounds pertussis vaccine. The most thorough investigation into this problem is published as a report of the Committee of the National Institute of Medicine of the Unites States to review the adverse effects of pertussis and rubella vaccines (Howson et al 1991). The Committee found that the evidence favored the rejection of a causal relation between DPT vaccine and encephalomyelitis (Stratton et al 1994). Case reports and case series offered no consistent evidence for a clinically distinct pertussis vaccine-induced encephalomyelitis. Encephalomyelitis is also known to occur during the natural course of pertussis and the excess risk with pertussis vaccine is 0–10 per million immunizations. There is insufficient evidence to indicate a causal relation between DPT vaccine and permanent neurological damage. No animal model for seizure and DPT vaccine has been developed. The Therapeutic and Technology Assessment Committee of the American Neurological Association concluded in 1992:
– DPT immunization is an important public health measure. Acute reactions warrant development of improved vaccines.
– Case reports raise the question of association between pertussis vaccine and chronic neurological disorders. Controlled studies have failed to prove such an association.
– At present there is no means by which diagnosis of pertussis vaccine encephalomyelitis can be established in an individual case.

Miller et al (1993) conducted a 10-year follow-up of children in the National Childhood Encephalopathy study in the United Kingdom. They concluded that illnesses leading to death or brain damage after DPT vaccine are extremely rare. In view of the high mortality and morbidity that results from unmodified natural pertussis, the use of DPT is recommended subject to observance of appropriate contraindications. In view of the rising incidence of pertussis, the continued use of available pertussis vaccines is recommended pending development and licensure of less reactive and well characterized acellular pertussis vaccines for infants (Rabinovich and Robbins 1994).

Camfield (1992) has reviewed this subject and concluded that there is no evidence of brain damage from pertussis vaccine. In the largest population-based study, no statistically significant increased risk of onset of serious acute neurological illness was found occurring within 7 days following DPT vaccine in young children (Gale et al 1994).

Measles. A causal relationship between measles-containing vaccines and encephalitis may exist but it is very rare. Claims data submitted to the National Vaccine Injury Compensation program contain 40 cases of acute encephalitis followed by permanent brain injury and 8 cases of death 2–15 days after receiving the first dose of measles containing vaccines between 1970 and 1993 (Weibel et al 1998). None of these cases involved a monovalent measles vaccine.

Influenza. There is one case reported so far of a rapidly progressive multifocal leukoencephalopathy in an elderly patient following influenza vaccination (Ory et al 1994).

Hepatitis B Vaccine. Recombinant hepatitis B vaccine has been reported to be associated with Guillain-Barre Syndrome, optic neuritis, and transverse myelitis. Herroelen et al (1991) described two patients, one with known multiple sclerosis and the other with no history of neurological disease, who developed encephalopathy after immunization with recombinant hepatitis B vaccine, and in whom MRI showed demyelination of the CNS. Another patient was reported with severe demyelination after recombinant hepatitis B vaccine and recovered after treatment with adrenocorticotrophin (Kaplanski et al 1995). One case of leukoencephalitis was reported in a patient two weeks after the second dose of recombinant hepatitis B vaccine (Manna et al 1996). She presented with weakness, paresthesias and loss of vision in her right eye. MRI showed multiple areas of impaired signal in the white matter of cerebral hemispheres. She improved after treatment with intravenous methyl-prednisolone and mannitol.

All the four cases quoted above had a HLA B7 haplotype which might have made them susceptible to immune mechanisms than can induce leukoencephalitis.

Japanese B Encephalitis Vaccine. Acute disseminated encephalomyelitis (ADEM) after Japanese B encephalitis vaccine is rare (< 1:1,000,000 vaccinations). The clinical pattern consists of an acute illness in the second or third week following the vaccination. Ohtaki et al (1995) reported two cases of ADEM after Japanese B encephalitis vaccine with components derived from mice actively infected with virus. The most striking feature was the combination of white matter lesions and abnormal intensity signals from the thalami. Similar findings have been reported in naturally occurring Japanese B encephalitis. The patient was treated with oral prednisolone with improvement of clinical and MRI findings. Ohtaki et al (1995) stated that the incidence of ADEM within one month after receiving Japanese B encephalitis vaccine was less than 1 in 1,000,000 vaccinees. This appears to be an underestimation because from 1982–1996, three cases of ADEM occurred in Denmark out of approximately 175,000 vaccinees (Plesner et al 1996).

Syndromes with Encephalopathy in which Drugs are Implicated

Two syndromes will be considered in this section: Reye's syndrome and toxic encephalopathy of the newborn.

Reye's Syndrome

It is a rare sporadic disorder of childhood of unknown origin characterized by hepatic dysfunction and metabolic encephalopathy. Excellent reviews have been presented by Trauner (1982) and Mowat (1987). The syndrome is named after Reye et al (1963) who described 21 children between the ages of 5 months and 9 years. The outstanding clinical features were profound disturbances of consciousness, vomiting, disturbances of respiratory rhythm, convulsions and coma. There were abnormalities of liver function tests. Seventeen of these patients died and the main autopsy findings were brain swelling and fatty accumulation in the liver and the kidneys. The prodrome is viral infection. Viruses most often associated with the syndrome are influenza B and varicella. In 1980s this syndrome received prominent attention because of its link to salicylate intoxication.

Pathogenesis of this syndrome is unknown. Genetic predisposition is recognized and several metabolic abnormalities have been identified. Both experimental and epidemiologic studies suggest that Reye's syndrome is a stereotypic reversible reaction in mitochondria arising from an interaction of viral, toxic and genetic factors. Transient mitochondrial dysfunction possibly limited to the hepatocytes and increased tissue metabolism account for most of the biochemical changes reported in Reye's syndrome. Aspirin, particularly in subjects deficient in L-carnitine, may compromise detoxification and lead to accumulation of toxic products and precipitate the onset of symptoms. Aspirin is the drug most often associated with Reye's syndrome. The evidence for this along with criticisms is as follows:

– *Epidemiological studies*. Four studies from various parts of North America have shown that patients with Reye's syndrome had taken aspirin more frequently, prior to, or early in, the illness than had controls with prodromal illnesses that were similar (Starko et al 1980; Waldman et al 1982; Halpin et al 1982). These studies were criticized because of bias in case control selection and data collection (Brown et al 1983).

– *Histopathological evidence*. Apparent similarities between liver changes in Reye's syndrome and those associated with salicylate poisoning have not been confirmed (Partin et al 1984).

– *Elevated serum levels of salicylates*. The report of these findings in Reye's syndrome was based on non-specific technology and has not been confirmed (Partin et al 1982).

– *Long-term salicylate therapy*. The syndrome was reported among children on long-term salicylate therapy for connective tissue disorders and the reported reduction in incidence now is attributed to decrease in use of salicylates in the United States (Hurwitz et al 1987). However, studies from Japan failed to confirm any such association.

In conclusion, Reye's syndrome is still an enigma and challenge for further research. It indicates the range of metabolic responses to exogenous agents, some of which will modify the body's response to viral infection.

Toxic Encephalopathy in the Newborn

Most cases of neonatal encephalopathy are secondary to hypoxia, ischemia, major malformations and infection. Toxic encephalopathy refers to disorders of cerebral function due to extraneous toxins including drugs. Exposure to drugs is usually via the mother through placenta in the prenatal period and through breast milk in the postnatal period. A discussion of congenital malformations induced by drugs is beyond the scope of this work. Drugs involved in toxic encephalopathies of the newborn have been reviewed by Mast (1993) and are shown in Table 3.8.

Most of the neurological manifestations in the newborn of a mother exposed to these drugs during pregnancy are those of withdrawal or abstinence with the exception of non-barbiturate anticonvulsants. Chronically drug effects are mostly manifested by a static encephalopathy, probably secondary to teratogenic effects of the drugs on the developing nervous system. Such infants may be obviously retarded or may have developmental retardation which may not be diagnosed till a few years later.

Table 3.8. Drugs involved in the toxic encephalopathies of the newborn.

Drug abuse by the mother
  opiates
  cocaine
  amphetamines
  phencyclidine
  marijuana
  alcohol
Prescription drugs used during pregnancy
  Anticonvulsants
  Antidepressants
  Barbiturates
  Benzodiazepines
  Codeine
  Propoxyphene
Drug exposure through breast milk

During breast feeding drugs which are excreted in the milk are ingested by the infant and may produce direct neurotoxicity. Drugs such as diazepam and chlorpromazine taken by the nursing mother can produce drowsiness of the infant.

Exposure to drugs via the mother is an important factor to be considered in the evaluation of an infant with encephalopathy.

References

Adams JH, Haller L, Boa FY, et al: Human African trypanosomiasis: a study of 16 fatal cases of sleeping sickness with some observations on the acute reactive arsenical encephalopathy. Neuropathol Appl Neurobiol 1986; 12: 81–94.

Agarwal K, Manas DM, Hudson M: Terbinafine and fulminant hepatic failure. N Engl J Med 1999; 340: 1292–1293.

Agosti R, Yasargil G, Egli M, et al: Neuropathology of a human hippocampus following long-term treatment with vigabatrin: lack of microvacuoles. Epilepsy Res 1990; 6: 166–170.

Alfrey AC, Froment DC: Dialysis encephalopathy. In DeBroe ME, Coburn JW (Eds.): Aluminum and renal failure, Dordrecht, Kluwer, 1990, pp 249–257.

Allen LJC: The neurotoxicity of cisplatin. In Rottenberg DA (Ed.): Neurological complications of cancer treatment, Butterworth, Boston, 1991, pp 135–142.

Antonini G, Morino S, Fiorelli M, et al: Reversal of encephalopathy during treatment with amphotericin-B. J Neurol Sci 1996; 144: 212–213.

Aoki N: Reversible leukoencephalopathy caused by 5-fluouracil derivatives, presenting as akinetic mutism. Surg Neurol 1986; 25: 279–282.

Arieff AI: Management of hyponatremia. BMJ 1993; 307: 305–308.

Arroz JOL: Melarsoprol and reactive encephalopathy in Trypanosoma brucei rhodesiense. Trans Roy Soc Trop Med 1987; 81: 192.

Asato R, Akiyama Y, Ito M, et al: Nuclear magnetic resonance abnormalities of the cerebral white matter in children with acute lymphoblastic leukemia and malignant lymphoma during and after central nervous system prophylactic treatment with intrathecal methotrexate. Cancer 1992; 70: 1997–2004.

Averbruch-Heller L: Valproate encephalopathy and hypocartininemia in diabetic patients. J Neurol 1994; 241: 567–569.

Barbui T, Rambaödi A, Parenzan L, et al: Neurological symptoms and coma associated with doxorubicin administration during chronic cyclosporin therapy. Lancet 1992; 339: 1421–1422.

Basile AS, Hughes RD, Harrison PM, et al: Elevated brain concentrations of 1,4-benzodiazepines in fulminant hepatic failure. NEJM 1991; 325: 473–478.

Bauer J, Elger CE: Die akute Valproinsäure-Enzephalopathie. Akt Neurol 1993; 20: 16–21.

Beales P, Almond NK, Kwan JTC: Acyclovir neurotoxicity following oral therapy: prevention and treatment in patients on hemodialysis. Nephron 1994; 66: 362–363.

Beck WT, Kuttesch JF: Neurological symptoms associated with cyclosporin plus doxorubicin. Lancet 1992; 340: 496–497.

Bem JL, Kerr L, Stuerchler D: Mefloquine prophylaxis: an overview of spontaneous reports of severe psychiatric reactions and convulsions. J Trop Med Hyg 1992; 95: 167–179.

Berden JHM, Hottsma AJ, Merx JL, et al: Severe central nervous system toxicity associated with cyclosporin. Lancet 1985; i: 219–220.

Berger JR, Pall L, McArthur J, et al: A pilot study of recombinant α 2a interferon in the treatment of AIDS-related progressive multifocal leukoencephalopathy (abstract). Neurology 1992; 42 (suppl 3): 257.

Bernard JT, Ameriso S, Kempf RA, et al: Transient focal neurologic deficits complicating interleukin-2 therapy. Neurology 1990; 40: 154–155.

Bernini JC, Fort DW, Griener JC, et al: Aminophylline for methotrexate-induced neurotoxicity. Lancet 1995; 345: 544–547.

Beuzeboc P, Dorval T, Garcia-Giralt E, et al: Encephalopathy caused by an ifosfamide/mesna combination. Presse Med 1988; 17: 591–592.

Biarez O, Marsepoil T, Caillard G, et al: Acute encephalopathy during lithium-neuroleptic combined treatment (letter). Therapie 1989; 44: 303–304.

Bocci V: Central nervous system toxicity of interferons and other cytokines. J Biol Regul Homeost Agents 1988; 3: 107–118.

Bond CR, Curry SC: Dimethysulphoxide-induced encephalopathy (letter). Lancet 1989; i: 1134–1135.

Boogerd W, Sande JJ, Moffie D: Acute fever and delayed leukoencephalopathy following low doses intraventricular methotrexate. JNNP 1988; 51: 1277–1283.

Broussolle E, Setiey A, Moene Y, et al: Reversible Creutzfeldt-Jakob like syndrome due to lithium toxicity. JNNP 1989; 52: 686–687.

Brown AK, Fikrig S, Findberg L: Aspirin and Reye's syndrome. J Pediatr 1983; 102: 157–178.

Bruck W, Heise E, Friede RL: Leukoencephalopathy after cisplatin therapy. Clin Neuropathol 1989; 8: 263–265.

Burkhalter EL, Starzl TE, Van Thiel DH: Severe neurological complications following orthotopic liver transplantation in patients receiving FK506 and prednisone. J Hepatology 1994; 21: 572–577.

Burns R, Thomas DW, Barron VJ: Reversible encephalopathy possibly associated with bismuth subgallate ingestion. BMJ 1974; i: 220–223.

Cain MS, Burton GV, Holcombe RF, et al: Fatal leukoencephalopathy in a patient with non-hodgkin's lymphoma treated with CHOP chemotherapy and high dose steroids. Am J Med Sci 1998; 315: 202–207.

Cales P: Propranolol et risque d'encéphalopathie hépatique chez le cirrhotique. Ann Gastroenterol Hepatol (Paris) 1989; 25: 315–317.

Camfield P: Brain damage from pertussis immunization. AJDC 1992; 146: 327–331.

Cantu TG, Korek JS: Central nervous system reactions to histamine-2 receptor blockers. Ann Int Med 1991; 114: 1027–1034.

Cantwell BMJ, Idle M, Millward MJ, et al: Encephalopathy with hyponatremia and inappropriate arginine vasopressin secretion following an intravenous ifosfamide infusion. Ann Oncol 1990; 1: 232.

Cerny T, Küpfer A: The enigma of ifosfamide encephalopathy. Ann Oncol 1992; 3: 679–681.

Ceylan S, Baykal S, Kuzeyli K, et al: A case of acute encephalopathy after iohexal lumbar myelography. Clin Neurol Neurosurg 1993; 95: 45–47.

Chen TC, Hinton DR, Leichman L, et al: Multifocal inflammatory leukoencephalopathy associated with levamisole and 5-fluorouracil: case report. Neurosurgery 1994; 35: 1138–1143.

Cheson BD, Vena DA, Foss FM, et al: Neurotoxicity of purine analogs: a review. J Clin Oncol 1994; 12: 2216–2228.

Cho SG, Moon H, Lee JH, et al: Behenoyl cytarabine-associated reversible encephalopathy in a patient with acute myelogenous leukemia. J Korean Med Sci 1999; 14: 89–92.

Choy DS, Weiss A, Lin PT, et al: Progressive multifocal leukoencephalopathy following treatment for Wegner's granulomatosis. JAMA 1992; 268: 600–601.

Cilio MR, Danhaive O, Gadisseux JF, et al: Unusual cyclosporin related neurological complications in recipients of liver transplants. Arch Dis Child 1993; 68: 405–407.

Cocito L, Maffini M: Vigabatrin edema (letter). Neurology. 1995; 45: 2115–2116.

Cohen IJ, Stark B, Kaplinsky C, et al: Methotrexate-induced leukoencephalopathy is treatable with high-dose folinic acid: a case report and analysis of the literature. Pediatr Hematol Oncol 1990; 7: 79–87.

Cohen RB, Abdallah JM, Gray JR, et al: Reversible neurologic toxicity in patients treated with standard-dose fludarabine phosphate for mycosis fungoides and chronic lymphocytic leukemia. Arch Int Med 1993; 118: 114–116.

Cohen RJ, Cuneo RA: Transient left homonymous hemianopsia and encephalopathy following treatment of testicular carcinoma with cisplatin, vinblastine, and bleomycin. J Clin Oncol 1983; 1: 392–393.

Cohen W, Cohen N: Lithium carbonate, haloperidol, and irreversible brain damage. JAMA 1974; 230: 1283–1287.

Coleman AE, Norman DJ: OKT3 encephalopathy. Ann Neurol 1990; 28: 837–838.

Cooke DEM, Glasstone MA: Baclofen poisoning in children. Veterinary and Human Toxicology 1994; 36: 448–450.

Crawford SM, Rustin GJS, Bagshawe KD: Acute neurological toxicity of intrathecal cytosine arabinoside: a case report. Cancer Chemother Pharmacol 1986; 16: 306–307.

Danesh MM, De Giorgio C, Beydoun SR, et al: Ifosfamide encephalopathy. Clin Toxicol 1989; 27: 293–298.

De Groen PC, Aksamit AJ, Rakela J, et al: Central nervous system toxicity after liver transplantation: the role of cyclosporin and cholestrol. NEJM 1987; 317: 861–866.

De Groen PC: Cyclosporin, low density lipoprotein, and cholestrol. Mayo Clin Proceed 1988; 63: 1012–1021.

De Klippel N, De Keyser J, De Greve J, et al: A Wernicke's encephalopathy-like syndrome induced by erbulozole. Neurology 1991; 4: 762–763.

De Klippel N, Sennesael J, Lamote J, et al: Cyclosporin leukoencephalopathy induced by intravenous lipid solution. Lancet 1992; 339: 1114.

De Leeuw P, Lefebvre C, Tomasi JP, et al: Severe hepatitis with encephalopathy induced by acetylsalicylic acid in a case of lupus erythematosus disseminatus. Gastroenterol Clin Biol 1992; 16: 359–361.

del Rio Fernandez M, Plagaro Cordero ME, de Frutos Arribas JF, et al: Hepatic encephalopathy related to omeprazole. Rev Esp Enferm Dig 1997; 89(7): 574–575.

del Rosario M, Werlin SL, Lauer SJ: Hyperammonemic encephalopathy after chemotherapy. Survival after treatment with sodium benzoate and sodium phenylacetate. J Clin Gastroenterol 1997; 25: 682–684.

Delanty N, Vaughan C, Frucht S, et al: Erythropoietin-associated hypertensive posterior leukoencephalopathy. Neurology 1997; 49: 686–689.

Delhaas EM, Brouwers JRBJ: Intrathecal baclofen overdose: report of 7 events in 5 patients and review of the literature. Int J Clin Pharmacol Ther Toxicol 1991; 29: 274–280.

Devinsky O, Lemann W, Evans AC, et al: Akinetic mutism in a bone marrow transplant recipient following total body irradiation and amphotericin B chemoprophylaxis: a positron emission tomographic and neuropathologic study. Arch Neurol 1987; 44: 414–417.

Devuyst O, Goffin E, van Ypersele de Stribou C: Recurrent hemiparesis under amphotericin B for Candida albicans peritonitis. Nephrology Dialysis Transplantation 1995; 10: 699–701.

Dhodapkar M, Goldberg SL, Tefferi A, et al: Reversible encephalopathy after cryopreserved peripheral blood stem cell infusion. Am J Hematol 1994; 45: 187–188.

Dobashi N, Kuraishi Y, Hattori S, et al: A case report of leukoencephalopathy caused by 5FU with 5-day continuous infusion against rectal cancer. Nippon Gan Chiryo Gakkai Shi 1994; 29: 310 (abstract).

Donaghy M, Fletcher A, Schott GD: Encephalopathy after iohexal myelography. Lancet 1985; 2: 887.

Donat JF, Bochini JA, Gonzalez E, et al: Valproic acid fatal hepatitis. Neurology 1979; 29: 273–274.

Donnet A, Dufour H, Regis H, et al: Encephalopathie toxique a la carbamazepine. Ann Med Int (Paris) 1991; 142: 391–392.

Douglas MA, Quandt CM, Stanley DA, et al: Ceftazidime-induced encephalopathy in a patient with renal impairment (letter). Arch Neurol 1988; 88: 936–937.

Duval L, Hautecoeur P, Mahieu M: Cimetidine-induced hyperammonemic encephalopathy. Presse Med 1999; 28: 582–583.

Ellis EG, Bencken E, LeCouteur RA, et al: Neurotoxicity of amphotericin B methyl ester in dogs. Toxicol Pathol 1988; 16: 1–9.

Ellis WG, Sobel RA, Nielsen SL: Leukoencephalopathy in patients treated with amphotericin B methyl ester. J Infect Dis 1982; 146: 125–137.

El-Mallakh: Acute lithium neurotoxicity. Psychiatr Dev 1986; 4: 311–328.

Ene L, Géhénot M, Horsmans Y, et al: Transient blurred vision after interferon for chronic hepatitis C. Lancet 1994; 344: 827–828.

Engel, Cruz ME, Shapiro B: Phenytoin encephalopathy? Lancet 1971; 2: 824–825.

Epstein R: Wernicke's encephalopathy following lithium-induced diarrhea. Am J Psychiatry 1989; 146: 806–807.

Estol CJ, Faris AA, Martinez J, et al: Central pontine myelinolysis after liver transplantation. Neurology 1989a; 39: 493–498.

Estol CJ, Lopez O, Brenner RP, et al: Seizures after liver transplantation: A clinicopathologic study. Neurology 1989b; 39: 1297–1301.

Ettinger J, Feiden W, Hübner G, et al: Progressive Multifokale Leukoenzephalopathie bei Wegener'scher Granulomatose unter Therapie mit Cyclosporin A. Klin Wochenschr 1989; 67: 260–264.

Fassas ABT, Gattani AM, Morgello S: Cerebral demyelination with 5-fluorouracil and levamisole. Cancer Investigation 1994; 12: 379–383.

Filley CM, Graff-Radford JR, Lacy MA, et al: Neurologic manifestations of podophyllin neurotoxicity. Neurology 1982; 32: 308–311.

Fraser CL, Arieff AI: Epidemiology, pathophysiology, and management of hyponatremic encephalopathy. Am J Med 1997; 102: 67–77.

Fuji Y, Mizuno Y, Hongo T, et al: Serial spectral EEG analysis in a patient with non-Hodgkin's lymphoma complicated by leukoencephalopathy induced by high dose methotrexate. Gan To Kagaku Ryoho 1988; 15: 713–717.

Galassi G, Tassone G, Sintini M, et al: 5-Fluorouracil- and levamisole-associated multifocal leukoencephalopathy. Eur Neurol 1996; 36: 244–6.

Gale JH, Thapa PB, Wassilak SGF, et al: Risk of serious acute neurological illness after immunization with diphtheria-tetanus-pertussis vaccine. JAMA 1994; 271: 37–41.

Gay CT, Bodensteiner JB, Nitschke R, et al: Reversible treatment-related leukoencephalopathy. J Child Neurol 1989; 4: 208–213.

Ghalie R, Fitzsimmons WE, Bennett D, et al: Cortical blindness: a rare complication of cyclosporine therapy. Bone Marrow Transplantation 1990; 6: 147–149.

Ghosn M, Carde P, LeClerq B, et al: Ifosfamide/mesna related encephalopathy: a case report with a possible role of phenobarbital in enhancing neurotoxicity. Bull Cancer 1988; 75: 391–392.

Gil-Paraiso A, Sierra M, Huarte E, et al: Encephalopathy caused by acyclovir in hemodialysis. Neurology Dialysis Transplantation 1994; 9: 1515.

Gobel R, Gortzen A, Braunig P: Encephalopathies caused by valproate. Fortschr Neurol Psychiatr 1999; 67: 7–11.

Gomez Campdera FJ, Verde E, Vozmediano MC, et al:

More about acyclovir neurotoxicity in patients on haemodialysis. Nephron 1998; 78: 228–229.

Gopal AK, Thorning DR, Bacl AL: Fatal outcome due to cyclosporine neurotoxicity with associated pathological findings. Bone Marrow Transplantation 1999; 23: 191–193.

Gordon MF, Abrams RI, Rubin DB, et al: Bismuth subsalicylate toxicity as a cause of prolonged encephalopathy with myoclonus. Mov Disord 1995; 10: 220–222.

Gorman DJ, Kefford R, Stuart-Harris Jr: Focal encephalopathy after cisplatin therapy. Med J Australia 1989; 150: 399–401.

Greenway JR, Abuaisha A, Bramble MG: Digoxin toxicity presenting as encephalopathy. Postgraduate Medical Journal 1996; 72: 367–368.

Gregorios JB, Soucy D: Effects of methotrexate on astrocytes in primary culture: light and electron microscopic studies. Brain Res 1990; 516: 20–30.

Guerrero A, Pérez-Simon JA, Guttierrez N, et al: Neurological complications after autologous stem cell transplantation. Eur Neurol 1999; 41: 48–50.

Guilhem I, Charasse C, Gary J, et al: Neurotoxicity of acyclovir in peritoneal dialysis apropos of 1 case. Nephrologie 1991; 12: 241–243.

Gütling E, Landis T, Kleihues P: Akinetic mutisms in bilateral necrotizing leukoencephalopathy after radiation and chemotherapy: electrophysiological and autopsy findings. J Neurol 1992; 239: 125–128.

Haan J, Muller E, Gerhard L: Spongiose Leukodystrophie nach Drogenmissbrauch. Nervenarzt 1983; 54: 489–490.

Halpin TJ, Holthauser TJ; Campbell RJ, et al: Reye's syndrome and medication use. JAMA 1982; 248: 687–691.

Hanston P, Mahieu P, Gersdorff M, et al: Encephalopathy with seizures after use of aluminum-containing bone cement (letter). Lancet 1994; 344: 1647.

Harkness K, Howell SJL, Davies-Jones DAB, et al: Encephalopathy associated with intravenous immunoglobulin treatment for Guillain-Barré syndrome. JNNP 1996; 60: 586–598.

Hata T, Sano A, Nakagawa M, et al: A case of reversible leukoencephalopathy caused by tegafur. No To Shinkei 1992; 44: 173–175.

Hayashi R, Hanyo N, Kitahara A: Leukoencephalopathy induced by tegafur: serial studies of somatosensory evoked potentials and cerebrospinal fluid. Int Med 1992; 31: 828–831.

Hennessy MJ, Wiles CM: Lamotrigine encephalopathy. Lancet 1996; 347: 947–948.

Herishanu YO, Zlotnik M, Mosttoslavsky M, et al: Cefuroxime-induced encephalopathy. Neurology 1998; 50: 1873–1875.

Hernandez E, Praga M, Moreno F, et al: Acute renal failure induced by oral acyclovir. Clin Nephrol 1991; 36: 155–156.

Herroelen L, De Keyser J, Ebinger G: Central nervous system demyelination after immunization with recombinant hepatitis B vaccine. Lancet 1991; 338: 1174–1175.

Hildebrand J (Ed.): Neurological adverse reactions to drugs, New York, Springer-Verlag, 1990.

Himmelsbach FA, Köhler E, Zanker B, et al: Baclofenintoxikation bei chronischer Hämodialyse und Nierentransplantation. Dtsch Med Wschr 1992; 117: 733–737.

Hinchey J, Chaves C, Appignani B, et al: A reversible posterior leukoencephalopathy syndrome. NEJM 1996; 334: 494–500.

Hitchins RN, Thomson DB: Encephalopathy following cisplatin, bleomycin and vinblastine therapy for nonseminomatous germ cell tumours of the testis. Aust NZ J Med 1988; 18: 67–68.

Hoefnagels WAJ, Gerritsen EJA, Brouwer OF, et al: Cyclosporin encephalopathy associated with fat embolism induced by the drug's solvent. Lancet 1988; ii: 901

Hoffman DL, Howard JR, Sarma R, et al: Encephalopathy, myelopathy, optic neuropathy, and anosmia associated with intravenous cytosine arabinoside. Clin Neuropharmacol 1993; 16: 258–262.

Hook IJC, Kimmel DW, Kvols LK, et al: Multifocal inflammatory leukoencephalopathy with 5-fluorouracil and levamisole. Ann Neurol 1992; 31: 262–267.

Hormes JT, Benarroch EE, Rodriguez M, et al: Periodic sharp waves in baclofen-induced encephalopathy. Arch Neurol 1988; 45: 814–815.

Howson CP, Howe CJ, Fineberg HV (Eds.): Adverse effects of pertussis and rubella vaccines, Washington, National Academy Press, 1991, pp 86–118.

Hunter CA, Jennings FW, Adams JH, et al: Sub-curative chemotherapy may underlie the fatal post-treatment reactive encephalopathies in human African trypanosomiasis. Lancet 1992a; 339: 956–958.

Hunter CA, Jennings FW, Kennedy PGE, et al: The use of azathioprine to ameliorate post-treatment encephalopathy associated with African trypanosomiasis. Neuropathol Appl Neurobiol 1992b; 18: 619–625.

Hurst EW: The lesions produced in the central nervous system by certain organic arsenical compounds. J Pathol Bact 1959; 77: 523–534.

Hurwitz ES, Barrett MJ, Bregman D, et al: Public health service study of Reye's syndrome and medications. JAMA 1987; 257: 1905–1911.

Hurwitz RL, Mahoney DH, Armstrong DL, et al: Reversible encephalopathy and seizures as a result of conventional vincristine administration. Med Pediatr Oncol 1988; 18: 228–230.

Idilman R, De maria N, Kugelmans M, et al: Immunosuppressive drug-induced leukoencephalopathy in patients with liver transplant. Eur J Gastroenterol Hepatology 1998; 10: 433–436.

Ifergane G, Masalha R, Zigulinski R: Acute encephalopathy associated with vigabatrin monotherapy in patients with mild renal failure. Neurology 1998; 51: 314–315.

Iizuka H, Amano N, Izeki E, et al: A case of antirabies inoculation encephalitis with a long clinical course. Jpn J Psychiat Neurol 1993; 47: 603–608.

Ito Y, Niwa H, Iida T, et al: Post-transfusion reversible posterior leukoencephalopathy syndrome with cerebral vasoconstriction. Neurology 1997; 49: 1174–1175.

Jackson G, Berkovic S: Ceftazidime encephalopathy: absence status and hallucinations (letter). JNNP 1992; 55: 333–334.

Jacobs P, Rutherford GS, King HS, et al: Methotrexate encephalopathy. Eur J Cancer 1991; 27: 1061–1062.

Jones EA, Basile AS: Does ammonia contribute to increased GABA-ergic neurotransmission in liver failure? Metab Brain Dis 1998; 13(4): 351–360.

Jones GL, Matsuo F, Baringer JR, et al: Valproic acid-associated encephalopathy. West J Med 1990; 153: 199–202.

Joss DV, Barrett AJ, Kendra JR, et al: Hypertension and convulsions in children receiving cyclosporin A. Lancet 1982; i: 906.

Jungreis AC, Schaumburg HH: Encephalopathy from abuse of bismuth subsalicylate (Pepto-bismol). Neurology 1993; 43: 1265.

Kajita M, Iwase K, Matsumoto M, et al: Clinical and biochemical studies in a case of acute encephalopathy associated with calcium hopanthenate administration (Japanese). No To Hattatsu 1990; 22: 267–273.

Kalaawi MH, Auger LT, Carroll JE, et al: Encephalopathy and brain stem dysfunction in an infant with non-accidental carbamazepine intoxication. Clin Pediatr 1991; 30: 385–386.

Kamata H, Murakami A, Miyagawa N, et al: A case of leukoencephalopathy caused by HCFU. Gan No Rinsho 1988; 34: 783–786.

Kamen BA: Methotrexate folate and the brain. Neurotoxicology 1986; 7: 209–216.

Kaplanski G, Retornaz F, Durand JM, et al: Central nervous system demyelination after vaccination with hepatitis B and HLA haplotype. JNNP 1995; 58: 758–759.

Karp BI, Yaang JC, Khorsand M, et al: Multiple cerebral lesions complicating therapy with interleukin-2. Neurology 1996; 47: 417–424.

Kastrup O, Diener HC: Granulocyte-stimulating factor filgrastim and molgramostim induced recurring encephalopathy and focal status epilepticus. J Neurol 1997; 244: 274–275.

Kawada T, Satomi K, Kambara K, et al: An autopsied case of leukoencephalopathy seemingly induced by tegafur. Gann No Rinsho 1991; 37: 1790–1794.

Kendel K, Schäffer S: Chronische Wismuthintoxikation mit Enzephalopathie und Demenz. Dtsch Med Wschr 1993; 118: 221–224.

Kessel JB, Verghese C, Simpson GM: Neurotoxicity related to lithium and neuroleptic combinations? A retrospective review. J Psychiatr Neurosci 1992; 17: 28–30.

Kimmel DW, Wijdicks EFM, Rodriguez M: Multifocal inflammatory leukoencephalopathy associated with levamisole therapy. Neurology 1995; 45: 374–376.

Kimmel DW, Schutt AJ: Multifocal leukoencephalopathy: occurrence during 5-fluorouracil and levamisole therapy and resolution after discontinuation of therapy. Mayo Clin Proc 1993; 68: 363–365.

Kirkland JL: Propylthiouracil-induced hepatic failure and encephalopathy in a child. DICP Ann Pharmacother 1990; 24: 470–471.

Kitching AR, Fagg D, Hay NM, et al: Neurotoxicity associated with acyclovir in end stage renal failure. N Z Med J 1997; 110: 167–169.

Kondo K, Fujiwara M, Murase M, et al: Severe acute metabolic acidosis and Wernicke's encephalopathy following chemotherapy with 5-fluorouracil and cisplatin: case report and review of the literature. Jpn J Clin Oncol 1996; 26: 234–236.

Kornblau SM, Cortes-Franco J, Estey E: Neurotoxicity associated with fluarabine and cytosine arabinoside chemotherapy for acute leukemia and myelodysplasia. Leukemia 1993; 7: 378–383.

Kriegelstein AR, Armitage BA, Kim PY: heroin inhalation and progressive espongiform leukoencephalopathy. NEJM 1997; 336: 589–590.

Kubo M, Azuma E, Arai S, et al: Transient encephalopathy following a single exposure of high dose methotrexate in a child with acute lymphoblastic leukemia. Pediatr Hematol Oncol 1992; 9: 157–165.

Küpfer A, Aeschlimann C, Wermuth B, et al: Prophylaxis and reversal of ifofamide encephalopathy with methylene blue. Lancet 1994; 343: 763–764.

Kutlay P, Sava S, Yalcin P, et al: Central nervous system toxicity of cyclosporin. A treatment in rheumatoid arthritis. British Journal of Rheumatology 1997; 36: 397–399.

Kwee IL, Nakada. Wernicke's encephalopathy induced by tolazamide. N Engl J Med 1983; 309(10): 599–600.

Lam CW, Lau CH, Williams JC, et al: Mitochondrial myopathy, encephalopathy, lactic acidosis and stroke-like episodes (MELAS) triggered by valproate therapy. Eur J Pediatr 1997; 156: 562–664.

Lazarus HM, Herzig RH, Herzig GP, et al: Central nervous system toxicity of high dose systemic cytosine arabinoside. Cancer 1981; 48: 2577–2582.

Lazzarino LG, Nicolai A, Valassi F: Acute transient cerebral intoxication induced by low doses of baclofen. Ital J Neurol Sci 1991; 12: 323–325.

Leào M: Valproate as a cause of hyperammonemia in heterozygotes with ornithine-transcarbamylase deficiency. Neurology 1995; 45: 593–594.

Lee TH, Chen SS, Su SL, et al: Baclofen intoxication: report of four cases and review of literature. Clin Neuropharmacol 1992; 15: 56–62.

Leikin JB, Shicker L, Orlowski J, et al: Hemodialysis removal of acyclovir. Veterinary and Human Toxicology 1995; 37: 233–236.

Lewin S, Rao SD, Chandrasekhara MK, et al: Phenytoin toxic encephalopathy. Indian Pediatr 1993; 30: 79–80.

Liaw CC, Wang HM, Wang CH, et al: Risk of transient hyperammonemic encephalopathy in cancer patients who received continuous infusion of 5-fluorouracil with the complication of dehydration and infection. Anticancer Drugs 1999; 10: 275–281.

Lipsy RJ, Fennerty B, Fagan TC: Clinical review of histamine$_2$-receptor antagonists. Arch Int Med 1990; 150: 745–751.

Lopez Gaston JI, Carod Artal FJ: Recurrent acute encephalopathy induced by isoniazide. Medicine Clinica 1994; 102: 756–757.

Lucia P, Pocek M, Passacantando A, et al: Multifocal leukoencephalopathy induced by levamisole (letter). Lancet 1996; 348: 1450.

Lyass O, Lossos A, Hubert A, et al: Cisplatin-induced non-convulsive encephalopathy. Anti-Cancer Drugs 1998; 9: 100–104.

Lye WC, Leong SO: Neurotoxicity associated with intraperitoneal ceftazidime therapy in a CAPD patient. Peritoneal Dialysis International 1994; 14: 408–409.

MacDiarmaid-Gordon AR, O'Connor M, Beaman M, et al: Neurotoxicity associated with oral acyclovir in patients undergoing dialysis. Nephron 1992; 62(3): 280–283.

Maegaki Y, Koeda T, Kawahara H, et al: Two cases of theophylline-associated encephalopathy in childhood: clinical and CT findings (Japanese). No To Hattatsu 1993; 25: 277–282.

Manna R, De Sanctis A, Oliviero A, et al: Leukoencephalitis after recombinant hepatitis B vaccine. Journal of Hepatology 1996; 24: 764–765.

Margolin KA, Rayner AA, Hawkins MJ, et al: Interleukin-2 and lymphokine-activated killer cell therapy of solid tumors: analysis of toxicity and management of guidelines. J Clin Oncol 1989; 7: 486–498.

Martin-Bouyer G, Foulon G, Guerbois H, et al: Aspects epidemiologiques des encephalopathies apres administration de bismuth par voie oral. Therapie 1980; 35: 307–313.

Mast J: Toxic encephalopathy in the newborn. Sem Neurol 1993; 13: 66–72.

Mataix AL, Duarte J, Revuelta K, et al: Oral acyclovir and neurologic adverse effects in endstage renal disease. Ann Pharmacother 1994; 28: 961–962.

Mathy I, Gille M, Van Raemdonck F, et al: Neurological complications of intravenous immunoglobulin (IVIg) therapy: an illustrative case of acute encephalopathy following IVIg therapy and a review of the literature. Acta Neurol Belg 1998; 98(4): 347–351.

McAlpine D: Acute disseminated encephalomyelitis. Lancet 1931; i: 846–852.

McCormick PA, Kennedy F, Curry M, et al: COX 2 inhibitor and fulminant hepatic failure. Lancet 1999; 353(9146): 40–41.

McLean J, Manchip S: Wernicke's encephalopathy induced by magnesium depletion. Lancet 1999; 353: 1768.

McManus RP, O'Hair DP, Schweiger J, et al: Cyclosporin-associated central neurotoxicity after heart transplantation. Ann Thorac Surg 1992; 53: 326–327.

Meanwell CA, Blake AE, Kelly KA, et al: Prediction of isosfamide/mesna associated encephalopathy. Eur J Cancer Clin Oncol 1986; 22: 815–819.

Meanwell CA, Blake AE, Latief TN, et al: Encephalopathy associated with ifosphamide/mesna therapy. Lancet 1985; i: 406–407.

Mendelowitz PC, Hoffman RS, Weber S: Bismuth absorption and myoclonic encephalopathy during bismuth subsalicylate therapy. Ann Int Med 1990; 112: 140–141.

Menegaux F, Keeffe EB, Andrews BT, et al: Neurologic complications of liver transplantation in adult versus pediatric patients. Transplantation 1994; 58: 447–450.

Merimsky O, Loewenstein A, Chaitchik S: Cortical blindness—a catastrophic side effect of vincristine. Anti-Cancer Drugs 1992; 3: 371–373.

Merimsky O, Reider I, Merimsky E, et al: Interferon-related leukoencephalopathy in a patient with renal cell carcinoma. Tumori 1991; 77: 361–362.

Merimsky O, Reider-Groswasser I, Wigler N, et al: Encephalopathy in ifosfamide-treated patients. Acta Neurol Scand 1992; 86: 521–525.

Meyers CA, Obbens EAM, Schiebel RS, et al: Neurotoxicity of intraventricularly administered α-interferon for leptomeningeal disease. Cancer 1991; 68: 88–92.

Meyers JD, Flournoy N, Sanders JE, et al: Prophylactic use of human leukocyte interferon after allogeneic marrow transplantation. Ann Intern Med 1987; 107: 809–16.

Michon A, Sereni C, Gauthier C, et al: Encephalopathy caused by bromide salts (letter in French). Presse Med 1989; 18: 228.

Miller D, Madge N, Diamond J, et al: Diphtheria, tetanus and pertussis vaccine. BMJ 1993; 307: 1171–1176.

Miller F, Menninger J: Lithium-neuroleptic neurotoxicity is dose-dependent. J Clin Psychopharmacol 1987; 72: 89–91.

Miller LJ, Eaton VE: Ifosamide-induced neurotoxicity: a case report and review of the literature. Ann Pharmacother 1992; 26: 183–187.

Millot F, Chastagner P, Dhondt J, et al: Substitutive therapy in a case of methotrexate neurotoxicity. Eur J Cancer 1992; 28A: 1935.

Min DI, Fallo SA: Encephalopathy associated with muromonab-CD3. Clin Pharm 1993; 12: 610–612.

Mitsuyama Y, Hashiguchi H, Murayama T, et al: An autopsied case of interferon encephalopathy. Japanese Journal of Psychiatry 1992; 46: 741–748.

Miyazaki C, Matsuyama K, Ichikawa M, et al: Effect of sodium valproate on cerebral amino acids: mechanism of γ-aminobutyric acid (GABA) elevation and possible causal relation of VPA-induced encephalopathy and glutamine level. Chem Pharm Bull 1988; 36: 3589–3594.

Moitinho E, Salmeron JM, Mas A, et al: Severe hepatotoxicity of tuberculostatic agents. Increase in the incidence. Gastroenterol Hepatol 1996; 19: 448–451.

Molina JA, Calandra L, Bermejo F: Myoclonic encephalopathy due to bismuth salts: treatment with dimercaprol and analysis of CSF transmitters. Acta Neurol Scand 1989; 79: 200–203.

Monteiro L, Almeida-Pinto J, Rocha N, et al: Case report: Cyclosporin A-induced neurotoxicity. Brit J Radiol 1993; 66: 271–272.

Mott SH, Packer RJ, Vezina LG, et al: Encephalopathy with parkinsonian features in children following bone marrow transplantations and high-dose amphotericin B. Ann Neurol 1995; 37: 810–814.

Mowat AP: Reye's Syndrome—a continuing enigma. Adv Drug React Pois Rev 1987; 4: 211–230.

Mueller AR, Platz KP, Bechstein WO, et al: Neurotoxicity after orthotopic liver transplantation. Transplantation 1994; 58: 155–169.

Muller-Schwefe G, Penn RD: Physostigmine in the treatment of intrathecal baclofen overdose. J Neurosrg 1989; 71: 273–275.

Murphy CP, Cox RL, Harden DA, et al: Encephalopathy and seizures induced by intravesical alum irrigations. Bone Marrow Transplantation 1992; 10: 383–385.

Murphy JVK, Marquardt K: Asymptomatic hyperammonemia in patients receiving valproic acid. Arch Neurol 1982; 39: 591–592.

Nadel AM: Wernicke's encephalopathy and high-dose nitroglycerin. Ann Intern Med 1985; 102: 134.

Naganuma M, Shima K, Matsumoto A, et al: A case of autonomic dysfunction and leukoencephalopathy occurring during administration of l5-fluouracil derivative tegafur. Rinsho Shinkeigaku 1988; 28: 1058–1064.

Nakamura M, Fuchinoue S, Sato S, et al: Clinical and radiological features of two cases of tacrolismus-related posterior leukoencephalopathy in liver transplantation. Transplantation Proceedings 1998; 30: 1477–1478.

Nakanishi T, Funahashi S, Shimizu A, et al: Urinary organic acids in elderly Japanese patients with ketosis and encephalopathy who have taken panto-yl-gamma-aminobutyrate, calcium salt (calcium hopantetate, HOPA). Clinica Chimica Acta 1990; 188: 85–90.

Netter JC, Dhondt JL, Rance F, et al: Neurotoxicite precoce du mehtotrexate a haute dose et deficit en tetrahydrobiopterine. Arch Fr Pediatr 1991; 48: 719–722.

Neu IS, Ober H: Multifokale Leukoenzephalopathie nach adjuanter Therapie mit Fluouracil und Levamisol. DMW 1992; 117: 1379.

Neufeld MY: Periodic triphasic waves in levodopa-induced encephalopathy. Neurology 1992; 42: 444–446.

Ng THK, Chan YW, Yu YL, et al: Encephalopathy and neuropathy following ingestion of a chinese herbal broth containing podophyllin. J Neurol Sci 1991; 101: 107–113.

Noble-Jamieson CM, Reger R, Silverman M: Dexamethasone in neonatal chronic lung disease. Eur J Pediatr 1989; 148: 365–367.

Noda S, Hartake J, Sasaki A, et al: Acute encephalopathy with hepatic steatosis induced by pantothenic acid antagonist calcium hopantenate, in dogs. Liver 1991; 11: 134–142.

Nunez JC, Alonso MD, Santafe C, et al: Encefalopatia por fenotoina. Med Clin (Madrid) 1992; 98: 60.

Oechsner M, Steen C, Sturenburg HJ, et al: Hyperammonaemic encephalopathy after initiation of valproate therapy in unrecognised ornithine transcarbamylase deficiency. J Neurol Neurosurg Psychiatry 1998; 64: 680–682.

Ohtaki E, Matsuishi T, Hirano Y, et al: Acute disseminated encephalomyelitis after treatment with japanese B encephalitis vaccine. JNNP 1995; 59: 316–317.

Ortiz A, Martin-Llonch N, Garron MP, et al: Cefazolin-induced encephalopathy in uremic patients. Rev Infect Dis 1991; 13: 772–773.

Ory JP, Wiest F, Delacour JL, et al: Rapidly progressive multifocal leukoencephalitis after vaccination. A case report. Revue de Medecine Interne 1994; 15(suppl 3): 424.

Osterman JD, Truaner DA, Reznik VM, et al: Transient hemiparesis associated with monoclonal CD3 antibody (OKT3) therapy. Pediatric Neurology 1993; 9: 482–484.

Pakalnis AM, Drake ME, Denio L: Valproate-associated encephalopathy. J Epilepsy 1989; 2: 41–44.

Pandit MK, Burke J, Gustafson AB, et al: Drug-induced disorders of glucose tolerance. Ann Int Med 1993; 118: 529–539.

Partin JS, Daugherty CC, McAdams AJ, et al: A comparison of liver ultrastructure and salicylate intoxication in Reye's syndrome. Hepatology 1984; 4: 687–690.

Partin JS, Partin JC, Schubert WK, et al: Serum salicylate concentration in Reye's disease. A study of 130 biopsy-proven cases. Lancet 1982; 1: 191–194.

Peces R, de la Torre M, Alcazar R: Acyclovir-associated encephalopathy in haemodialysis. Nephrol Dial Transplant 1996; 11: 752.

Pepin J, Milord F, Guern C, et al: Trial of prednisolone for prevention of melarsoprol-induced encephalopathy in Gambiense sleeping sickness. Lancet 1989; i: 1246–1250.

Pepin J, Milord F: African trypanosomiasis and drug-induced encephalopathy: risk factors and pathogenesis. Trans Roy Soc Trop Med Hyg 1991; 85: 222–224.

Perazella M, Brown E: Acute aluminum toxicity and alum bladder irrigation in patients with renal failure. Am J Kidney Dis 1993; 21: 44–46.

Phillipi W, Manon-Espaillat R, Spiegel P, et al: Clinical and electroencephalographic manifestations of baclofen-induced encephalopathy: review of the literature. Neurology 1990; 40: 134.

Phillips PC, Reinhardt CS: Antipyrimidine neurotoxicity: cytosine arabinoside and 5-fluorouracil. In Rottenberg DA (Ed.): Neurological complications of cancer treatment, Boston, Butterworth, 1991, pp 97–114.

Phillips PC: Methotrexate neurotoxicity. In Rottenberg DA (Ed.): Neurological complications of cancer treatment, Boston, Butterworth, 1991: 115–130.

Pialoux G, Kernbaum S, Vachon F: Arsenical-induced encephalopathy. Bull Soc Pathol Exot Filiales 1988; 81: 555–556.

Playford RJ, Mathews CH, Campbell MJ, et al: Bismuth-induced encephalopathy caused by tri potassium dilcitrato bismuthate in a patient with chronic renal failure. GUT 1990; 31: 359–360.

Plesner A-M, Arlien-Soborg P, Herning M: Neurological complications and Japanese B encephalitis vaccination. Lancet 1996; 348: 202–203.

Quesada JR: Toxicity and side effects of interferons. In Baron S, et al (Eds.): Interferon: principals and medical applications, Galveston, University of Texas Medical Branch, 1992: 427–432.

Rabinovich R, Robbins A: Pertussis vaccines—a progress report. JAMA 1994; 271: 68–69.

Raichle ME, Kutt H, McDowell F: Neurotoxicity of intravenously administered penicillin G. Arch Neurol 1971; 25: 232–239.

Rangel RJ, Warner JJ, Wilder BJ: Valproic acid encephalopathy. J Epilepsy 1988; 1: 197–202.

Rao JK, Katsetos CD, Herman MM, et al: Experimental aluminum encephalomyelopathy. Relationship to human neurodegenerative disease. Clin Lab Med 1998; 18: 687–698.

Rashiq S, Briewa L, Mooney M, et al: Distinguishing acyclovir neurotoxicity from encephalomyelitis. J Int Med 1993; 234: 507–511.

Reboli AC, Mandler HD: Encephalopathy and Psychoses associated with sulfadiazine in two patients with AIDS and CNS toxoplasmosis. Clin Infect Dis 1992; 15: 556–557.

Reece DE, Frei-Lahr DA, Shepherd JD, et al: Neurologic complications in allogeneic bone marrow transplant patients receiving cyclosporin. Bone Marrow Transplantation 1991; 8: 393–401.

Renard JL, Felten D, Bèquet D: Post-otoneurosurgery aluminum encephalopathy. Lancet 1994; 344: 63–64.

Resar LMS, Phillips PC, Kastan MB, et al: Acute neurotoxicity after intrathecal cytosine arabinoside in two adolescents with acute lymphoblastic leukemia of B-cell type. Cancer 1993; 71: 117–123.

Reusche E, Gerke P, Kruger S, et al: A long-term organic brain syndrome and brain stem symptoms in an undiagnosed dialysis-associated encephalopathy. Dtsch Med Wochenschr 1999; 124: 176–181.

Reusche E, Rohwer J, Forth W, et al: Ionomeric cement and aluminium encephalopathy. Lancet 1995; 345: 1633–1634.

Reye RDK, Morgan G, Baral J: Encephalopathy and fatty degeneration of the viscera: a disease entity in childhood. Lancet 1963; 2: 749–752.

Rfidah EI, Findlay CA, Beattie TJ: Reversible encephalopathy after intravenous ciprofloxacin therapy. Pediatric Nephrology 1995; 9: 250–255.

Ricart C, Higes F, Mallada J: Encefalopatia cronica por fenitoina. Med Clin (Madrid) 1991; 97: 635.

Robin E, Lebrec D, Hammel P, et al: Hepatic encephalopathy after injection of lanreotide, a somatostatin analog. Gastroenterol Clin Biol 1996; 20: 1014–1016.

Rohatiner AZS, Färkkilä M: Neurotoxicity of interferon therapy. In Smith RA (Ed.): Interferon treatment of neurologic disorders, New York, Marcel Dekker, 1988, pp 135–143.

Rosenberg B: Fundamental studies with cisplatin. Cancer 1985; 55: 2303–2316.

Rosenberg SA, Lotze MT, Yang JC, et al: Experience with the use of high dose interleukin-2 based therapies in the treatment of 652 patients with cancer. Ann Surg 1989; 210: 274–285.

Rosendahl L, Friis ML: Metabolic encephalopathy: oxcarbazepine-induced hyponatremia. Ugeskr Laeger 1991; 153: 2637–2638.

Ross JF, Sahenk Z, Hyser C, et al: Characterization of a murine model for human bismuth encephalopathy. Neurotoxicology 1988; 9: 581–586.

Rouveix B, Bricaire F, Michon C, et al: Mefloquine and an acute brain syndrome. Ann Int Med 1989; 110: 577–578.

Saitoh H, Shinohara Y, Fujita H, et al: A case of carmofur-induced leukoencephalopathy: MR images and CT findings. Tokai J Exp Clin Med 1989; 14: 357–360.

Salcman M, Pippenger CE: Acute carbamazepine encephalopathy. JAMA 1975; 231: 915.

Sälke-Kellermann A, Baier H, Rambeck B, et al: Acute encephalopathy with vilgabatrin. Lancet 1993; 342: 185.

Sasaki T, Minagawa M, Yamamoto T, et al: A case of Rett syndrome with acute encephalopathy induced during calcium hopantenate treatment. Brain Dev 1991; 13: 52–55.

Sasazaki Y, Asami K, Utsumi J: Transient subacute encephalopathy induced by high dose methotrexate treatment in children with acute lymphoblastic leukemia and malignant lymphoma. Gan To Kagaku Ryohu 1992; 19: 1851–1857.

Savarese DM, Gordon J, Smith TW, et al: Cerebral demyelination syndrome in a patient treated with 5-fluorouracil and levamisole. Cancer 1996; 77: 387–394.

Schinkel AH, Wagenaar E, Mol CA, et al: P-glycoprotein in the blood-brain barrier of mice influences the brain penetration and pharmacological activity of many drugs. J Clin Invest 1996; 97: 2517–2524.

Schneider F: Progressive multifocal leukoencephalopathy as a cause of neurologic symptoms in Sharp syndrome. Z Rheumatol 1991; 50: 222–224.

Schoenide SE, Dana WJ: Ifosfamide and mesna. Clin Pharm 1990; 9: 179–191.

Schoonjans R, Mast A, Abeele GVD, et al: Sulfasalazine-associated leukoencephalopathy in a patient with Crohn's disease. Am J Gastroenterol 1993; 88: 1416–1420.

Schou M: Adverse lithium neuroleptic interactions—are there permanent effects? Human Psychopharmacol 1990; 5: 263–265.

Schulz PE, Weiner SP, Haber LM, et al: Neurological complications from fat embolism. Ann Neurol 1994; 35: 628–630.

Seddigh S: Ifosfamideinduzierte Enzephalopathie. Akt Neurol 1993; 20: 214–215.

Seifer DB, Sandberg EC, Ueland K, et al: Water intoxication and hyponatremic encephalopathy from the use of oxytocin nasal spray. J Reproduct Med 1985; 30: 225–228.

Seltzer HS: Severe drug-induced hypoglycemia: a review. Comp Ther 1979; 5: 21–29.

Sempere AP, Posada I, Ramo C, et al: Spongiform leukoencephalopathy after inhaling heroin. Lancet 1991; 338: 320.

Sharief MK, Sander JWA, Shorvon SD: Acute encephalopathy with vigabatrin. Lancet 1993; 342: 619.

Sharma RR, Cast IP, Redfern RM, et al: Extradural application of bismuth iodoform paraffin paste causing relapsing bismuth encephalopathy: a case report with CT and MRI studies. J Neurol Neurosurg Psychiatry 1994; 57: 990–3.

Shihab F, Barry JM, Bennett WM, et al: Cytokine-related encephalopathy induced by OKT3: incidence and predisposing factors. Transplantation Proceedings 1993; 25: 564–565.

Simonioan NA, Gilliam FG, Chiappa KH: Ifosfamide causes a diazepam-sensitive encephalopathy. Neurology 1993; 43: 2700–2702.

Sivenius J, Paljärvi V, Vapalahti M, et al: Vigabatrin: neuropathologic evaluation in 5 patients. Epilepsia 1993; 34: 193–196.

Slikkerveer A, De Wolff FA: Bismuth: biokinetics and neurotoxicity. In De Wolff FA (Ed.): Handbook of clinical neurology, vol 20 (64): Intoxications of the nervous system, Amsterdam, Elsevier, 1994, pp 331–351.

Small SL, Fukui MB, Bramblett GT, et al: Immunosuppression-induced leukoencephalopathy from tacrolimus (FK506). Ann Neurol 1996; 40: 575–580.

Smedley H, Katruk M, Sikora K, et al: Neurological effects of recombinant human interferon. BMJ 1983; 286: 262–264.

Smith CR: Encephalomyelopathy as an idiosyncratic reaction to carbamazepine: a case report. Neurology 1991; 41: 760–761.

Smith SJM, Kocen RS: A Creutzfeldt-Jakob like syndrome due to lithium toxicity. JNNP 1988; 51: 120–123.

Soriano-Soriano C, Jimenez-Jimenez FJ, Edigo-Harero JA, et al: Acute encephalopathy following lumbar myelography with iohexal. Acta Neurol (Napoli) 1992; 14: 127–129.

Sriram S, Steinman L: Postinfectious and postvaccinial encephalomyelitis. Neurol clin 1984; 2: 341–353.

Starko KM, Ray CG, Dominguez LB, et al: Reye's syndrome and salicylate use. Pediatrics 1980; 66: 859–864.

Steiner I, Brenner T, Mizrachi-Kol R, et al: Development of experimental allergic encephalomyelitis during steroid administration. Isr J Med Sci 1991; 27: 365–368.

Stephan F, Etienne MC, Wallays C, et al: Fatal encephalopathy and tumor lysis syndrome: case report. Am J Med 1995; 99: 685–688.

Stommel EW: Carbamazepine encephalopathy. Neurology 1992; 42: 705.

Stratton KR, Howe CJ, Johnston RB: Adverse effects associated with childhood vaccines other than pertussis and rubella. JAMA 1994; 271: 1602–1605.

Suter CC, Westmoreland BF, Sharbrough FW, et al: Electro- encephalographic abnormalities in interferon encephalopathy: a preliminary report. Mayo Clin Proc 1984; 59: 847–850.

Swartz CM, Dolinar LJ: Encephalopathy associated with rapid decrease of high levels of lithium. Annals of Clinical Psychiatry 1995; 7: 207–209.

Takimoto CH, Lu ZH, Zhang R, et al: Severe neurotoxicity following 5-fluorouracil-based chemotherapy in a patient with dihydropyrimidine dehydrogenase deficiency. Clin Cancer Res 1996; 2: 477–481.

Tartara AR, Manni R: Sodium valproate "encephalopathy": report of three cases with generalised epilepsy. Ital J Neurosci 1985; 6: 93–95.

Taylor R, Arze R, Gokal R, et al: Cephaloridine encephalopathy. BMJ 1981; 283: 409–410.

Theodorou AA, Barton LL, Rice SA, et al: Trimethoprim-Sulfamethoxazole-associated central nervous system disease. Pediatric Infectious Disease Journal 1995; 14: 76–78.

Therapeutics and Technology Assessment Committee, American Academy of Neurology: DTP vaccination. Neurology 1992; 42: 471–472.

Thompson GB, June CH, Sullivan KM, et al: Association between cyclosporin neurotoxicity and hypomagnesemia. Lancet 1984; ii: 1116–1120.

Trauner DA: Reye's syndrome. Curr Prob Ped 1982; 12: 1–31.

Truwit CL, Denaro CP, Lake JR, et al: MR imaging of reversible cyclosporin A-induced neurotoxicity. AJNR 1991; 12: 651–659.

Tsiouris J, Tsiouris N: Hemiplegia as a complication of treatment of childhood immune thrombocytopenic purpura with intravenously administered immunoglobulin. J Pediatrics 1998; 133: 717.

Usui S, Komiya T, Imai H, et al: Metrizamide encephalopathy in a child with hydrocephalus. No To Shinkei 1988; 40: 1075–1080.

Vass K, Heininger K, Schäfer B, et al: Interferon-g potentiates antibody-mediated demyelination in vivo. Ann Neurol 1992; 32: 198–206.

Vecht CJ, Keohane C, Menon RS, et al: Acute fatal leukoencephalopathy after interleukin-2 therapy. Lancet 1990; 323: 1146–1147.

Vesikaril T, Nuutila A, Cantell K: Neurologic sequelae following interferon therapy of juvenile laryngeal papilloma. Acta Pediatr Scand 1988; 77: 619–622.

Vial T, Descotes J: Clinical toxicity of interleukin-2. Drug Safety 1992; 7: 417–433.

Vial T, Descotes J: Clinical toxicity of the interferons. Drug Safety 1994; 10: 115–150.

Visticot F, Montreul G: Stuporous encephalopathy induced by sodium valproate. Revue de Medecine Interne 1994; 15: 365–366.

Von Bose MJ, Zaudig M: Encephalopathy resembling Creutzfeldt-Jakob disease following oral, prescribed doses of bismuth nitrate. Br J Psychiatry 1991; 158: 278–80.

Wagner T: Ifosfamide clinical pharmacokinetics. Clin Pharmacokinet 1994; 26: 439–456.

Wainer V, Ducharme J, Granvil CP, et al: Ifosfamide stereoselective dichloroethylation and neurotoxicity (letter). Lancet 1994; 343: 982–983.

Waldman RJ, Hall WN, McGee H, et al: Aspirin as a risk factor in Reye's syndrome. JAMA 1982; 247: 3089–3094.

Walker RW, Rosenblum MC: Amphotericin-B associated leukoencephalopathy. Neurology 1992; 42: 2005–2010.

Warkin SW, Husband DJ, Green JA, et al: Ifosfamide encephalopathy: a reappraisal. Eur J Cancer Clin Oncol 1989; 25: 1303–1310.

Weibel RE, Caserta V, Benor DE, et al: Acute encephalopathy followed by permanent brain injury or death associated with further attenuated measles vaccines: a review of claims submitted to the National Vaccine Injury Compensation Program. Pediatrics 1998; 101: 383–387.

Welge-Lüssen UC, Gerhartz HH: Late onset of neurotoxicity with cyclosporin (letter). Lancet 1994; 343: 293.

Wijdicks EFM, Wieser RH, Krom RAF: neurotoxicity in liver transplant recipients with cyclosporine immunosuppression. Neurology 1995; 45: 1962–1964.

Winick N, Kamen B, Lester C, et al: Effect of chronic methotrexate treatment on tissue levels of folate and methotrexate polyglutamates. Cancer Drug Delivery 1987; 4: 25–31.

Wolters EC, Wijngaarden GK, Stan FC, et al: Leukoencephalopathy after inhaling "heroin" pyrolysate. Lancet 1982; ii: 1233–1237.

Worthley SG, McNeil JD: Leukoencephalopathy in a patient taking low dose oral methotrexate therapy for rheumatoid arthritis. J Rheumatology 1995; 22: 335–337.

Wothman F, Türker T, Müller AR, et al: Progressive multifocal encephalopathy after orthotopic liver transplantation. Transplantation 1994; 57: 1268–1271.

Yamada T, Okamura S, Okazaki T, et al: Leukoencephalopathy following treatment with carmofur: a case report and review of the Japanese literature. Asia-Oceania J Obstet Gynecol 1989; 15: 161–168.

Yap HY, Lau CP: Hyponatremic encephalopathy complicating thiazide reserpine preparation. Postgrad Med J 1992; 68: 149–153.

Yeh KH, Cheng AL: High-dose 5-fluorouracil infusional therapy is associated with hyperammonaemia, lactic acidosis and encephalopathy. Br J Cancer 1997; 75(3): 464–465.

Yellowlees P, Greenfield C, McIntyre N: Dimethylsulfoxide induced toxicity. Lancet 1980; ii: 1004–1006.

Yoshimoto K, Saima S, Echizen H, et al: Famotidine-associated central nervous system reactions and plasma and cerebrospinal drug concentrations in neurosurgical patients with renal failure. Clin Pharmacol Ther 1994; 55: 693–700.

Young CL: Acute encephalopathy associated with sulfadiazine in a patient with AIDS-related complex (letter). J Infect Dis 1989; 160: 163–164.

Zabernigg A, Maier H, Thaler J, et al: Late onset fatal neurological toxicity of fludarabine. Lancet 1994; 344: 1780.

Zheng R, Zhang X, Lin Z, et al: Clinical features and diagnosis of delayed encephalopathy induced by anthelminthic imidazoles: clinical analysis of 202 cases. Pharmacoepidemiol Drug Safety 1994; 3 (suppl 1): 119.

Zulian GB, Tullen E, Maton B, et al: Methylene blue for ifosfamide associated encephalopathy (letter). NEJM 1995; 332: 1239–1240.

Chapter 4
Drug-Induced Disorders of Consciousness

Introduction

Various drugs impair consciousness. Consciousness is usually defined as a state of awareness of the self and the surroundings. Drug-induced altered stated of consciousness are described in this chapter. *Delirium* or clouding of consciousness is described in Chapter 5 along with altered state of consciousness which involve cognitive functions. *Syncope* is a transient loss of consciousness. *Stupor* is defined as unresponsiveness from which the patient can be aroused only by vigorous stimuli. *Coma* is unarousable unresponsiveness. *Drowsiness* is a state between full alertness and stupor.

Syncope

Syncope is defined as sudden transient loss of consciousness with loss of postural tone usually lasting no more than 15 seconds. Presyncope, which can be characterized as near fainting, light-headedness, or extreme dizziness, may be a part of a continuum that leads to syncope or may occur as an isolated event. Syncope is a common presenting complaint accounting for 1% to 6% of hospital admissions and 3% of visits to the emergency departments. Nearly half of the population may suffer at least one episode of syncope during their life time.

Etiology. Causes of syncope have been reviewed by Kapoor (1992) and are summarized with approximate range of frequencies as follows:

- Vagovasal. 1% to 29%
- Orthostatic hypotension. 4% to 12%
- Organic cardiac disease. 3% to 11%
- Cardiac arrhythmias. 5% to 30%
- Situational syncope; micturition, cough, etc. 1% to 8%
- Psychogenic syncope; anxiety and panic disorders. < 5%
- Glossopharyngeal and trigeminal neuralgias. < 5%
- Cerebrovascular ischemia. Transient ischemic attacks. < 5%
- Carotid sinus syncope. < 1%
- Drug-induced syncope. 2% to 9%.

Diagnosis. In various reported studies, cause of syncope could not be diagnosed in 13% to 47% of the patients. In patients with structural heart disease, ECG can be helpful in establishing the diagnosis. Although vagovasal reactions are considered to be a frequent cause of syncope in the absence of heart disease, it is difficult to substantiate this diagnosis. Neurally mediated hypotension and bradycardia are believed to be the common causes of syncope but studies of the hemodynamic profiles of vagovasal reactions have shown that heart rate and arterial pressure frequently increase before the onset of symptoms. Increase of concentration of circulating catecholamines before the syncope suggests that this may paradoxically enhance the susceptibility to bradycardia and hypotension. Isoproterenol (exogenous catecholamine) infusion in conjunction with upright tilt test can reproduce neurally mediated syncope and identify the subjects susceptible to it (Almquist et al 1989).

Syncope should be differentiated from seizures and other states of altered consciousness. Epileptic seizures are associated with such features as blue face, frothing at mouth, loss of consciousness more than 5 minutes, and disorientation after the event. Syncope is usually associated with nausea and sweating before the event and maintenance of orientation after the event which is an important point of distinction from a seizure. Occasionally syncope may be accompanied by myoclonic jerks and micturition disturbances which may give the impression of the patient having a seizure. Sometimes, it is difficult to differentiate between a syncope and a seizure. A thorough history and electrophysiological studies, particularly EEG and ECG may be helpful in ascertaining the cause of unknown episodes of brief loss of consciousness.

Syncope and falls are often two concomitant adverse effects of drugs reported in elderly patients. An overlap between syncope and falls is becoming increasingly acknowledged. In the elderly, determining the cause of a fall can be difficult. A patient may be unable to recall documented falls some months later and a witness account for syncopal events is often unavailable. In one study, in almost 40% of patients in whom an attributable diagnosis of carotid sinus syndrome was made, the only presenting symptoms were falls alone or falls with dizziness; syncope was denied (Shaw and Kenny 1997).

Drug-Induced Syncope

Syncope is reported as an adverse event with several drugs. Because it is a common event, its relation to the drug is difficult to determine in most of the cases. The act of injection itself may provoke a vasovagal syncope regardless of the medication contained in it. In one study, using a standardized adverse drug reaction algorithm, nine (13%) of 70 patients were rated as having probable drug-related syncope or presyncope (Hanlon et al 1990).

Epidemiology. Syncope occurs in approximately 20% to 50% of the population. In one study, using a standardized adverse drug reaction algorithm, nine (13%) of 70 patients with syncope were rated as having probable drug-related syncope or presyncope (Hanlon et al 1990). Epidemiology of hypotension is also relevant to syncope. Hypotension is common in the elderly and

in 10% of the individuals above 71, blood pressure values were found to be ≤ 122 mm Hg systolic and ≤ 68 mm Hg diastolic (Busby et al 1994). An association between hypotension and drugs was found in this study.

Drugs Related to Syncope. Drugs reported to be associated with syncope are shown in Table 4.1.

Table 4.1. Drugs reported to be associated with syncope.

Analgesics
  – Non-steroidal anti-inflammatory drugs
  – Opioid analgesics
Antineoplastic drugs: vincristine
Cytokines: interferon-α
Digitalis
Drugs that produce postural hypotension (see Table 4.2)
Drugs and combinations which prolong Q-T interval / torsades de pointes (see Table 4.3)
Hypnotic-sedative drugs (depressants of CNS)
  – Barbiturates
  – Benzodiazepines
  – Niaprazine (Sarda et al 1996)
Hypoglycemic drugs
  – Insulin
  – Oral hypoglycemics
  – Vaccines
Miscellaneous drugs
  – Gamma hydroxy butyrate (Schwartz 1998)
  – Local anesthetics
  – Meglumine antimonate (antileishmaniasis antimony compound)
  – Topical ophthalmic preparations
    – Levobunolole ointment
    – Betaxolol ophthalmic solution
Xanomeline (in treatment of AD if M_1 receptor activity has been restored)

Only a few published reports of individual drug-induced syncope are available. Syncope is sometimes listed along with more serious adverse effects such as seizures in the same patient and is not significant for assessment.

Katz et al (1988) reported two children treated with interferon-α who experienced confusion, somnolence and syncope, associated with transient EEG abnormalities. Symptoms abated with discontinuation of the therapy and EEG normalized. Readministration of interferon-α at a lower dose did not produce any adverse effects.

Tricyclic antidepressants are known to produce cardiac arrhythmias as adverse effects and are associated with syncope. Fluoxetine, a sero-tonin reuptake inhibitor, has been considered to be free of anticholinergic and cardiovascular adverse effects. However, a syncopal episode with EEG changes has been reported with fluoxetine (McAnally et al 1992). Carbamazepine, an antiepileptic drug structurally related to tricyclic antidepressants is associated with cardiac conduction disturbances and syncope.

Syncope is a common adverse effect of vaccination. Braun et al (1997) have described the individual characteristics, clinical features, and morbidity associated with syncope following immunization. From 1990 to 1995, 697 cases of syncope after vaccination were reported to the National Vaccine Adverse Event Reporting System in the United States.Most of the subjects were younger than 20 years and syncope occurred within one hour or less after vaccination. Tonic or clonic movements, which have been associated with the anoxia of vasovagal syncope, were reported in 30.4% of syncopal episodes occurring 15 minutes or less after and in 12.8% of those occurring 15 minutes or longer after vaccination. It was recommended that patients exhibiting presyncopal signs and symptoms around the time of immunization need to be evaluated carefully and may need to be assisted to sit or lie down after immunization until free of symptoms.

Pathomechanism of Drug-Induced Syncope

Important causes of drug-induced syncope are postural hypotension and cardiac rhythm and conduction disorders.

Postural Hypotension. This is an important cause of syncope (Mets 1995). Drugs which produce postural hypotension as an adverse effect are shown in Table 4.2.

Significant hypotension is drop of at least 20 mm Hg in systolic pressure or 10 mm Hg in diastolic pressure within 3 minutes on standing up. Recent evidence from animal experimental studies suggests that the site for induction of postural hypotension by passive upright tilt may lie in the forebrain region, whereas the primary center for the induction of postural hypotension lies

Table 4.2. Drugs that produce postural hypotension.

Drugs used to treat hypertension
ACE inhibitors
Beta-blockers
Calcium antagonists
Diuretics
Drugs which have hypotension as an adverse effect
Antidepressants: MAO inhibitors
Antiparkinsonian drugs
Levodopa
Bromocriptine
Selegeline (deprenyl)
Anticholinergics.
Antipsychotics
Phenothiazines
Butyrophenones
Vasodilators
Nitrates

in the brain stem (Park et al 1990). Critical lower limit of cerebral perfusion lies at or close to 50% below baseline supine (horizontal) mean cerebral blood flow velocity. At this level of cerebral hypoperfusion, unconsciousness ensues in 80% of subjects (Njemanze 1992). This indicates impaired autoregulation and there may be a yet unknown clinical predisposition to this condition.

Most antihypertensive medications produce syncope due to postural hypotension. However, other mechanisms may also play a part. A case is reported of a patient who developed cough after start of treatment of hypertension with ACE inhibitor enalapril and developed a cough syncope (Jayarajan and Prakash 1993). No hypotension was reported. The patient recovered from cough on discontinuation of enalapril.

A significant association between the use of potassium-sparing diuretics, dopaminergic antiparkinsonian drugs and butyrophenone antipsychotics and low blood pressure in the elderly was found in a Swedish study (Passare et al 1998). Orthostatic hypotension is often associated with hyponatremia and is found in one-fifth of the elderly who take diuretics. A slight decrease in sodium levels induced by diuretics results in marked orthostatic hypotension in the healthy elderly persons whereas it does not affect younger adults. Nitrates dilate arterial and venous smooth muscle and reduce cardiac output by pooling blood in the periphery. This leads to fall in blood pressure and this risk is higher in the elderly. Levodopa produces orthostatic hypotension in patients with late-onset Parkinson's disease who are prone to it because of autonomic dysfunction.

Oral formulation of the selective M_1 agonist xanomeline used for the treatment of Alzheimer's disease is associated with an increased incidence of syncope. Alzheimer's patients, who presumably lack M_1 receptor activity, usually have a reduced risk of tilt-induced syncope compared with normal subjects. Both groups, however, have enhanced susceptibility to hypotension and syncope when M_1 receptor activity is pharmacologically increased such as by xanomeline administration (Medina et al 1997).

An isoproterenol-mediated increase in cardiomotor tone and a decrease in afterload contribute to the induction of vasovagal syncope. Contrary to conventional belief, a significant decrease in preload is not observed immediately before isoproterenol-induced syncope (Shen et al 1997). Syncope after an antihypertensive drug is not always due to postural hypotension. β-blockers may produce bradycardia in addition to hypotension. Paradoxically, beta-blockers are also used in the treatment of syncope. In one case the patient developed cough syncope as a result of prolonged coughing as an adverse reaction to the ACE-inhibitor enalapril used for the treatment of hypertension (Jayarajan and Prakash 1993).

Paradoxical hypotension due to suppression of vasomotor outflow may occur after amphetamine intoxication. A case is reported of recurrent syncopes with postural hypotension in a young healthy female after ingestion of 20 mg of amphetamine (Smit et al 1996).

Postural hypotension is the most frequent, and at times treatment limiting, side effect encountered with MAO inhibitors. The pathomechanism of MAO inhibitor-induced postural hypotension is not known. It probably results from inhibition of normal breakdown of dietary tyramine. The excess tyramine undergoes α-hydroxylation to form a "false neurotransmitter" resulting in diminished sympathetic outflow (McDaniel 1986).

Nitrates are commonly used sublingually for relief of angina pectoris. Hypotension is a known effect of nitrates. A case is reported of a 65-year old woman who experienced a syncope after taking 5 mg of isosorbide dinitrate sublingually in a sitting position (Chong et al 1998). The patient had no hypotension, bradycardia or autonomic symptoms after subjecting her to a postural change without isosorbide but she had a syncope after she was placed again in a sitting position 15 minutes after taking isosorbide dinitrate. This incident points out the importance of the patient being in a supine position when taking nitrates and a lower dose is recommended for elderly patients.

Cardiac Arrhythmias and Conduction Disturbances. CNS drugs such as antidepressants may produce cardiac arrhythmias which is a

Table 4.3. Drugs reported to cause syncope by inducing arrhythmias and conduction disturbances including torsades de pointes.

Single drugs
Antiarrhythmic drugs
  Amiodarone (Winters et al 1997)
  Disopyramide
  Procainamide
  Quinidine
  Sotalol
Antihistaminic drugs: astemizole, terfenadine
Antimalarial or antiprotozoal: chloroquine, halofantrine, mefloquine, pentamidine, quinine
Antimicrobials: erythromycin, trimethoprim-sulfa methoxazole
Atropine
Cisapride (cytochrome P450 3A4 substrate), for the treatment of gastrointestinal motility disorders)
Encainide
Flecainide
Psychoactive drugs
  Chloral hydrate
  Haloperidol
  Lithium (Terao et al 1996)
  Phenothiazines
  Pimozide
  Tricyclic antidepressants
Miscellaneous drugs
  Amantadine
  Probucol
  Tacrolismus
  Trimetaphan
  Vasopressin
Combination of drugs
– cisapride and diltiazem (Thomas et al 1998)
– cisapride and ranitidine (Valdes et al 1997)
– clozapine and cocaine (Hameedi et al 1996)
– clozapine and enalapril (Aronowiltz et al 1994)
– fluoxetine and ranitidine (McAnally et al 1992)
– terfenadine and itraconazole (Lekkerkerker and Broekmans 1997; Romkes et al 1997)
– terfenadine and erythromycin
– terfenadine and astemizol (Zechnich et al 1994)

known cause of syncope. Atropine is widely used as a parasympatholytic agent during diagnostic and therapeutic procedures. Syncope has been observed an unexpected paradoxical response to atropine after cardiac transplantation. Various degrees of atrioventricular block has been documented in these patients. Although the underlying mechanism is not clear, these findings suggest that atropine may paradoxically cause high-degree AV block in patients after transplantation (Brunner La-Rocca et al 1997).

Syncope has been reported during dobutamine stress echocardiography (Lanzarini et al 1996). At a dobutamine dosage of 20 µg/kg for 2 minutes, a 60-year old patient lost consciousness during a cardiac asystole. She was given an intravenous bolus of atropine 1 mg and recovered sinus rhythm and consciousness.

Antiarrhythmic drugs may produce syncope through the development of torsades de pointes.

Torsades de pointes. This is a life-threatening disorder characterized by polymorphic, "twisting" ventricular tachycardia (Raehl et al 1985). It is characterized by polymorphic QRS complexes that change in amplitude and cycle length and may be preceded by Q-T prolongation. Torsades de pointes may result from acquired medical and genetic disorders but it is often induced by drugs as shown in Table 4.3.

Management of Drug-Induced Syncope

In a patient with suspected drug-induced syncope, the drug in question should be discontinued. When assessing orthostatic hypotension in the elderly, drug treatment should always be reviewed. Whenever possible, antihypertensive drugs should be discontinued, and the dosages of essential drugs should be reduced (Verhaeverbeke and Mets 1997). Wearing elastic stockings sometimes corrects orthostatic hypotension. If non-pharmacological measures are not adequate, drug treatment may be considered. Fludrocortisone (0.1 to 0.4 mg/day) is recommended. A prostaglandin inhibitor such as indomethacin may be useful at a dose of 25 to 150 mg/day.

Patients with cardiac rhythm and conduction disturbances requires care in a cardiology unit. Drug management is complicated by the fact that several of the drugs used for the treatment of cardiac arrhythmias also have syncope as a side effect. Several drugs are used for the treatment of syncope but if syncope is drug-induced, there may be complications and interactions if the offending drug therapy is maintained.

Drowsiness. It is variously reported as lethargy, somnolence and semistuporous state as a side effect of several drugs. This sometimes overlaps with excessive sleepiness reported as an adverse effect and which is discussed in Chapter 19. Drugs which are more likely to induce drowsiness belong to the therapeutic groups shown in Table 4.4.

Lethargy may be due to overdose of drugs which do not produce any impairment of consciousness in therapeutic doses. Certain metabolic disturbances as an adverse reaction to drugs predispose to drowsiness. An example is hyperammonemia as a complication of valproic acid therapy which can lead to drowsiness. Another predisposing factor for drowsiness is aging and brain damage. Drowsiness is usually a side effect of tricyclic antidepressants but stupor has been reported as a complication of paroxetine (specific serotonin reuptake inhibitor) in a patient with mental retardation (Lewis et al 1993).

Baclofen, an antispastic agent, inhibits polysynaptic nociceptive reflexes through an action on GABA$_B$ medullary interneurons. Because it can cross the BBB it can be given by systemic route but may result in drowsiness and respiratory depression. To avoid this, it is given by intrathecal route. However, side effects can still

Table 4.4. Drugs associated with drowsiness.

Antidepressants
Antiepileptics
Antihistaminics
Baclofen
Neuroleptics
Omeprazole
Opioid analgesics
Sedative-hypnotics
   Barbiturates
   Benzodiazepines
   Miscellaneous
Terbutaline

develop by this route because of an action on supraspinal centers leading to drowsiness and occasionally coma along with other neurological complications. These central effects are potentiated by benzodiazepines and can be counteracted by benzodiazepine antagonist flumazenil (Saissy et al 1992).

Sedation is a common adverse effect of neuroleptics and antiepileptics at start of therapy. Most patients develop a tolerance to this effect with prolonged use of the drug. Some of this effect can be avoided by giving the drug at bed time.

Omeprazole, a selective inhibitor of hydrogen-potassium ATPase in parietal cells of the stomach, is sued for reducing gastric acidity. The side effects are predominantly gastrointestinal but CNS side effects such as reduced consciousness, confusion and agitation have also been reported. A case is reported where a 64-year old man experienced drowsiness after start of therapy with omeprazole for reflux esophagitis (Meeuwisse et al 1997). He improved after discontinuation of the drug but had recurrent episodes of drowsiness after resuming therapy. The mechanism of this adverse effect is not understood.

Somnolence has been reported in some studies with terbutaline, a β_2-sympathomimetic drug and may be characteristic for this drug occurring in some 25% of patients.

Drowsiness is not always an undesirable side effect. Antihistaminics are sometimes used to induce sleep. However, daytime use leads to reduced alertness and would be a dangerous for those operating machinery or vehicles.

Drug-Induced Coma

Coma or loss of consciousness induced by drugs is a serious condition and a medical emergency. A basic concept of mechanism of consciousness is essential for discussing the pathophysiology of drug-induced impairment of consciousness.

Mechanism of Consciousness. The maintenance of consciousness depends on the integrity of the reticular activating system (RAS). During normal sleep, the RAS is inhibited by caudal reticular formation structures and this is reversed by sensory stimulation and awakening. Electrical stimulation of the RAS produces marked cortical activation which wakes up a sleeping animal. Damage to the RAS by surgery, disease, or drugs causes loss of consciousness even if the cortex is intact. This state is irreversible until function of the RAS is restored.

Pathomechanism of Drug-Induced Coma. Drug-induced coma may be due to direct effect of drugs on the brain or indirect effect due to disturbances of other systems.

– *Direct effect of drugs on the brain.* This is usually due to drugs which act mainly on the nervous system such as sedative hypnotics. However, overdose of drugs not normally acting on the CNS. e. g., propranolol may also induce coma.

Coma may be reversible or irreversible if there is significant structural damage to the brain such as in leukoencephalopathy (see Chapter 3).

– *Indirect effect on the brain by drug-induced disorders of other systems.* Examples of this are hepatic and renal failure, and drug-induced hypoglycemia. Drug-induced respiratory or circulatory failure can also depress the RAS leading to coma.

Table 4.5. Drug-induced coma.

Direct effect from prolonged use
Barbiturates
Benzodiazepines
Opioids
Tricyclic antidepressants
Valproic acid
Vigabatrin
Drug-induced hypoglycemia
Insulin
Oral hypoglycemic agents
Pentamidine
Salicylates
Drug-induced hyperosmolar coma due to drug-induced diabetes inspidus
Lithium (MacGregor et al 1995)
Drug-induced hyperosmolar non-ketotic diabetic coma
Prednisone (Yang et al 1995)
Somatostatin (Vandercam et al 1995)
Drug-induced hepatic encephalopathy (see Chapter 3)
Drug-induced hyponatremia (see Chapter 25)

Coma is associated with several drug-induced encephalopathies and the pathomechanism of these has been discussed in Chapter 3. Discussion of drug overdose is beyond the scope of this book. Normal doses of some drugs may produce overdose effect in some circumstances such as drug interactions and renal failure impairing excretion of the drug. Drugs associated with coma are shown in Table 4.5 and mechanism of action of some common of these is described in the following text.

Benzodiazepines. Distribution of benzodiazepines in the brain and their enhancement of GABA activity at specific sites accounts for the clinical features of benzodiazepine-induced coma to a large extent. These drugs can cause decrease in CBF and cerebral metabolism, the distribution of which correlates with density of benzodiazepine binding sites. Endozepines, the ligands for benzodiazepine recognition sites on $GABA_A$ receptors in the CNS, are elevated in idiopathic recurring stupor which can be reversed by use of benzodiazepine antagonist flumazenil (Rothstein et al 1992).

The major site of action of the benzodiazepines is the RAS but in high doses generalized cortical depression may occur which contributes to stupor. Unlike barbiturates, even high doses of benzodiazepines rarely produce severe depression of vital brainstem centers. However, benzodiazepines potentiate the effects of other CNS depressants. Benzodiazepine-induced coma can be rapidly reversed by the antagonist flumazenil.

Barbiturates. At high concentrations barbiturates dissolve in lipid membranes and interfere with ionic transfer and calcium uptake by nerve cell membrane . They cause a dose-dependent decrease in CBF and glucose utilization.

Barbiturates act mainly at GABA synapses where they enhance inhibition and suppress excitation. Hypnotic and sedative effects of barbiturates may depress other brain structures in addition to the RAS. Depression of the cerebral cortex can lead to confusion and intellectual impairment. a state of anesthesia supervenes as dosage increases above the hypnotic range.

Antidepressants. Tricyclic antidepressants inhibit the high affinity, energy dependent uptake of monoamines into the cytoplasmic stores in the presynaptic membranes in the CNS. Most of these drugs produce some drowsiness as a side effect. In moderate overdose it may proceed to stupor and severe overdose may lead to coma and this may be attributed to their anticholinergic action. Slow waves on EEG indicate that the CNS depression is due to inhibitory effects of these drugs on the RAS whereas simultaneously fast activity indicates stimulating effect in other areas of the brain (Itil and Soldatos 1980).

Other antidepressants have different modes of action but the clinically they can produce the sedative effect. Mianserin has no effect on monoamine uptake, no sympathomimetic activity, and no significant cholinergic effect in therapeutic dosage. There is some evidence that it blocks presynaptic α_2-adrenoreceptors, thus inhibiting the negative feedback on noradrenaline release and increases noradrenaline turnover (Fludder and Leonard 1979). Trazodone inhibits serotonin uptake but blocks central serotonin receptors. Both these drugs have marked sedative action.

Valproic Acid (VPA). Several cases of stupor and coma due to therapeutic use of valproic acid in epilepsy as well as to its overdose have been reported in literature (Koskiniemi and Hakimies 1979). Most of the patients are on multiple antiepileptics. The frequency of occurrence is about 1 per 100,000 patients treated with valproic acid. Various explanations have been given for this VPA-induced coma and some of these are:

- *Overdose.* Pedersen and Juul-Jensen (1984) described a case of intentional overdose in a epileptic patient whose seizures were well controlled with VPA monotherapy. EEG became flat without any activity but the patient was treated successfully by hemodialysis. Another case of overdose with prolonged coma recovered slowly with residual neurological deficits (Bigler 1985).
- *Polytherapy.* Most of the cases of stupor have been described in patients on polytherapy with antiepileptic drugs where the dose of VPA was increased (Gentile et al 1991). This led to the conjecture that coma may result from drug interaction after addition of VPA as evidenced by recovery after discontinuation

of VPA or other antiepileptic drugs (Sackellares et al 1979). However, stupor has been reported in patients on VPA monotherapy as well (Zaccara et al 1984)

– *Carnitine deficiency.* Low serum carnitine levels may predispose patients to impairment of consciousness when treated with VPA (Triggs et al 1990).

– *Carbamyl phosphate synthetase-1 deficiency.* This has been discovered in a patient after VPA-induced coma (Verbiest et al 1992). This patient recovered but had cerebral atrophy shown on CT scan.

– *Hyperammonemia.* The role of hyperammonemia in VPA-induced coma was pointed out in earlier reports (Coulter and Allen 1980; Kulick and Kramer 1993) but elevation of ammonia is also a common asymptomatic finding in patients undergoing VPA treatment. As a precaution, however, hyperammonemia in patients being treated with phenytoin or phenobarbital when VPA is administered concomitantly should be monitored clinically and VPA should be discontinued immediately if drowsiness or lethargy occurs (Duarte et al 1993). VPA-induced coma has been reported in a patient where VPA was used for mania and blood ammonia level was elevated to 134 µg/dL with normal liver function tests (Settle 1995). The patient improved after discontinuation of VPA.

– In case overdose with valproic acid there may be increase concentration of inhibitory neurotransmitter GABA in the brain. Such a drowsy state has been shown to respond to naloxone (Alberto et al 1989).

– *Neurosurgery.* Unexplained impairment of consciousness has been reported in neurosurgical patients given prophylactic VPA for prevention of seizures. An incidence of 2% in this patient population (8 cases out of about 400 treated with VPA) has been reported by Landau et al (1993). EEG changes in these cases were diffuse high voltage triphasic complexes mixed with regular delta waves, interrupted by short flattenings. There was no evidence of epileptiform activity and these patients recovered after discontinuation of VPA. Blood VPA and ammonia levels in these patients were within the normal range. The authors speculated that this increased sensitivity of the neurosurgical patients to VPA may be due to increased permeability of the blood brain barrier, due to operative injury, allowing toxic levels of VPA to enter brain tissue despite normal levels in the serum.

Drugs Producing Hypoglycaemia. Glucose is the only nutrient that brain cells can utilize in sufficient quantity to meet their energy requirements. Fall of blood glucose level to 20–50 mg/dL range (normal 80–100 mg/dL) can produce convulsions and coma. The most likely cause of it is insulin overdose but several other drugs can produce hypoglycaemia in non-diabetic patients.

Drugs Producing Hyponatremia. Several drugs produce hyponatremia which can lead to coma. One example is oxcarbazepine which can produce hyponatremia (serum sodium level 115 mmol/L) leading to coma (Steinhoff et al 1992).

Differential Diagnosis of Drug-Induced Coma

Drug-induced coma should be differentiated from coma due to structural lesions of the brain and metabolic encephalopathies. There are no hard and fast rules because drug-induced coma may resemble metabolic encephalopathy on one hand and may induce structural lesions in the brain. It is helpful to keep in mind a few rules of classical neurology while investigating a patient with possible drug-induced coma.

– History of drug ingestion is the most valuable piece of information.

– Coma due to structural lesions usually progresses while toxic or metabolic coma is usually stable or improves.

– Structural brain lesions have focal or localizing features and the manifestations are asymmetrical. Toxic and metabolic lesions usually present with symmetrical neurological signs. but can also asymmetrical features.

– Abnormal movements often accompany coma due to toxic-metabolic causes, whereas coma

due to structural lesions is accompanied by abnormal posturing.
- Reflex eye movements are usually intact in toxic-metabolic coma except with overdosage of some drugs such as phenytoin.
- Pupil reactivity is usually spared in toxic-metabolic coma with exception of drugs such as atropine which dilate the pupils.
- Raised intracranial pressure and papilledema is more likely in intracranial space-occupying lesions. Occasionally these findings may be drug-induced.
- Response to emergency therapy is helpful in the differential diagnosis. Response by recovery after intravenous glucose indicates hypoglycemic coma, response to naloxone usually indicates opiate drug overdose and response to flumazenil indicates benzodiazepine overdose.
- Laboratory aids to diagnosis. Blood toxicology screen helps to identify the levels of various drugs. Brain imaging studies such as CT scan and MRI help to differentiate the causes of lesions in the CNS.

References

Alberto G, Erickson T, Popei R, et al: Central nervous system manifestations of a valproic acid overdose responsive to naloxone. Ann Emerg Med 1989; 18: 889–891.

Almquist A, Goldenberg IF, Milstein S, et al: Provocation of bradycardia and hypotension by isoproterenol and upright posture in patients with unexplained syncope. NEJM 1989; 320: 346–351.

Aronowitz JS, Chakos,MH, Safferman AZ, et al: Syncope associated with the combination of clozapine and enalapril (letter). J Clin Psychopharmacol 1994; 14: 429–430.

Bigler D: Neurological sequelae after intoxication with sodium valproate. Acta Neurol Scand 1985; 72: 351–352.

Braun MM, Patriarca PA, Ellenberg SS: Syncope after immunization. Arch Pediatr Adolesc Med 1997; 151(3): 255–259.

Brunner La-Rocca-HP, Kiowski W, Bracht C, et al: Atrioventricular block after administration of atropine in patients following cardiac transplantation. Transplantation 1997; 63: 1838–1839.

Busby WJ, Campbell AJ, Robertson MC: Is low blood pressure in elderly people just a consequence of heart disease and frailty? Age Ageing 1994; 23: 69–74.

Cherin P, Colvez A, Deville-de-Periere G, et al: Risk of syncope in the elderly and consumption of drugs: a case-control study. J Clin Epidemiol 1997; 50: 313–320.

Chong Y, Yamamoto T, Hayashi J, et al: Syncope in a 65-year-old woman after nitrate ingestion. Fukuoka Igaku Zasshi 1998; 89: 282–286.

Coulter DL, Allen RJ: Secondary hyperammonemia: a possible mechanism for valproate encephalopathy. Lancet 1980; i: 1310–1313.

Duarte J, Macias S, Coria IF, et al: Valproate-induced coma: case report and literature review. Ann Pharmacother 1993; 27: 582–583.

Fludder JM, Leonard BE: Chronic effects of mianserin on noradrenaline metabolism in the rat brain. Psychopharmacology 1979; 64: 329–332.

Gaggioli G, Bottoni N, Mureddu R, et al: Effects of chronic vasodilator therapy to enhance susceptibility to vasovagal syncope during upright tilt testing. Am J Cardiol 1997; 80: 1092–1094.

Gentile S, Buffa C, Ravetti C, et al: State of stupor from valproic acid during chronic treatment: case report. Ital J Neurol Sci 1991; 12: 215–217.

Grubb BP, Samoil D, Kosinski D, et al: Cerebral syncope: loss of consciousness associated with cerebral vasoconstriction in the absence of systemic hypotension. Pacing Clin Electrophysiol 1998; 21: 652–658.

Hameedi FA, Sernyak MJ, Navui SA, et al: Near syncope associated with concomitant clozapine and cocaine use (letter). J Clin Psychiatry 1996; 57: 371–372.

Hanlon JT, Linzer M, MacMillan JP, et al: Syncope and presyncope associated with probable adverse drug reactions. Arch Int Med 1990; 150: 2309–2312.

Itil TM, Soldatos C: Clinical neurophysiological properties of antidepressants. In Hoffmeister F, Stille G (Eds.): Psychotropic agents part I: Antipsychotics and antidepressants, Springer-Verlag, Berlin, 1980: 437–469.

Jayarajan A, Prakash O: Cough syncope induced by enalapril. Chest 1993; 103: 327–328.

Kapoor WN: Evaluation and management of the patient with syncope. JAMA 1992; 268: 2553–2560.

Katz JA, Mahoney DH, Steuber CP, et al: Human leukocyte α interferon-induced transient neurotoxicity in children. Investigational New Drugs 1988; 6: 115–120.

Koskiniemi M, Hakimies L: Valproic acid and coma. Neurology 1979; 29: 1430.

Kulick SK, Kramer DA: Hyperammonemia secondary to valproic acid as a cause of lethargy in a postictal patient. Ann Emerg Med 1993; 22: 610–612.

Landau J, Baulac M, Durand G, et al: Impairment of consciousness induced by valproate treatment following neurosurgical operations. Acta Neurochir 1993; 125: 92–96.

Lanzarini L, Previtali M, Diotallevi P: Syncope caused by cardiac asystole during dobutamine test. Heart 1996; 75: 320–321.

Lekkerkerker JF, Broekmans-AW: Syncopes with simultaneous use of terfenadine and itraconazole. Drug Monitoring Board (letter). Ned Tijdschr Geneeskd 1997; 141: 1753–1754.

Lewis J, Braganza J, Williams T: Psychomotor retardation and semistuporous state with paroxetine. BMJ 1993; 306: 1169.

MacGregor DA, Baker AM, Appel RG, et al: Hyperosmolar coma due to lithium-induced diabetes inspidus. Lancet 1995; 346: 413–417.

McAnally LA, Threlkeld KR, Dreyling CA: Case report of a syncopal episode associated with fluoxetine. Ann Pharmacother 1992; 26: 1090–1091.

McAnnally LE, Threlked KR, Dreyling CA: Case report of a syncopal episode associated with fluoxetine. Ann Pharmacother 1992; 26: 1090–1091.

McDaniel KD: Clinical pharmacology of monoamine oxidase inhibitors. Clin Neuropharmacol 1986; 9: 207–234.

Medina A, Bodick N, Goldberger AL, et al: Effects of central muscarinic-1 receptor stimulation on blood pressure regulation. Hypertension 1997; 29: 828–834.

Meeuwisse EJM, Groen FC, Dees A, et al: Lethargy with omeprazole. BMJ 1997; 314: 481.

Mets TF: Drug-induced orthostatic hypotension in older patients. Drugs and Aging 1995; 6: 219–228.

Njemanze PC: Critical limits of pressure—flow relation in the human brain. Stroke 1992; 23: 1743–1747.

Park KH, Long JP, Cannon JG: Evaluation of the central and peripheral components for induction of postural hypotension by guanethidine, clonidine, dopamine$_2$ receptor agonists and 5-hydroxytryptamine$_{1A}$ receptor agonists. J Pharmacol Exp Ther 1990; 255: 240–247.

Passare G, Guo Z, Winblad B, et al: Drug use and low blood pressure in the elderly: a study of data from Kungsholmen project. Clin Drug Invest 1998; 15: 487–506.

Pedersen B, Juul-Jensen P: Electroencephalographic alterations during intoxication with sodium valproate: a case report. Epilepsia 1984; 25: 121–124.

Raehl CL, Patel AK, LeRoy M: Drug-induced torsade de pointes. Clin Pharmacol 1985; 4: 675–690.

Romkes JH, Froger CL, Wever EF, et al: Syncopes during simultaneous use of terfenadine and itraconazole. Ned Tijdschr Geneeskd 1997; 141: 950–953.

Rothstein JD, Guidotti A, Tinuper P, et al: Endogenous benzodiazepine receptor ligands in idiopathic recurring stupor. Lancet 1992; 340: 1002–1004.

Sackellares JC, Lee SI, Dreifuss FE. Stupor following administration of valproic acid to patients receiving other antiepileptic drugs. Epilepsia 1979; 20: 697–703.

Saissy JM, Vitris M, Demaziere J, et al: Flumazenil counteracts intrathecal baclofen-induced central nervous system depression in tetanus. Anesthesiology 1992; 76: 1051–1053.

Sarda H, Benkhelifa S, Housset C, et al: Syncope after niaprazine (Nopron) (letter). Arch Pediatr 1996; 3: 90.

Schwartz RH: Gamma-hydroxy butyrate (letter). Am Fam Physician 1998; 57: 2078, 81.

Settle EC: Valproic acid-associated encephalopathy with coma. Am J Psychiatry 1995; 152: 1236–1237.

Shaw FE, Kenny RA: The overlap between syncope and falls in the elderly. Postgrad Med J 1997; 73: 635–639.

Shen WK, Fenton AM, Lohse CM, et al: Hemodynamic analysis during isoproterenol-induced vasovagal syncope. Am J Cardiol 1997; 80: 817–822.

Smit AAJ, Wieling W, Voogel AJ, et al: Orthostatic hypotension due to suppression of vasomotor outflow after amphetamine intoxication. Mayo Clin Proc 1996; 71: 1067–1070.

Steinhoff BJ, Stoll KD, Stodiek SRG, et al: Hyponatremic coma under carbamazepine therapy. Epilepsy Res 1992; 11: 67–70.

Terao T, Abe H, Abe K: Irreversible sinus node dysfunction induced by resumption of lithium therapy. Acta Psychiatr Scand 1996; 93: 407–408.

Thomas AR, Chan LN, Bauman JL, et al: Prolongation of the QT interval related to cisapride-diltiazem interaction. Pharmacotherapy 1998; 18: 381–385.

Triggs WJ, Bohan TP, Lin SN, et al: Valproate-induced coma with ketosis with carnitine deficiency. Arch Neurol 1990; 47: 1131–1133.

Valdes L, Champel V, Olivier C, et al: Syncope with long QT interval in a 39 day-old infant treated with cisapride. Arch Pediatr 1997; 4: 535–537.

Vandercam B, Hermans MP, Coumans P, et al: Non-ketotic hyperosmolar coma in a patient with AIDS: case report. Presse Medicale 1995; 24: 1389–1390.

Verbiest HBC, Straver JS, Colombo JP, et al: Carbamyl phosphate synthetase-1 deficiency discovered after valproic acid-induced coma. Acta Neurol Scand 1992; 86: 275–279.

Verhaeverbeke I, Mets T: Drug-induced orthostatic hypotension in the elderly: avoiding its onset. Drug Safety 1997; 17: 105–118.

Winters SL, Sachs RG, Curwin JH: Nonsustained polymorphous ventricular tachycardia during amiodarone therapy for atrial fibrillation complicating cardiomyopathy. Management with intravenous magnesium sulfate. Chest 1997; 111: 1454–1457.

Yang JY, Cui XL, He XJ: Non-ketotic hyperosmolar coma complicating steroid treatment in childhood nephrosis. Pediatr Nephrol 1995; 9: 621–622.

Zaccara G, Paganini M, Campostrini R, et al: Hyperammonemia and valproate induced alterations of consciousness. Eur Neurol 1984; 23: 104–112.

Zechnich AD, Hedges JR, Eiselt-Proteau D, et al: Possible interactions with terfenadine or astemizole. West J Med 1994; 160: 321–325.

Chapter 5
Drug-Induced Neuropsychiatric Disorders

Introduction

Neuropsychiatric adverse effects are included in this book because of the close relation between neurology and psychiatry. Psychiatric adverse effects constitute 30% of adverse drug reactions seen in a general practice. In a study of 25,947 intensively monitored hospitalized patients with no history of psychiatric disorders, there were 147 (0.6%) who developed psychoses, depression, and hallucinations thought to be drug-induced (Danielson et al 1981). It is difficult to follow the standard classification of psychiatric disorders because of lack of precise psychiatric diagnosis in most of the adverse drug reaction reports. The classification shown in Table 5.1 will be used for discussing the neuropsychiatric dis-

Table 5.1. Classification of drug-induced neuropsychiatric disorders.

Behavioral toxicity of drugs
 – Behavioral disinhibition
Psychiatric disorders
 – Delirium
 – Depression
 – Mania and hypomania
 – Hallucinations as the main feature (may be part of psychosis)
 – Catatonia
 – Psychoses; paranoia, delusions, and includes hallucinations as well
Cerebral insufficiency (decline of mental function)
 – Cognitive impairment: non-specific or global
 – Psychomotor disturbances
 – Memory disorders
 – Intellectual impairment
 – Dementia
Mental disorders secondary to adverse drug reactions involving other systems of the body

orders induced by drugs. There is overlap of some manifestations in various categories.

Behavioral Toxicity

Behavioral toxicity is defined as a fundamentally reversible pharmacological, drug-induced disruption of neuropsychological processes controlling behavior (Ramaekers 1998). This is a broad definition and includes side effects such as sedation which affect the behavior. Theoretically it covers the psychiatric side effects but is a less pejorating term than "neuropsychiatric" side effects. Currently the strongest evidence supporting this concept comes from epidemiological studies of relationship between falls and psychoactive drugs, between traffic accidents and use of sedatives, and occupational accidents attributable to use of medications in work environments. Empirical evidence is provided by the spontaneous reports of such events associated with the use of drugs.

Falls. Drug-related falls which occur mostly in the elderly are a major health problem and have multiple causes. These include neurological

Table 5.2. Drugs associated with falls.

Antidepressants
 Tricyclic antidepressants
Antiepileptic drugs
Antihistaminics
Anxiolytics
Antipsychotics
Sedative-hypnotics
 Benzodiazepines
Opioid analgesics
Vasodilators

causes such as stroke and Parkinson's disease as well as bone and joint disorders. Various drugs associated with falls are shown in Table 5.2. Most of these these drugs are associated with behavioral toxicity and have several adverse effects including sedation. Psychotropics have been most frequently linked to falls and the most compelling evidence is for the association with antidepressants (Cumming 1998). The only drug category not linked to behavioral toxicity is that of vasodilators which produce a tendency to fall by producing postural hypotension or syncope.

Psychoactive Drugs and Motor Vehicle Accidents. Psychoactive drugs as well as old age are considered to be risk factors for injurious motor vehicle accidents. The ability of an older person to drive a vehicle safely may be affected by decrease in sensory cognitive and motor function. An epidemiological study has shown that among drivers over the age of 65, the relative risk of injurious crashes for current users of psychoactive drugs was 1.5 (95% confidence interval (CI) 1.2–1.9). This relative increase was confined to users of benzodiazepines and tricyclic antidepressants (Ray et al 1992). Another study showed that brief or extended periods of exposure to long-half-life benzodiazepines are associated with an increased risk of motor vehicle crash involvement in the elderly population but there was no such elevated risk for short-half-life benzodiazepines. (Hemmelgarn et al 1997).

Behavioral "Disinhibition." This is a non-specific term applied to a wide range of behaviors and implies loss of restraint over some form of behavior (Bond 1998). It may mean socially inappropriate behavior or behavior that is unpredictable or uncharacteristic of an individual. Symptoms that are reported to occur in association with behavioral disinhibition include irritability, euphoria, impulsive acts and hyperactivity. As drug-induced reactions, manifestations of behavior disinhibition are difficult to evaluate.

Social behavior is affected by psychotropic drugs and a classical example of social disinhibition is that resulting from use of alcohol. Behavioral disinhibition has been reported with a number of therapeutic drugs such as antipsychotics, benzodiazepines and antidepressants. Mechanism of disinhibition has been hypothetically divided into four stages (Patterson and Newman 1993; Bond 1998) and this helps to explains the drug-induced behavioral disinhibition.

1. *Appetitive learning.* This is a motivational state in which goal-directed behavior is likely to take place. It is associated with behavioral activation system and is influenced by the mesolimbic dopamine transmission. Antipsychotics decrease appetitive learning and reduce disinhibition at the first stage.
2. *Arousal.* The strength of this depends on the individual's response to the aversive events. Benzodiazepines reduce the activity of behavioral disinhibition at this as well as the next stage.
3. *Behavioral coping response.* The arousal increment enables an effortful adaptive switch to a passive information-gathering set. Drugs which facilitate this switch are benzodiazepines and lithium.
4. *Retrospective reflection.* Causal associations are formed between behaviors and their consequences. Benzodiazepines impair the formation of causal associations at this stage and produce disinhibition.

This chapter will not discuss behavioral toxicity or behavioral disinhibition further as such but various adverse effects will be discussed under clinically familiar symptoms, signs and diseases which are usually included under the term of neuropsychiatric disorders.

Pathomechanisms

Drugs acting on the central nervous system (CNS) are more likely to produce neuropsychiatric adverse effect than are drugs designed to treat diseases of other systems but the latter may cross the BBB and affect the CNS. Generally accepted basic mechanisms of adverse reactions to psychotropic drugs and factors influencing them are shown in Table 5.3.

Assessment of cause-effect relationship in case of an individual drug requires a knowledge of mode of action of the drug and the biologic

Table 5.3. Basic mechanisms and factors influencing adverse reactions to psychotropic drugs.

Factors related to the drug
Extension of primary action of the drug
  – Excessive stimulation
  – Excessive sedation
Secondary pharmacologic effects
Pharmacokinetics
  – Speed of brain penetration
  – Elimination half time
Drug interactions
Toxicity due to overdose or altered response to normal
  dose

Factors related to the patient
Brain damage leading to impaired cognitive function
Genetic aberrations of drug metabolism
Old age
Idiosyncratic reactions
Development of tolerance or drug-dependance
Drug withdrawal effects
Hepatic and renal disease affecting drug metabolism
  and clearance

basis of the action of the drug on the disease being treated and on other underlying disorders including those of the psyche. Drugs with high lipid solubility such as benzodiazepines, β-blockers, tricyclic antidepressants, and central α-agonist antihypertensives are more likely to produce CNS disturbances.

Drugs intended for treatment of non-CNS disorders may have side-effects involving the CNS. It would be difficult to conceive of a drug, which would not affect the CNS under some circumstances. Even severe allergic reactions to drugs involve some disturbances of CNS. Psychiatric disturbances may be due to indirect effects of both CNS and non-CNS drugs, e. g., vitamin B_{12} and folate deficiency.

There are several predisposing factors for drug-induced psychiatric reactions. Old age and brain damage increase the susceptibility to such adverse reactions. Another ill-defined factor is presence of occult (subclinical) psychiatric disorders which are precipitated by drugs. Adverse effects based on biochemical disturbances may be reversible whereas effects of structural damage to the CNS by drugs may not be reversible. Pathomechanisms will be discussed according to specific psychiatric reaction and as well as according to the drug categories.

Delirium

Delirium is now the accepted term for acute, transient, global organic disorder of higher nervous system function involving impaired consciousness and attention. It has also been described as "brain failure." There are more than 30 synonyms for delirium of which exogenous psychoses, reversible toxic confusional state, toxic delirious reaction, toxic encephalopathy and toxic psychosis would closely resemble the concept of drug-induced delirium (Carter et al 1996). The term substance-induced delirium can be due to exposure to a medication, toxin or drug of abuse as well as withdrawal from these.

Delirium is characterized by a reduction of the level of consciousness manifested clinically by disorientation and sometimes referred to as cognitive impairment. Cognitive impairment should be distinguished from the broader term of cognitive disorders which includes decline of cognitive functions or cerebral insufficiency which id discussed in a later section in this chapter. Clinical features are listed in DSM-IV criteria for the diagnosis of substance intoxication delirium (Table 5.4).

Manifestations of delirium include short-term memory deficits, misinterpretation of the surroundings and language difficulties. In addition to fluctuations of consciousness and cognition, the affective and psychotic features may vary a

Table 5.4. DMS-IV Criteria for Substance Intoxication Delirium (American Psychiatric Association 1994),

A. Disturbances of consciousness (i. e., reduced clarity of awareness of the environment) with reduced ability to focus, sustain or shift attention.
B. A change in cognition (such as memory deficit, disorientation, language disturbance) or the development of a perceptual disturbance that is not better accounted for by a preexisting, established, or evolving dementia.
C. The disturbance develops over a short period of time (usually hours to days) and tends to fluctuate during the course of the day.
D. There is evidence from the history, physical examination, or laboratory findings of either (1) or (2).
  (1) the symptoms in criteria A and B developed during substance intoxication.
  (2) medication use is etiologically related to the disturbance.

great deal from time to time. Other features include insomnia, difficulty in concentration, restlessness, irritability, hypersensitivity to lights and sounds and nightmares. Physical signs of delirium may include autonomic system activation but these are blunted in elderly patients.

Incidence and Prevalence. Accurate data on incidence, prevalence and mortality of delirium are difficult to obtain and evaluate because of differences in definitions and methodology. Most of the information is based on hospitalized patients but one community study, Eastern Baltimore Mental Survey, found a point prevalence rate of 0.4% in the adult population, rising to 1.1% in those aged 55 or over (Folstein et al 1991).

In contrast to the low prevalence rate in the community, 10% of all hospitalized patients meet criteria for delirium at some point during their stay (Lipowski 1980). This would make it the mental disorder with the highest incidence. In a prospective study of 1500 hospital neurological consultations, delirium accounted for 7% of all cases and 19% of all iatrogenic neurological disorders (Moses and Kadan 1986). Delirium was drug-induced in 17% of cases and drugs were suspected to have contributed to delirium in 47% of the cases in which no single cause was identified.

Drugs Associated with Delirium. Bowen and Larson (1993) who have reviewed drug-induced cognitive impairment state this to be a common cause of delirium. The drugs have been reported to be associated with delirium are listed in Table 5.5 and some of these are described in the following text.

Table 5.5. Drugs associated with delirium

Anticancer drugs
  – Chemotherapeutics
  – Cytokines: Interferons*
Anticholinergic agents*
Anticonvulsants
Antidepressants
  – Tricyclic antidepressants
  – Fluoxetine
Antimalarials: Chloroquine, Mefloquine
Antimicrobials

Table 5.5 continued

  – Acyclovir
  – Amphotericin
  – Ciprofloxacin (Jay and Fitzgerald 1997)
  – Gentamicin
  – Nalidixic acid
  – Ofloxacin
  – Sulfonamides
  – Tobramycin
Antiparkinsonian drugs
  – Levodopa
  – Benzatropine
  – Trimethobenzamide
Antipsychotics
  – Chlorpromazine
  – Clozapine
  – Lithium
  – Perphenazine
  – Risperidone
  – Thioridazine
  – Trifluoperazine
Benzodiazepines*
Cardiovascular drugs
  – Antihypertensives
      Beta-blockers
      Clonidine
  – Antiarrhythmics
  – Diuretics
  – Digitalis
  – Quinidine
CNS stimulants
Drug abuse
Drug interactions
  – clozapine and lorazepam (Jackson et al 1995)
  – fluoxetine and clarithromycin (Pollack et al 1995)
  – ibuprofen and tacrine (Hooten and Pearlson 1996)
  – lithium and risperidone (Chen and Cardasis 1996)
  – paroxetine and zolpidem (Katz 1995)
  – tranylcypromine and disulfiram (Blansjaar and Egberts 1995)
Corticosteroids
Histamine H_2-receptor antagonists*
Hypnotics-sedatives
Non-steroidal anti-inflammatory drugs*
Opioid analgesics*
Miscellaneous drugs
  – Baclofen
  – Bromides
  – Cyclobenzaprine
  – Disulfiram
  – Fentanyl transdermal (Kuzma et al 1995)
  – Metrizamide
  – Methazolamide (Cyr et al 1997)
  – Niridazole
  – Podophyllin
  – Procaine derivatives
  – Sodium nitroprusside (Harmon and Wohlreich 1995)

*denotes established and frequent association.

Antiparkinsonian drugs. A variety of neuropsychiatric disturbances (psychoses, hallucinations, delirium, etc.) occur as a complication of drug treatment of Parkinson's disease. All drug categories including anticholinergic drugs, levodopa, and dopaminergic agonists have the potential to produce delirium. Older patients with dementia are particularly at risk when on anticholinergic drugs.

Benzodiazepines. There is an increased risk of delirium in older hospitalized patients receiving benzodiazepines (Foy et al 1995). Delirium may also occur in long-term users of benzodiazepines as a result of withdrawal. Short-acting agents such as alprazolam are more likely to produce withdrawal reactions.

Interferons. Neuropsychiatric symptoms are a prominent feature of interferon syndrome. Thirty case reports published in Japan, covered 49 cases that refer to psychiatric symptoms accompanying interferon (IFN), therapy were reviewed (Nozaki et al 1997). Ten of these patients had delirium and the symptoms of delirium appeared soon after IFN was administered whereas the symptoms of psychotic disorders appeared later. The patients with delirium displayed many neurological abnormalities, which were improved by discontinuing IFN therapy.

Drug abuse. Cocaine-related delirium has become common and is likely due to disruption of dopaminergic function. An outbreak of deaths from cocaine-induced delirium in Dade County, Florida between 1979 and 1990 has been analyzed from a registry of all cocaine-related deaths in that area (Ruttenber et al 1997). The epidemiologic findings are most consistent with the hypothesis that chronic cocaine use disrupts dopaminergic function and, when coupled with recent cocaine use, may precipitate agitation, delirium, aberrant thermoregulation, rhabdomyolysis, and sudden death.

Histamine H_2-receptor antagonists. All drugs of this class have the potential to cause delirium (Cantu and Korek 1991). Cimetidine has the largest number of reported cases because it was the first drug of this class to enter the market. CNS toxicity generally occurs during the first 2

weeks of therapy and is seen most commonly in the intensive care patients, particularly those with renal land hepatic failure. The reaction usually resolves within a few days of drug withdrawal. Six cases of delirium associated with famotidine have been reported (Catalano et al 1996) adding to two cases reported previously. In five of these, delirium resolved after famotidine was switched to sucalfate. The six patient was switched to ranitidine (another H_2-receptor antagonist) and had recurrence of delirium.

Non-steroidal anti-inflammatory drugs. There are several reports of association of NSAIDs with delirium (Morgan and Clark 1998). Because these are the most commonly used drugs, the cognitive impact is considerable. Toxicity from aspirin frequently manifests as delirium.

Opioid analgesics. Meperidine (pethidine) poses the greatest risk for delirium because of the accumulation of its metabolite norpethidine which has anticholinergic properties. Because the clearance is by the kidney, the metabolite is more likely to accumulate in elderly subjects with impaired renal function.

Risk Factors. Various risk factors for the development of delirium are shown in Table 5.6.

A review of 7 prospective studies of risk factors identified advanced age, pre-existing cognitive impairment, severe chronic illness and functional impairment as common risk factors (Inouye 1994). Lipowski (1990) identified three main risk factors for delirium: advanced age, brain damage, and addiction to alcohol or other drugs. Age is a significant risk factor for drug-induced delirium. Elderly patients taking multi-

Table 5.6. Risk factors for development of drug-induced delirium.

Advanced age
Brain damage
Dementia
Psychiatric disorders
Addiction to alcohol or drugs
Polypharmacy
Severe general illness: fever or infection
Low serum albumin level
Surgery and immobilization
Stress
Sensory under- or overstimulation

ple psychotropic drugs are at increased risk for developing delirium because of cholinergic effects of these drugs. Meperidine and benzodiazepines given in the postoperative period are considered to have a significant association with delirium (Marcantonio et al 1994). In a study of 25 most commonly prescribed drugs for the elderly, 14 were associated with detectable anticholinergic levels as measured by radioreceptor assay (Tune et al 1992). Age-associated changes or diseases of liver and kidney may interfere with drug clearance. Drug interactions such as those between disulfiram and tranylcypromine can cause delirium (Blansjaar and Egberts 1995). Brain magnetic resonance imaging studies have shown that patients with basal ganglia lesions are more vulnerable to antidepressant-induced delirium (Figiel et al 1989). There is little data available as to which drugs are most commonly associated with delirium. Among hospitalized patients, the leading causes in descending order are as follows (Francis et al 1990):
- Opioid analgesics
- Benzodiazepines
- Anticholinergics
- Non-steroidal anti-inflammatory drugs
- Sedative withdrawal

Pathomechanism of Drug-Induced Delirium.
Drugs can induce delirium in several ways such as:
- Toxic concentrations of drugs as a result of overdose or impaired clearance.
- Pharmacodynamic changes may result in increased sensitivity to normal concentrations of centrally acting drugs.
- Drug-disease interaction such as in patients with dementia where is risk of delirium is enhanced due to diminished "cognitive reserve."
- Drug-drug interactions in case of polypharmacy.

The actual mechanism by which drugs cause delirium are poorly because the pathophysiology of delirium itself is not well understood. Delirium is a diffuse brain disturbance that involves both cortical and subcortical structures. Although multiple neurotransmitters are involved, most of the current evidence points to cholinergic failure. Anticholinergic medications produce classical delirium which can be reversed with cholinesterase inhibitors and clinical conditions such as thiamine deficiency and hypoglycemia which cause delirium also impair acetylcholine synthesis. Radioreceptor assays which measure muscarinic binding enable a more precise determination of mechanism of drug-induced delirium. Acute confusion can correlated with increased serum anticholinergic activity (Mach et al 1995). Several of the drugs that are not traditional anticholinergics but cause delirium show measurable cholinergic receptor binding by this assay (Tune et al 1992). Other neurotransmitters (GABA, serotonin, dopamine) may be involved in delirium but their role is supported by experimental evidence.

Pathomechanism of delirium may be related to biochemical pathways involved in inflammatory states. Endogenous cytokine activation is postulated to cause delirium in conditions such as sepsis (Bolton et al 1993) and following cardiac surgery (Stephano et al 1994). This might explain why cytokines have a well known adverse effect on cognitive function.

Prevention. There are no studies of primary or secondary prevention of drug-induced delirium. Some preventive measures are:
- Anticholinergic, sedative-hypnotic and opioid medications should be used sparingly in the elderly.
- Acutely ill elderly patients should have a brief mental test on admission to detect early features of delirium.
- Avoid combination of drugs suspected to cause delirium. The combination of benzodiazepines and clozapine should be avoided if possible, and if they are used in combination, it should be with great caution.

Management. Delirium usually clears up on removal of the offending medication. General principles of clinical management of delirium are:
- Early recognition of the condition
- Identification and treatment of the underlying cause, e. g., offending medication
- Management of agitation
- General supportive care

The most important measure is recognition and discontinuation of the offending drug. Nonpharmacological treatment is empirical and includes appropriate sensory input, no interruption of sleep, clear communication and encouragement of self-care.

Anticholinergic delirium. This is the only form of delirium for which specific pharmacotherapy is available. Anticholinergic delirium is best managed by physostigmine, a cholinesterase inhibitor (Lipowski 1990). It can reverse delirium due to anticholinergic toxicity for up to one hour following a 1–2 mg intravenous dose. The short duration of action and potential for serious cholinergic side effects, which requires close monitoring, are major limitations to its use. It can potentiate toxicity of tricyclic antidepressant overdose.

Non-specific pharmacotherapy. There are few controlled studies of pharmacological management of delirium. The major reported methods of treatment are antipsychotics or benzodiazepines. If the patient is aggressive or dangerous, intravenous diazepam may be used until the patient is fully sedated. Parenteral antipsychotics that have been used in this situation include haloperidol, trufluoperazine and thiothixine. The major advantage of haloperidol is the lack of anticholinergic activity. Risperidone may prove to be an effective alternative to haloperidol in delirious patients, especially the elderly and the severely medically ill, who are more prone to adverse effects (Sipahimalani and Masand 1997).

Depression

The term depression describes a continuum of phenomena starting from mood changes (which affect everyone from time to time) and progressing to a severe disorder. A central feature of all depressive conditions is sadness and lowering of mood which may be severe and accompanied by lack of ability to take interest or pleasure in one's usual activities. Depression may become more pronounced and pathological to reach the level of a psychiatric disorder.

Drug-induced depressive disorders were classified in DSM-III-R as organic mood syndrome, depressed type which is considered in the differential diagnosis of depressive symptoms. These diagnostic criteria are not adequate for application in studies of drug-induced depression. DSM-IV criteria include a requirement for depressive symptoms to emerge during on within a month of intoxication or withdrawal from a drug. This appears to be more applicable to depression induced by psychoactive substances rather than drugs used in medical therapy. Depressive reactions to drugs may manifest by mood changes, insomnia, and loss of interest.

Depression may be due to interaction of multifocal causes. Drug-induced depression may lead to socioeconomic complications which may further aggravate depression (Harper et al 1989). Depression is known to worsen the course of medical illness thus increasing the requirement for further medications and increasing the chances for drug-induced depression. Drug-induced depression may present atypically. Lability of mood and physical symptoms of depression such as sleep and motility disorders are more common than psychological symptoms (Paykel et al 1982). Drugs may unmask depression due to other causes due to other causes and finally drug interactions may interfere with the effect of antidepressants and recovery from depression. Drugs usually precipitate depression only in susceptible patients. Depression following withdrawal of drug therapy may be more insidious in onset and may not be apparent for months. Depression may be overlooked in patients who complain only of lack of sleep or decline of mental function which may not be identified as a manifestation of depression.

Pathomechanism. Pathomechanism of drug-induced depression is related to neurotransmitters. Brain biological amines are important in the etiology of depression and are basic consideration for the pharmacotherapy of depression. Of the various neurotransmitters, norepinephrine and serotonin are the most closely associated with depression. Of these two systems, serotonergic neurons are more important as they have an influence on the noradrenergic neurons. If these neurons are destroyed, synthesis of serotonin is blocked. Depressive disorders seem to be associated with dysfunction of 5-HT receptors. Suicidal depression is also linked with low cerebro-

Table 5.7. Drugs associated with depression.

ACE inhibitors
  – Enalapril
Anabolic steroids*
Antimicrobials
  – Amphotericin B
  – Isoniazid
Antiepileptic drugs
  – Carbamazepine (Gardner & Cowdry 1986)
  – Phenytoin
  – Phenobarbital (Brent et al 1990)
  – Tiagabine
  – Topiramate
  – Vigabatrin
Antihistaminics
  – Cimetidine
  – H$_2$-antagonists
Antihypertensives
  – Clonidine
  – Reserpine
Antineoplastic drugs
  – L-asparaginase
  – Vincristine
Antiviral agents
  – Acyclovir
  – α-interferon
β-blockers
  – Nadolol
  – Propmanolol
  – Timolol
Baclofen (Sommer and Petrides 1992)
Calcium antagonists*
  – Diltiazem
  – Nifedipine
  – Verapamil
Cholesterol-lowering drugs
  – HMG-CoA reductase inhibitors
Corticosteroids*
Digitalis*
Diuretics: thiazides
Levodopa
Mefloquine
Metoclopramide
Neuroleptic drugs
Non-steroidal anti-inflammatory drugs
  – Indomethacin
  – Naproxen
Oral contraceptives
Retinoids
  – Isoretinoin (Hazen et al 1983, Scheinman et al 1990)
  – Etretinate (Henderson and Highet 1989).
Sedative-Hypnotics: barbiturates, benzodiazepines*
Withdrawal effect: antidepressants, psychostimulants*

*Frequently reported.

spinal fluid levels of 5-hydroxyindolacetic acid (5-HIAA), a metabolite of serotonin following its degradation by monoamine oxidase. Drugs which deplete serotonin may be liable to induce depression.

Antidepressants and Suicide. A question has been raised if antidepressants increase the suicidality. A detailed discussion of this topic is beyond the scope of this book. Jick et al (1995) found that after controlling for the various factors for suicide, the risk of suicide was similar among 10 antidepressants tested. Patients treated with tricyclic antidepressantsmay be at no greater overall risk of suicide than those treated by newer antidepressants which are considered to be safer (Edwards 1995). It has been estimated that half of all patients who commit suicide suffer from major depression and a quarter of patients with major depression attempt suicide in a lifetime. Antidepressant prescriptions may provide the patients with a means to commit suicide by using overdose of these medications. Conclusions of the consensus statement on this topic by the American Council for Neuropharmacology (ACNP 1993) are:
– Antidepressants are effective treatment for depression, and, in the vast majority of patients, result in substantial improvement or total remission of suicidal ideation.
– It is a good clinical practice to monitor patients receiving antidepressants for emergence of suicidal ideation.
– New generation, low toxicity antidepressants, may carry a lower risk of suicide than older tricyclic compounds, possibly because of lower toxicity with overdose.

Several drugs have been reported to be associated with depression are listed in Table 5.7. The evidence is suggestive but not conclusive for most of the drugs.

ACE Inhibitors

Angiotensin converting enzyme (ACE) inhibitors were associated with depressive disorders in patients treated with those agents for congestive heart failure or for hypertension (Patten et al

1996). This is the first reported epidemiological evidence of an association between ACE inhibitors and depressive disorders but it does not prove any causal relationship. Hallas (1996) analyzed the exposure histories of 11,244 incident antidepressant users, using the Odense University Pharmaco-Epidemiologic Database. The initial screening showed nonsymmetrical prescription orders for a wide range of cardiovascular drugs. After adjustment for an increasing incidence of antidepressant prescribing, the author found a depression-provoking effect of ACE inhibitors (rate ratio = 1.29; 95% confidence interval = 1.08–1.56).

Anabolic Steroids

Depression has been identified as a complication of anabolic steroids in a cross-sectional studies (Perry et al 1990). Pope and Katz (1988) performed structured interviews of 41 body builders and football players who had used steroids. Nine subjects (22%) displayed a full affective syndrome. Depression may manifest during withdrawal from anabolic steroids. The level of testosterone appears to be positively associated with aggressive behavior and withdrawal from these drugs can lead to depression (Uzych 1992). The relative contribution of pharmacologic and psychosocial factors to the etiology of depression in these cases remains to be determined.

Antihypertensives

The association between antihypertensive medications and depression has been recognized for several years. Manifestations of depression such as fatigue, lassitude, and sleep disorders are manifestations of several antihypertensive medications as well. A knowledge of the role of neurotransmitters in the etiology of depression enables us to understand how antihypertensive drugs cause depression. Biogenic amine depletion can cause depression and many of the drugs used to treat hypertension interfere with this system. Guanethidine, clonidine, hydralazine, and prazosin appear to pose little risk in causing de-

pression, although rare occurrences have been reported.

Methyldopa. Cases of depression associated with methyldopa have been reported by Beers and Passman (1990). The incidence of depression caused by methyldopa is lower than that due to reserpine but higher than that caused by other antihypertensive drugs.

Reserpine. This drug has been used extensively in the treatment of hypertension but its use has diminished due to adverse effects on the CNS. One of the most serious adverse effects is depression (Gerber and Nies 1990). Symptoms of depression due to reserpine differ from those of endogenous depression and the term "pseudodepression" has been used to describe these symptoms. Depression due to reserpine appears to be dose-related.

All patients receiving medication to treat hypertension should be evaluated periodically for depression, and if depression occurs, medication should be suspected as playing a role in its etiology (Beers and Passman 1990). Large scale studies, however, that depression due to antihypertensive medications is rare and is an idiosyncratic reaction. β-blockers, calcium channel blockers, and ACE inhibitors are discussed separately as they are used for other indications besides hypertension.

β-Blockers

Propmanolol and other β-blockers have reported to be associated with depression (Pollack et al 1985; Kurtz et al 1993) whereas other studies have failed to identify this association (Sorgi et al 1992; Schleifer et al 1991). From individual case reports, it appears that β-blockers induced depression occurs in those patients who have a pre-existing vulnerability to depression (Ganzini et al 1993a). One double-blind, randomized, crossover study has reported lower depression scores in glaucoma patients treated with topical betaxalol than in those treated with timolol (Duch et al 1992).

Depression as an adverse effect of β-blockers is widely accepted in medical literature because of the biological plausibility of association.

Long-term exposure to β-blockers reduces the density of β-adrenergic receptors in a variety of tissues. Goble (1992) has described a syndrome in patients on β-blocker therapy characterized by certain typical depressive symptoms such as loss of drive and interest but without sadness, guilt or self-accusation. This author suggests that the syndrome does not meet the DSM-IIIR criteria for major depression and calls this syndrome by the name of "blockade malade."

A recent systematic review of published literature has concluded that β-blockers may have been unjustly associated with depression and their use avoided for that reason (Ried et al 1998). It is recommended that future studies into the association between depression and β-blocker use should evaluate whether the association is affected by case definition and study design characteristics, including disease, dose-response, bias, measurement error, or ability to precisely measure the length of the exposure.

Management. Measures to prevent and manage this adverse effect of β-blockers are as follows (Yudofskyy 1992):

1. β-blockers should be avoided in patients with family or past history of depression.
2. If depression develops during the use of a β-blocker, the drug should be replaced by another drug. If no alternative is available a more lipophilic β-blocker may be substituted.
3. Antidepressant drugs may be combined with β-blockers if necessary.

Ca-Channel Blockers

There is considerable evidence supporting the causal relationship of flunarizine (and the related drug cinnarizine) with depression (Centonze et al 1990; Sorensen et al 1991; D'Allessandro 1986). Interference with dopaminergic transmission is a potential pathomechanism. Use of Ca-channel blockers should be avoided in patients with past history of depression. However, this depression responds well to antidepressants. Hallas (1996), using prescription sequence symmetry analysis, found a depression-provoking effect calcium channel blockers (rate ratio = 1.31; 95% confidence interval = 1.14–1.51).

Antineoplastic Drugs

Evaluation of depression in cancer patients during antineoplastic therapy is difficult. Isolated reports have described depression in association with various antineoplastic agents, e. g., fluorouracil (Milstein 1980).

Cholesterol-Lowering Drugs

Increase in depressive symptoms may occur after lowering of cholesterol (Davidson et al 1996). There are single case reports of association of depression with pravastatin (Lechleitner et al 1992; Kassler-Taub et al 1993) and simvastatin (Duits and Bos 1993). There is a potential link between lowered cholesterol and risk of suicide (Young 1993).

Corticosteroids

Depression is a feature of several diseases treated with corticosteroids such as multiple sclerosis and systemic lupus erythematosus. Depressive symptoms induced by corticosteroids have been described in several reports (Grigg 1989; Lewis and Smith 1983) and reviews (Ling et al 1981; Kershner and Wang-Chen 1989). Association between corticosteroids and depression appears to be biologically plausible because of the overlap between Cushing's syndrome and major depression (Dubrovsky 1993). No definite guidelines are available for prevention and treatment of corticosteroid-induced depression.

Digitalis

Strong evidence of association of digitalis with depression was noted in a prospective study of post-myocardial infarction patients (Schleifer et al 1991). Digoxin was found to be a statistically significant predictor of depression at 3 to 4 months post-myocardial infarction.

Histamine H₂-Antagonists

Case reports have described depressive episodes associated with cimetidine (Billings et al 1981; Pierce 1983) and ranitidine (Billings and Stein 1986). In a randomized, placebo-controlled, double-blind prospective study of duodenal ulcer patients, no elevations in scores of Hamilton Depression Rating Scale was identified in patients receiving ranitidine (Robins et al 1984).

Review of published literature suggests that a family history of affective disorder is a risk factor for depression induced by cimetidine (Klysner et al 1992). The evidence, however, is not strong enough to regard family history of depression as a contraindication for the use of H₂-antagonists.

Interferon-α (IFN-α)

An organic affective syndrome has been described as one of the adverse effects of IFN-α (Renault et al 1987). Several cases have been reported of depressive symptoms in association with cognitive dysfunction in recipients of IFN-α (Merimsky et al 1990; Meyers et al 1991). Severe depression has been reported in clinical trials of IFN-α (Arthur and Ma 1993; Thomas and Ibanez 1993). The pathomechanism of depression has not been elucidated but it is speculated to be induced by interaction of interferon with neurotransmitter systems (Okada 1995). Depression due to IFN-α can be treated with fluoxetine (Levenson and Fallon 1993).

Levodopa

Depression has been reported as an adverse effect of levodopa but it is difficult to confirm this because depression is also a feature of Parkinson's disease (Cummings 1992). However, a higher prevalence of depression has been reported in patients on levodopa therapy than in those treated with anticholinergic agents or amantadine (Mindham et al 1976). It may be advisable to use an alternative antiparkinsonian drug in patients with history of depression. Although anti-depressants have been used in the management of Parkinson's disease, one potential complication of these drugs is drug-induced parkinsonism.

Mefloquine

Depression has been reported as an adverse reaction of mefloquine (Caillon et al 1992). Bem et al (1992) reported 12 cases of depression from the data base of the manufacturer.

Metachlopramide

This is a dopamine D₂ receptor antagonist and is used as an antiemetic drug. Cases have been reported of its association with depression (Bottner and Tullio 1985; Feder 1987). No epidemiological studies have been done. The symptoms usually resolve after discontinuation of the medication.

Oral Contraceptives (OCs)

Earlier reports after introduction of OCs suggested an association with depression. In 9 out of 16 studies, oral contraceptives were believed to have caused depression in 16–56% of patients (Slap 1981). Depression associated with oral contraceptives may differ significantly from non-organic major depressive episodes. Low-dose OCs are not associated with complaints of depression (Kay 1984).

Sedative-Hypnotic Drugs

Several reports in literature describe the association of sedative hypnotic drugs with depression (Buckner and Mandell 1990).

Benzodiazepines (BZD). The drugs of this class are usually believed to cause depression although a few BZDs are used as antidepressants (Tiller and Schweitzer 1992). Depression has been described as a paradoxical reaction to BZD (Hall and Zisook 1981).

BZDs are prescribed for anxiety and insomnia which are commonly associated with depression and would confound assessment of depression as an adverse reaction to BZD. No controlled studies have been done to settle this issue.

Withdrawal Effect

Withdrawal from antidepressants can be associated with aggravation of depression.

Psychostimulants. Drugs of this class are used for the treatment of attention deficit disorders (methylphenidate, and pemoline), as nasal decongestants (phenylpropanolamine), or as anorexiants (fenfluramine). Depressive symptoms have been reported after withdrawal of psychostimulants, e. g., pemoline (Brown et al 1985) and fenfluramine (Steel and Briggs 1972). Gradual tapering of the dose of psychostimulants may prevent the emergence of depression.

Anxiety and Panic Disorders

Syndromes of anxiety include general anxiety disorders (GAD), panic disorder and social phobia. Panic disorder is a specific type of anxiety characterized by abrupt onset and rapid crescendo peak of prominent autonomic symptoms, often seeming to "come out of the blue." It has an association with depression as the depressed patients are 12 times more likely to present with comorbid panic disorder than should occur by chance. Panic disorder can be differentiated from GAD by diagnostic criteria of DSM-IV. Panic disorder is diagnosed when an individual experiences recurrent panic attacks along with fearful anticipation of panic or of frightening consequences or implication of these attacks. These patients do not want to be in places or situations, where they believe they could be physically or socially trapped, or alone and unable to get help. Thus the syndrome of panic disorder has three components:
1. Panic attacks
2. Anticipatory anxiety
3. Phobic symptoms

Panic attacks can be rarely precipitated by drugs particularly in patients with history of anxiety or previous panic attacks. These drugs are shown in Table 5.8 and some of them are described in the following text.

Table 5.8. Drugs that precipitate anxiety states and panic attacks.

Antiparkinsonian drugs
Amantadine
Levodopa
Benzodiazepine-receptor antagonists such as flumazenil
Caffeine in high doses
Catecholamine infusions
Desmopressin (von Gontard and Lehmkuhl 1996)
Lactate infusions (Lader and Bruce 1986)
Naltrexone
Yohimbine

Naltrexone. Treatment for bulimia nervosa with naltrexone precipitated a panic attack in a patient with history of anxiety which was relieved with alprazolam but recurred on readministration of naltrexone (Maremmani et al 1998). The predisposing factor in this case was considered to be overactivity of endogenous opioids.

Amantadine. Panic attack has been reported in a patient with Parkinson's disease after starting amantadine therapy (Noveske 1996). This patient had a past history of panic attacks which were controlled with alprazolam and the dose of this drug was increased with control of panic in spite of continued amantadine therapy. The catacholamine effect of amantadine may have precipitated panic attack in this patient.

Levodopa. Panic attacks have also been reported in Parkinson's disease patients on levodopa therapy and these were not related directly to pharmacologic properties of levodopa but to the alterations in the noradrenergic system in the brain (Vazquez et al 1993).

Yohimbine. Yohimbine induced panic attacks in 1 of 20 healthy volunteers whereas it aggravated panic attacks in 37 of 68 patients with previous panic disorders (Charney et al 1987). In the healthy volunteers, yohimbine did not significantly increase plasma cortisol levels whereas such an effect could be observed in those who experienced a panic attack after yohimbine administration.

The management is mainly pharmacologic. Various medications that are used include benzodiazepines, monoamine oxidase inhibitors, tricyclic antidepressantsand SSRIs

Mania and Hypomania

The main clinical feature of mania is elevated mood which is more marked and prolonged than usual. Hypomania is a lesser degree of mania. Elevated or changed mood accompanied by impairment of concentration and attention may persist for several days. Annual incidence of the first episode of mania in the general population is estimated to be 2.6/100,000 (Leff et al 1976).

Secondary Mania

Mania resulting from organic causes including drugs is termed secondary mania by Krauthammer and Klerman (1978) who described the following criteria for its diagnosis:
– A prominent and persistent elevated or expansive mood.
– Presence of two of the following symptoms: hyperactivity, flight of ideas, grandiosity, poor sleep, lack of concentration, easy distractibility, and risk-taking behavior.
– No previous history of affective disorder.
– No frank confusion
– Duration of at least one week.

Various causes of secondary mania include metabolic disturbances, seizures, drugs, degenerative and vascular diseases. Cognitive impairment is common in organic mania. Clinically it is important to differentiate mania from delirium. Both have disorganized thinking, psychomotor agitation, delusions and hallucinations. The important distinguishing feature is impairment of consciousness in delirium. Mania has a narrow range of drug-induced causes whereas episodes of delirium are usually multifactorial.

Drug-Induced Mania

Drug-induced mania is difficult to diagnose. Case reports of drug-induced mania have a predominance of patients with a history of mood disorder. These patients were excluded from the classification of secondary mania by Krauthammer and Klerman. Diagnostic criteria for drug-induced mania are shown in Table 5.9 and various drugs reported to induce mania are listed in Table 5.10.

Anabolic Steroids

Adverse behavioral effects of anabolic steroids are described in the section of drug-induced psychoses. One of the 20 volunteers in the study reported by Su et al (1993) developed hypomania and another became manic. In a more recent study, 10% of the subjects using anabolic steroids experienced hypomania and 5% experienced mania (Pope and Katz 1994). When not taking steroids, only 1% of the subjects experienced mania and none of the control subjects developed this complication. High doses of anabolic steroids can induce mania and this should be should be suspected in athletes who present with manic symptoms.

Antidepressants

Mania Versus Depression. Mania is at the end opposite to that of depression in the spectrum of

Table 5.9. Criteria for diagnosis of drug-induced mania (modified from DMS-IV, 1994).

Abnormally elevated mood with 3 or more of the following criteria:
 – increased activity
 – inflated self-esteem
 – more talkative than usual
 – flight of ideas
 – decreased need to sleep
 – excessive risk-taking behavior
Evidence from history, physical examination, or laboratory tests of use or withdrawal of a drug known to induce mood disorders
Exclusion of other causes of mania and delirium

Table 5.10. Drugs that have been reported to induce mania.

ACE inhibitors
  Lisinopril (Skop and Masterson 1995)
  Captopril (Gajula and Berlin 1993)
Anabolic steroids*
Antidepressants*
  Tricyclic antidepressants
  Selective serotonin reuptake inhibitors: fluoxetine, paroxetine, sertraline
  Mirtazapine
  Nefazodone
  Trazodone
  Bupropion
Antiparkinsonian drugs: amantadine, bromocriptine, levodopa*
Antipsychotics
  Risperidone (Lane et al 1998; Barkin et al 1997)
  Olanzapine (London 1998)
Baclofen
Benzodiazepines
Captopril
Chloroquine (Akhtar & Mukherjee 1993)
Corticosteroids*
Cyclobenzaprine
Cyclosporine
Drug abuse: phencyclidine, cannabis*
Histamine H$_2$-antagonists: ranitidine, cimetidine (Hubain et al 1982; Titus 1983)
Interferon-α-2a (Takahashi et al 1993)
Isoniazid
Lisuride
Quinacrine
Sympathomimetic drugs: amphetamine, phenylpropanolamine*
Thyroid hormones
Vasodilator: inositol (Levin et al 1996)
Yohimbine alkaloids (Price et al 1984)

*More frequently reported.

affective disorders. A mixed form where patient develops mania while remaining severely depressed has been described (Spitzer et al 1987; Dilsaver and Swann 1995). The term "bipolar" means that the patient can change from depression to mania and vice versa in different phases of the disorder. Such a switch from depression to mania has been reported in 14 out of 70 hospital admissions of 30 patients with bipolar affective disorder treated with antidepressants (Solomen et al 1990). Such a switching has been reported in 21.5% of a larger series of patients treated with amitriptyline (Koszewska and Puzynski 1991). These results point to a role of cholinergic

system in the pathophysiology of switching out of depression into mania. A surge in CNS noradrenergic transmission has been postulated by Bunney et al (1972). However, fluvoxamine, a specific serotonin reuptake inhibitor affecting 5 HT$_2$ receptors has been reported to unmask maniac behavior in a series of 8 patients (Dorevitch et al 1993). Stanley and Stanley (1990) propose that antidepressant-induced mania involves further disruption of an already dysregulated serotonergic system. The destabilizing effect of antidepressants is not corrected by the addition of mood stabilizers and often requires the withdrawal of the drug (Hurowitz and Liebowitz 1993).

Mania as an Adverse Reaction to Antidepressants. Manic reactions may occur as an effect of excessive stimulation of the brain such as may occur with non-specific MAOIs inhibition. Antidepressants may precipitate such a reaction in depressive phase of bipolar illness. This would not meet the criteria of secondary mania. In a prospective study of patients with recurrent depression treated with imipramine, 2.6% developed hypomania during the first 6 months and none experienced mania (Kupfer et al 1988). Mania as an adverse reaction is not confined to the treatment of depression with antidepressants. A recent study in patients with other indications for the use of antidepressant drugs reached the following conclusions (Levy et al 1998):

– Patients with anxiety disorders, obsessive compulsive disorder and Parkinson's disease also suffer manic episodes with antidepressant treatment.

– Several chemically different antidepressants have been implicated in these patients.

– Borderline personality disorders contribute to behavioral dyscontrol in these patients.

Serotonin reuptake inhibitors can induce mania (Lennhof 1987; Howland 1996). Selective serotonin reuptake inhibitors (SSRIs) have less adverse effects than tricyclics but mania has been reported. Mania were described as an adverse effect of fluoxetine for various invocations: post-stroke depression (Kulisevsky and Berthier 1997), adolescents treated for obsessive compulsive disorder (Go et al 1998) and adolescents with attention deficit hyperactivity disorder (Venkataraman et al 1992). Other SSRIs associated with mania include sertraline (Heimann and March 1996) and paroxetine (Christensen 1995). Other antidepressants reported to precipitate mania include trazodone (serotonin reuptake inhibitor), bupropion (noradrenaline/dopamine reuptake inhibitor) and mirtazapine which is a noradrenergic and specific serotonergic antidepressant (De Leon et al 1999) and nefazodone, a dual-action serotonin and norepinephrine reuptake inhibitor (Dubin et al 1997).

Peet (1994) attempted to resolve the controversy regarding antidepressant induced mania by pooling all available clinical trial data for tricyclic antidepressants, selective serotonin reuptake inhibitors and placebos. He found that rate of mania was less than 1% in patients with predominantly unipolar depression, and that differences between drugs and placebo were statistically but not clinically significant. In bipolar depression, manic switch occurred more frequently with tricyclic antidepressants(11.2%) than with serotonin reuptake inhibitors (11.2%) or placebo (4.2%).

Antiparkinsonian Drugs

Patients with parkinson's disease usually suffer from depression and manic episodes are rare. Dopaminergic drugs, however, can precipitate mania. Hypomania was reported in 1.5% of patients treated with levodopa (Goodwin 1971). Use of levodopa in non-parkinsonian patients with bipolar depression was reported to precipitate mania in 6 out of 7 cases and the symptoms resolved within 48 hours of discontinuation of the drug (Murphy et al 1971). Milder manic disturbances following levodopa usually resolve without specific therapy. Others may improve by dosage reduction or changing over to another antiparkinsonian drug.

Bromocriptine was reported to induce mania in 2 out of 10 depressed parkinsonian patients without any previous history of manic episodes or use of antidepressants (Jouvent et al 1983). Mania has also been reported with the use of bromocriptine for pituitary tumors (Turner et al 1984) and for suppression of lactation in postpartum women (Lake et al 1987).

Corticosteroids

Psychiatric manifestations occur in 5% of patients treated with corticosteroids and about one-third of these are develop mania (Lewis and Smith 1983). Milder mental disturbances caused by corticosteroids usually resolve spontaneously. Dosage reduction or discontinuation of the drug may be required in some cases. In severe episodes of mania where continuation of the corticosteroid treatment is medically necessary, phenothiazines have been found to be an effective treatment. Lithium is effective for the prophylaxis of corticosteroid-induced mania in a patient with previous history of such episodes.

Management of Drug-Induced Mania

As a preventive measure, Dilsaver and Swann (1995) do not treat bipolar patients with tricyclic antidepressantsbut with a combination of carbamazepine and lithium. The following are some of the recommendations for management of drug-induced mania (Ganzini et al 1993b).

- Drug-induced mania usually resolves with discontinuation of the medication.

- Low potency neuroleptics such as thioridazine and chlorpromazine should be used in the younger patients and haloperidol in the elderly to avoid anticholinergic and hypotensive complications.

- Because drug-induced mania is short-lived treatment with antipsychotics should not be longer than 2 weeks to avoid extrapyramidal complications.

- Antipsychotic drugs should be used with extreme caution in patients with Parkinson's disease because of risk of worsening the parkinsonism.

- Lithium is usually less effective in the treatment of drug-induced mania than in bipolar affective disorders.

- CBZ is used for the treatment of mania but manic reactions have been reported after treatment of seizures with CBZ (Reiss and O'Donnell 1984; Drake and Peruzzi 1986).

Drug-Induced Hallucinations

Hallucination is defined as a perception without any external source. This can involve any sensory modality but visual hallucinations are the commonest type. Hallucinations can occur in various conditions such as schizophrenia, seizures, dementia, or may be drug-induced. Drugs which have been reported to be associated with hallucinations are listed in Table 5.11.

Pathomechanism. The anatomical substrate of hallucinations lies in the visual and auditory-associated cortices as demonstrated by increase of rCBF by PET during hallucinations in a schizophrenic patient (Silbersweig et al 1995). The pathomechanism of drug-induced visual hallucinations is not known. The hallucinogenic properties of LSD-25, the classical psychedelic drug derives from its ability to interfere with serotonergic and dopaminergic transmission (Freedman and Halaris 1978). The hallucinogenic properties of some β-blockers may be due to a derangement in the output form, i. e., the balance between some aminergic mechanisms (Koella 1985).

Possible 5-HT$_2$ receptor stimulation has been suggested as an explanation of hallucinations seen in fluoxetine-dextromethorphan interaction (Achamallah 1992). Serotonergic depletion in Parkinson's disease can possibly produce 5-HT$_2$ hypersensitivity and this may explain hallucinations produced by fluoxetine (a serotonin reuptake blocker) in a patient with Parkinson's disease (Lauterbach 1993).

Fisher (1991a) has studied in detail the phenomenon of visual hallucinations in a patient with atropine toxicity. He postulated that the hallucinations originated in sleep-dream system of the brainstem. Fisher (1991b) reported a similar case of visual hallucinations experienced by a patient only after eye closure following local anesthesia with lidocaine. There are three case reports of complex visual hallucinations following cyclosporin administration (Steg and Garcia 1991; Noll and Kulkarni 1984; Katirji 1987). The pathomechanism is not known but this adverse effect is dose-related and reversible after discontinuation of the drug. Visual and auditory hallucinations may be the sole or the first manifestation of neurotoxicity of ifosfamide Di Mag-

Table 5.11. Drugs associated with hallucinations.

Antimicrobial drugs
- acyclovir
- amoxicillin
- cephalosporins
- clarithromycin
- gentamicin
- sulfonamides

Antineoplastic drugs
- chlorambucil
- ifosfamide

Antiparkinsonian drugs
- anticholinergics,
- bromocriptine
- levodopa*
- pergolide

Cardiovascular drugs
- β-blockers: propranolol*
- captopril
- clonidine
- digitalis*
- diltiazem
- prazosin

Psychotropic drugs
- antidepressants*
- barbiturates
- benzodiazepines*
- ephedrine*
- lithium (Hambrecht 1995)
- methylphenidate*
- promethazine
- zolpidem*

Miscellaneous
- antihistaminics: H$_2$-antagonists*
- baclofen
- β-agonists inhaler (excessive use)
- chloroquine
- mefloquine*
- corticosteroids
- cyclosporine
- epoietin-alfa (Steinberg et al 1996)
- iopromide (non-ionic radio contrast medium)
- ketamine
- lidocaine
- metrizamide
- talwin*

*Frequently reported.

gio et al 1994). Hallucinations are the most frequently reported adverse reactions to benzodiazepines (Patten and Love 1994). This may be a paradoxical reaction. Among the β-blockers more lipid soluble drugs such as propranolol are likely to induce hallucinations as compared to hydrophilic drugs such as metoprolol (White and Riotte 1982). Excessive use of solbutamol (a β-agonist) by inhalation was reported to induce hallucinations in a 8 year old child (Schnapf and Santeiro 1994). This was attributed to fluorocarbon propellant in the inhaler.

Some examples of drug-induced hallucinations are described in the following paragraphs.

Levodopa-Induced Hallucinations. Visual hallucinations are among the most common of drug-induced disorders in patients with Parkinson's disease approaching 30% of the treated individuals. Chronic exposure to dopamine agonists can cause hypersensitivity of dopamine receptors. Levodopa produces an increased turnover of serotonin into its major metabolite 5HIAA (5-hydroxyindolacetic acid) in the rat brain (Melamed et al 1993). These authors have proposed that overstimulation of the central serotonergic (5-HT$_3$) receptors results from levodopa-induced elevations in serotonin release and concluded that this mechanism is, in part, responsible for levodopa-induced hallucinations. Moser et al (1996) have positively correlated urine salsolinol (tetrahydroquinoline derivative) levels to homovanillic acid/3-O-methyldopa ratio in the CSF which reflects dopamine metabolism in Parkinson's disease patients. In patients with levodopa-induced visual hallucinations, mean salsolinol ratio was increased to 3-times that in similar patients without hallucinations. This was considered to be due to an overloaded dopaminergic pathway with an imbalance between dopaminergic and serotonergic systems. Thus salsolinol appears to be a predictor for hallucinations in Parkinson's disease.

Management. Clozapine in low doses is effective in the treatment of levodopa-induced delusions and hallucinations (Rabey et al 1995). Risperidone, a benzisoxazole derivative with 5-HT$_2$ antagonism, has been shown to control these hallucinations (Meco et al 1994). Ondansetron has also been found to be a safe and effective therapy for hallucinations (Zoldan et al 1993). A more detailed description of levodopa-induced psychoses is given in the section of drug-induced psychoses.

Antimicrobial Drugs. Hallucinations are known as an adverse reaction to penicillin. Several cases of amoxicillin-induced hallucinations have been reported (Stell and Ojo 1996) and these are considered to be a variant of Hoigne's syndrome which is a pseudo-anaphylactic reactions induced by intramuscular administration of procaine penicillin G. This complication, characterized by acute psychological and neurological manifestations. The distinction is important from a therapeutic viewpoint since Hoigne's syndrome allows continuation of treatment, whereas it is absolutely contraindicated in anaphylactic shock. Clarithromycin has been reported to be associated with visual hallucination in a patient with renal failure which impaired the elimination and increased serum levels of this drug (Steinman and Steinman 1996). Visual hallucinations and abnormal bodily sensations were reported after triazolam or nitrazepam and concomitant erythromycin administration (Tokinaga et al 1996).

Antidepressants. Hallucinations are well documented as an adverse effect of various antidepressants. In case of tricyclic antidepressantssuch as imipramine, hallucinations may be related to the anticholinergic effect (Terao 1995).

Zolpidem. This belongs to a new class of hypnotic agents, chemically distinct from the pre-existing ones, and believed to act exclusively at the benzodiazepine omega 1 receptor. Clinically, zolpidem is indicated for the short term treatment of insomnia. Several cases have been reported of visual hallucinations with zolpidem (van Puijenbroek et al 1996; Markowitz et al 1997). Most of these are of short duration and occurred in women in whom peak plasma zolpidem concentrations are 40% than in men. Elko et al (1998) reported five patients who experienced visual hallucinations lasting from 1–7 hours soon after taking zolpidem. Most had been taking zolpidem for less than a week and all five were concurrently taking an antidepressant: sertraline, desipramine, fluoxetine, bupropion, or venlafaxine. The precise mechanism of zolpidem-associated hallucinations remains unknown but it is possible that a pharmacodynamic interaction between serotonin reuptake inhibition and zolpidem may lead to prolonged zolpidem-associated hallucinations in susceptible individuals.

Catatonia

Classic clinical signs of the catatonic syndrome include catalepsy, muscular rigidity, waxy flexibility, mutism, mannerism, and bizarre behavior. This can occur spontaneously as a variant of psychotic illness or may be drug-induced. Drugs usually implicated are neuroleptics (Ayd 1983). Bahro et al (1999) reported a patient who developed severe catatonia under medication with a serotonergic/dopaminergic neuroleptic, risperidone. The catatonic disorder was dose-dependent and subsided immediately after switching the medication to another atypical antipsychotic, clozapine. Catatonia has also been described due to disulfiram toxicity in the alcoholic patient (Fisher 1989) who proposed the action of disulfiram as an inhibitor of dopamine β-decarboxylase for this toxic effect. Intravenous lorazepam has been reported to be effective in reversing neuroleptic-induced catatonia (Fricchione et al 1983).

Drug-Induced Psychoses

Drugs have been reported to induce various forms of psychoses some of which resemble schizophrenia and include hallucinations, delusions and paranoid states. Drugs reported to be associated with psychoses are listed in Table 5.12.

Pathomechanism

The pathomechanism of drug-induced psychoses is not clearly understood. One example is the psychosis resulting from reserpine withdrawal which may be due to mesolimbic system hypersensitivity and differs from the recurrence of pre-existing psychoses after withdrawal of neuroleptics (Kent and Wilber 1982). The pathomechanism of psychosis associated with various drugs wherever it is known or postulated is described in this section.

Table 5.12. Drugs associated with psychoses.

Anabolic steroids*
Anticholinergics
Antidepressants
Antiepileptics*
 – carbamazepine
 – clonazepam
 – ethosuximide
 – felbamate
 – lamotrigine
 – phenytoin
 – tiagabine
 – topiramate
 – valproic acid
 – vigabatrin
Antihistaminics
Antimalarials
 – chloroquine
 – mefloquine
 – quinacrine
Antimicrobials
 – cephalexin
 – ciprofloxacin
 – cycloserine
 – sulfonamides
Antineoplastic drugs
Antiparkinsonian drugs*
 – bromocriptine
 – levodopa
Antipsychotics
 – clozapine
 – risperidone
Baclofen
Benzodiazepines*
Cardiovascular drugs
 – antihypertensives
 – β-blockers
 – digitalis
Clomifene
CNS stimulants*
 – methylphenidate
 – amphetamines
Corticosteroids*
Cyclobenzaprine
Cytokines
Disulfiram
Doxazosin
Drugs of abuse*
Ganciclovir (Hansen et al 1997)
Metronidazole
Melatonin (Force et al 1997)
Neuroleptics
Non-steroidal anti-inflammatory drugs
Oral contraceptives
Radiologic contrast media
Zolpidem

*Frequently reported.

Anabolic Steroids

In humans, the anabolic androgenic steroids comprise a group of chemicals that are structurally related to cholesterol. Most of the anabolic steroids are synthetic androgens, that have a greater growth-promoting activity relative to masculinizing effect as compared with androgens. They are indicating in the management of certain debilitating chronic illnesses but are also abused by some athletes. Adverse behavioral effects have been shown in a placebo-controlled prospective trial with methyltestosterone in healthy male volunteers (Su et al 1993). These consisted of negative mood changes and cognitive impairment. To assess the frequency of neuropsychiatric disorders in athletes using anabolic steroids, Pope and Katz (1988) performed structured interviews of 41 body builders and football players who had used steroids and found that five (12%) displayed psychotic symptoms.

Anabolic steroids may be used in combination with other drugs such as ethyl alcohol and cocaine — a practice that may contribute to the increase in aggressive behavior. There is need for better understanding of the pathomechanism of this type of drug abuse and brain imaging with MRI, PET has been combined with brain electrical activity mapping and behavioral pharmacological procedures to understand the CNS effect of various drugs and drug combinations on the brain (Lukas 1996). Such an understanding may lead to better approaches to management of these problems.

Anticholinergic Drugs

In addition to atropine and related alkaloids, several other drugs have anticholinergic action. These include synthetic quaternary ammonium compounds, antiparkinsonian agents, antihistaminics, tricyclic antidepressants, and phenothiazines. Profound behavioral disturbances produced by anticholinergic drugs are termed "anticholinergic syndrome" (see Chapter 18). Psychotoxicity can occur after systemic absorption of anticholinergic ophthalmic ointment (Barker and Solomen 1990).

Antidepressants

Many of the adverse effects of tricyclic antidepressantsare related to their anticholinergic action. The role of antidepressants in causing a switch from depression to mania has been discussed under the topic of pathomechanism of drug-induced mania. Serotonin (5-HT) reuptake inhibitors can exacerbate paranoia (Lauterbach 1991). Interaction of fluoxetine with concomitantly used amphetamines can produce psychotic reactions (Barrett et al 1996). Psychosis has been described following withdrawal of phenelzine, a MAO inhibitor (Liskin et al 1985).

Antiepileptic Drugs

There is a complex relationship between epilepsy and psychiatric disorders which makes it difficult to assess the neuropsychiatric effects of antiepileptic drugs. This issue is further complicated by the use of antiepileptic drugs for psychiatric disorders. Behavioral disturbances and psychotic reactions are commoner in epileptics than in the general population and all antiepileptic drugs are associated with psychotic reactions although they occur rarely. Schizophrenia-like psychoses have been reported to be associated with anticonvulsant drug toxicity and brain-damaged persons are more sensitive to marginally raised concentrations of these drugs (Franks and Richter 1979). Psychosis has been reported to be precipitated in epileptic patients after withdrawal of antiepileptic medications and recovery followed reinstitution of the drugs (Demers-Desrosiers et al 1978). The role of "forced normalization" to emergence of psychoses under antiepileptic therapy has been discussed by Trimble (1986). Forced normalization is an old term applied to suppression of seizures by antiepileptic drugs with normalization of EEG and occurrence of a psychotic state. Discontinuation of the medication leads to recurrence of seizures and disappearance of psychosis. In patients with temporal lobe EEG abnormalities, a hypothetical relationship between psychosis and epilepsy states that the mesolimbic dopaminergic system and kindling of this system with epileptic discharge in temporal-limbic circuits could induce a florid psychotic state in some patients (Pakalnis et al 1987). This biochemical relationship to schizophrenia with heightened dopamine activity would also explains the amelioration of antiepileptic drug-induced psychosis with neuroleptic agents which act by antagonizing this increased dopaminergic outflow state.

– *Carbamazepine (CBZ).* There are structural similarities between CBZ and tricyclic antidepressants. Reported psychiatric adverse effects of CBZ include schizophrenia-like psychoses and delusions. A non-specific psychotic state has been described in a patient treated with CBZ for trigeminal neuralgia (Mizukami et al 1990). Acute psychosis has been reported after seizure control with CBZ (Pakalnis et al 1987) and psychosis has been reported to be precipitated by the addition of valproic acid in a patient on CBZ therapy (McKee et al 1989). Abrupt withdrawal of carbamazepine following intoxication has been reported in a patient with trigeminal neuralgia where epilepsy and psychiatric disorders were excluded (Darbar et al 1996).

– *Clonazepam.* This is a benzodiazepine and its use has been reported to be associated with personality changes in the form paranoid psychoses during treatment (White et al 1982) or after withdrawal (Jaffe and Gibson 1986).

– *Ethosuximide.* Episodes of psychosis during treatment with ethosuximide have been describe several years ago (Roger et al 1968; Fischer et al 1965). There are more recent reports where psychotic symptoms emerged in patients with no previous psychiatric history and after normalization of EEG abnormalities following ethosuximide therapy (Pakalnis et al 1987).

– *Felbamate.* Seven cases of psychoses have been reported in patients with refractory seizure disorders on felbamate therapy (McConnel et al 1996). Five of these were on concomitant valproic acid (and other agents). Anergia, apathy, bradyphrenia, and increased irritability were prominent. One patient on felbamate monotherapy had a new-onset psychosis. Felbamate's NMDA receptor antagonism and GABA potentiation (perhaps enhanced by valproic acid use) are considered as possible mechanisms of these side effects.

– *Lamotrigine.* An epileptic patient was reported to develop psychosis with behavioral disturbances after start of lamotrigine monotherapy (Martin et al 1995). The symptoms cleared up after discontinuation of lamotrigine and treatment with antipsychotic medications. In a placebo-controlled study of lamotrigine, psychosis occurred in 2.8% of the patients and was the most commonly reported adverse effect that led to withdrawal of lamotrigine (Matsuo et al 1993).

– *Phenytoin.* The spectrum of neuropsychiatric reactions to phenytoin includes delirium accompanied by visual and tactile hallucinations, somatic delusions, paranoid reactions (McDanal and Bolman 1975), or schizophrenia-like psychoses (Franks and Richter 1979).

– *Valproic Acid.* It increases the brain levels of GABA and is able to provoke dose-related delirium, visual hallucinations, and hyperactivity, particularly in children (Chadwick 1985). Exacerbation of schizophrenia has been reported (Meldrum 1982).

– *Vigabatrin.* This is a new antiepileptic drug and psychosis has been reported following its use. Sander et al (1991) reported 14 patients with epilepsy who developed psychosis following the prescription of vigabatrin. Nine of these patients had no previous history of psychiatric illness. In all cases the psychosis resolved after discontinuation of the drug. Psychotic reaction was reported in a 7-year old boy after dose escalation with vigabatrin (Martinez et al 1995). This resolved after discontinuation of vigabatrin and substitution by carbamazepine. A review of the literature revealed that severe abnormal behavior develops in 3.4% of the adults and 6% of the children in controlled clinical trials with vigabatrin in epilepsy (Ferrie et al 1996). Results of a retrospective study suggest that psychosis as a treatment emergent effect of vigabatrin is seen in patients with more severe epilepsy, compared with those patients who never develop psychopathology, and those developing an affective disorder (Thomas et al 1996). The psychosis was related to a right-sided EEG focus, and suppression of seizures as 64% of these patients became seizure free.

The following measures are recommended to reduce the risk of psychoses with vigabatrin:
- The drug should be introduced slowly and dose should be raised to that required for control of seizures.
- This drug should be used with caution in patients with a history of psychiatric illness.
- Avoid use of vigabatrin if possible in patients with idiopathic generalized epilepsy.
- Therapy should be withdrawn slowly.

Antihistaminics

Histamine H_1-blocker agents are used for treatment of various allergic disorders. Many of them have anticholinergic properties and produce neuropsychiatric disturbances. Histamine H_2-blocker agents are associated with neuropsychiatric reactions: delirium, psychoses, hallucination, and mental changes (Cantu and Korek 1991). Ranitidine associated adverse effects such as delirium occur more often in elderly patients with renal disease (Slugg et al 1992). Cimetidine, another histamine H_2-receptor blocker has been reported to be associated with psychosis (Schentag 1980).

Antimalarials

Chloroquine and atabrine, originally antimalarials, but used for other indications as well are associated with paranoid hallucinatory psychoses sometimes with manic features (Torrey 1968). Mefloquine has also been reported to be associated with neuropsychiatric adverse effects and there are isolated case reports of psychoses (Bjorkman 1989; Stuiver et al 1989; Folkerts and Kuhs 1992; Marsepoil et al 1993; Meszaros 1996). In a review of adverse reactions since the introduction of the drug in 1985 till 1991, Bem et al (1992) reported 20 psychotic episodes. In a study in Germany, it was estimated that one out of 13,000 mefloquine users for prophylaxis suffers from neuropsychiatric reactions as compared with one of 215 therapeutic users (Weinke et al 1991). Neuropsychiatric side effects of me-

floquine have also been reported among Africans (Sowunmi et al 1993). Piening and Young (1996) reported the case of a man with no history of psychiatric disorder who developed a psychosis after receiving both mefloquine and primaquine. The manifestations were elevated mood, racing thoughts, distractability, psychomotor agitation with paranoia and delusions. He was treated with haloperidol and diazepam and recovered with no further recurrences of the episode.

Mefloquine should not be used in patients with history of psychiatric disorders. The drug should be discontinued early at the onset of neuropsychiatric symptoms. The treatment is symptomatic and most of the patients recover.

Antimicrobials

Neuropsychiatric complications of antimicrobials are rare, i. e., approximately 2 per 10,000 (Ricci et al 1986). Psychoses have been reported with older sulfonamides compounds such as trimethoprim-sulfamethoxazole (Mermel et al 1986). Over 100 acute non-anaphylactic reactions with psychiatric features have been reported with injections of procaine penicillin during the past 40 years. The psychiatric reactions are attributed to inadvertent intravascular injection of procaine moiety and affecting the limbic region of the brain. The profile of this adverse reaction is summarized as follows (Ilechukwu 1990):
- Reaction within one minute of injection
- Hallucinations
- Depersonalization and perceptual changes in the body image
- Absence of anaphylactic features
- Condition subsides with reassurance or sedation
- Usually does no recur on subsequent injections.

Psychoses have also been reported with the use of amoxicillin (Beal et al 1986) and erythromycin (Cohen and Weitz 1981; Umstead and Neumann 1986). Rarely, psychiatric reactions have been reported with streptomycin, gentamycin, ofloxacin, and ceftazidime. Acute psychosis has been reported with ciprofloxacin (James and Demian 1998; Zabala et al 1998). Isoniazid is associated with several psychiatric reactions. The explanation is the structural similarity of isoniazid to niacin (vitamin B_1) and the induction of pellagra-like syndrome by induction of deficiency of pyridoxine coenzymes.

Cycloserine is associated with a long list of psychiatric symptoms. It tends to activate schizophrenic patients, increasing agitation and hallucinations and inducing disorientation (Simeon et al 1970).

Psychiatric reactions have been reported to be associated with the antiviral drugs, amantadine and acyclovir (Jones and Beier-Hanratty 1986).

Antineoplastic Drugs

Several drugs used for the treatment of cancer have adverse neuropsychiatric effects. Neuropsychiatric effects may be due either to the remote effects of cancer on the CNS or direct involvement of the CNS by cancer. Some of these effects may be secondary to leukoencephalopathy caused by anticancer drugs.

Antiparkinsonian Drugs

Drug-induced psychosis represents one of the more serious side effects of therapy for Parkinson's disease. These occur with dopaminergic agents such as levodopa. Of patients treated with dopaminergic agents, 30% develop visual hallucinations, 10% exhibit delusions, 10% have euphoria, 15% experience increased anxiety, and 15% have confusional periods. Visual hallucinations and paranoid psychosis are major and increasingly common complications of long-term levodopa therapy in patients with Parkinson's disease (Nausieda et al 1984; Klawans 1988). Anticholinergic drugs have a greater tendency to produce confusional states than dopaminergic compounds. Risk factors for the development of psychosis are:
- Patients with Parkinson's disease who develop psychosis while receiving levodopa have an increased odds ratio for dementia.
- A previous history of psychiatric illness is an additional risk factor for the development of psychosis.

- The incidence of psychosis increases with increasing age.
- High dose of drugs

Pathophysiology. The exact pathophysiological basis of drug-induced psychosis in Parkinson's disease is not established. Dopamine replacement may have different effects on the basal ganglia and the cortex because dopamine levels in the former exceed those in the latter by a factor of 1:30. Excessive stimulation of dopamine receptors in the mesolimbic/mesocortical pathways may result in symptoms similar to those of schizophrenia. The number of striatal dopamine receptors in the brains of patients with Parkinson's disease, who had suffered drug-induced psychoses, are found to be increased at postmortem examination. This is considered to be due to denervation hypersensitivity resulting from loss of presynaptic dopaminergic neurons which is characteristic of Parkinson's disease. Stimulation of these hypersensitive receptors may result in hallucinations.

Management. An approach to the management of drug-induced psychosis in a patient with Parkinson's disease is shown in Figure 5.1. Dosage reduction is one of the strategies in management. The most likely offending agent should be tapered first. Anticholinergic agents should be considered first unless the symptoms are clearly related to another drug. Selegeline, amantadine, dopamine agonists and levodopa should be considered for tapering in that order (Young et al 1997). The followings methods have been used for management of psychoses:
- *Atypical antipsychotics.* Psychoses have been treated successfully with clozapine which is unlikely to aggravate extrapyramidal symptoms (Kahn et al 1991; Wolk and Douglas 1992; Rosenthal et al 1992; Greene et al 1993; Factor et al 1994; Gonski 1995; Rabey et al 1995). A randomized, double-blind, placebo-controlled study has shown that low dose clozapine (50 mg or less) is safe and significantly improves drug-induced psychosis without worsening parkinsonism (The Parkinson Study Group 1999). Clozapine has also been shown to resolve bromocriptine-induced psychosis in Parkinson's disease (Al-Semaan et

al 1997). Other atypical antipsychotics that have been found to be useful for treatment of psychoses in parkinson's disease are: risperidone (Cohen 1994) and quetiapine (Fernandez et al 1999).

- *Ondansetron.* This is an antagonist of 5-HT$_3$ receptors and is approved for the management of chemotherapy-induced emesis and postanesthetic vomiting. It has also been found to produce moderate to marked improvement in drug-induced psychosis (Zoldan et al 1995).
- *Non-pharmacological approaches.* These include electroconvulsive therapy (ECT) and surgery, particularly median pallidotomy. This is receiving increasing attention for the treatment of motor symptoms such as dyskinesias and may enable reduction of levodopa dose with amelioration of psychiatric symptoms. Surgery is often contraindicated in the pres-

ence of psychosis as it has not been shown to be beneficial in this population of patients with parkinson's disease (Mendis et al 1996).

Baclofen

Patients with chronic baclofen intoxication have been reported to present with hallucinations, impaired memory, catatonia, and acute mania (Lee et al 1992; Pauker and Brown 1986; Yassa and Iskander 1988; Roy and Wakefield 1986; Wolfe et al 1982). A case of frontal lobe syndrome with perseveration was reported by Liu et al (1991) and resolved after discontinuation of the medication. Most psychiatric reactions to baclofen seem to occur from doses greater than 60 mg or on withdrawal of the medication. Manifestations of baclofen withdrawal include psychoses and

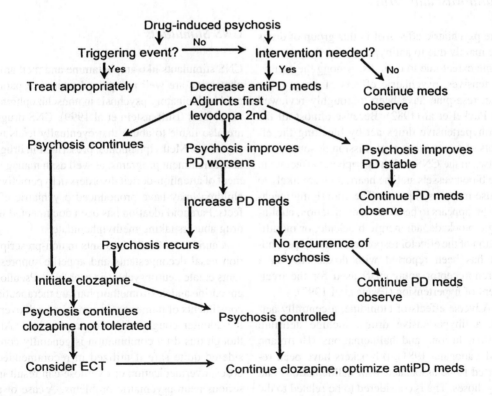

Figure 5.1. Flow diagram for the treatment of drug-induced psychoses in Parkinson's disease (PD). From Factor SA, et al: Parkinson's disease: drug-induced psychiatric states. In Weiner WJ and Lang AE (Eds.) Behavioral Neurology of Movement Disorders. Advances in Neurology vol 65. New York, Raven Press, 1995:115–138 (by permission of publisher). ECT = electroconvulsive therapy.

hallucination (Riva et al 1993). Patients with renal failure and pre-existing brain damage are at risk of baclofen-induced psychosis (Himmelsbach et al 1992).

Benzodiazepines

Increased aggressive, violent, and impulsive behavior states have been reported during the use of benzodiazepines (Mathew et al 1993). Psychosis can occur on withdrawal from these medications.

A case of psychosis has been described on withdrawal of triazolam in a patient addicted to this drug and this was managed by used of lorazepam, another benzodiazepine (Heritch et al 1989).

Cardiovascular Drugs

The psychiatric effects of in this group of drugs are mainly due to antihypertensive drugs and to some extent due to digitalis. Among the antihypertensives, psychiatric effects of drugs other than reserpine have been thoroughly reviewed ba Paykel et al (1982). Because almost all the antihypertensive drugs act by blocking the effects of sympathetic transmission at some point between the CNS and the peripheral effectors in the blood vessels and the heart, they are likely to cause mental symptoms. The underlying mechanism appears to be either central action, cholinergic blockade, adrenergic blockade, or modification of the effector response. A case of psychosis has been reported with doxazosin (an a adrenoreceptor antagonist) used for the treatment of hypertension (Evans et al 1997).

Adverse effects of clonidine, a centrally acting antihypertensive drugs, include delirium with delusions and hallucinations (Hoffmann and Ladogana 1981). β-blockers have been reported to be associated with hallucinations and psychoses. The is considered to be related to the degree of lipophilicity of these compounds. In randomized, double-blind cross-over studies, metaprolol which is lipophilic was responsible for more CNS complications than atenolol and

propranolol which are hydrophilic (Westerlund 1985).

The cardiac glycoside digoxin is well known for such effects as delirium, hallucinations, and psychosis. Neuropsychiatric side effects of digitalis can be used as an early indicator of digitalis toxicity (Cooke 1993).

Clomiphene

Clomiphene, a fertility treatment, has been associated with psychoses in a few cases (Siedentopf and Kentenich 1998; Oyffe et al 1997; Kapfhammer et al 1990; Cashman and Shephard 1982). The pathogenetic role of clomiphene is supported by comparable findings in certain post-partum psychoses. Women with a history of psychiatric instability have a greater risk of developing this adverse effect.

CNS Stimulants

CNS stimulants like amphetamine and methamphetamine are well recognized to induce paranoid hallucinatory psychosis in nonschizophrenic subjects (Buffenstein et al 1999). CNS drugs are also liable to abuse that eventually leads to psychosis. Methylphenidate, prescribed in drug-abuse treatment programs, as well as in management of attention-deficit disorders in hyperactive children, may have pronounced psychiatric effects. Paranoid ideation has been documented in drug abusers taking methylphenidate.

A number of CNS stimulants in non-prescription nasal decongestants and appetite suppressants create neuropsychiatric problems. Pseudoephedrine and dextromethorphan are therapeutic constituents of numerous commonly used, over-the-counter cough and cold preparations. Although this drug combination is generally considered quite safe if utilized in recommended doses, overmedication or overdose can result in serious neuropsychiatric problems. A case of a 2-year-old child who developed hyperirritability and psychosis after ingestion of such a cough syrup has been reported (Roberge et al 1999). Various mental disturbances including hallucinatory-paranoid states have been reported in 44 patients abusing "BRON"—a Japanese over-the-counter cough suppressant containing codeine, caffeine, methylephedrine, and chlorpheniramine (Ishigooka et al 1991).

Withdrawal from use of CNS stimulants also produces psychotic states. Experimental studies in animals suggest that lasting enhancement of methamphetamine-induced dopamine release in the striatum is related to the development and expression of brain vulnerability to schizophrenic symptoms (Sato et al 1992). A schizophrenia-like psychosis can persist after discontinuation of methamphetamine.

Corticosteroids

The most widely recognized review of side effects of corticosteroids is that compiled by the Boston Collaborative Drug Surveillance Program (1972). In this study 676 hospitalized patients treated with corticosteroids were analyzed. Of these 3.1% developed acute psychiatric reactions and there was a dose-response relationship. Only 1.3% of the 463 patients receiving less than 40 mg of prednisone per day demonstrated significant psychiatric disturbances in contrast to 4.6% of 175 patients receiving 41–80 mg, and 18.4% of 38 patients receiving more than 80 mg. This study indicates that psychiatric disturbances occur with high-dose and not low-dose corticosteroid therapy.

A study by Hall et al (1979) suggested that patients receiving greater than 40 mg of prednisone or its equivalent, are at greater risk of developing steroid psychosis with symptoms ranging from affective through schizophrenia-like to those of an organic brain syndrome. The patients responded to phenothiazines but were aggravated by tricyclic antidepressants.

Patients with SLE are more prone to develop psychotic symptoms during treatment with corticosteroids. A case of mania triggered by a steroid nasal spray in a patient with stable bipolar disorder has been reported (Goldstein and Preskorn 1989). However, generally speaking, preexisting psychiatric disturbances do not increase the likelihood of steroid psychoses in adults,

emotional instability in children predisposes them to steroid-related psychological problems (Milgrom and Bender 1993). A steroid-induced acute psychosis has been reported in a child with asthma (Dawson and Carter 1998). Women are liable to develop postpartum psychosis if they have received antepartum steroids (Brockington and Brownell 1997;

Prevention. In most cases psychiatric side-effects can be avoided by keeping the prednisone dose below 40 mg/day. When patients do develop psychosis, the steroid dose should be reduced to physiologic replacement levels, provided the underlying disease remains under control. Abrupt cessation may result in rebound depression, therefore, the dose reduction should be carried out over several days. Hassanyeh et al (1991) presented a case where adrenocortical suppression, accompanied by neuropsychiatric disturbances, persisted for a year after discontinuation of prednisone. The patient recovered after resumption of low dose prednisone therapy. Prophylactic therapy with lithium has been shown to prevent psychiatric complications of ACTH therapy for multiple sclerosis.

Cytokines

Psychiatric side effects have been reported during treatment of viral and malignant disorders with recombinant interferon-α (McDonald et al 1987; Renault et al 1987). The side-effects are not due to any contaminants, they seem to be dose-related, and are reversed by stopping the interferon treatment. Various neuropsychiatric manifestations are:

– Confusion
– Thought blockage
– Memory disturbance
– Hallucinations
– Visuospatial disorientation.

Pathomechanism of CNS effects of interferons are discussed in Chapter 3. An interesting observation is that interferon-α, possibly synthesized in the brain, is the cause of psychosis in patients with SLE (Shiozawa et al 1992). Psychotic reactions to interferon-α-2b have been reported

(Heeringa et al 1998). Neuropsychiatric side effects have also been reported with interleukin-2 (Fenner et al 1993a; Buter et al 1993).

Metronidazole

A number of psychotic adverse reactions have been reported after the use of metronidzole (Schreiber and Spernal 1997; Uhl and Riely 1996). This drug is used for the treatment of portosystemic encephalopathy in patients with cirrhosis of the liver. In patients who signs of psychosis without obvious or precipitating cause, metronidazol should be discontinued.

Neuroleptics

This group of drugs includes phenothiazines, haloperidol and atypical neuroleptics which are used in the treatment of schizophrenia and disturbed behavior due to other causes.

Withdrawal symptoms for typical antipsychotics are generally mild, self-limited and do not include development of psychotic symptoms. In contrast, withdrawal symptoms for clozapine can be severe with rapid onset of agitation and psychotic symptoms (Stanilla et al 1997). The withdrawal symptoms usually resolve rapidly with resumption of low doses of clozapine. Severe withdrawal symptoms can probably be avoided by slowly tapering clozapine and/or simultaneously substituting another psychotropic with high anticholinergic activity, such as thioridazine.

Neuroleptic withdrawal can precipitate schizophrenia-like psychosis even in manic-depressive patients and this is attributed to dopamine-receptor hypersensitivity (Witschy et all 1984). Sandel et al (1993) have reported a patient with brain injury who developed a delusional state after administration of chlorpromazine.

Non-Steroidal Anti-Inflammatory Drugs (NSAID)

These are among the most commonly prescribed medications. About a quarter of all adverse reac-

tions reported are attributed to these medications. Neuropsychiatric events are the third most common adverse reactions to these drugs (Clark and Ghose 1992). Psychiatric reactions include delirium, depression, hallucinations and psychoses. Chronic salicylate intoxication may present with delirium, paranoia, and hallucinations (Gittelman 1993).

Psychoses have been reported most commonly with indomethacin and sulindac (Hoppmann et al 1991). These should be suspected in any patient who has begun a regimen of indomethacin and who acutely develops disorientation, paranoia or hallucinations. Indomethacin-induced psychoses can be controlled by chlorpromazine even when the NSAID therapy is not discontinued (Gotz 1978).

Opioid Analgesics

Morphine oversedation can lead to paranoid thinking and hallucinations. Pentazocine and methadone, synthetic opioid analgesics, are associated with a variety of psychiatric effects. Withdrawal from opioids also produces psychiatric problems. Opioid administration suppresses endorphin production and withdrawal produces a temporary relative deficiency of endogenous opioids which is relevant to the psychiatric manifestations. The development of an organic mood syndrome is a common occurrence in patients undergoing slow detoxification from methadone maintenance treatment and is associated with a poor outcome (Kanof et al 1993).

Oral Contraceptives

Various neuropsychiatric adverse effects of the hormonal oral contraceptives have been reported. These include affective changes, phobic anxiety and psychotic reactions (Taubert and Kuhl 1981). Most of the reports of psychosis associated with oral contraceptives appeared in the literature of the 1960s and 1970s. No psychoses have been reported with the modern versions of oral contraceptives.

Radiologic Contrast Media

Water soluble non-ionic contrast media used for myelography are safer than ionic media which produce complications such as arachnoiditis. Nonetheless, neuropsychiatric disturbances have been reported following the use of non-ionic contrast media due to intracranial diffusion following intraspinal administration. Metrizamide has ben shown to produce neuropsychiatric disturbances (Galle and Arnold 1984).

Zolpidem

Zolpidem is reported to be a safe and effective hypnotic agent for the short-term treatment of insomnia. There are several case reports of zolpidem causing psychotic reactions in patients with no history of psychosis (Ansseau et al 1992; Pitner et al 1997). Markowitz and Brewerton (1996) report two additional cases in which zolpidem was implicated in psychotic reactions characterized by auditory and visual hallucinations as well as delusional thinking. Both patient's symptoms resolved with the discontinuation of zolpidem use.

Most of the reported cases were female, there appeared to be some dose dependency involved, and the adverse event resolved fairly quickly upon zolpidem discontinuation. Zolpidem should be used at the lowest effective dose for the least amount of time as necessary. Female patients may possibly require smaller doses. In patients manifesting new-onset or unexplained psychotic symptoms, zolpidem use should be considered in the differential diagnosis.

Drug-Induced Cerebral Insufficiency

Cerebral insufficiency is a general term indicating decline of mental function (Jain 1990). It does not specify the cause but the clinical effects which may be mild moderate or severe (dementia). The frequently used term cognitive impairment refers to disturbances of information processing. It covers the acquisition, storage, retrieval and use of information. Cognitive processes involved in acquisition of information are linked to consciousness and cognitive disturbances thus include delirium described earlier in this chapter. Cognitive disorders also include disturbances of memory and intellect as well as behavioral disturbances.

Drug-Induced Cognitive Disturbances

Non-specific cognitive disturbances have been reported with drugs shown in Table 5.13.

Table 5.13. Drugs associated with non-specific cognitive disturbances.

Antidepressants
Antiepileptics
Antihypertensives
Antineoplastics
Corticosteroids
Cytokines: interleukin-2, interferon-$\alpha2$
Lithium
Opioid analgesics
Neuroleptics
Non-steroidal anti-inflammatory drugs

Antidepressants

Several antidepressant medications have been reported to produce cognitive impairment. Cognitive impairment is more likely to occur with tricyclic antidepressants. Amitriptyline produces noticeable and significant impairment of cognition and psychomotor function whereas moclobemide is relatively free from these adverse effects (Hindmarch and Kerr 1992). This is due to selective MAOI action and lack of anticholinergic effects of moclobemide (Allain et al 1992). Amoxapine, an antidepressant with neuroleptic effect, has been associated with cognitive impairment (Burns and Tune 1987).

Antiepileptic Drugs (AEDs)

Effect of antiepileptic drugs on cognitive function is a controversial issue. Four AEDs are commonly used: carbamazepine (CBZ), phenytoin

(PHT), valproic acid (VPA) and phenobarbital (PB). There are few studies about the neuropsychiatric effects of new antiepileptic drugs such as vigabatrin. Some of the comments apply to all of the AEDs and will be discussed first. Discussion of individual AEDs and comparative studies are described later.

According to Dodrill (1992) problems in assessment of cognitive effects of AEDs include subject selection factors, statistical difficulties, choice of cognitive tests, and the impact of seizures on psychological performance. After an extensive review of literature, Trimble (1987) suggested that AEDs impair cognitive function and that maximum impairment is seen in patients receiving polytherapy. Maximum cognitive deficits were seen with phenytoin, while phenobarbital and valproic acid induced moderate disturbances, and carbamazepine had the least toxic effect. Thompson (1992) noted that newly diagnosed cases and those on monotherapy had fewer cognitive effects. Evaluation of memory function in most studies was limited and where effects were recorded they were possibly secondary to changes in the level of attention or speed of mental processing.

Comparative Studies of AEDs. In a review, Vining (1987) stated that PB impairs memory and concentration, PHT affects attention, problem solving ability, and performance of visuomotor tasks. In contrast CBZ may affect only concentration, while VPA may have a minimal effect on cognition. Meador et al (1990) investigated the neuropsychological effects of CBZ, PB, and PHT in 15 patients with complex partial seizures treated with each drug for 3 months, using a randomized double-blind, triple crossover design. Their data showed that all patients had comparable neuropsychological performance on most measures. Their results suggest that differential cognitive effects of AEDs may be subtle. Little difference in cognitive effects was found in a single randomized double-blind study of the cognitive effects of VPA and PHT in elderly epileptics (Craig and Tallis 1994).

Another approach to study of cognitive effects of AEDs is after withdrawal of these medications. In a double-blind, prospective placebo-controlled study of discontinuation of PHT, VPA, and CBZ, it was noted that all of them affected the motor functions adversely but PHT did so more than the others (Duncan et al 1990). In another study, improvement after discontinuation of AEDs was limited to psychomotor speed with some suggestion that PHT treated patients had more impairment on tests of motor and mental speed (Aldenkamp et al 1993). In a more elaborate study of the cognitive effects of antiepileptic drug discontinuation, Gallassi et al (1992) found that patients receiving CBZ did not differ from controls at any time, those receiving PB had significant differences only at full dose when compared to normal matched controls. Patients on VPA and PHT had some differences at full dose but these disappeared 1 year after discontinuation.

Most of the comparative studies involve two most widely use drugs: CBZ and PHT. Gilham et al (1990) found that psychomotor performance is more selectively affected by CBZ whereas memory is impaired by PHT. Some studies have concluded that PHT affects cognitive function more than CBZ (Gallassi et al 1988; Andrews et al 1986; Aldenkamp et al 1994; Pulliainen and Jokelainen 1994). Most of these studies are on patients with idiopathic epilepsy. Kirschner et al (1991) found no difference between PHT and CBZ in treating patients with seizures due to blunt head injury. Dodrill and Troupin (1991) reported that if patients with high serum PHT levels are excluded there is no difference between the psychological profiles of PHT and CBZ.

To eliminate the confounding effect of epilepsy and also because AEDs are used for non-epileptic indications as well some studies have been done in healthy volunteers. Meador et al (1991) investigated the neuropsychological effects of CBZ and PHT in 21 healthy adults using a randomized, double-blind, double-crossover design and treating each subject with each drug for 1 month, separated by a 1 month washout. Their results show that differences in the cognitive effects of CBZ and PHT are not clinically significant.

Oxcarbazepine, a derivative of CBZ has also been compared with PHT in epileptic patients and no significant differences were found in neuropsychological effects (Äikia et al 1992). However, a recent study by Curran and Java (1993) has shown that oxcarbazepine improves performance on a focused attention task and increases manual writing speed in healthy volunteers. Some reports on the use of these AEDs as monotherapy are as follows:

- *Phenytoin.* A study on normal volunteers reported deleterious effect of PHT on several important measures of cognition, including memory, concentration, and mental as well as motor speed (Thompson et al 1981). PHT has been shown to produce cognitive impairment in patients with head injury when it was used as a prophylaxis for seizures (Dikmen et al 1991).
- *Carbamazepine.* Poor psychomotor performance in patients on CBZ therapy is significantly associated with high CBZ plasma concentration (O'Dougherty et al 1987). In another study, children performed better shortly after peak plasma CBZ concentration (Aman et al 1990).
- *Valproic Acid.* The effects of VPA on cognition are considered to be minimal but some adverse effects on psychomotor performance were observed but reversed after withdrawal of the drug (Gallassi et al 1990).
- *Phenobarbital.* Long-term phenobarbital therapy induces a significant impairment in learning ability (Calandre et al 1990). PB depresses cognitive performance in children treated for febrile seizures but this disadvantage which may outlast the administration of the drug by several months, is not offset by the benefits of seizure prevention (Farwell et al 1990).
- *Vigabatrin.* This GABA analog is not free from cognitive adverse effects on cognition. Vigabatrin was associated with a significant reduction in a measure of motor speed and overall score on a design learning test in a randomized, placebo-controlled, double-blind trial (Grünewald et al 1994).

Antihypertensive Drugs

Cognitive side effects are common with antihypertensive drugs. These effects are rarely clear cut and involve various neuropsychologic func-

tions. Literature on this topic has been reviewed by Dimsdale (1992) who has pointed out the difficulties of any comparisons across studies due to lack of standardized methods. The patient is a relatively poor observer of these changes and even those on placebo experience these adverse effects.

Antineoplastics

Cognitive deficits in the areas of visual-motor performance and attention have been shown in children with acute lymphocytic leukemia treated by chemotherapeutic agents (Brown et al 1992). CNS prophylactic chemotherapy in such patients before the age of 15 years produces a decline of cognitive functions quantified as decline of IQ scores (Giralt et al 1992; Kingsma et al 1993). Previous treatment with biologic modifiers in cancer patients is associated with a 53% incidence of cognitive abnormalities as compared with only 18% in such patients never treated before with such agents (Meyers and Abbruzzese 1992). A frontal lobe syndrome has been reported in a patient following treatment with carmofur (a masked compound of 5-fluouracil) and was correlated with structural changes due to leukoencephalopathy induced by the drug (Suzuki et al 1990).

Corticosteroids

Excessive circulating levels of endogenous and exogenous corticosteroids, such as occur in Cushing's syndrome, are frequently associated with cognitive impairment as manifested by difficulties with attention, concentration, and memory. Wolkowitz et al (1990) have reviewed several studies on this topic and pointed out the importance of recognition of corticosteroid-related cognitive pathology as well as its separation from cognitive deficits related to the patient's primary pathology. Milgram and Bender (1993) have reviewed studies about the psychologic effects of steroids in children. Corticosteroids have been shown to have detrimental cognitive effects in children with asthma.

Cytokines

Cognitive changes have been reported with interleukin-2 (IL-2), interferon (IFN)-α, and tumor necrosis factor (TNF).

Interferon. Intramuscular therapy with interferon has been reported to be associated with cognitive and behavioral changes (Adams et al 1984). In another report (Meyers et al 1991), fourteen cancer patients showed evidence of persistent cognitive changes after the discontinuation of IFN-α therapy. The pattern of deficits was consistent with frontal-subcortical dysfunction. Follow-up was available only in four cases: two improved and two had deteriorated indicating, that IFN toxicity is not always reversible.

The CNS side effects associated with interferon-α (IFN-α) therapy, including cognitive changes, can compromise otherwise effective immunotherapy. A syndrome of mood disturbance with memory impairment, cognitive slowing, and impaired executive function is common with IFN-α therapy and is consistent with mild subcortical dementia. Cognitive deficits and mood disorder may occur independently, and in some cases depression is a reactive phenomenon. Risk factors for development of IFN-α neurotoxicity include duration of treatment, high-dose therapy, and prior cranial irradiation or neurologic illness. Possible pharmacologic interventions to decrease the neurotoxicity associated with IFN-α therapy include antidepressants, psychostimulants, and opioid antagonists. Preliminary clinical and research experience suggests that it is possible to effectively palliate IFN-α toxicity (Valentine et al 1998).

IL-2. Of the 44 patients with metastatic cancer treated with intravenous bolus injections of IL-2, 22 (50%) developed severe cognitive changes (Denicoff et al 1987). All of these patients recovered from cognitive impairment after discontinuation of treatment. In a larger series of 101 patients treated with combination of subcutaneous IL-2 and IFN-α-2b, one-third developed minor or major cognitive difficulties (Fenner et al 1993). The authors considered this to be due to cytokine-induced capillary leak syndrome causing increase of brain water content which can be demonstrated by MRI (see Chapter 3). Meyers

et al (1994) described a case of cognitive deficits resulting from IL-2 and TNF treatment in a patient with renal carcinoma. Cognitive deficits as well as frontal lobe perfusion deficits (demonstrated by SPECT) resolved one month following completion of treatment.

Lithium

The extensive literature on lithium-induced cognitive dysfunction has been reviewed by Marchand (1985). The pathomechanism of this effect is the same as for lithium-induced encephalopathy (see Chapter 5).

Neuroleptics

There is a great deal of variability and inconsistency in various reports dealing with the effects of neuroleptics on cognitive and psychomotor functions. Psychopharmacological invention may impair cognitive function especially in a brain-damaged person. King (1990) has reviewed various studies on this topic and some of his conclusions are as follows:

1. Sedative phenothiazines depress psychomotor function and sustained attention but higher cognitive functions are relatively unaffected.

2. Controls show neuroleptic-induced cognitive impairments whereas schizophrenic patients show cognitive improvement.

Further review (King 1994) has failed to demonstrate any consistent effects of typical or atypical neuroleptics on psychomotor or cognitive function in schizophrenic patients. Better methods and study designs are required, and healthy volunteer studies are necessary to control for variables due to schizophrenic psychopathology. Eye movements are a sensitive and reliable measure of attention and arousal. These are impaired by neuroleptics but it is not possible to distinguish this from similar effect of benzodiazepines.

Non-Steroidal Anti-Inflammatory Drugs

This subject has been reviewed by Hoppmann et al (1991). In a retrospective study, Goodwin and Regan (1982) were able to eight out of fifty elderly patients who developed cognitive dysfunction while on treatment with ibuprofen or naproxen. None of these patients had any neuropsychiatric problems prior to start of treatment with NSAIDs and the cognitive changes cleared up after discontinuation of the drugs. In a prospective study, Wysenbeek et al (1988) assessed cognitive dysfunction by standardized tests in 12 elderly patients treated with naproxen. The authors concluded that naproxen-induced changes were mild and of questionable clinical significance. The small number of patients and lack of self-assessment limits the value of this study. Better studies are need on this subject before any firm conclusions can be drawn but simple bedside tests should be done to detect cognitive changes in the elderly on NSAIDs for early detection of any changes.

Opioid Analgesics

Morphine and other opioid analgesics may interfere with normal cognition and motor function when these drugs are used for long periods for treatment of pain. Morphine has been shown to interfere with cognitive performance at plasma drug concentrations within the usual therapeutic range (Kerr et al 1991). Danziger et al (1994) reported the case of man with hepatic dysfunction who developed agitation and delirium after several days of pethidine (meperidine) for postoperative pain. He did not respond to intravenous haloperidol and lorazepam but the symptoms resolved after discontinuation of pethidine. The patient had recurrence of this adverse reaction after rechallenge with pethidine. Portenoy has suggested the following measures for the management of patients who develop cognitive disturbances during use of opioids for pain relief:

– Eliminate non-essential drugs which may exacerbate adverse effects

– Reduce the opioid dose by 25–50% if analgesia is sufficient
– Add a nonopioid analgesic such as NSAID to enable a dose reduction of opioid
– Try another opioid preparation

Psychomotor Disturbances

Psychomotor performance involves coordination of certain muscular movements in response to stimulation of the CNS. Impairment of psychomotor performance have been reported with drugs shown in Table 5.14.

Table 5.14. Drugs producing psychomotor disturbances.

Antidepressants
Antihistaminics
Calcium antagonists
Clonidine
Morphine
Neuroleptics

Antidepressants, morphine, and neuroleptics have been discussed under the heading of general cognitive dysfunction where psychomotor impairment has been mentioned.

Antihistaminics

Drowsiness and impairment of psychomotor performance are well known effects associated with the use of antihistaminics (Clark and Nicholson 1978). The mechanism of this is not clear. The problem of impaired psychomotor performance with the older antihistaminics does not apply to terfenadine (Aaronson 1993).

Calcium Antagonists

Effects of calcium channel blockers, verapamil and nifedipine, was tested on psychomotor performance and higher mental functions in human volunteers (Jaguste et al 1991). Placebo and diazepam (5 mg) were used as negative and positive controls respectively. Psychomotor tests performed were arithmetic ability, visual and auditory reaction time, letter (alphabet) cancellation, rapid fire arithmetic deviation and short term memory for playing cards. Verapamil, both in 40 and 80 mg dose, was found to impair the performance of subjects to a significant extent in auditory reaction time, letter cancellation and short term memory. These effects were similar to those observed with administration of diazepam. With nifedipine, impairment in performance was observed only in rapid arithmetic deviation test. It was concluded that calcium channel antagonists, specially verapamil, impaired psychomotor performance of human subjects in our study. Nifedipine, verapamil and diltiazem were shown to impair recognition ability in a study on volunteers (Saieed and Hassan 1996). Three hours after administration of the calcium antagonists, recognition reaction times significantly increased compared to the values after placebo administration.

The results of the studied quoted above have not been confirmed by others. Gerrard et al (1995) conducted a study to evaluate the central effects of single doses of the beta-adrenoceptor antagonist atenolol and the calcium antagonist nifedipine retard, alone and in combination, in normal subjects. Twelve normal males received single oral doses of atenolol 100 mg, nifedipine retard 20 mg, atenolol 100 mg and nifedipine retard 20 mg in combination, diazepam 5 mg (active control), and each of two matching placebos in a double-blind, randomized fashion. Psychomotor performance was assessed using digit symbol substitution, letter cancellation (LCT), continuous attention, choice reaction time, finger tapping, immediate recall and short-term memory. Two flash fusion and critical flicker fusion thresholds were measured and subjective assessments made using visual analogue scales. Diazepam 5 mg significantly worsened LCT scores at 4 h, significantly impaired alertness at 2 h and 4 h, and tended to increase reaction time and impair continuous attention and physiological measurements. Atenolol 100 mg alone significantly reduced alertness at 2 h and 4 h, and also tended to impair physiological measurements. Nifedipine retard 20 mg produced no significant psychomotor effects. Combined atenolol and nifedipine retard administration produced a small

but significant improvement in continuous attention and a reduction in body sway, with no adverse effects being evident on performance or subjective awareness. The results suggest that no significant adverse effects on psychomotor performance are produced by single doses of atenolol 100 mg and nifedipine retard 20 mg when given together in normal subjects

Calcium channel blockers, added to a stable regimen of neuroleptic medication, have been shown to enhance learning and memory in schizophrenic patients with tardive dyskinesia (Schwartz et al 1997). Nifedipine improved performance in the rotary pursuit test and conceptual abilities in the dementia scale compared with placebo, but only for patients who first were exposed to the tests during the placebo condition.

Clonidine

Clonidine impairs psychomotor performance of young human volunteers (Kugler et al 1980). Clonidine has been shown to impair the ability of aged monkeys to perform a microcomputer-controlled delayed response test in a dose-dependent manner (Davis et al 1988).

Drug-Induced Memory Disturbances

Memory is not a unitary process but consists of disturbances of various components. These may be affected differentially by both the illnesses and the drugs which may impair or improve the memory function. A number of commonly used medications as well as a some of the recreational drugs are known to produce memory disturbances. The focus of this section is on medications-induced memory disturbances but studies with drugs of abuse, both experimental and clinical, serve to throw some light on the pathomechanisms of drug-induced memory loss.

Mechanisms of memory are complex and are beyond the scope of this work. Various disturbances of memory are defined as follows:

– *Amnesia* refers to pathological loss of memory.

- *Amnestic syndrome* is isolated memory loss. The diagnostic criteria are:
  - Both short-term memory impairment (inability to learn new information) and long-term memory impairment (inability to remember information that was known in the past) are the predominant clinical features.
  - No clouding of consciousness, as in delirium and intoxication, or general loss of major intellectual abilities, as in dementia.
  - Evidence, from history, physical examination, or laboratory tests, of a special organic factor that is judged to be etiologically related to the disturbance.
- *Retrograde amnesia* refers to difficulty in recalling events that have occurred in the premorbid period.
- *Anterograde amnesia* implies difficulty in registering new information.
- *Transient global amnesia* is characterized by sudden onset of severe anterograde amnesia from which the patient usually recovers in a few hours except for the memory gap for the duration of the attack.

Pathomechanisms. The exact mechanism if not clear but some of the known pathomechanisms of drug-induced memory disturbances are as follows:

- The basal forebrain cholinergic system plays an important role in memory. Patients with Alzheimer's disease often show degeneration of central cholinergic system. Anticholinergic drugs are known to impair memory.
- Drug-induced seizures may be followed by an amnesic syndrome. Status epilepticus was followed by amnesia in two patients with theophylline-induced seizures (O'Riordan et al 1993).
- The hippocampi, essential for episodic memory function, are targets of MDMA neurotoxicity in experimental animals (Green et al 1995).
- Glucocorticoids whether administered or generated in response to stress have been shown to have an adverse effect on the rodent brain, particularly in the hippocampus, a structure vital to learning and memory and also a location of high concentration of receptors for glucocorticoids (Sapolsky 1996). Hippocampal atrophy has been attributed to glucocorticoid overproduction in patients with Cushing's syndrome and posttraumatic stress disorder. these observations imply that high-dose corticosteroid therapy can produce hippocampal atrophy in humans and explains the memory impairment.
- Dopaminergic mechanisms are possibly involved in morphine-induced memory impairment. The interaction between the non-competitive NMDA receptor antagonist MK-801 and morphine in memory consolidation as well as the involvement of dopamine mechanisms in this interaction has been studied in mice (Cestari and Castellano 1997). Memory consolidation impairment exerted by MK-801 was potentiated by the administration of the a D_1 dopamine receptor antagonist. Administration of a dose of MK-801, ineffective by itself, potentiated the memory impairment exerted by morphine. Similar ineffective doses of a D_1 DA receptor agonist antagonized the impairment of memory consolidation produced by MK-801 and morphine in combination, suggesting the involvement of dopaminergic mechanisms.
- Calcium channel-mediated processes are involved in immediate memory recall. Lanthanum chloride, a calcium channel antagonist, has been shown to induce a transient loss of memory retrieval in day-old chicks (Summers et al 1996). There is, however, no convincing evidence of memory impairment caused by calcium channel blockers used clinically for the treatment of hypertension.
- Memory storage is believed to be initiated by neuronal transmission increasing Ca^{2+} influx via NMDA receptors. The key phenomenon is long term potentiation (LTP) which is an electrophysiological manifestation of a long-lasting increase in the strength neuronal synapse that has been stimulated in an appropriate fashion. The main evidence supporting LTP as a memory mechanism is the blocking of hippocampal NMDA receptors by 2-amino-5-phosphonopentanoate which prevents spatial learning in rodents (Morris et al 1987). Gene targeting approaches for the study of memory and learning suggest that hippocampal long

term depression (LTD) could be the basis for memory storage (Tonegawa 1994). LTD is similar to LTP in that it depends on NMDA receptors and Ca^{2+} influx but it is a long-lasting reduction of synaptic efficacy. Reduced dorsal hippocampal glutamate release has been shown to correlate significantly with the spatial memory deficits produced by benzodiazepines and ethanol in a rat model of amnesia (Shimizu et al 1998).

– GABA is a major inhibitory neurotransmitter in the brain. The classical BDZs potentiate GABA-stimulated chloride flux (Ramaekers 1998). The mechanism of benzodiazepine-induced amnesia is discussed in the following section.

Drug-induced amnesia as a tool for memory research. Drug-induced amnesia has implications for cognitive neuropsychological investigations of memory. Healthy volunteers were enrolled in a double-blind placebo-controlled study to evaluate the amnestic effects of orally administered lorazepam (Mac et al 1985). The subjects were tested for immediate and delayed recall, using a word recall memory task. The subjects taking lorazepam did not differ from subjects receiving placebo on immediate recall. However, the delayed recall scores of lorazepam subjects were significantly lower compared to the placebo group The effects of lorazepam on encoding, remembering and awareness have been assessed in a study on healthy volunteers (Curran et al 1995). Drug-induced deficits at encoding persisted regardless of the level at which information was initially processed.

Cholinergic drugs have been used as tools to manipulate the functional state of the cerebral cortex based on the theory that cholinergic system controls the functional state of the cortex (Warburton and Rusted 1993). Cholinergic blockage by scopolamine impairs performance on tasks involving sustained and selective attention. It also reduces the working memory capacity and argues for a cholinergic modulation of a common, resource-limited, information processing system.

Quinolinic acid, a NMDA receptor agonist, has been infused into the cerebral ventricles of rats and produced a short-term working memory deficit in the T-maze (alternation) but no change in reversal

learning in the same test (Misztal et al 1996). The working memory deficit in the T-maze was progressive and persisted for at least for 3 weeks after the termination of the infusion. Histological examination revealed a modest decrease in the number of cells in the nucleus basalis magnocellularis but not in the striatum, entorhinal cortex, or hippocampus. Subchronic infusion of quinolinic acid may serve as a model of progressive deterioration of cognitive functions.

Epidemiology. No figures are available about the incidence of drug-induced amnesia. Attempts to design studies for determining the incidence of memory disturbances are problematic because is not a unitary phenomenon within cognitive disorders and tests of neuropsychologic function may vary as a function of sensitivity and selectivity among tests of similar functions (Meador 1998). Various clinical variable that affect the results are drug dosage, blood levels, underlying disease, comedications, clinical response and age of the patient.

Drugs have been reported to be the primary cause or contribute to cognitive impairment in 10% of the patients evaluated for dementia (Larson et al 1987). The risks are increased by polypharmacy, with relative odds increasing from 2.7 with two or three drugs to 9.3 with four or five drugs and to 13.7 with more than six drugs.

Prevention. The following are general measures for prevention of drug-induced memory problems:

– Avoidance of drugs known to cause memory disturbances if possible
– Avoidance of polypharmacy
– Careful use of psychotropic drugs in the elderly subjects

Management. Discontinuation of the medication causing memory disturbance is usually sufficient and the patient may recover spontaneously. Memory training exercises may accelerate the recovery but there are no controlled studies in patients with drug-induced memory disturbances.

Benzodiazepine overdose can produce severe amnesia due to sedative and hypnotic effects. Flumazenil, a competitive benzodiazepine antagonist, is indicated in the management, but its role in the routine reversal of endoscopic conscious sedation has not been defined (Kankaria et al 1996).

The use of antidotes is anticholinergic-induced memory deficits is somewhat tricky because these are neurotransmitter specific. Amphetamine can reduce the sedative effect of scopolamine but makes the memory deficits worse. Scopolamine-induced memory deficits can be ameliorated by anticholinesterase physostigmine but not by a benzodiazepine antagonist (Preston et al 1989).

Drugs that Impair Memory

Memory impairment has been reported with the drugs shown in Table 5.15.

Anesthesia

Memory impairment has been assessed in children following the two most common variants of general anesthesia—fluothane and ketamine (Egorov et al 1996). Impairment of long-term memory persisted for 2 weeks after fluothane anesthesia and for 1–2 months after ketamine anesthesia but was reversible.

Antineoplastic Agents

Various drugs used for treatment of cancer can directly affect the CNS and cause acute as well as chronic cognitive disturbances. Examples of these treatment are cytokines and chemotherapy.

Cytokines. Interferon-α and interleukin-2 are known to produce cognitive disturbances. Memory disturbances are a part of interferon-α-induced interferon syndrome (see Neurobase article on drug-induced dementia). Duration of therapy is an important determinant of cognitive effects of cognitive effects of interferon-α. One study, impairment of learning, recall of verbal material and efficiency of cognitive processing were impaired in patients with chronic myelogenous leukemia, who were treated with interferon-α for 6 months (Pavol et al 1995).

Table 5.15. Pharmaceuticals reported to impair memory.

Alcohol
Anesthesia: fluothane and ketamine
Antineoplastic agents
  – cytokines
  – intrathecal chemotherapy
Anticholinergic drugs
Antidepressants
Antihypertensives
Antiepileptic drugs
Antiparkinsonian drugs
Baclofen (Lee et al 1992).
Benzodiazepines
  – alprazolam
  – clorazepate
  – diazepam
  – lorazepam
  – triazolam
Beta-blockers and similar drugs
  – atenolol
  – propafenone
Corticosteroids
Drug abuse
  – amphetamine dependence
  – marijuana
  – MDMA (ecstasy)
Gonadotropin-releasing hormone agonist
Hypnotics
  – barbiturates
  – zolpidem
Iohexol: contrast medium for cerebral angiography
Lithium
Mefloquine
Non-steroidal anti-inflammatory drugs
  – ibuprofen
  – naproxen
Opioid analgesics

Chemotherapy. Seventy-five percent of patients with breast cancer who received chemotherapy consisting of cyclophosphamide, methotrexate and 5-fluorouracil was found to perform 2 standard deviations below expectation on at least one of the measures of information processing speed, memory and visuospatial functioning (Wienke and Dienst 1995). Childhood survivors of lymphoblastic leukemia who have been treated with intrathecal chemotherapy have shown memory deficits on Wide Range Assessment of Memory and learning Test as compared to matched controls without cancer (Hill et al 1997). Deficits were mostly in visual-spatial tasks whereas verbal learning range was normal.

Anticholinergic Drugs

Several drugs with anticholinergic properties are used in medical practice. Symptoms of the "anticholinergic syndrome" (see Chapter 18) produced by these drugs include confusion, impaired memory, delirium, hallucinations and psychosis. Anticholinergics impair memory retrieval, especially free recall. Atropine is the classical drug of this series and is known to impair memory in normal subjects which can be reversed by physostigmine. Scopolamine has been shown to impair working memory in healthy volunteers (Rusted and Warburton 1988). Even over-the counter H_1 antihistaminics, which have anticholinergic effects, can impair cognitive performance. Other cholinergic drugs such as benzotropine used in the treatment of Parkinson's disease can impair memory (Van Putten et al 1987). In a double-blind cross-over study, patients receiving amantadine performed better on memory tests than those receiving trihexyphenidyl for drug-induced extrapyramidal symptoms (Fayen et al 1988). There was an inverse correlation between ventricular size and memory indicating that patients with brain pathology are more susceptible to memory-disrupting effect of trihexyphenidyl. Elderly patients are particularly susceptible to loss of memory while on anticholinergic drugs (Molloy and Brooymans 1989). Cholinergic drugs improve memory in Alzheimer's disease whereas anticholinergic drugs aggravate it.

Antidepressants

Depression is a cause of cognitive impairments and antidepressants generally reduce cognitive deficits. The available evidence suggests that antidepressants can have a negative impact on memory functions both directly and indirectly. One difficulty in evaluating these studies is that depression *per se* has a negative effect on memory processes. Amitriptyline, mianserin, and trazodone have been reported to have an effect on a range of cognitive processes including memory. Detrimental effect of these drugs on memory is more marked following acute administration

and the effects wear off with prolonged use. Because relief of depression improves memory, the adverse effect on memory in patients is less marked than that observed in healthy volunteers during short-term administration.

The central cholinergic effects of tricyclic antidepressantsare the primary cause of cognitive effects in these agents. Compounds with anticholinergic effects such as amitriptyline have a more pronounced effect on long-term memory than on short-term memory. In healthy elderly subjects, amitriptyline has been shown to disrupt verbal recall and produces noticeable and significant impairment of cognition and psychomotor function, whereas moclobemide is relatively free from these adverse effects (Hindmarch and Kerr 1992). This is due to selective MAOI action and lack of anticholinergic effects of moclobemide (Allain et al 1992). In a placebo-controlled study evaluating choice reaction time and short-term memory, amitriptyline, mianserin and trazodone produced a significant impairment but bupropion, fluoxetine, sertraline and paroxetine did not (Hindmarch 1990).

Newer compounds such as fluoxetine (a selective serotonin reuptake inhibitor) are devoid of anticholinergic effects and usually do not impair memory. However, Bangs et al (1994) have described a 14-year-old male patient who complained of memory problems during treatment with fluoxetine for major depression. The patient showed impairments on all five scales of the Wechsler Memory Scale-Revised during fluoxetine treatment. Three of the scales, Verbal Memory, Visual Memory, and General Memory, showed statistically significant improvements after fluoxetine was discontinued. This case represents the first time memory deficits related to fluoxetine were quantitated with a standardized memory test. It points to cognitive side effects that need to be understood.

Antiepileptic Drugs

Because AEDs reduce neuronal irritability, it is suspected that they may reduce neuronal excitability and impair cognitive function. Most of the cognitive effects of AEDs are dose-related.

Assessment of effects of AEDs on cognitive function, however, is a controversial issue because of problems of subject selection, genetic factors, statistical difficulties, choice of cognitive tests, and the impact of seizures on psychological performance. Evaluation of memory function in most studies is limited and where effects are recorded they are possibly secondary to changes in the level of attention or speed of mental processing. Long-term phenobarbital therapy induces a significant impairment in learning ability (Calandre et al 1990). Randomized, double-blind, crossover studies in patients and healthy volunteers have shown moderately greater cognitive effects for phenobarbital compared to other AEDs but no significant differences between phenytoin, carbamazepine and valproate (Meador et al 1990; Meador et al 1991; Craig and Tallis 1994). Few cognitive side effects have been reported in studies of newer AEDs.

Antihypertensive Medications

A number of centrally acting antihypertensive drugs have been alleged to impair memory among other cognitive and neuropsychiatric effects. Because hypertension *per se* produces cognitive changes, it is difficult to evaluate these reports. In a pilot study, verbal memory impairment was present in hypertensive and normotensive patients taking methyldopa or propranolol (a β-adrenergic receptor blocker), while hypertensive patients receiving only a diuretic did not show this effect (Solomen et al 1983). Fisher (1992) reported the case of an elderly women who developed an amnestic syndrome as an adverse reaction to propranolol. At its height, the clinical picture resembled that of Alzheimer's disease.

Antiparkinsonian Drugs

Mental slowness (bradyphrenia) has been considered to be a feature of Parkinson's disease and has been linked to mesocorticolimbic dopamine deficiency and to respond to levodopa therapy.

Poewe et al (1991) have shown that levodopa can adversely affect the high-speed memory scanning in Parkinson's disease patients, possibly as a result of dopaminergic stimulation, thus questioning the concept of dopaminergic deficiency as a cause of bradyphrenia. Variations in plasma dopamine level associated with "wearing off" phenomenon in levodopa-carbidopa treated patients with Parkinson's disease can produce a state-dependent memory impairment, i. e., the recall occurs under the same circumstances in which the encoding takes place (Huber et al 1989).

There are several new antiparkinsonian drugs which have minimal neuropsychiatric side effects. Among the older medications, anticholinergic drugs are still in use for these patients. Administration of trihexyphenidyl chronically to patients with Parkinson's disease was shown to cause a decrease in performance on recent but not immediate memory tests (Koller 1984).

Benzodiazepines (BZD)

BZDs are used for a number of indications besides their use as hypnotics. An example of this is alprazolam which has been used as an anxiolytic in minor surgical procedures but it produces memory impairment at the dosages necessary to produce clinically significant anxiolysis during oral surgery (Coldwell et al 1997).

Pathophysiology of BZD-Induced Amnesia. Drugs of this category affect the encoding stage of memory by disturbing attention and impair the transference of material from the short-term storage to long-term memory. Another possible mechanism is that long-term memory deficit could be the result of failure of memory consolidation during rapid sleep onset. A neuroanatomical/neurophysiological model based on 3-stage concept of memory has been proposed to explain the selective effect of BZD on memory function (Barbee et al 1992). Neuroanatomically, the subcortical structures appear to play an important role in the consolidation of newly learned information. Pharmacologically BZD potentiate the effect of GABA, a major inhibitory neurotransmitter. GABA facilitation is likely to impair the function of these structures in the consolidation process. At a neurophysiological level, the disruption of consolidation that occurs in these structures may be mediated through the effect of GABA on LTP, a phenomenon in which relatively short periods of electrical stimulation result in enduring changes in the synaptic efficiency. Thus BZD, as GABA agonists, may impair LTP and cause deficits both in the acquisition and retention of information through their immediate and long-term effects upon consolidation.

In long-term administration of BZD, the acquisition phase of the memory may be affected and delayed recall may be impaired for the material learned during the intoxication period. BZD dependence in the elderly can cause memory impairment which can persist into the early drug-free period (Rummans et al 1993). Amnestic effects of BZD are mediated by the BZD receptor and can be blocked by specific BZD receptor antagonists in the animals model (Gamzu 1987).

Frequency and severity of cognitive resulting from use of BZDs has been correlated with pharmacokinetic and pharmacodynamic factors. Elimination half-life, receptor binding affinity, effects on the locus coeruleus-norepinephrine and hypothalamic-pituitary-adrenal axis, and the interaction of these factors appear to be the major determinants of frequency and severity of these untoward reactions (Vgontzas et al 1995).

Triazolam. This is a short-acting BZD and has been most in the news because of its adverse neuropsychiatric effects which have led to its ban in some countries. Some of the anecdotal reports are:
- Travellers' amnesia—transient global amnesia secondary to triazolam (Morris and Estes 1987). Three neuroscientist who took triazolam to minimize jet lag suffered this complication but they had also imbibed alcoholic drinks. The role of triazolam as a cause of amnesia is difficult to assess in these cases.
- Triazolam syndrome in the elderly (Patterson 1987). Five elderly patients suffered a syndrome characterized by reversible delirium, anterograde amnesia, and automatic movements causally associated with triazolam used as a hypnotic.

- Triazolam, handwriting, and amnestic state— 2 cases (Boatwright 1987). These individuals negotiated and signed complicated agreements after the use of triazolam and had no recollection of the events afterwards. There was no change in handwriting.
- Triazolam-induced nocturnal binging with amnesia (Menkes 1992).
- Anterograde amnesia in triazolam overdose despite use of flumazenil (Hung et al 1992).

The following studies have also been reported:
- Juhl et al (1984): Next day anterograde amnesia was more frequent in the flurazepam than in the triazolam group.
- Bixler et al (1991). Double-blind parallel group study of triazolam versus temazepam/ placebo. Next day impairment of memory was seen only in triazolam group in 5 out of 6 subjects.
- Kirk et al (1990). Double-blind, balanced, cross-over study of effects of placebo, triazolam, and pentobarbital. Both triazolam and pentobarbital quantitatively impaired the acquisitional processes involved in short-term recall.

Rothschild (1992) reviewed the literature on adverse effects of triazolam and remarked that there were no adequately controlled studies to show that triazolam was associated with memory problems any more than other BZD.

Lorazepam. This is an intermediate-acting BZD used intravenously to induce preoperative anterograde amnesia. Placebo-controlled studies on healthy subjects have shown that oral doses of lorazepam produced an anterograde amnesia (Scharf et al 1983; Curran et al 1987). Other studies in human volunteers have shown that lorazepam produces dose-related deficits in verbal secondary memory (Preston et al 1988) and impairment of information acquisition and recall (Shader et al 1986). File et al (1992) reported that memory impairment with lorazepam was independent of increased sedation. In contrast to deficits in episodic memory with sedatives, there were no lorazepam-induced impairments on tests of semantic memory.

Clorazepate. This is a long-acting BZD and no

significant impairment of immediate or delayed recall was found in geriatric patients (Scharf et al 1985).

Diazepam. This is an anxiolytic BZD. Acute administration of diazepam is known to produce anterograde amnesia for both verbal and visual information. Intravenous diazepam impairs free recall significantly in a dose-dependent manner (Anthenelli et al 1991).

β-*Blockers and Similar Drugs*

Lipophilic β-blockers such as propranolol are known to cause cognitive impairment. Hydrophilic β-blockers such as atenolol can also cause neuropsychiatric side effects. Drugs with structural similarities to β-blocker agents can also produce neurological adverse effects.

Atenolol. There is one case report of a hypertensive man who developed memory impairment after 14 year therapy with atenolol (Ramanathan 1996). Other causes of memory impairment were ruled out and atenolol was replaced with amiloride/hydrochlorthiazide combination. One month later the patient showed 75% recovery, thus confirming atenolol as the cause of memory impairment.

Propafenone is an antiarrhythmic drug with structural similarities to β-blocker agents. Reported CNS effects include seizures, psychoses, confusion, dizziness, ataxia, headaches, tremor and depression. Five anecdotal cases of memory disturbances have been reported to the manufacturer. One case of transient global amnesia has been published (Jones et al 1995).

Corticosteroids

Endogenous steroids also modulate memory processes (McGaugh 1989). Dexamethasone administration to normal volunteers has been shown to lead to increase of intrusion errors and decreased free recall (Wolkowitz et al 1993). These changes in memory were correlated with decrease of serum cortisol, plasma ACTH, noradrenaline, beta endorphin, and somatostatin.

Chronic treatment with corticosteroid can produce neuropsychiatric disturbances and can produce memory disturbance during treatment of patients with systemic diseases without brain lesions. Pulsed methylprednisolone has been shown to induce reversible impairment of memory in patients with relapsing-remitting multiple sclerosis (Olivieri et al 1998).

Drug Abuse

Abuse of recreational drugs is associated with memory impairment. Some examples are.

Amphetamine. Drugs are this category are associated with cerebral vasculitis and intracerebral as well as subarachnoid hemorrhage. Cognitive function impairment in illicit amphetamine users has been tested by a neuropsychological test battery (Wechsler Memory Scale-revised) and severity of amphetamine dependence was found to be associated with poor performance on memory as well as attention/concentration indices (McKetin and Mattick 1997).

MDMA (Ecstasy). This is an amphetamine derivative which has become increasingly popular as a recreational drug in recent years and is assumed to be relatively safe. There are several reports of neuropsychiatric disturbances as well as cerebral infarctions following MDMA use. Review of various disturbances includes reports of memory disturbances (McCann et al 1996). One case is reported of a pure amnestic syndrome in a young women who had taken no other drugs except MDMA (Spatt et al 1997). Two months after the event she still had retrograde amnesia for about a week and anterograde memory problems. MRI three weeks after the onset showed bilateral hyperintensity lesions in the globus pallidus and these lesions partially disappeared at 2 months following the acute episode.

Marijuana. Several studies have examined the residual effects of cannabis on neuropsychological performance. In one study on college students, heavy users displayed significantly greater impairment that light users on attentional/executive function as evidenced by reduced learning and recall of visual and visuospatial information (Pope and Yurgelun-Todd 1996). The question as to whether this impairment is due to a residue of the drug in the brain, withdrawal effect from the drug or a direct neurotoxic effect of the drug, remains unanswered. Functional brain imaging can show altered brain function after marijuana but the regions showing these abnormalities have not been localized.

Gonadotropin-Releasing Hormone Agonist

GnRH-a treatment is used for women with endometriosis and infertility. Its effect on memory has been assessed in a randomized prospective study (Newton et al 1996). Moderate to marked impairment of perceived memory functioning was reported by 44% of women. Prospective memory was most affected and withdrawal of GnRH-a treatment resulted in a return to normal memory functioning. Memory disturbances were temporary and were considered likely a result of rapid estrogen depletion.

Hypnotics

Barbiturates as well as non-barbiturate hypnotics affect memory. There is a dose-dependent selective impairment of input encoding processes required for memory tasks in daily human activity. This has been shown for secobarbital (Rundell et al 1978) and for methaqualone (Smith et al 1988).

Zolpidem is a non-benzodiazepine hypnotic of the imidazopyridine class. It acts by modulation of a subunit of $GABA_A$ receptor chloride channel macromolecular complex. Reported CNS adverse effects include cognitive impairment, confusion. psychoses and vertigo. Two cases have been reported or amnesia of events which occurred following ingestion of normal doses of the drug as a hypnotic (Canaday 1996). Both patients had been awakened at night and had prolonged telephone conversations but had no recollection of these the following morning.

Iohexol

Brady et al (1993) reported two patients who developed transient global amnesia after cerebral angiography with iohexol used as a contrast medium. In both of the patients the procedure was performed by catheter technique under local anesthesia. Both of them had minor transient neurological disturbances but amnesia persisted for a day in each case. This is a rare occurrence and the pathomechanism is not known.

Lithium

Lithium has been implicated in the impairment of short-term memory (STM), long-term memory (LTM), and inability to transfer information from the STM to the LTM (Reus et al 1979). However, when variable such as serum lithium levels, psychopathology, age of patient, and physical illnesses of the patient are controlled, no association was noted between memory function and duration of treatment with lithium (Ghadirian et al 1983). Ananth et al (1987) reviewed systemic clinical studies suggesting memory and cognitive impairment in patients suffering from unipolar and bipolar disorders as well as in healthy subjects. A number of studies failed to demonstrate lithium-induced memory deficits. Methodological and design problems were noted in several studies. Use of prospective studies to test the effect of lithium on memory using refined memory tests was emphasized. Shaw et al (1987) used an off-on design and administered a battery of psychological tests to outpatients with affective disorders in remission, both during lithium treatment and blind placebo substitutions. These authors reported a significant detrimental effect on memory and motor speed. Performance improved after discontinuation of lithium and declined after reintroduction of lithium. In view of this controversy, Engelsman et al (1992) have discussed the difficulties inherent in blind studies and in matched group designs, examining the effect of lithium on memory. They pointed out the advantages of a prospective within-subject design with repeated testing in which patients serve as their own control. There are no published results of such a study.

Nonsteroidal Antiinflammatory Drugs

Various forms of cognitive dysfunction, e. g., memory deficit and inability to concentrate, have been associated with NSAID use in retrospective studies involving ibuprofen and naproxen. This topic is controversial because some epidemiological studies also support the view that NSAIDs may have a protective role in Alzheimer's disease (Morgan and Clark 1998).

Drug-Induced Dementia

The Committee on Geriatrics of the Royal College of Physicians of the United Kingdom (1981) defined dementia as "a global impairment of higher cortical functions, including memory, the capacity to solve the problems of everyday living, the performance of learned perceptual motor skills and the correct use of social skills and the control of emotional reactions, in the absence of gross clouding of consciousness. DSM-IV diagnostic criteria for substance-induced persisting dementia are shown in Table 5.16.

Various terms have been used to describe dementia associated with drugs—usually according to the name of the drug, e. g., valproic acid (or valproate)-induced dementia, Dilantin (phenytoin) dementia and interferon dementia which is a part of interferon syndrome (see Chapter 3). Drug-induced dementias also come under the broad category of pseudodementias to differentiate them from dementia associated with degenerative neurological disorders and also under the category of reversible dementias implying that the manifestations improve following discontinuation of the offending drug. Dementia is the most severe form of cognitive deficit and is sometimes referred to as brain failure. Drug-induced dementia has no characteristic features except in the situations where it is accompanied by other drug-induced symptoms. Anticholinergic drugs used to treat parkinsonism may mimic or exacerbate the clinical signs of Alzheimer's disease.

Epidemiology. No definite epidemiological

Table 5.16. Diagnostic criteria for substance-induced persisting dementia.

A. The development of multiple cognitive deficits manifested by both
   (1) memory impairment (impaired ability to learn new information or to recall previously learned information)
   (2) one or more of these cognitive disturbances
      (a) aphasia (language disturbance)
      (b) apraxia (impaired ability to carry out motor activities despite intact motor function)
      (c) agnosia (failure to recognize or identify objects despite intact sensory function)
      (d) disturbances in executive functioning (i. e., planning, organization, sequencing, abstracting)

B. The cognitive deficits in criteria A1 and A2 each cause significant impairment in social or occupational functioning and represent a significant decline from a previous level of functioning.

C. The deficits do not occur exclusively during the course of a delirium and persist beyond the usual duration of substance intoxication or withdrawal.

D. There is evidence from the history, physical examination, or laboratory findings that the deficits are etiologically related to the persisting effects of substance intoxication or withdrawal.

studies are available for the incidence or prevalence of drug-induced dementia. In a review of 516 cases in literature, toxic effect of medications accounted for 2.7% of the cases whereas cerebral atrophies (including Alzheimer's disease and unknown causes) constituted 52.1% of the cases (Mumenthaler 1987).

Pathomechanism of Drug-Induced Dementia. Drugs may induce dementia by a number of different mechanisms only a few of which are understood. Some of basic mechanisms are (Starr and Whalley 1994):
- Anticholinergic drugs block the cholinergic neurotransmission and produce a condition similar to dementia of Alzheimer's disease
- Noradrenergic transmission is also important for cognitive function. Antihypertensive drugs adversely affecty cognitive function through central noradrenergic system.
- Impairment of calcium and intracellular messenger systems. Neurotransmitter release is calcium-dependent. Calcium channel block-

ers can have an inhibitory influence on neurotransmission. Protein kinase C (PKC) is a calcium dependent enzyme which is inhibited by lithium.

- Increased permeability of the blood brain barrier (BBB). Cyclosporine, by increasing BBB permeability, may explain the aluminum-induced dementia in a renal transplant patient (Bertoli et al 1988).
- Modification of cytokine action. IL-2 has an adverse effect on cognition. It may act by the following mechanisms:
  · by increasing the BBB permeability
  · activation of inappropriate central neuropeptidergic systems that impair memory
  · direct neurotoxic effect
- Binding to high affinity sites of GABA$_A$ receptors. Benzodiazepine-induced cognitive impairment may be by this mechanism. GABA$_A$ is the main cortical inhibitory neurotransmitter activating chloride channels. This mechanism, therefore involves several cognitive domains producing global cognitive impairment as compared with anticholinergics which produce selective deficits of attention and memory.

Apart from pharmacological and toxic effects, therapeutic materials may cause transmission of Creutzfeldt-Jakob disease, a neurogenerative dementing condition. This will be discussed later in this section.

Drugs that Induce Dementia

All the drugs which cause cognitive impairment and severe loss of memory can lead to dementia. Drug-induced dementia should be differentiated from the degenerative dementias such as that of Alzheimer's disease. Most of the drug-induced dementias are reversible if the medication is discontinued. However, if the medications cause a structural lesion, dementia may not be reversible. Medications may also aggravate a moderate degree of pre-existing cerebral insufficiency and result in a demented state. Another important differential diagnosis is from delirium which also results in cognitive impairment with impairment of level of consciousness whereas consciousness is not impaired in dementia.

Table 5.17. Drugs associated with dementia.

Anticholinergic drugs
Antihypertensives
Antiepileptics
Antipsychotics (neuroleptics)
Benzodiazepines
Corticosteroids
Cytokines: interferons and interleukins
Desferoxamine
Drugs associated with iatrogenic Creutzfeldt-Jakob disease (see Table 5.18)
Tryptophan: eosinophilia myalgia syndrome (Armstrong et al 1997)

Drugs are the leading cause of dementia in the elderly (Lowenthal and Nadeau 1991). Adverse drug reactions are commonly associated with global cognitive impairment (dementia) in elderly persons on polypharmacy (Larson et al 1987). Drugs reported to be associated with dementia are shown in Table 5.17.

Anticholinergic Drugs

Anticholinergic drugs are known to impair cognitive function. In one study patients with probable Alzheimer's disease showed deterioration at serum levels of anticholinergic drugs which caused no impairment in psychogeriatric patients without dementia (Thienhaus et al 1990). Anticholinergic drugs used to treat parkinsonism may mimic or exacerbate the clinical signs of Alzheimer's disease and should be withdrawn if such a situation arises (Kurlan and Como 1988). In a comparative study of anticholinergics alone, in combination with levodopa, and levodopa alone, it was shown that there was deterioration of mental function in patients treated with anticholinergics, alone or in combination, whereas patients treated with levodopa did not show any decline of mental function. Nishiyama et al (1993) reported five cases of chronic dementia in patients with Parkinson's who had been treated for over 6 months with anticholinergic drugs and had no other adverse reactions. All these patients improved after discontinuation of anticholinergics and the improvement was documented by neuropsychological testing as well as SPECT and PET scans. In another investigation benzhexol (anticholinergic drug) was shown to aggravate memory impairment in patients with Parkinson's disease (Miller et al 1987).

Pathomechanism. Anticholinergic drugs block the cholinergic neurotransmission and produce a condition similar to dementia of Alzheimer's disease. Long-term anticholinergic therapy in patients with Parkinson's disease causes intellectual impairment which is correlated with bilateral diffuse glucose hypometabolism demonstrated by PET (Nishiyama et al 1995).

Acetylcholinesterase (ACh) inhibitors should theoretically benefit dementia and this is the basis of most of the therapeutic agents currently available for treatment of Alzheimer's disease— a condition in which there is damage to cholinergic pathways. AChE inhibitors may decrease the cholinergic tone as a delayed effect which can be exacerbated by stress and this may disrupt cognition (Kaufer et al 1998). Both stress and AChE inhibitors increase the postsynaptic concentration of calcium in the cytosol. This causes a rapid induction of the transcription factor c-Fos. This has been offered as an explanation of neuropsychological features of the "Gulf War syndrome" in soldiers who were given AChE inhibitors as prophylactic against some of the poisonous war gases under stressful conditions.

Antihypertensive Drugs

Two important categories of drugs for this purpose are calcium channel blockers and adrenergic antagonists. Noradrenergic transmission is also important for cognitive function. Antihypertensive drugs adversely affect cognitive function through central noradrenergic system. Calcium channel blockers can have an inhibitory influence on neurotransmission by impairment of calcium and intracellular messenger systems. Neurotransmitter release is calcium-dependent.

Antiepileptic Drugs

Valproic acid. Reversible valproic acid (VPA)-induced dementia in a patient with epilepsy has been reported (Zaret and Cohen 1986). Three pathomechanisms were proposed to explain this:
1. A direct toxic effect of valproic acid on the CNS.
2. An indirect CNS toxic effect mediated by valproic acid-induced hyperammonemia.
3. A paradoxical epileptogenic effect secondary to valproic acid.

Reversible VPA-induced pseudoatrophy of the brain. Several cases of cerebral atrophy have been reported in patients on VPA treatment. One case of pseudoatrophy of the brain, documented by CT and accompanied by cognitive deficits, occurred in a patients who had been on VPA therapy (McLachlan 1987). Within two weeks of discontinuation of valproic acid and its substitution by carbamazepine, the neuropsychological functions of the patient improved and CT scan done four months later showed no abnormality. Reversible cerebral atrophy documented by radiologic correlates was reported in a case of valproate-induced parkinsonism-dementia syndrome (Shin et al 1992). An 10-year old girl developed dementia and cerebral atrophy documented by MRI after two years of VPA therapy (Guerrini et al 1998). Her condition improved after discontinuation of VPA. The relation between valproate, brain atrophy and dementia is likely to be exceedingly complex and no explanation of the pathomechanism was offered in two children who developed dementia and atrophy during valproate therapy but recovered following discontinuation of the drug (Papazian et al 1995).

Phenytoin. Patients on long-term phenytoin (Dilantin) therapy have been reported to deteriorate intellectually in the absence of any signs of oversedation, a condition termed Dilantin dementia by Rosen (1968). All of the patients improved after discontinuation of the drug. Phenytoin intoxication of subacute onset may occur in non-epileptic patients who receive phenytoin for cardiac arrhythmias and a case with cerebellar dysfunction and dementia has been reported (Tindall and Willersen 1978). Withdrawal of phenytoin led to slow improvement of the neurological status.

Lamotrigine. Treatment with lamotrigine at a

dose of 100 mg twice daily with serum lamotrigine level of 13.6 mg/l (normal < 4 mg/l) was reported to induce dementia in a 69-year woman (Bouman et al 1997). Discontinuation of lamotrigine lead to recovery and restarting the medication at lower dose (25 mg twice daily) did not produce any recurrence of this adverse effect.

Antipsychotics (Neuroleptics)

Lifetime use of neuroleptics has been considered to be possibly related to reduction of brain density in the posterior areas as determined by CT scan (Lyon et al 1981). A case of dementia with cerebral atrophy was reported in a patient on long-term therapy with multiple neuroleptics was reported by Federico et al (1992). The patient improvement after discontinuation of the drugs. Neuroleptic use has been observed to be associated with more rapid cognitive decline in the following conditions.

- The elderly are more susceptible to this adverse effect because drug metabolism and clearance is slowed down with aging and target cells in the CNS may become more sensitive and vulnerable to drugs due to altered metabolism or cellular loss.
- Carriers of apolipoprotein E e4 allele have a more rapid cognitive decline during antipsychotic therapy as compared to patients without this allele (Holmes et al 1997).
- A two-year prospective, longitudinal study has shown that patients with dementia have a more rapid cognitive decline while on antipsychotic therapy (McShane et al 1997). In other words, antipsychotic therapy given to manage the behavioral of dementia accelerates the progression of dementia.
- Multi-infarct dementia. Repetitive sharp EEG discharges, reversible upon withdrawal of neuroleptic drugs, are reported in clinical multi-infarct dementia (van Sweden 1984). The EEG changes have been correlated with dysfunction of the adrenergic transmission.
- Previous leucotomy. Welch (1993) has reported a case of dementia following neuroleptic malignant syndrome (NMS) in an elderly patient who has previous electroconvulsive ther-

apy and bilateral leucotomy. The IQ was, however, normal before the development of NMS. NMS is usually not accompanied by dementia (see Chapter 23). Dementia persisted after resolution of NMS. It was postulated that bilateral leucotomy involving destruction of subcortical structures may have predisposed the patient to dementia.

Benzodiazepines (BZD)

Benzodiazepine-induced cognitive impairment may occur by binding of BZDs to high affinity sites of $GABA_A$ receptors. $GABA_A$ is the main cortical inhibitory neurotransmitter activating chloride channels. This mechanism, therefore involves several cognitive domains producing global cognitive impairment as compared with anticholinergics which produce selective deficits of attention and memory.

Corticosteroids

Steroid-induced psychosis is well recognized but steroid-induced impairment of cognitive function is rare. Corticosteroid-induced dementia has been described in six patients all of whom recovered after discontinuation of the corticosteroids (Varney et al 1984). Four of these patients never showed symptoms of steroid psychosis; the remaining two continued to show steroid dementia well after their steroid psychosis had resolved.

Cytokines

Cytokines, particularly interleukin-2 (IL-2) and interferon-α are associated with neuropsychiatric disturbances when given systemically. Meyers and Yung (1993) have reported a patient treated with intraventricular IL-2 for leptomeningeal disease who developed progressive cognitive dysfunction. The deterioration started 3 months post-treatment and worsened over the ensuing 4 years to develop into a subcortical dementia. MRI showed white matter changes that were not present before the treatment with IL-2.

Five out of 38 patients (13%) with metastatic renal cell carcinoma were reported to develop dementia 3 weeks to 13 months after the start of treatment with recombinant interferon-α-C (Merimsky et al 1990). Paraneoplastic changes, metastatic spread to the brain and other causes of dementia were ruled out. No cerebral atrophy was seen on CT scan and discontinuation of treatment led to improvement of mental status. Dementia in these cases was considered to be possibly due to neurotoxic effect of interferon. The mode of action of interferon on the CNS is not fully understood (see Chapter 3). Possible mechanisms include competition on the membrane receptors with neurotropic hormones. Meyers et al (1993) examined the neurological test profiles of 16 patients with chronic myelogenous leukemia treated with interferon-α and found cognitive impairments consistent with the diagnosis of subcortical dementia.

Pathomechanism. Cytokines are being used increasingly in therapeutics. Interleukins and interferons are considered to have neurotoxic effects. Possible mechanisms include competition on the membrane receptors with neurotropic hormones. The pathomechanisms of CNS toxicity of cytokines may involve possible direct interaction of these proteins at level of the circumventricular organs (area postrema, hypothalmic neurosecretory centers, vascular organ of the lamina terminalis) but appears unlikely to be on cortical neurons. IL-2 has an adverse effect on cognition. It may act by the following mechanisms:
- By increasing the BBB permeability
- Activation of inappropriate central neuropeptidergic systems that impair memory
- Direct neurotoxic effect

Desferoxamine

This chelating agent has been found to be useful for treatment of aluminum intoxication as a complication of renal failure. Desferoxamine has been reported to precipitate dialysis dementia in patients with chronic renal failure (Sherrard et al 1988). The pathomechanism is not known but patients are at high risk for development of this complication if they demonstrate very high levels of aluminum either before or after the standard desferoxamine infusion test. Direct desferoxamine CNS toxicity is unlikely but desferoxamine-aluminum complex has a relatively low molecular weight and may cross the BBB more readily than the naturally occurring serum aluminum which is bound to serum albumin.

Tryptophan

Eosinophilia myalgia syndrome (EMS) due to a contaminant in tryptophan is described in Chapter 20. A patient with EMS was reported to develop cognitive deficits suggestive of subcortical dementia and high signal lesions in the white matter were demonstrated on MRI (Lynn et al 1992). The patient did not recover despite the discontinuation of tryptophan although there was some improvement with methylprednisone suggesting a role of autoimmune mechanisms in the pathogenesis of this adverse drug reaction.

Iatrogenic Creutzfeldt-Jakob Disease (CJD)

CJD is a transmissible spongiform encephalopathy characterized by a long incubation period which precedes clinical symptoms related to the degeneration of the CNS resulting in dementia. The nature of the etiologic agents prions remains unknown. The prion hypothesis suggests a key role for the host derived protein (the prion protein, PrP) as the transmissible agent. Although supported by numerous experimental data, the prion only hypothesis has not yet been convincingly demonstrated (Dormont 1999).

Various therapeutic procedures that have been reported to be associated with iatrogenic CJD are shown in Table 5.18. These include corneal transplants, dural grafts, neurosurgical instrumentation, stereotactic placement of EEG electrodes, pharmaceutical preparations containing material of bovine origin, and administration of cadaver pituitary-derived human growth hormone (Brown et al 1992).

Human Growth Hormone (hGH). CJD, has been reported following the use of human pitu-

Table 5.18. Therapeutic substances associated with Creutzfeldt-Jakob Disease (CJD).

Transmission of CJD
Human growth hormone from cadaver pituitary
Dural grafts (human)
Corneal grafts (human)
Bovine somatotrophine (equivalent of HGH used in France)*
Pharmaceutical preparations containing bovine material
Blood for transfusion and blood products obtained from patients with CJD

Cause of Creutzfeldt-Jakob-like syndrome
Lithium monotherapy
Lithium combined with the following drugs:
  Chlorpromazine and levomepromazine
  Levodopa
  Lorazepam
  Nortriptyline
  Phenobarbitone
  Trihexyphenidyl

---

*This drug was banned in 1992.

itary-derived growth hormone (Powell-Jackson et al 1985; Mills et al 1990; Markus et al 1992; Zachman 1993). Seven neuropathologically confirmed cases of CJD were detected during epidemiological follow-up of 6284 recipients of hGH in 1991 (Fradkin et al 1991). All seven cases occurred among 700 recipients of hGH before 1970. Contaminated hGH-induced CJD is similar to the iatrogenic transmission of CJD during neurosurgical procedures in the 1970s. The brains of CJD-infected cadavers contain particles of an abnormal form of prion protein which is highly resistant to most common sterilization procedures. A preparation of one batch of hormone requires several thousand pituitary glands, it is not unlikely that a batch could become contaminated. This problem has been eliminated for the future by the current use of recombinant human growth hormone but cases of CJD may still show up years after the treatment with contaminated growth hormone. The United States and United Kingdom banned the use of cadaver-derived pituitary growth hormone in 1985 but France continued to allow the use of the hormone from this source until 1993 provided it had been treated with urea, a procedure known to deactivate the prion. There were cases of CJD in France due to distribution of potentially contaminated after it was forbidden to do so.

Cases of iatrogenic CJD are rare considering the large number of subject treated with hGH. This has been explained by genetic susceptibility to prion infection. Molecular genetic studies in two patients with CJD done by and 10 other cases from literature showed that 9 out of 12 had the valine 129 homozygous genotype (Masson et al 1994). The prevalence of this codon in the general population is only 9%.

Somatotrophine. This is the bovine equivalent of hGH and has been prescribed as intramuscular injection for "tissue repairs" in France since 1951. It has a lipolytic and protein anabolic effect but has no effect on growth. It has been banned as a precautionary measure since 1992. There is one case of new variant of CJD reported in France which might be due to injections of somatotrophine contaminated with bovine spongiform encephalopathy (Verdrager 1998).

Creutzfeldt-Jakob-Like Syndrome

This syndrome is induced by drugs but the symptoms resemble CJD. EEG is also similar to CJD but this returns to normal when the patient recovers. Lithium is the best documented of the drugs which induce this syndrome.

Lithium. Two patients with a syndrome resembling CJD as a result of lithium toxicity were first reported in 1988 (Smith and Kocen 1988). EEG was similar to that seen in CJD and the patients recovered after discontinuation of lithium. Subsequently, 8 more cases have been reported either due to lithium alone or lithium combined with other drugs such as levodopa and nortriptyline (Casanova et al 1996). One case was reported due to a combination of lithium, levopromazine and phenobarbitone (Kikyo and Furukawa 1999).

Lithium can induce dementia by inhibiting protein kinase C which is a calcium-dependent enzyme. It is important to recognize the lithium-induced CJD-like syndrome and to avoid the costly and unnecessary investigative procedures for CJD. This syndrome clears up after discontinuation of lithium.

References

Aaronson DW: Effects of terfenadine on psychomotor performance. Drug Safety 1993; 8: 321–330.

Achamallah NS: Visual hallucination after combining fluoxetine and dextromethorphan. Am J Psychiatry 1992; 149: 14406.

ACNP: Suicidal behavior and psychotropic medication. Neuropharmacology 1993; 8: 177–183.

Adams F, Queseda JR, Gutterman JU: Neuropsychiatric manifestations of human leukocyte interferon therapy in patients with cancer. JAMA 1984; 252: 938–941.

Äikia M, Kälviäinen R, Sivenius J, et al: Cognitive effects of oxcarbazepine and phenytoin monotherapy in newly diagnosed epilepsy: one year follow-up. Epilepsy Res 1992; 11: 199–203.

Aldenkamp AP, Alpherts WCJ, Blennow G, et al: Withdrawal of antiepileptic medication in children—effects on cognitive function. Neurology 1993; 43: 41–50.

Aldenkamp AP, Alpherts WCP, Diepman L, et al: Cognitive side effects of phenytoin compared with carbamazepine in patients with localization-related epilepsy. Epilepsy Research 1994; 19: 37–43.

Allain H, Lieury A, Brounet-Bourgin C, et al: Antidepressants and cognition: comparative effects of moclobemide, viloxazine and maprotiline. Psychopharmacology 1992; 106: S56–S61.

Al-Semaan YM, Clay HA, Meltzer H: Clozapine in the treatment of bromocriptine-induced psychosis. J Clin Psychopharmacol 1997; 17: 126–128.

Aman MLG, Werry JS, Paxton JS, et al: Effect of carbamazepine on psychomotor performance in children as a function of drug concentration, seizure type, and time of medication. Epilepsia 1990; 31: 51–60.

American Psychiatric Association: Diagnosis and statistical manual of mental disorders, 4th ed., Washington, DC, American Psychiatric Association, 1994: 317–391.

Ananth J, Gadirian AM, Engelsmann F: Lithium and memory: a review. Can J Psychiatry 1987; 32: 312–316.

Andrews DG, Bullen JG, Tomlinson L, et al: A comparative study of the cognitive effects of phenytoin and carbamazepine in new referrals with epilepsy. Epilepsia 1986; 27: 128–134.

Ansseau M, Pitchot W, Hansenne M, et al: Psychotic reactions to zolpidem. Lancet 1992; 339: 809.

Anthanelli RM, Monteiro MG, Blunt B, et al: Amnestic effects of intravenous diazepam in healthy young men. Am J Drug Alcohol Abuse 1991; 17: 129–136.

Armstrong C, Lewis T, D'Esposito M, et al: Eosinophilia-myalgia syndrome: selective cognitive impairment, longitudinal effects, and neuroimaging findings. J Neurol Neurosurg Psychiatry 1997; 63(5): 633–41.

Arthur CK, Ma DD: Combined interferon α-2a and cytosine arabinoside as first-line treatment for chronic myeloid leukemia. Acta Haematol 1993; 89(suppl 1): 15–21.

Ayd FJ: Neuroleptic-induced catatonia: further report. Int Drug Ther News 1983; 18: 89–12.

Bahro M, Kampf C, Strnad J: Catatonia under medication with risperidone in a 61-year-old patient. Acta Psychiatr Scand 1999; 99(3): 223–226.

Bangs ME, Petti TA, Janus MD: Fluoxetine-induced memory impairment in an adolescent. J Am Acad Child Adolesc Psychiatry 1994; 33(9): 1303–6.

Barbee JG, Black FW, Todorov AA: Differential effects of alprazolam and buspirone upon acquisition, retention, and retrieval processes in memory. J Neuropsychiat Clin Neurosci 1992; 4: 308–314.

Barker DB, Solomen DA: The potential for mental status changes associated with systemic absorption of anticholinergic ophthalmic medications: concerns for the elderly. DICP Ann Pharmacother 1990; 24: 847–850.

Barkin JS, Pais VM, Gadffney MF: Induction of mania by risperidone resistant to mood stabilizers. J Clin Psychopharmacol 1997; 17: 57–58.

Barrett J, Meehan O, Fahy T: SSRI and sympathominetic interaction. Br J Psychiatry 1996; 168: 253.

Beal DM, Hudson B, Zaiac M: Amoxicillin-induced psychosis. Am J Psychiatry 1986; 143: 155–256.

Beers MH, Passman LJ: Antihypertensive medications and depression. Drugs 1990; 40: 792–799.

Bem JL, Kerr L, Stuerchler D: Mefloquine prophylaxis and overview of spontaneous reports of severe psychiatric reactions and convulsions. J Trop Med Hyg 1992; 95: 167–179.

Bertoli M, Romagnoli GF, Margreiter R, et al: Reversible dementia following cyclosporine therapy in a renal transplant patient. Nephron 1988; 49: 433–434.

Billings R, Tang SW, Rafkoff VM: Depression associated with cimetidine. Can J Psychiatry 1981; 26: 260–261.

Billings RF, Stein MB: Depression associated with ranitidine. Am J Psychiatry 1986; 143: 915–916.

Biriell C, McEwen J, Sanz E: Depression associated with diltiazem. BMJ 1989; 299: 796.

Bixler EO, Kales A, Manfredi RL, et al: Next-day memory impairment with triazolam use. Lancet 1991; 337: 827–831.

Bjorkman A: Acute psychosis following mefloquine prophylaxis. Lancet 1989; 2: 865.

Blansjaar BA, Egberts TCG: Delirium in a patient treated with disulfiram and tranylcypromine (letter). Am J Psychiatry 1995; 152: 296.

Boatwright DE: Triazolam, handwriting, and amnestic states: two cases. J Forensic Sci 1987; 32: 1118–1124.

Bolton CF, Young GB, Zochodne DW: The neurological complications of sepsis. Ann Neurol 1993; 33: 94–100.

Bond AJ: Drug-induced behavioral disinhibition. CNS Drugs 1998; 9: 41–57.

Boston Collaborative Drug Surveillance Program: Acute adverse reactions to prednisone in relation to dosage. Clin Pharmacol Therap 1972; 13(5): 694–8.

Bottner RK, Tullio CJ: Metoclopramide and depression. Ann Int Med 1985; 103: 482.

Bouman WP, Pinner G, Johnson H: Cognitive impairment associated with lamotrigine. Brit J Psychiat 1997; 170: 388–389.

Bowen JD, Larson EB: Drug-induced cognitive impairment. Drugs and Aging 1993; 3: 349–357.

Brady AP, Hough DM, Lo R, et al: Transient global amnesia after cerebral angiography with iohexal. Canad Assoc Radiol J 1993; 44: 450–452.

Breitbart W, Marotta R, Platt MM, et al: A double-blind trial of haloperidol, chlorpromazine, and lorazepam in the treatment of delirium in hospitalized AIDS patients. Am J Psychiatry 1996; 153: 231–237.

Brent DA, Crumrine PK, Varma R, et al: Phenobarbital treatment and major depressive disorder in children with epilepsy: a naturalistic follow-up. Pediatrics 1990; 85: 1086–1091.

Brockington IF, Brownell LW: Steroid-induced prepartum psychosis. Br J Psychiatry 1997; 170: 90.

Broussolle E, Setiey A, Trielett M, et al: Reversible Creutzfeldt-Jakob like syndrome induced by lithium plus levodopa treatment. JNNP 1989; 52: 686–687.

Brown lRT[??], Madan-Swain A, Pais R, et al: Chemotherapy for acute lymphocytic leukemia: cognitive and academic sequelae. J Pediatr 1992; 121: 885–889.

Brown P, Preece MA, Will RG: "Friendly fire" in medicine: hormones homografts, and Creutzfeldt-Jakob disease. Lancet 1992; 340: 24–27.

Brown RT, Borden KA, Spunt Al, et al: Depression following pemoline withdrawal in a hyperactive child. Clin Paed 1985; 24: 174.

Buckner JC, Mandell W: Risk factors for depressive symptomatology in a drug-using population. Am J Pub Health 1990; 80: 580–585.

Buffenstein A, Heaster J, Ko P: Chronic psychotic illness from methamphetamine. Am J Psychiatry 1999; 156(4): 662.

Bunney WE, Goodwin FK, Murphy DL, et al: The "switch" process in manic-depressive illness II: relationship to catecholamines, REM sleep and drugs. Arch Gen Psychiatry 1972; 27: 304–309.

Burns A, Tune L: Amoxapine-induced cognitive impairment lin two patients. J Clin Psychiatry 1987; 48: 166–167.

Buter J, De Vries EGE, Sleijfer DT, et al: Neuropsychiatric symptoms during treatment with interleukin-2. Lancet 1993; 341: 628–629.

Caillon E, Schmitt L, Moron P: Acute depressive symptoms after mefloquine treatment. Am J Psychiatry 1992; 149: 712.

Calandre EP, Dominguez-Granados R, Gomez-Rubio M, et al: Cognitive effects of long-term treatment with phenobarbital and valproic acid in school children. Acta Neurol Scand 1990; 81: 504–506.

Canaday BR: Amnesia possibly associated with zolpidem administration. Pharmacotherapy 1996; 16: 687–689.

Cantu TG, Korek JS: Central nervous system reactions to histamine H₂-receptor blockers. Ann Int Med 1991; 115: 658.

Carter GL, Dawson AH, Lopert R: Drug-induced delirium. Drug Safety 1996; 15: 291–301.

Casanova B, de Entrambasaguas M, Gomez-Siurana E, et al: Lithium-induced Creutzfeldt-Jakob syndrome. Clinical Neuropharmacol 1996; 19: 356–359.

Cashman FE, Sheppard R: Clomiphene citrate as a possible cause of psychosis. Can Med Assoc J 1982; 126(2): 118.

Catalano G, Catalano MC, Alberts VA: Famotidine-asso-

ciated delirium. A series of six cases. Psychosomatics 1996; 37: 349–355.

Centonze V, Magrone D, Vino M, et al: Flunarizinee in migraine prophylaxis: efficacy and tolerability of 5 mg and 10 mg dose levels. Cephalalgia 1990; 10: 17–24.

Cestari V, Castellano C: MK-801 potentiates morphine-induced impairment of memory consolidation in mice: involvement of dopaminergic mechanisms. Psychopharmacology (Berl) 1997; 133: 1–6.

Chadwick DW: Concentration-effect relationship valproic acid. Clin Pharmacokinetics 1985; 10: 155.

Charney DS, Woods SW, Goodman WK, et al: Neurobiological mechanisms of panic anxiety: biochemical and behavioral correlates of yohimbine-induced panic attacks. Am J Psychiatry 1987; 144: 1030–1036.

Chaves MLF, Bianchin MM, Peccin S, et al: Chronic use of benzodiazepines and cognitive deficit complaints: a risk factor study. Ital J Neurosci 1993; 14: 429–435.

Chen B, Cardassis W: Delirium induced by lithium and risperidone combination. American Journal of Psychiatry 1996; 153: 1233–1234.

Christensen RC: Paroxetine-induced psychotic mania. Am J Psychiatry 1995; 152: 1399–1400.

Clark CH, Nicholson AN: Performance studies with antihistamines. Br J Clin Pharmacol 1978; 6: 31–35.

Clark DW, Ghose K: Neuropsychiatric reactions to nonsteroidal anti-inflammatory drugs. Drug Safety 1992; 7: 460–465.

Cohen IJ, Weitz R: Psychiatric complications with erythromycin. Drug Intell Clin Pharm 1981; 15: 388.

Cohen LJ: Risperidone. Pharmacotherapy 1994; 14: 253–265.

Coldwell SE, Milgrom P, Getz T, et al: Amnestic and anxiolytic effects of alprazolam in oral surgery patients. J Oral Maxillofac Surg 1997; 55: 1061–1070.

Cole MG, Primeau FJ: Prognosis of delirium in elderly hospital patients. Canad Med Assoc J 1993; 149: 41–46.

Committee on Geriatrics of the Royal College of Physicians of the United Kingdom: Organic mental impairment in the elderly. Implications for research, education and the provision of services. J R Coll Physicians Lond 1981; 15: 141–67

Cooke DM: The use of central nervous system manifestations in the early detection of digitalis toxicity. Heart Lung 1993; 22: 477–481.

Craig I, Tallis R: Impact of valproate and phenytoin on cognitive functions in elderly patients: results of a single-blind randomized comparative study. Epilepsia 1994; 35: 381–390.

Cumming RG: Epidemiology of medication-related falls and fractures in the elderly. Drugs & Aging 1998; 12: 43–53.

Cummings JL: Depression and Parkinson's disease: a review. Am J Psychiatry 1992; 149: 443–454.

Curran HV, Allen D, Lader M: The effects of single doses of alpidem and lorazepam on memory and psychomotor performance in normal humans. J Psychopharmacol 1987; 2: 81–89.

Curran HV, Barrow S, Weingartner H, et al: Encoding, remembering and awareness in lorazepam-induced amnesia. Psychopharmacology (Berl) 1995; 122: 187–193.

Curran HV, Java R: Memory and psychomotor effects of oxcarbazepine in healthy human volunteers. Eur J Clin Pharmacol 1993; 44: 529–533.

Cyr M, Laizure SC, daCunha CM: Methazolamide-induced delirium. Pharmacotherapy 1997; 17: 387–389.

D'Allessandro R, Benassi G, Morganti G: Side effects of flunarizine. Lancet 1986; 2: 4663.

Danielson DA, Porter JB, Lawson DH, et al: Drug-associated psychiatric disturbances in medical patients. Psychopharmacology 1981; 74: 105–108.

Danziger LH, Martin SJ, Blum RA: Central nervous system toxicity associated with meperidine use in hepatic disease. Pharmacotherapy 1994; 14: 235–238.

Darbar D, Connachie AM, Jones AM, et al: Acute psychosis in an elderly patient: case report. Br J Clin Practice 1996; 50: 350–351.

Davidson KW, Reddy S, McGrath P, et al: Increases in depression after cholesterol-lowering drug treatment. Behav Med 1996; 22(2): 82–84.

Davis RE, Callahan MJ, Downs DA: Clonidine disrupts aged-monkey delayed response performance. Drug Development Research 1988; 12: 279–286.

Dawson KL, Carter ER: A steroid-induced acute psychosis in a child with asthma. Pediatr Pulmonol 1998; 26(5): 362–4.

De Leon OA, Furmaga KM, Kaltsounis J: Mirtazapine-induced mania in a case of poststroke depression. J Neuropsychiatry Clin Neurosci 1999; 11(1): 115–6.

Demers-Desrosiers LA, Nestoros JN, Vaillancourt P: Acute psychosis precipitated by withdrawal of anticonvulsant medications. Am J Psychiatry 1978; 135: 981–982.

Denicoff KD, Rubinow DR, Papa MZ, et al: The neuropsychiatric effects of treatment with interleukin-2 and lymphokyne-activated killer cells. Ann Int Med 1987; 107: 293–300.

Dikmen SS, Temkin NR, Miller B, et al: Neurobehavioral effects of phenytoin prophylaxis of posttraumatic seizures. JAMA 1991; 265: 1271–1277.

Dilsaver SC, Swann AC: Mixed mania: apparent induction by a tricyclic antidepressant in five consecutively treated patients with bipolar depression. Biol Psychiatry 1995; 37: 60–62.

Di Maggio JR, Brown R, Baile WF, et al: Hallucinations and ifosfamide-induced neurotoxicity. Cancer 1994; 73: 1509–1514.

Dimsdale JE: Reflections on the impact of antihypertensive medications on mood, sedation, and neuropsychologic functioning. Arch Int Med 1992; 152: 35–39.

Dodrill CB, Troupin AS: Neuropsychological effects of carbamazepine and phenytoin: a reanalysis. Neurology 1991; 41: 141–143.

Dodrill CB: Problems in assessment of cognitive effects of antiepileptic drugs. Epilepsia 1992; 33(suppl 6): S29–S32.

Dorevitch A, Frankel Y, Bar-Halpern A, et al: Fluvoxamine associated manic behavior: a case series. Ann Pharmacother 1993; 27: 1455–1457.

Dormont D: Agents that cause transmissible subacute spongiform encephalopathies. Biomed Pharmacother 1999; 53(1): 3–8.

Drake ME, Peruzzi WT: Manic state with carbamazepine therapy of seizures. J National Med Assoc 1986; 78: 1105–1107.

Dubin H, Spier S, Giannandrea P: Nefazodone-induced mania. Am J Psychiatry 1997; 154; 578–579.

Dubrovsky B: Effects of adrenal cortex hormones on limbic structures: some experimental and clinical correlations related to depression. J Psychiatr and Neurosci 1993; 18: 4–16,

Duch S, Duch C, Past L, et al: Changes in depressive status associated with topical β-blockers. Int Ophthalmol 1992; 16: 331–335.

Duits N, Bos FM: Depressive symptoms and cholesterol lowering drugs. Lancet 1993; 341: 114.

Duncan JLS, Shorvon SD, Trimble MR: Effects of removal of phenytoin, carbamazepine, and valproate on cognitive functions. Epilepsia 1990; 31: 584–591.

Edwards JG: Suicide and antidepressants (editorial). BMJ 1995; 310: 205–206.

Egorov VM, Verbuk AM, Verbuk VM: Comparative characterization of damaging mental effect of general anesthesia using fluothane and ketamine in surgery of the face in children with congenital facial and palatal clefts. Anesteziol Reanimatol 1996; 6: 31–33.

Elko CJ, Burgess JL, Robertson WO: Zolpidem-associated hallucinations and serotonin reuptake inhibition: a possible interaction. J Toxicol Clin Toxicol 1998; 36(3): 195–203.

Engelsman F, Ghadirian AM, Grof P: Lithium treatment and memory assessment: methodology. Neuropsychobiology 1992; 26: 113–119.

Evans M, Perera PW, Donoghue J: Drug induced psychosis with doxazosin. BMJ 1997; 314: 1869.

Factor SA, Brown D, Mohlo ES, et al: Clozapine: a 2-year open trial in Parkinson's disease patients with psychosis. Neurology 1994; 44: 544–546.

Farwell JR, Lee YJ, Hirtz DG, et al: Phenobarbital for febrile seizures—effect on intelligence and on seizure recurrence. NEJM 1990; 322: 364–369.

Fayen M, Goldman MB, Moulthrop MA, et al: Differential memory function with dopaminergic anticholinergic treatment of drug-induced extrapyramidal symptoms. Am J Psychiatry 1988; 145: 483–486.

Feder R: Metoclopramide and depression. J Clin Psychiatry 1987; 48: 38.

Federico A, Palmeri S, Malandrini A, et al: Dementia, myoclonus, peripheral neuropathy, and lipid-like material in skin biopsy during psychotropic drug treatment. Biol Psychiatry 1992; 32: 721–727.

Fenner M, Schomberg A, Menzel T, et al: Neuropsychiatric effects of treatment with subcutaneous interleukin-2 and interferon-α₂ in metastatic renal cancer. Quality of Life Research 1993a; 2: 52–53.

Fenner MH, Hänninen EL, Kirchner HH, et al: Neuropsychiatric symptoms during treatment with interleukin-2 and interferon-α. Lancet 1993b; 341: 372.

Fernandez HH, Friedman JH, Jacques C, et al: Quetiapine for the treatment of drug-induced psychosis in Parkinson's disease. Mov Disord 1999; 14(3): 484–487 .

Ferrie CD, Robinson RO, Panayiotopoulos CP: Psychotic

and severe behavioral reactions with vigabatrin. Acta Neurol Scand 1996; 93: 1–8.

Figiel GS, Krishnan KRR, Nemeroff CB: Radiologic correlates of antidepressant-induced delirium: the possible significance of basal ganglia lesions. J Neuropsychiatry Clin Neurosci 1989; 1: 188–190.

File SE, Sharma R, Shaffer J: Is lorazepam-induced amnesia specific to the type of memory or to the task used to assess it? J Psychopharmacol 1992; 6: 76–80.

Finelli PF: Drug-induced Creutzfeldt.Jakob like syndrome. J Psychiatr Neurosci 1992; 17: 103–105.

Fischer M, Korskjaer G, Pedersen E: Psychotic episodes in Zarondan treatment. Effects and side-effects in 105 patients. Epilepsia 1965; 6(4): 325–334.

Fisher CM: "Catatonia" due to disulfiram toxicity. Arch Neurol 1989; 46: 798–804.

Fisher CM: Amnesic syndrome associated with propranolol toxicity: a case report. Clin Neuropharmacol 1992; 15: 397–403.

Fisher CM: Visual hallucinations and racing thoughts on eye closure after minor surgery. Arch Neurol 1991b; 48: 1091–1092.

Fisher CM: Visual hallucinations on eye closure associated with atropine toxicity: a neurological analysis and comparison with other hallucinations. Canad J Neurosci 1991a; 18: 18–27.

Folkerts H, Kuhs H: Psychotic episode caused by prevention of malaria with mefloquine. A case report. Nervenarzt 1992; 63(5): 300–302.

Folstein MF, Bassett SS, Romanoski AJ, et al: The epidemiology of delirium in the community: the Eastern Baltimore Mental Health Survey. Int Psychogeriatr 1991; 3: 169–176.

Force RW, Hansen L, Bedell M: Psychotic episode after melatonin. Ann Pharmacother 1997; 31: 1408.

Foy A, O'Connell D, Henry D, et al: Benzodiazepine use as a cause of cognitive impairment in elderly hospital inpatients. J Gerontol 1995; 50: 99–106.

Fradkin JE, Schonberger LB, Millis JS, et al: Creutzfeldt-Jakob disease in pituitary growth hormone recipients in the United States. JAMA 1991; 165: 880–884.

Francis J, Martin D, Kapoor WN: A prospective study of delirium in hospitalized elderly. JAMA 1990; 263: 1097–1101.

Francis J: Drug-induced delirium. CNS drugs. 1996; 5: 103–114.

Franks RD, Richter AJ: Schizophrenia-like psychosis associated with anticonvulsant toxicity. Am J Psychiatry 1979; 136: 973–974.

Freedman DX, Halaris AE: Monoamines and the biological mode o action of LSD at synapses. In Lipton MA, et al (Eds.): Psychopharmacology, Raven Press, New York, 1978, pp 347–359.

Fricchione GL, Cassem NH, Hooberman D, et al: Intravenous lorazepam in neuroleptic-induced catatonia. J Clin Psychopharmacol 1983; 3: 338–342.

Friedman DL, Kastner T, Plummer AT, et al: Adverse behavioral effects in individuals with mental retardation and mood disorders treated with carbamazepine. Am J Ment Retard 1992; 96: 541–546.

Gajula RP, Berlin RM: Captopril-induced mania. Am J Psychiatry 1993; 150(9): 1429–430.

Gallassi R, Morreale A, Di Sarro R, et al: Cognitive effects of antiepileptic drug discontinuation. Epilepsia 1992; 33(suppl 6): S41–S44.

Gallassi R, Morreale A, Lorusso S, et al: Carbamazepine and phenytoin. Arch Neurol 1988; 45: 892–894.

Gallassi R, Morreale A, Lorusso S, et al: Cognitive effects of valproate. Epilepsy Res 1990; 5: 160–164.

Galle G, Arnold K: Psychopathometric demonstration and quantification of mental disturbances following myelography with metrizamide and iopamidol. Neuroradiology 1984; 26: 229–233.

Gamzu ER: The role of benzodiazepines in amnesia: laboratory predictors. J Clin Psychiatry Monogr 1987; 5: 8–13.

Ganzini L, Miller SB, Walsh JR: Drug-induced mania in the elderly. Drugs & Aging 1993b; 3: 428–435.

Ganzini L, Walsh JR, Miller SB: Drug-induced depression in the aged. Drugs & Aging 1993a; 3: 147–158.

Gardner DL, Cowdry RW: Development of melancholia during carbamazepine treatment in borderline personality disorder. J Clin Pharmacol 1986; 6: 236–239.

Gerber JG, Nies AS: Antihypertensive agents and drug therapy of hypertension. In Gilman, Gordman and Gilman' The pharmacological basis of therapeutics, 8th ed, New York, Pergamon Press, 1990, pp 784–813.

Gerrard L, Wheeldon NM, McDevitt DG: Effect of combined atenolol and nifedipine administration on psychomotor performance in normal subjects. Eur J Clin Pharmacol 1995; 48(3–4): 229–33.

Ghadirian AM, Engelsman F, Ananth J: Memory functions during lithium therapy. J Clin Psychopharmacol 1983; 3: 313–315.

Gilham RA, Williams N, Wiedman KD, et al: Cognitive function in adult epileptic patients established on anticonvulsant therapy. Epilepsy Res 1990; 7: 219–225.

Giralt J, Ortega JJ, Olive T, et al: Long-term neuropsychologic sequelae of childhood leukemia: comparison of two CNS prophylactic regimens. Int J Radiat Oncol Biol Phys 1992; 24: 49–53.

Gittelman DK: Chronic salicylate intoxication. Southern Med J 1993; 86: 683–685.

Go FS, Malley EE, Birmaher B, et al: Manic behaviors associated with fluoxetine in three 12- to 18-year-olds with obsessive-compulsive disorder. J Child Adolesc Psychopharmacol 1998; 8(1): 73–80.

Goble AJ: β-blocker treatment and depression. Arch Int Med 1992; 152: 649.

Goldstein ET, Preskorn SH: Mania triggered by a steroid nasal spray in a patient with stable bipolar disorder. Am J Psychiatry 1989; 146: 8.

Goodwin FK: Psychiatric side effects of levodopa in man. JAMA 1971; 218: 1915–1920.

Gonski P: Clozapine in Parkinson's disease. Lancet 1995; 345: 516.

Goodwin JS, Regan M: Cognitive dysfunction associated with naproxen and ibuprofen in the elderly. Arthritis Rheum 1982; 25: 1013–5.

Gotz V: Paranoid psychosis with indomethacin (letter). BMJ 1978; 1: 49.

Green AR, Cross AJ, Goodwin GM: A review of the pharmacology and clinical pharmacology of 3,4-methylenedioxymethamphetamine (MDMA or "Ecstasy"). Psychopharmacology 1995; 119: 247–260.

Greene P, Cote L, Fahn S, et al: Treatment of drug-induced psychosis in Parkinson's disease with clozapine. In Narabayashi H, et al (Eds.) Parkinson's disease: from basic research to treatment (Advances in neurology, vol 60), New York, Raven Press, 1993, pp 703–706.

Grigg JR: Prednisone mood disorder with associated catatonia. J Geriatric Psychiatry & Neurology 1989; 2: 41–44.

Grünewald RA, Thompson PJ, Corcoran R, et al: Effects of vigabatrin on partial seizures and cognitive function. JNNP 1994; 57: 1057–1063.

Guerrini R, Belmonte A, Casalini C, et al: Reversible pseudoatrophy of the brain and mental deterioration associated with valproate treatment. Epilepsia 1998; 39: 27–32.

Hall RCW, Popkin MK, Stickney SK, et al: Presentation of steroid psychosis. J Nerv Ment Dis 1979; 167: 229–236.

Hall RCW, Zisook S: Paradoxical reaction to benzodiazepines. J Clin Pharmacol 1981; 11: 99S–104S.

Hallas J: Evidence of depression provoked by cardiovascular medication: a prescription sequence symmetry analysis. Epidemiology 1996; 7: 478–484.

Hambrecht M: Lithium and pseudohallucinations: a rare side effect. Biol Psychiatria 1995; 37: 120–121.

Hansen BA, Greenberg KS, Richter JA: Ganciclovir-induced psychosis. N Engl J Med 1996; 335: 1397.

Harmon C, Wohlreich MM: Sodium nitroprusside-induced delirium. Psychosomatics 1995; 36: 83–85.

Harper CM, Newton PA, Walsh JR: Drug-induced illness in the elderly. Postgrad Med 1989; 86: 245–256.

Hassanyeh F, Murray RB, Rodgers H: Adrenocortical suppression presenting with agitated depression, morbid jealousy, and a dementia-like state. Br J Psychiatry 1991; 159: 870–872.

Hazen PG, Carney JF, Walker AE, et al: Depression— a side effect of 13-*cis*-retinoic acid therapy. J Am Acad Dermatol 1983; 9: 278–279.

Heeringa M, Honkoop P, de Man RA: Major psychiatric side effects of interferon-α-2b. Ned Tijdschr Geneeskd 1998; 142(28): 1618–21.

Heimann SW, March JS: SSRI-induced mania. J Am Acad Child Adolesc Psychiatry 1996; 35: 4.

Hemmelgarn B, Suissa S, Huang A, et al: Benzodiazepine use and the risk of motor vehicle crash in the elderly. JAMA 1997; 278(1): 27–31.

Henderson CA, Highet AS: Depression induced by etretinate. BMJ 1989; 298: 964.

Heritch AJ, Capwell R, Roy-Byrne PP: A case of psychosis and delirium following withdrawal from triazolam. J Clin Psychiatry 1989; 48: 168–169.

Hill DE, Ciesielski KT, Sethre-Hofstad L, et al: Visual and verbal short-term memory deficits in childhood leukemia survivors after intrathecal chemotherapy. J Pediatr Psychol 1997; 22: 861–70.

Himmelsbach FA, Kohler E, Zanker B, et al: Baclofen intoxication in chronic hemodialysis and kidney transplantation. Dtsch Med Wochenschr 1992; 117(19): 733–737.

Hindmarch I: Antidepressants: the implications of the cognitive and psychomotor effects in the elderly. Int Clin Psychopharmacol 1990; 5(suppl 3): 57–60.

Hindmarch I, Kerr J: Behavioral toxicity of antidepressants with particular reference to moclobemide. Psychopharmacology 1992; 106: S49–S55.

Hoffmann WF, Ladogana L: Delirium secondary to clonidine therapy. NY State Med J 1981; 81: 382.

Holmes C, Fortenza O, Powell J, et al: Do neuroleptic drugs hasten cognitive decline in dementia? Carriers of apolipoprotein E epsilon 4 allele seem particularly susceptible to their effects. BMJ 1997; 314: 1411–1412.

Honer WG, Prohovnik I, Smith G, et al: Scopolamine reduces frontal cortex perfusion. J Cerebral Blood Flow Metabolism 1988; 8: 635–641.

Hooten WM, Pearlson G: Delirium caused by tacrine and ibuprofen interaction. Am J Psychiat 1996; 153: 842.

Hoppmann RA, Peden JG, Ober SK: Central nervous system side effects of nonsteroidal anti-inflammatory drugs. Aseptic meningitis, psychosis, and cognitive dysfunction. Arch Intern Med 1991; 151(7): 1309–13.

Hoppmann RA, Peden JG, Ober SK: Central nervous system side effects of non-steroidal anti-inflammatory drugs. Arch Int Med 1991; 151: 1309–1313.

Howland RH: Induction of mania with serotonin reuptake inhibitors. J Clin Psychopharmacol 1996; 16: 425–448.

Hubain P, Sobolski J, Mendlewicz J: Cimetidine induced mania. Neuropsychobiology 1982; 8: 223–224.

Huber SJ, Shulman HG, Paulson GW, et al: Dose-dependent memory impairment in Parkinson's disease. Neurology 1989; 39: 438–440.

Hung DZ, Tsai WJ, Deng JF: Anterograde amnesia in triazolam overdose despite flumazil treatment: a case report. Human Exp Toxicol 1992; 11: 289–290.

Hurowitz GI, Liebowitz MR: Antidepressant-induced rapid cycling: six case reports. J Clin Psychopharmacol 1993; 13: 52–56.

Ilechukwu STC: Acute psychotic reactions and stress response syndromes following intramuscular aqueous procaine penicillin. Br J Psychiatry 1990; 156: 554.

Inouye SK: The dilemma of delirium: clinical and research controversies regarding diagnosis and evaluation of delirium in hospitalized elderly medical patients. Am J Med 1994; 97: 278–288.

Ishigooka J, Yoshidaa Y, Murasaki M: Prog Neuropsychopharmacol Biol Psychiatry 1991; 15: 513–521.

Jackson CW, Markowitz JS, Brewerton TD: Delirium associated with clozapine and benzodiazepine combinations. Ann Clin Psychiatry 1995; 7: 139–141.

Jaffe R, Gibson E: Clonazepam withdrawal psychosis. J Clin Psychopharmacol 1986; 6: 193.

Jaguste VS, Dadkar VN, Dhar HL: Effects of verapamil and nifedipine on psychomotor performance in human subjects. J Assoc Physicians India 1991; 39(6): 457–462.

Jain KK: Cerebral insufficiency. Year Book Medical Publishers, Chicago, 1990.

James EA, Demian AZ: Acute psychosis in a trauma patient due to ciprofloxacin. Postgrad Med J 1998; 74: 189–190.

Jay GT, Fitzgerald JM: Ciprofloxacin-induced delirium. Ann Pharmacother 1997; 31: 252.

Jick SS, Dean AD, Jick H: Antidepressants and suicide. BMJ 1995; 310: 215–218.

Johnson I: Steroid-induced prepartum psychosis. Br J Psychiatry 1996; 169(4): 522.

Jones PG, Beier-Hanratty SA: Acyclovir: neurologic and renal toxicity. Ann Int Med 1986; 104: 892.

Jones RJ, Brace SR, Vander Tuin EL: Probable propafenone-induced transient global amnesia. Ann Pharmacother 1995; 29: 586–590.

Jouvent R, Abensour P, Bonnet AM, et al: Antiparkinsonian and antidepressant effects of high doses of bromocriptine. J Affect Disord 1983; 5: 141–145.

Juhl RP, Daugherty VM, Kroboth PD: Incidence of next day anterograde amnesia caused by flurazepam hydrochloride and triazolam. Clin Pharm 1984; 3: 622–625.

Kahn N, Freeman A, Juncos JL, et al: Clozapine is beneficial for psychosis in Parkinson's disease. Neurology 1991; 41: 1699–1700.

Kankaria A, Lewis JH, Ginsberg G, et al: Flumazenil reversal of psychomotor impairment due to midazolam or diazepam for conscious sedation for upper endoscopy. Gastrointest Endosc 1996; 44: 416–421.

Kanof PD, Aronson MJ, Ness R: Organic mood syndrome associated with detoxification from methadone maintenance. Am J Psychiatry 1993; 150: 423.428.

Kapfhammer HP, Messer T, Hoff P: Psychotic illness during treatment with clomifen. Dtsch Med Wochenschr 1990; 115(24): 936–9.

Kassler-Taub K, Woodward T, Markowitz JS: Depressive symptoms and pravastatin. Lancet 1993; 341: 371–372.

Katirji MB: Visual hallucinations and cyclosporine. Transplantation 1987; 43: 768–769.

Katz IR, Parmelee P, Brubaker K: Toxic and metabolic encephalopathies in long-term care patients. Int Psychogeriatr 1991; 12: 21–29.

Katz SE: Possible paroxetine-zolpidem interaction. Am J Psychiat 1995; 152: 1689.

Kaufer D, Friedman A, Seldman S, et al: Acute stress facilitates long-lasting changes in cholinergic gene expression. Science 1998; 393: 373–377.

Kay CR: The Royal College of General Practitioners Oral Contraceptive Study: some recent observations. Clinics in Obstetrics Gynaecology 1984; 11: 759–786.

Kent TA, Wilber RD: Reserpine withdrawal psychosis: the possible role of denervation supersensitivity of the receptors. J Nerv Ment Dis 1982; 170: 502–504.

Kerr BR, Hill H, Coda B, et al: Concentration-related effects of morphine on cognition and motor control in human subjects. Neuropsychopharmacology 1991; 5: 157–166.

Kershner P, Wang-Chen R: Psychiatric side-effects of steroid therapy. Psychosomatics 1989; 30: 135–139.

Kikyo H, Furukawa T: Creutzfeldt-Jakob-like syndrome induced by lithium, levomepromazine, and phenobarbitone. JNNP 1999; 65: 802–803.

King DJ: Psychomotor impairment and cognitive disturbances induced by neuroleptics. Acta Psychiatr Scand 1994; 89(suppl 380): 53–58.

King DJ: The effect of neuroleptics on cognitive and psychomotor function. Br J Psychiatry 1990; 157: 799–811.

Kingsma A, Mooyart EL, Kamps WA, et al: Magnetic resonance imaging of the brain and the neuropsychological evaluation in children treated for acute lymphoblastic leukemia at a young age. Am J Pediatr Hematol Oncol 1993; 15: 231–238.

Kinsey RE: Psychosis due to sulfonamides. Ann Int Med 1943; 19: 795–798.

Kirk T, Roache JD, Griffiths RR: Dose-response evaluation of the amnesic effects of triazolam and pentobarbital in normal subjects. J Clin Psychopharmacol 1990; 10: 161–168.

Kirschner KL, Sahgal V, Armstrong KJ, et al: A comparative study of the cognitive effects of phenytoin and carbamazepine in patients with blunt head injury. J Neurol Rehab 1991; 5: 169–174.

Klawans HL: Psychiatric side effects during the treatment of Parkinson's disease. J Neural Trans 1988; 27(suppl): 117–122.

Klysner R: Drug induced depression. Pharmacology and Toxicology 1992; 71(suppl): 107–112.

Koella WP: CNS-related ((side-)effects of β-blockers with special reference to mechanism of action. Eur J Clin Pharmacol 1985; 28(suppl): 55–63.

Koller WC: Disturbance of recent memory function in parkinsonian patients on anticholinergic therapy. Cortex 1984; 20: 307–311.

Koszewska I, Puzynski S: Transition from the depressive state to manic stage during the treatment with antidepressant drugs. Psychiatr Pol 1991; 25: 76–82.

Krauthammer C, Klerman GL: Secondary mania: manic syndromes associated with antecedent physical illness or drugs. Arch Gen Psychiatry 1978; 35: 1333–1339.

Kugler J, Seus R, Krauskopf R, et al: Differences in psychic performance and guanfacine and clonidine in normotensive subjects. Br J Clin Pharmacol 1980; 10: 71S–80S.

Kulisevsky J, Berthier ML: A new case of fluoxetine-induced mania in post-stroke depression. Clin Neuropharmacol 1997; 20: 180–181.

Kupfer DJ, Carpenter LL, Frank E: Possible role of antidepressants in precipitating mania and hypomania in recurrent depression. Am J Psychiatry 1988; 145: 804–808.

Kurlan R, Como P: Drug-induced alzheimerism. Arch Neurol 1988; 45: 356–357.

Kurtz S, Ashkenazi I, Melamed S, et al: Major depressive episodes secondary to antiglaucoma drugs. Am J Psychiatry 1993; 150: 524–525.

Kusumo KS, Vaughan M: Effects of lithium salts on memory. Br J Psychiatry 1977; 131: 451–457.

Kuzma PJ, Klein MD, Stamatos JM, et al: Acute toxic delirium: an uncommon reaction to transdermal fentanyl. Anesthesiology 1995; 83: 869–871.

Lader M, Bruce M: States of anxiety and their induction by drugs. Br J Clin Pharmacol 1986; 22: 251–261.

Lake CR, Reid A, Martin C, et al: Cyclothymic disorder and bromocriptine: predisposing factors for postpartum mania? Can J Psychiatry 1987; 32: 693–694.

Lane HY, Lin YC, Chang WH: Mania induced by risperidone: dose related? J Clin Psychiatry 1998; 59: 85–86.

Larson EB, Kukull WA, Buchner D, et al: Adverse drug reactions associated with cognitive impairment in elderly persons. Ann Int Med 1987; 107: 169–173.

Larson EB, Kukull WA, Buckner D, et al: Adverse drug reactions associated with global cognitive impairment in elderly persons. Ann Int Med 1987; 107: 169–173.

Lauterbach EC: Dopamine hallucinosis with fluoxetine in Parkinson's disease. Am J Psychiatry 1993; 150: 1750.

Lauterbach EC: Serotonin reuptake inhibitors, paranoia, and the ventral basal ganglia. Clin Neuropharmacol 1991; 14: 547–555.

Lechleitner M, Hoppichler F, Konwalinka G, et al: Depressive symptoms in hypocholestremic patients treated with pravastatin. Lancet 1992; 340: 910.

Lee TH, Chen SS, Su SL, et al: Baclofen intoxication: report of four cases and review of literature. Clin Neuropharmacol 1992; 15: 56–62.

Leff JP, Fischer M, Bertelsen A: A cross-national epidemiological study of mania. Br J Psychiatry 1976; 129: 428–442.

Lennhof M: Trazodone-induced mania. J Clin Psychiatry 1987; 48: 423.

Levenson JL, Fallon HJ: Fluoxetine treatment of depression caused by interferon-α. Am J Gastroenterol 1993; 88: 760–761.

Levine J, Witzum E, Greenberg BD, et al: Inositol-induced mania? Am J Psychiatry 1996; 153: 839.

Levy D, Kimhi R, Barak Y, et al: Antidepressant-associated mania: a study of anxiety disorders patients. Psychopharmacology 1998; 136: 243–246.

Lewis DA, Smith RE: Steroid induced psychiatric syndromes. A report of 14 cases and a review of the literature. J Affective Disorders 1983; 5: 319–332.

Ling MHM, Perry PJ, Tsuang MT, et al: Side effects of corticosteroid therapy. Arch Gen Psychiatry 1981; 38: 471–477.

Lipowski Z: Delirium: acute confusional states, Oxford University Press, New York, 1990.

Lipowski ZJ: Delirium: acute brain failure in man, Springfield, Illinois, Charles C Thomas, 1980.

Liskin B, Roose SP, Walsh BT, et al: Acute psychosis following phenelzine discontinuation. J Clin Psychopharmacol 1985; 5(1): 46–47.

Liu HC, Tsai SC, Liu TY, et al: Baclofen-induced frontal lobe syndrome. case report. Paraplegia 1991; 29: 554–556.

London JA: Mania associated with olanzapine. J Am Acad Child Adolesc Psychiatry 1998; 37(2): 135–136.

Lowenthal DT, Nadeau SE: Drug-induced dementia. South Med J 1991; 84(suppl 1): S24–S31.

Lukas SE: CNS effects and abuse liability of anabolic-androgenic steroids. Annu Rev Pharmacol Toxicol 1996; 36: 333–357.

Lynn J, Rammohan KW, Bornstein RA, et al: Central nervous system involvement in the eosinophilia-myalgia syndrome. Arch Neurol 1992; 49: 1082–1085.

Lyon K, Wilson LJ, Golden LCJ, et al: Effects of long-term neuroleptic use on brain density. Psychiatry Res 1981; 5: 33–37.

Mac DS, Kumar R, Goodwin DW: Anterograde amnesia with oral lorazepam. J Clin Psychiatry 1985; 46: 137–138.

Mach JR, Dysken MW, Kuskowski M, et al: Serum anticholinergic activity in hospitalized older persons with delirium: a preliminary study. J Am Geriatr Soc 1995; 43: 491–495.

Marcantonio ER, Juarez G, Goldman L, et al: The relationship of postoperative delirium with psychoactive medications. JAMA 1994; 272: 1518–1522.

Marchand MP: Lithium et fonctions cérébrales. L'Encephale 1985; 11: 235–246.

Maremmani I, Marini G, Fornai F: Naltrexone-induced panic attacks. Am J Psychiatry 1998; 155: 447.

Markowitz JS, Brewerton TD: Zolpidem-induced psychosis. Ann Clin Psychiatry 1996; 8: 89–91.

Markowitz JS, Rames LJ, Reeves N, et al: Zolpidem and hallucinations. Ann Emerg Med 1997; 29(2): 300–301.

Markus HS, Duchen LW, Parkin EM, et al: Creutzfeldt-Jakob disease in recipients of human growth hormone in the United Kingdom. Quart J Med 1992; 82: 43–51.

Marsepoil T, Petithory J, Faucher JM, et al: Encephalopathy and memory disorders during treatments with mefloquine. Rev Med Interne 1993; 14(8): 788–91.

Martin M, Munoz-Blanco JL, Lopez-Ariztegui N: Acute psychosis induced by lamotrigine. Epilepsia 1995; 36(suppl 3): 118.

Martinez AC, Baines JPO, Marquez MB, et al: Vigabatrin-associated reversible acute psychosis in a child. Ann Pharmacotherapy 1995; 29: 1115–1117.

Masson C, Delalande I, Deslys JP, et al: Creutzfeldt-Jakob disease after pituitary-derived human growth therapy: two cases with valine 129 homozygous genotype. Neurology 1994; 44: 179–180.

Mathew VM, Dursun SM, Revely SM: Increased aggression, violent and more impulsive behavior rate in patients during chronic benzodiazepine use. J Psychopharmacol (Oxford) 1993; suppl A58.

Matsuo F, Bergen D, Faught E, et al: Placebo-controlled study of the efficacy and safety of lamotrigine in patients with partial seizures. Neurology 1993; 43: 2284–2291.

McCann UD, Slate SO, Ricaurte GA: Adverse reactions with 3,4-methylenedioxymethamphetamine (MDMA; "Ecstasy"). Drug Safety 1996; 15: 107–115.

McConnell H, Snyder PJ, Duffy JD, et al: Neuropsychiatric side effects related to treatment with felbamate. J Neuropsychiatry Clin Neurosci 1996; 8(3): 341–346.

McDanal CE, Bolman WM: Delayed idiosyncratic psychosis with diphenylhydantoin. JAMA 1975; 231: 1063.

McDonald EM, Mann AH, Thomas HC: Interferons as mediators of psychiatric morbidity. Lancet 1987; ii: 1175–1178.

McGaugh JL: Involvement of hormonal and neuromodulatory systems in regulation of memory storage. Annu Rev Neurosci 1989; 12: 255–287.

McKee RJW, Larkin JG, Brodie MJ: Acute psychosis with carbamazepine and sodium valproate. Lancet 1989; i: 167.

McKetin R, Mattick RP: Attention and memory in illicit

amphetamine users. Drug Alcohol Depend 1997; 48: 235–242.

McLachlan RS: Pseudoatrophy of the brain with valproic acid monotherapy. Canad J Neurosci 1987; 14: 194–296.

McShane R, Keene J, Gedling K, et al: Do neuroleptic drugs hasten cognitive decline in dementia? Prospective study with necropsy follow up. BMJ 1997; 314: 266–270.

Meador KJ, Loring DW, Allen ME, et al: Comparative cognitive effects of carbamazepine and phenytoin in healthy human adults. Neurology 1991; 41: 1537–1540.

Meador KJ, Loring DW, Huh K, et al: Comparative cognitive effects of antiepileptics. Neurology 1990; 40: 391–394.

Meador KJ: Cognitive side effects of medications. Neurological Clinics of North America 1998; 16: 141–155.

Meco G, Alessandria A, Bonifati V, et al: Risperidone for hallucinations inn levodopa-treated Parkinson's disease patients. Lancet 1994; 343: 1370–1371.

Melamed E, Zoldan J, Friedberg G, et al: Is hallucination in Parkinson's disease due to central serotonergic hyperactivity? Mov Disord 1993; 8: 406–407.

Meldrum B: GABA and acute psychosis. Psychol Med 1982; 12: 1–5.

Mendis T, Barclay CL, Mohr E: Drug-induced psychosis in Parkinson's disease. CNS Drugs 1996; 5: 166–174.

Menkes DB: Triazolam-induced nocturnal binging with amnesia. Austral NZ J Psychiatry 1992; 26: 320–321.

Merimsky O, Reider-Groswasser I, Inbar M, et al: Interferon-related mental deterioration and behavioral changes in patients with renal cell carcinoma. Eur J Cancer 1990; 26: 596–600.

Mermel LA, et al: Acute psychosis in patients receiving trimethoprim-sulfamethoxazole intravenously. J Clin Psychiatry 1986; 47: 269–270.

Meszaros K: Acute psychosis caused by mefloquine prophylaxis? Can J Psychiatry 1996; 41(3): 196.

Meyers CA, Abbruzzese JL: Cognitive functioning in cancer patients: effect of previous treatment. Neurology 1992; 42: 434–436.

Meyers CA, Mattis PJ, Pavol MA, et al: Pattern of neurobehavioral deficits associated with interferon-α neurotoxicity. Proc Am Assoc Cancer Res 1993; (84th meeting): 218.

Meyers CA, Scheibel RS, Forman AD: Persistent neurotoxicity of systemically administered interferon-α. Neurology 1991; 41: 672–676.

Meyers CA, Valentine AD, Wong FCL, et al: Reversible neurotoxicity of interleukin-2 and tumor necrosis factor: correlation of SPECT with neuropsychological testing. J Neuropsychiatry 1994; 6: 285–288.

Meyers CA, Yung WKA: Delayed neurotoxicity of intraventricular interleukin-2: a case report. J Neuro-Oncology 1993; 15: 265–267.

Milgrom H, Bender BG: Psychologic side effects of therapy with corticosteroids. Am Rev Resp Dis 1993; 147: 471–473.

Miller E, Berrios GE, Politynska B: The adverse effect of benzhexol on memory in Parkinson's disease. Acta Neurol Scand 1987; 76: 278–282.

Mills JL, Fradkin J, Schonberger L, et al: Status report on US human growth hormone recipient follow-up study. Horm Res 1990; 33: 116–120.

Milstein HG: Mental depression secondary to fluorouracil therapy for actinic keratosis. Arch Dermatology 1980; 116: 1100.

Mindham RHS, Marsden CD, Parkes JD: Psychiatric symptoms during levodopa therapy for Parkinson's disease and their relationship to physical disability. Psychological Medicine 1976; 6; 23–33.

Misztal M, Skangiel, Kramska J, et al: Subchronic intraventricular infusion of quinolinic acid produces working memory impairment—a model of progressive excitotoxicity. Neuropharmacology 1996; 35: 449–458.

Mizukami K, Naito Y, Yoshida M, et al: Mental disorders induced by carbamazepine. Jpn J Psychiatr Neurol 1990; 44: 59–63.

Molloy DW, Brooymans M: Anticholinergic medications and cognitive function. J Clin Exp Gerontology 1989; 10: 89–98.

Morgan A, Clark D: CNS adverse effects of nonsteroidal anti-inflammatory drugs. CNS Drugs 1998; 9: 281–290.

Morris HH, Estes ML: Traveler's amnesia. JAMA 1987; 258: 945–946.

Moser A, Siebecker F, Vieregge P, et al: Salsolinol, catecholamine metabolites, and visual hallucinations in L-dopa treated patients with Parkinson's disease. J Neural Transm 1996; 103: 421–432.

Moses H, Kadan I: Neurologic consultations in a general hospital. Am J Med 1986; 81: 955–958.

Mumenthaler M: Behebbare und vermeidbare Demenzen. Schweiz Med Wochenschr 1987; 117: 964–967, 1002–1008, 1040–1045.

Murphy DL, Brodie HKH, Goodwin FK, et al: Regular induction of hypomania by l-dopa in bipolar manic-depressive patients. nature 1971; 229: 135–136.

Nabeshima T, Noda Y: GABAergic modulation of memory with regard to passive avoidance and conditioned suppression tasks in mice. Psychopharmacology 1988; 94: 69–73.

Nausieda PA, Glanz R, Weber S, et al: Psychiatric complications of levodopa therapy of Parkinson's disease. Adv Neurol 1984; 40: 271–277.

Newton C, Slota D, Yuzpe AA, et al: Memory complaints associated with the use of gonadotropin-releasing hormone agonists: a preliminary study. Fertil Steril 1996; 65: 1253–1255.

Nishiyama K, Mizuno T, Sakuta M, et al: Chronic dementia in Parkinson's disease treated by anticholinergic agents. Adv Neurol 1993; 60: 479–483.

Nishiyama K, Momose T, Sugishita M, et al: Positron emission tomography of reversible intellectual impairment induced by long-term anticholinergic therapy. J Neurol Sci 1995; 132: 89–92.

Noll RB, Kulkarni R: Complex visual hallucinations and cyclosporine. Arch Neurol 1984; 41: 329–330.

Noveske FG: Breakthrough panic after amantadine treatment in a Parkinson's disease patient. J Clin Psychiatry 1996; 57: 374.

Nozaki O, Takagi C, Takaoka K, et al: Psychiatric manifestations accompanying interferon therapy for patients with chronic hepatitis C: an overview of cases in Japan. Psychiatry Clin Neurosci 1997 51: 175–180.

O'Dougherty M, Wright FS, Cox S, et al: Carbamazepine plasma concentration. Arch Neurol 1987; 44: 863–867.

Okada F: Interferon-induced depression. J Mol Med 1995; 73: 99–100.

Olivieri RL, Sibilia G, Valentino P, et al: Pulsed methylprednisolone induces a reversible impairment of memory in patients with relapsing-remitting multiple sclerosis. Acta Neurolog Scand 1998; 97: 366–369.

O'Riordan JI, Hutchinson J, Fitzgerald MX, et al: Amnesic syndrome following theophylline associated seizures. JNNP 1993; 56: 731.

Oyffe I, Lerner A, Isaacs G: Clomiphene-induced psychosis. Am J Psychiatry 1997; 154(8): 1169–70.

Pakalnis A, Drake ME Jr, John K, et al: Forced normalization. Acute psychosis after seizure control in seven patients. Arch Neurol 1987; 44(3): 289–292.

Pakalnis A, Drake ME, Kurvilla J, et al: Forced normalization: Acute psychosis after seizure control in seven patients. Arch Neurol 1987; 44: 289–292.

Papazian O, Canizales E, Alfonso I, et al: Reversible dementia and apparent brain atrophy during valproate therapy. Ann Neurol 1995; 38: 687–691.

Patten SB, Love EJ: Neuropsychiatric adverse drug reactions: passive reports to Health and Welfare Canada's Adverse Drug Reaction Database (1965–present). Int J Psychiatry 1994; 24: 45–62.

Patten SB, Williams JV, Love EJ, et al: Case-control studies of cardiovascular medications as risk factors for clinically diagnosed depressive disorders in a hospitalized population. Can J Psychiatry 1996; 41: 469–476.

Patterson CM, Newman JP: Reflectivity and learning from aversive events: towards a psychological mechanism for the syndromes of disinhibition. Psychol Rev 1993; 100: 716–736.

Patterson JF: Triazolam syndrome in the elderly. South Med J 1987; 80: 1425–1426.

Pauker SL, Brown R: Baclofen-induced catatonia. Psychopharmacology 1986; 6: 387.

Pavol MA, Meyers CA, Rexer JL, et al: Patterns of neurobehavioral deficits associated with interferon alfa therapy for leukemia. Neurology 1995; 45: 947–950.

Paykel ES, Fleminger R, Watson JP: Psychiatric side effects of antihypertensive drugs other than reserpine. J Clin Psychopharmacol 1982; 2: 14.

Peet M: Induction of mania with selective serotonin reuptake inhibitors and tricyclic antidepressants. Br J Psychiatry 1994; 164: 549–550.

Perry PJ, Yates WR, Anderseon KH: Psychiatric symptoms associated with anabolic steroids: a controlled retrospective study. Ann Clin Psychiatry 1990; 2: 11–17.

Piening RB, Young SA: Mefloquine-induced psychosis. Ann Emerg Med 1996; 27(6): 792–793.

Pierce JR: Cimetidine associated depression and loss of libido in a woman. Am J Med Sci 1983; 286: 31–34.

Pitner JK, Gardner M, Neville M, et al: Zolpidem-induced psychosis in an older woman. J Am Geriatr Soc 1997; 45: 533–4.

Poewe W, Berger W, Benke T, et al: High-speed memory scanning in Parkinson's disease: adverse effects of levodopa. Ann Neurol 1991; 29: 670–673.

Pollak PT, Sketris IS, MacKenzie SL, et al: Delirium probably induced by clarithromyciln in a patient receiving fluoxetine. Ann Pharmacother 1995; 29: 486–488.

Pollack MH, Rosenbaum JJF, Cassem NH: Propranolol and depression revisited: three cases and a review. J Nerv Ment Dis 1985; 173: 118–119.

Pope HG, Katz DL: Affective and psychotic symptoms associated with anabolic steroid use. Am J Psychiatry 1988; 145: 487–490.

Pope HG, Katz DL: Psychiatric and medical effects of anabolic-androgenic steroid use. Arch Gen Psychiatry 1994; 51: 375–382.

Pope HG, Yurgelun-Todd D: The residual cognitive effects of heavy marijuana use in college students. JAMA 1996; 275: 521–527.

Portenoy RK: Management of common opioid side effects during long-term therapy of cancer pain. Ann Acad Med Singapore 1994; 23: 160–170.

Powell-Jackson J, Weller RO, Kennedy P, et al: Creutzfeldt-Jakob disease after administration of human growth hormone. Lancet 1985; ii: 244–246.

Preston GC, Ward C, Lines CR, et al: Scopolamine and benzodiazepine models of dementia: cross reversals by Ro-1788 and physostigmine. Psychopharmacology 1989; 98: 487–494.

Preston GC, Broks P, Traub M, et al: Effects of lorazepam on memory, attention and sedation in man. Psychopharmacology 1988; 95: 208–215.

Price LH, Charney DS, Heniger GR: Three cases of manic symptoms following yohimbine administration. Am J Psychiatry 1994; 141: 1267–1268.

Pulliainen V, Jokelainen M: Effects of phenytoin and carbamazepine on cognitive function in newly diagnosed epileptic patients. Acta Neurol Scand 1994; 89: 81–86.

Rabey JM, Treves TA, Neufeld MY, et al: Low-dose clozapine in the treatment of levodopa-induced mental disturbances in Parkinson's disease. neurology 1995; 45: 432–434.

Rager P, Benezech M: Memory gaps and hypercomplex automatisms after single oral dose of benzodiazepines: clinical and medico-legal aspects. Ann Med Psychol (Paris) 1986; 144: 102–109.

Ramaekers JG: Behavioral toxicity of medicinal drugs. Drug Safety 1998; 18: 89–208.

Ramanathan M: Atenolol induced memory impairment: a case report. Singapore Medical Journal 1996; 37: 218–219.

Ray WA, Fought RL, Decker MD: Psychoactive drugs and the risk of injurious motor vehicle crashes in elderly drivers. Am J Epidemiol 1992; 136(7): 873–883.

Reiss AL, O'Donnell DJ: Carbamazepine-induced mania in two children: case report. J Clin Psychiatry 1984; 45: 272–274.

Renault PF, Hoofnagle JH, Park Y, et al: Psychiatric symptoms of long term interferon α therapy. Arch Int Med 1987; 147: 1577–1580.

Reus VI, Targum SD, Weingartner H, et al: Effect of lithium carbonate on memory processes of bipolar affectively ill patients. Psychopharmacology 1979; 63: 39–42.

Ricci S, Favero D, Longo VG: Central nervous system side effects of anti-infectious drugs. Drugs of Today 1986; 22: 283–300.

Ried LD, McFarland BH, Johnson RE, et al: β-blockers and depression: the more the murkier? Ann Pharmacother 1998; 32: 699–708.

Ritchie J, Steiner W, Abrahamowicz M: Incidence of and risk factors for delirium among psychiatric inpatients. Psychiatr Serv 1996; 47: 727–730.

Rivas DA, Chancellor MB, Hill K: Neurological manifestations of baclofen withdrawal. J Urol 1993; 150: 1903–1905.

Roberge RJ, Hirani KH, Rowland PL 3rd, et al: Dextromethorphan- and pseudoephedrine-induced agitated psychosis and ataxia: case report. J Emerg Med 1999; 17(2): 285–8.

Robins AH, McFayden ML, Lucke W, et al: Effect of the H_2 receptor antagonist ranitidine on depression and anxiety in duodenal ulcer patients. Postgrad Med J 1984; 60: 353–355.

Roger J, Grangeon H, Gueyj J, et al: Psychiatric and psychologic effects of ethosuximide treatment of epileptics. Encephale 1968; 57(5): 407–438.

Rosen JA: Dilantin dementia. Transac Am Neurol Assoc 1968; 93: 273.

Rosenthal SH, Fenton ML, Harnett DS: Clozapine for the treatment of levodopa-induced psychosis in Parkinson's disease. General Hospital Psychiatry 1992; 14: 285–286.

Rothschild AJ: Disinhibition, amnestic reactions, and other adverse reactions secondary to triazolam: a review of literature. J Clin Psychiatry 1992; 53(12, suppl): 69–79.

Roy CW, Wakefield IR: Baclofen pseudopsychosis: a case report. Paraplegia 1986; 24: 318–321.

Rummans TA, Davis LJ, Morse RM, et al: Learning and memory impairment in older, detoxified, benzodiazepine-dependent patients. Mayo Clin Proc 1993; 68: 731–737.

Rundell OH, Williams HLL, Lester BK: Secobarbital and information processing. Percept Motor Skills 1978; 46: 1255–1264.

Rusted JM, Warburton DM: The effects of scopolamine on working memory in healthy young volunteers. Psychopharmacology 1988; 96: 145–152.

Ruttenber AJ, Lawler-Heavner J, Yin M, et al: Fatal excited delirium following cocaine use: epidemiologic findings provide new evidence for mechanisms of cocaine toxicity. J Forensic Sci 1997; 42: 25–31.

Saieed WN, Hassan SM: Effect of three calcium antagonists, nifedipine, verapamil and diltiazem on psychomotor performance in humans. Medical Science Research 1996; 24: 427–428.

Sandel ME, Olive DA, Rader MA: Chlorpromazine-induced psychosis after brain injury. Brain Injury 1993; 7: 77–83.

Sander JWA, Hart YM, Trimble MR, et al: Vigabatrin and psychosis. JNNP 1991; 54: 435–439.

Sapolsky RM: Why stress is bad for your brain. Science 1996; 273: 7–8.

Sato M, Numachi Y, Hamamura T: Relapse of paranoid psychotic state in methamphetamine model of schizophrenia. Schizophr Bull 1992; 18: 115–122.

Scharf MB, Herschowitz J, Woods M, et al: Lack of amnestic effects of clorazepate on geriatric recall. J Clin Psychiatry 1985; 46: 518–520.

Scharf MB, Khosla N, Lysaght R, et al: Anterograde amnesia with oral lorazepam. J Clin Psychiatry 1983; 44: 362–364.

Scheinman PL, Peck GL, Rubinow DR, et al: Acute depression following isoretinoin. J Am Acad Dermatology 1990; 22: 1112–1114.

Schentag JJ: Cimetidine-associated mental confusion: further studies in 36 severely ill patients. Therapeutic Drug Monitoring 1980; 2: 133–142.

Schleifer SJ, Slater WR, Macari-Hinson MM, et al: Digitalis and β-blocking agents: effects on depression following myocardial infarction. Am Heart J 1991; 121: 1397–1402.

Schnapf BM, Santeiro ML: β-agonist inhaler causing hallucinations. Pediatric Emergency Care 1994; 10: 87–88.

Schreiber W, Spernal J: Metronidazole-induced psychotic disorder. Am J Psychiatry 1997; 154: 1170–1171.

Schwartz BL, Fay-McCarthy M, Kendrick K, et al: Effects of nifedipine, a calcium channel antagonist, on cognitive function in schizophrenic patients with tardive dyskinesia. Clin Neuropharmacol 1997; 20(4): 364–70.

Shader RI, Dreyfuss D, Gerrein JR, et al: Selective effects and impaired learning and recall after single oral doses of lorazepam. Clin Pharmacol Ther 1986; 39: 526–530.

Shaw ED, Stokes PE, Mann IJ, et al: effects of lithium carbonate on memory and motor speed of bipolar outpatients. Abnorm Psychol 1979; 63: 39–42.

Sherrard DJ, Walker JV, Boykin JL: Precipitation of dialysis dementia by desferoxamine treatment of aluminum-related bone disease. Am J Kidney Dis 1988; 12: 126–130.

Shimizu K, Matsubara K, Uenzono T, et al: Reduced dorsal hippocampal glutamate release significantly correlates with the spatial memory deficits produced by benzodiazepines and ethanol. Neuroscience 1998; 83: 701–706.

Shin C, Gray L, Armon C: Reversible cerebral atrophy: radiologic correlate of valproate-induced parkinsonism-dementia syndrome. Neurology 1992; 42(suppl 3): 277.

Shiozawa S, Kuroki Y, Kim M, et al: Interferon-α in lupus psychosis. Arthritis and Rheumatism 1992; 35: 417–422.

Siedentopf F, Kentenich H: Future use of clomiphene in ovarian stimulation. Psychic effects of clomiphene citrate. Hum Reprod 1998; 13(11): 2986–7.

Silbersweig DA, Stern E, Frith C, et al: A functional neuroanatomy of hallucinations in schizophrenia. Nature 1995; 378: 176–179.

Simeon J, Fink M, Itil TM, et al: D-cycloserine therapy for psychosis by symptom provocation. Compr Psychiatry 1970; 11: 80–88.

Sipahimalani A, Masand PS: Use of risperidone in delirium: case reports. Ann Clin Psychiatry 1997; 9: 105–107.

Skop BP, Masterson BJ: Mania secondary to lisinopril therapy. Psychosomatics 1995; 36(5): 508–509.

Slap G: Oral contraceptives and depression. J Adolesc Health Care 1981; 2: 53.

Slugg, Haug MT, Pippenger CE: Ranitidine pharmacokinetics and adverse central nervous system reactions. Arch Int Med 1992; 152: 2325–2329.

Smith LT, Williams HL, Rundell OH: Dose effects of methaqualone on stimulus encoding in a memory scanning task. Psychopharmacology 1988; 94: 126–132.

Smith SJM, Kocen RSK: A Creutzfeldt-Jakob like syndrome due to lithium toxicity. JNNP 1988; 51: 120–123.

Solomen RL, Rich CL, Darko DF: Antidepressant treatment and the occurrence of mania in bipolar patients. J Affect Disord 1990; 18: 253–257.

Solomen S, Hotchkiss E, Sarvay SM, et al: Impairment of memory function by antihypertensive medication. Arch Gen Psychiatry 1983; 40: 1109–1112.

Sommer BR, Petrides G: A case of baclofen-induced depression. J Clin Psychiatry 1992; 53: 211–212.

Sorensen PS, Larson BH, Rasmussen MJ, et al: Flunarizine versus metoprolol for migraine prophylaxis: a double-blind, randomized, parallel group study of efficacy and tolerability. Headache 1991; 31: 650–657.

Sorgi P, Ratey J, Knodler G, et al: Depression during treatment with β-blockers: results from double-blind, placebo-controlled study. Neuropsychiatry Clin Neurosci 1992; 4: 187–189.

Sowunmi A, Salako LA, Oduola AML, et al: Neuropsychiatric side effects of mefloquine in Africans. Trans Roy Soc Trop Med Hyg 1993; 87: 462–463.

Spatt J, Glawar B, Mamoli B: A pure amnestic syndrome after MDMA ("ecstasy") ingestion. JNNP 1997; 62: 418–419.

Spitzer RL, Endicott J, Robins E: Research diagnostic criteria for a selected group for functional disorders, 3rd edition, Biometrics Research Division, New York State Psychiatric Institute, 1987.

Stanilla JK, de Leon J, Simpson GM: Clozapine withdrawal resulting in delirium with psychosis: a report of three cases. J Clin Psychiatry 1997; 58(6): 252–255.

Stanley M, Stanley B: Post mortem evidence for serotonin's role in suicide. J Clin Psychiatry 1990; 51: 22–30.

Starr JM, Whalley LJ: Drug-induced dementia. Drug Safety 1994; 11: 310–317.

Steel JM, Briggs M: Withdrawal symptoms in obese patients after feenfluramine treatment. BMJ 1972; 3: 26–27.

Steg RE, Garcia EG: Complex visual hallucinations and cyclosporine neurotoxicity. Neurology 1991; 41: 1156.

Steinberg H, Saravay SM, Wadhwa N, et al: Erythropoietin and visual hallucinations in patients on dialysis. Psychosomatics 1996; 37(6): 556–563.

Steinman MA, Steinman TI: Clarithromycin-associated visual hallucinations in a patient with chronic renal failure on continuous ambulatory peritoneal dialysis. Am J Kid Dis 1996; 27: 143–146.

Stell IM, Ojo OA: Amoxycillin-induced hallucinations—a variant of Hoigne's syndrome? Br J Clin Pract 1996; 50(5): 279.

Stephano GB, Bilfinger TB, Fricchione GL: The immune- neuro-link and the macrophage: postcardiotomy delirium, HIV-associated dementia and psychiatry. Prog Neurobiol 1994; 42: 475–488.

Stuiver PC, Ligthelm RJ, Goud TJ: Acute psychosis after mefloquine. Lancet 1989; 2: 282.

Su TP, Pagliaro M, Schmidt PJ, et al: Neuropsychiatric effects of anabolic steroids in male normal volunteers. JAMA 1993; 269: 2760–2764.

Summers MJ, Crowe SF, Ng KT: Administration of lanthanum chloride following a reminder induces a transient loss of memory retrieval in day-old chicks. Brain Res Cogn Brain Res 1996; 4: 109–119.

Suzuki T, Koizumi J, Uchida K, et al: Carmofur-induced organic mental disorders. Jpn J Psychiat Neurol 1990; 44: 723–727.

Takahashi S, Ohnishi N, Tsukamato N: A case of mania associated with interferon treatment for chronic hepatitis type B. Seishin Igaku 1993; 35: 1219–1221.

Taubert HD, Kuhl HV: Kontrazeption mit Hormonen, Thieme, Stuttgart, 1981.

Terao T: Tricyclic-induced musical hallucinations and states of relative sensory deprivation. Biol Psychiatry 1995; 38: 192–193.

The Parkinson Study Group. Low-dose clozapine for the treatment of drug-induced psychosis in Parkinson's disease. NEJM 1999; 340: 757–763.

Thienhaus OJ, Allen A, Bennett JA, et al: Anticholinergic serum levels and cognitive performance. Eur Arch Psychiatry 1990; 240: 28–33.

Thomas L, Trimble M, Schmitz B, et al: Vigabatrin and behaviour disorders: a retrospective survey. Epilepsy Res 1996; 25(1): 21–27.

Thomas MA, Ibanez HE: Interferon α-2a in the treatment of subfoveal choroidal neovascularization. Am J Ophthalmol 1993; 115: 563–8.

Thompson P, Huppert F, Trimble M: Phenytoin and cognitive function: effects on normal volunteers and implications for epilepsy. Br J Clin Psychol 1981; 20: 155–162.

Thompson PJ: Antiepileptic drugs and memory. Epilepsia 1992; 33(suppl 6): S37–S40.

Tiller JWG, Schweitzer I: Benzodiazepines—depressants or antidepressants? Drugs 1992; 44: 165–169.

Tindall RSA, Willersen J: Subacute phenytoin intoxication syndrome. Arch Int Med 1978; 138: 1168–1169.

Titus J: Cimetidine-induced mania in depressed patients. J Clin Psychiatry 1983; 44: 267–268.

Tokinaga N, Kondo T, Kaneko S, et al: Hallucinations after a therapeutic dose of benzodiazepine hypnotics with co-administration of erythromycin Psychiatry Clin Neurosci 1996; 50(6): 337–379.

Tonegawa S: Gene targeting: a new approach to the analysis of mammalian memory and learning. Prog Clin Biol Res 1994; 390: 5–18.

Torrey EF: Chloroquine seizures: report of four cases. JAMA 1968; 204: 867–870.

Trimble MR: Anticonvulsant-induced psychiatric disorders. Drug Safety 1986; 15: 159–166.

Trimble MR: Anticonvulsant drugs and cognitive function: a review of the literature. Epilepsia 1987; 28(suppl 3): S37–S45.

Tune L, Carr S, Hoag E, et al: Anticholinergic effects of drugs commonly prescribed for the elderly: potential means of assessing risk of delirium. Am J Psychiatry 1992; 149: 1393–1394.

Turner TH, Cookson JC, Wass JAH, et al: Psychotic reactions during treatment of pituitary tumours with dopamine agonists. BMJ 1984; 289: 1101–1103.

Uhl MD, Riely CA: Metronidazole in treating portosystemic encephalopathy. Ann Int Med 1996; 124: 455.

Umstead GS, Neumann KH: Erythromycin ototoxicity and acute psychotic reactions in cancer patients with hepatic dysfunction. Arch Int Med 1986; 146: 897–899.

Uzych L: Anabolic androgenic steroids and psychiatric-related effects. Canad J Psychiatry 1992; 37: 23–28.

Valentine AD, Meyers CA, Kling MA, et al: Mood and cognitive side effects of interferon-α therapy. Semin Oncol 1998; 25(suppl 1): 39–47.

van Puijenbroek EP, Egberts AC, Krom HJ: Visual hallucinations and amnesia associated with the use of zolpidem Int J Clin Pharmacol Ther 1996; 34(7): 318.

Van Putten T, Gelenberg AJ, Lavori PW, et al: Anticholinergic effects on memory: benzotropine vs amantadine. Psychopharmacology Bull 1987; 23: 26–29.

van Sweden B: Drug-induced repetitive sharp EEG discharges in multi-infarct dementia. Gerontology 1984; 30: 397–402.

Vazquez A, Jimenez-Jimenez FJ, Garcia-Ruiz P, et al: "Panic attacks" in Parkinson's disease. Acta Neurol Scand 1993; 87: 14–18.

Varney NR, Alexander B, MacIndoe JH: Reversible steroid dementia in patients without steroid psychosis. Am J Psychiatry 1984; 141: 369–372.

Venkataraman S, Naylor MW, King CA: Mania associated with fluoxetine treatment in adolescents. J Am Acad Child Adolesc Psychiatry 1992; 31: 276–281.

Verdrager J: New variant Creutzfeldt-Jakob disease and bovine pituitary growth hormone. Lancet 1998; 351: 112–113.

Vgontzas AN, Kales A, Bixler EO: Benzodiazepine side effects. Role of pharmacokinetics and pharmacodynamics. Pharmacology 1995; 51: 205–223.

Vining EPG: Cognitive dysfunction associated with antiepileptic drug therapy. Epilepsia 1987; 28 (suppl 2): S18–S22.

von Gontard A, Lehmkuhl G: Desmopressin side effects. J Am Acad Child Adolesc Psychiatry 1996; 35: 129–130.

Warburton DM, Rusted JM: Cholinergic control of cognitive resources. Neuropsychobiology 1993; 28: 43–46.

Weinke T, Trautmann M, Held T, et al: Neuropsychiatric side effects after the use of mefloquine. Am J Trop Med Hyg 1991; 45: 86–91.

Welch JB: Dementia as a consequence of neuroleptic syndrome. Am J Psychiatry 1993; 150: 1561–1562.

Westerlund A: Central nervous system side-effects with hydrophilic and lipophilic β-blockers. Eur J Clin Pharmacol 1985; 28(suppl); 73–76.

White MC, Silverman JJ, Harrison JW: Psychosis associated with clonazepam therapy for blepharospasm. J Nerv Ment Dis 1982; 170: 117.

White WB, Riotte K: Propranolol and white rabbits. NEJM 1982; 307: 558–559.

Wienke MH, Dienst ER: Neuropsychological assessment of cognitive functioning following chemotherapy for breast cancer. Psycho-oncology 1995; 4: 61–66.

Witschy JK, Malone GL, Holden LD: Psychosis after neuroleptic withdrawal in a manic depressive patient. Am J Psychiatry 1984; 141: 105–106.

Wolfe ME, Almy G, Toll M, et al: Mania associated with the use of baclofen. Biol Psychiatry 1982; 17: 757–759.

Wolk SI, Douglas CJ: Clozapine treatment of psychosis in Parkinson's disease. J Clin Psychiatry 1992; 53: 373–376.

Wolkowitz OM, Reus VI, Weingartner H, et al: Cognitive effects of corticosteroids. Am J Psychiatry 1990; 147: 1297–1303.

Wolkowitz OM, Weingartner H, Rubinow DR, et al: Steroid modulation of human memory: biochemical correlates. Biol Psychiatry 1993; 33: 744–746.

Wysenbeek AJ, Klein Z, Nakar S, et al: Assessment of cognitive function in elderly patients treated with naproxen: a prospective study. Clin Exp Rheumatol 1988; 6: 399–400.

Yassa RY, Iskander HL: Baclofen-induced psychosis: two cases and a review. J Clin Psychiatry 1988; 499: 318–319.

Young BK, Camicioli R, Ganzini L: Neuropsychiatric adverse effects of antiparkinsonian drugs: characteristics, evaluation and treatment. Drugs and Aging 1997; 10: 367–383.

Young SN: Cholesterol, heart disease, and the brain: an opportunity in research and a disaster in public health education. J Psychiatry and Neurosciences 1993; 18: 1–3.

Yudofsky SC: β-blockers and depression: The clinician's dilemma. JAMA 1992; 267: 1826–1827.

Zabala S, Gascon A, Bartolome C, et al: Ciprofloxacin and acute psychosis. Enferm Infec Microbiol Clin 1998; 16: 42.

Zachmann M: Creutzfeldt-Jakob'sche Krankheit nach Behandlung mit aus menschlichen Hypophysen extrahiertem Wachstumhormon. Schweiz Ärztezeitung 1993; 74: 1744–1745.

Zaret BS, Cohen RA: Reversible valproic acid-induced dementia: a case report. Epilepsia 1986; 27: 234–240.

Zoldan J, Friedberg G, Goldberg-Stern H, et al: Ondasteron for hallucinosis in advanced Parkinson's disease. Lancet 1993; 341: 562–563.

Zoldan J, Friedberg G, Livneh M, et al: Psychosis in advanced Parkinson's disease: treatment with ondansetron, a 5-HT3 receptor antagonist. Neurology 1995; 45: 1305–8.

Chapter 6
Drug-Induced Headaches

Introduction

Headache is a common symptom in the general population and it is also one of the manifestations of several disorders, both neurological as well as non-neurological. Various drugs, including those used for treatment of headache, are also known to cause or trigger headache. Headache is also a manifestation of drug withdrawal. Headache is reported in clinical trials as a placebo effect. Onset of migraine may be a coincidental event because of its high prevalence. In an epidemiological study, the prevalence of mi-

graine was 16% with a male to female ratio of 1:3 (Rasmussen et al 1995).

The following subtypes of headache are usually recognized and their relationship to drugs is indicated:
- *Migraine*. It may be induced or exacerbated by drugs
- *Tension type headache*. This may be aggravated by drugs.
- *Chronic daily headache*. This may either be of chronic tension type or may be "transformed migraine," one subtype of which is drug-induced.

Table 6.1. Classification of drug-induced headache.

Headaches caused by direct pharmacological effects of drugs
    Acute
    Chronic
Secondary drug-induced headaches:
    Symptom of other drug-induced neurological disorder
        Benign intracranial hypertension (see Chapter 17)
        Aseptic meningitis (see Chapter 16)
        Encephalopathy (see Chapter 3)
        Depression (see Chapter 5)
        Drug-induced intracerebral hemorrhage (see Chapter 9)
    Symptoms of non-CNS adverse effects of drugs
        Hypertension
        Cervical myositis
Headaches due to drug /disease interaction where neither alone would cause it
Headache due to drug interaction where neither of the drugs alone would cause it
Drug withdrawal headache
    Recreational drugs
    Therapeutic drugs
Chronic daily headache due to drug misuse in headache patients (see Table 6.2)
    Transformed migraine
        with medication overuse
        without medication overuse
    Chronic tension type headache
        with medication overuse
        without medication overuse
    Hemicrania continua
        with medication overuse
        without medication overuse
Coincidental headaches not causally related to drugs

Classification

A classification of drug-induced headaches is shown in Table 6.1. Various terms have been used to describe the relationship to drugs to onset of headaches which include drug-associated headache, chronic daily headache (see Table 6.2) and drug-related headache. All of these terms have some limitations but the term "drug-induced headache" is broad in coverage and includes headache as a complication of drugs used for indications other than headache.

Table 6.2. Terms used to describe chronic daily headache associated with use of drugs.

Analgesic abuse headache (Lipman 1955)
Analgesic-induced headache (Diener et al 1989)
Analgesic rebound headache (Rapoport 1985)
Drug-abuse headache (Elkind 1989)
Drug-induced chronic daily headache (Mathew et al 1990)
Ergotamine headache (Wainscott et al 1974)
Ergotamine-induced headache (Andersson 1975)
Painkiller headache (Isler 1988)
Rebound headache (Granella et al 1975)
Transformed migraine (Mathew et al 1987)
Withdrawal headache (Diener et al 1988)

Table 6.3. Drugs used for the treatment of headaches which have been reported to induce headache.

Aminophenol derivatives: paracetamol, phenacetin
Antihistaminics
Barbiturates
Ergotamine
Intravenous immunoglobulin
Indomethacin
Opioids: codeine, oxycodone, propoxyphene, pethidine
  (meperidine)
Phenothiazines
Propranolol
Pyrazolone derivatives
Salicylates
Sumatriptan
Tranquilizers

Drugs and Other Substances Reported to Induce Headache

Headache can be induced by a variety of drugs (therapeutic as well as recreational), food items and other medical treatments. Drugs used for the treatment of headaches which have been report-

ed to induce headache are shown in Table 6.3 and drugs used for the treatment of other disorders are listed in Table 6.4. Headaches due to dietary

Table 6.4. Drugs used for the treatment of other disorders that cause headache.

Amphotericin B
Anthelminthic agents: piperazine, tetrachloroethylene
Antidepressants*
Atenolol
Benserazide (Polleri et al 1979)
Bromocriptine*
Captopril
Cimetidine*
Cromolyn sodium
Cyclosporine*
Dipyridamole
Glucanazole
Griseofulvin* (50% of patients) (Tester-Daldrup 1992)
Immunoglobulins*
Isoretinoin
Mefloquine* (frequency 30–50%; Harinasuta et al 1985)
Methyldopa
Metronidazole
Metoprolol
Nicotine*
Nifedipine
Ondansetron*
Oral contraceptives*
Piroxicam
Propranolol
Ranitidine
Sildenafil*
Terfenadine
Thalidomide (Garcia-Albia et al 1993)
Trimethoprim-sulfamethoxazole
Vasodilators*
  – glyceryl trinitrate
  – isosorbide dinitrates
Verapamil
Viloxazine (Barnes and Greenwood 1979)
Zimeldine

*Reported more frequently. This table does not include some of the drugs which produce headache by other adverse effects listed in Table 6.1.

Table 6.5. Dietary items, recreational drugs and other treatments.

Alcohol hangover
Aspartame*
Amphetamine
Caffeine withdrawal
Cranial radiation
Monosodium glutamate
Tyramine
Vitamin A abuse

items, recreational drugs and other treatments are listed in Table 6.5.

Clinical Features of Drug-Induced Headaches

Analgesic abuse is likely to aggravate headache in patients who use these for the treatment of headaches. Patients taking analgesics for pain in other body regions such as the back do not have such headaches. The association between analgesic abuse and headache was known in the seventeenth century in Europe and ergotamine-induced headache was described 50 years ago (Wolfson and Graham 1949). Analgesic-induced headache has been well documented in recent years by several authors (Bowdler et al 1988; Mathew 1990; Edmeads 1990; Elkind 1991). Overuse is defined as regular daily intake of simple analgesics, combination analgesics containing sedatives more often than four times a week, or opioid or ergotamine more often than twice a week. Overuse of analgesics has been known to worsen headache of migraine or tension type as well as mixed headache syndromes. This "paradoxical" effect of analgesics is also termed "rebound headaches" (Rapoport 1988) and refers to the following:

- Worsening of headache in three to four hours as the apparent analgesic effect of the medication wears off.
- The patient goes through a "withdrawal phase" after the medication is discontinued. It lasts 5 to 28 days or more corresponding to the washout period of the analgesic.

Excessive use of analgesic medications can cause episodic migraine or tension-type headache to evolve into a chronic daily headache with features of both episodic migraine and chronic tension-type headache, the so-called "mixed headache syndrome." Abrupt cessation of analgesics often causes head pain to intensify for 3 to 5 days. Features of drug-induced headache include the following (Mathew 1997):

- The headaches occur daily and vary in severity, type, and location.

- The threshold for headache is low. Physical or intellectual effort may bring on headache.
- Headaches are accompanied by asthenia, nausea and other gastrointestinal symptoms, restlessness, anxiety, irritability, memory problems, difficulty in intellectual concentration, and depression. Those consuming large quantities of ergot derivatives may exhibit cold extremities, tachycardia, paresthesias, diminished pulse, hypertension, light-headedness, muscle pain of the extremities, weakness of the legs, and depression.
- The headaches have a drug-dependent rhythmicity. Predictable early morning headaches are frequent, particularly in patients who use large quantities of analgesic, sedative, caffeine, or ergotamine combinations.

Risk Factors and Pathomechanism of Drug-Induced Headache

Risk Factors. The following are the risk factors for analgesic-induced headache:

- Patients who take analgesics for headache for prolonged periods. Persons taking daily analgesics are six times as likely to develop chronic daily headaches as those taking occasional analgesics (McGregor et al 1990).
- Patients with migraine are more prone. Iatrogenic worsening of migraine through analgesic abuse is known to be a major cause of migraine chronicity (Wallasch 1992; Rohr and Floch 1992).
- Use of combination analgesics, particularly those containing habit forming substances such as butabarbital or codeine are more likely to lead to addiction and "rebound headache."
- Analgesics containing caffeine are more likely to lead to caffeine withdrawal headaches.
- Patients with psychiatric disturbances such as depression are more likely to have analgesic abuse headaches.

Pathomechanism. The pathomechanism of analgesic abuse headache is not known. Obviously analgesics do not create the headache de novo in a previously headache-free individual (Lance et al 1988). Various pathomechanisms that have been proposed include the following:

– Headache may be a "rebound" effect with headache intensity inversely related to the blood concentration of the drug. More drug is consumed as the headache intensity increases. This starts a vicious cycle and if the amount of analgesic is not increased headache persists.

– Kindling has been proposed as a model for non-epileptic progressive disorders such as transformed migraine (Post and Silberstein 1994). The underlying mechanisms are not well established but may include alterations in gene expression.

– Rebound headaches may result from enhanced neuronal activity in the trigeminal nucleus caudalis as a result of fluctuating doses of ergots, analgesics, or narcotics which could result in resetting of the pain-control mechanisms in susceptible individuals. Central sensitization could be enhanced through NMDA receptors, or blocking adaptive antinociceptive changes (Silberstein and Lipton 1997).

– Chronic analgesic abuse may down-regulate a serotoninergically-mediated central anti-nociceptive system (Kudrow 1982). Discontinuation of drugs that stimulate 5-HT (serotonin) receptors may result in heightening of pain perception. This also interferes with the effect of serotoninergic antidepressants which may be used concomitantly for depression associated with muscle tension headache. Alterations of platelet serotonin are known to occur in migraine as well as muscle tension headache (Shimomura and Takahashi 1990).

Drug-induced headaches may be due to changes in diameter of cranial blood vessel by vasoconstrictor or vasodilator effect or may be serotonin-induced.

Diagnosis of Drug-Induced Headache

The diagnosis of drug-induced headache is made from the careful history of the patient. Other neurological conditions, particularly structural brain

Table 6.6. Diagnostic criteria for drug-related headaches (The International Headache Society, 1988).

Headache as chronic drug effect
  – Onset after a daily intake of a drug for at least 3 months.
  – A definite minimal dose should have been given.
  – Headache should be chronic (15 days or more per month).
  – Headache should disappear within a month after discontinuation of the drug.

Ergotamine headache
  – It is preceded by a minimal daily dose of ergotamine of 2 mg or rectal dose of 1 mg.
  – The headache is diffuse, pulsating and differs from the migraine attacks by the absence of headache or the accompanying symptoms.

Analgesic headache
One or more of the following conditions:
  – Minimal intake of 50 g aspirin per month or an equivalent amount of a comparable mild analgesic.
  – Minimum 100 tablets per month of a an analgesic combined with barbiturates or a non-narcotic substance.
  – One or more narcotic analgesic.

lesions, should be excluded by appropriate neurological investigations. Diagnostic criteria for various drug-related headaches are shown in Table 6.6.

Management of Drug-Induced Headache

The principles of the management of drug-induced headache is sudden or gradual withdrawal of the agent and management of withdrawal symptoms. This is followed by institution of prophylactic and therapeutic measures for the those who have a headache syndrome such as migraine requiring treatment. Using this approach 82% of the patients were reported to be free from pain four months after drug withdrawal (Edmeads et al 1997). Hering and Steiner (1991) treated 46 migraneurs with chronic daily headaches by abrupt withdrawal of the offending drugs. The supporting treatment was explanation of the disorder to the patient, amitriptyline and naproxen. At 6-month follow-up, 37 of these patients had relief from chronic headaches.

Treatment of Withdrawal. Serious withdrawal symptoms (e. g., delirium, seizures) may occur if the patient is overusing barbiturates, alcohol, and other benzodiazepines. Severe cases may need to be hospitalized. Various approaches used for the management of withdrawal are:
- Use of clonidine
- The Raskin (intravenous dihydroergotamine) protocol is effective for both analgesic rebound headache and ergotamine dependency (Raskin 1986).
- Sumatriptan may be as effective as repetitive intravenous dihydroergotamine (Diener et al 1991; Diener and Tfelt-Hansen 1993). Sumatriptan was found to be less effective In patients with muscle tension headache.
- Combined parenteral steroids and amitriptyline (Bonuccelli et al 1996).
- Ibudilast has been used successfully for the treatment of analgesic-induced headache (Shimomura et al 1991).
- Non-steroidal agents such as naproxen may decrease the severity of headache during the analgesic washout period. Hydroxyzine and similar antihistamines are believed not to cause rebound headache and are a useful substitute for butalbital-containing agents during the analgesic washout period.

Prevention. To avoid the development of drug-induced headache use of ergotamine tartrate for migraine should be restricted to no more than 2 usage days per week and total weekly dose should not exceed 10 mg (Silberstein and Young 1995). Preventive therapy, usually a tricyclic agent, is usually begun at the same time that the withdrawal process is initiated. Preventive therapy with the combination of a tricyclic agent and a β-blocker appears to be more effective than either agent alone. The effectiveness of preventive therapy can be further enhanced with nonpharmacologic measures such as biofeedback and relaxation training.

Mathew et al (1990) reached the following conclusions after study of 200 patients with drug-induced refractory headaches:
- Daily use of symptomatic relief medications led to chronic daily headache and discontinuation these medications resulted in improvement.
- Concomitant use of medications for symptomatic relief nullifies the effect of prophylactic medications and discontinuation these enhances the beneficial effect of prophylactic medications.
- Ancillary measures such as low tyramine and low-caffeine dietary instructions as well as biofeedback training are also useful.
- Detoxification should be carried out by rapid discontinuance rather than gradual reduction.

Headache Remedies that Induce Headaches

Some of the headache remedies associated with chronic daily headache are:

Ergotamine Headaches. Ergotamine has been used for the treatment of migraine since 1925. Ergotamine tartrate has alpha-adrenergic agonist and serotonergic agonist activity and vasoconstricting actions, stimulating arterial smooth muscles through serotonin receptors. It also constricts venous capacitance vessels. Dihydroergotamine (DHE) is a derivative of ergotamine tartrate. Both ergotamine tartrate and DHE are agonists at the serotonin $5-HT_{1B}$, $5-HT_{1D}$, and $5-HT_{1F}$ receptors (Peroutka 1990), and they interact with the $5-HT_2$, adrenergic and dopaminergic receptors. DHE is a safe and effective treatment for acute, severe migraine when given IV or IM or SC.

Ergotamine-induced migraine headaches usually occur in middle-aged women on moderate doses of ergotamine (10 to 14 mg/week) for less than 6 months and resolve within 2 weeks of stopping ergotamine (Rowell et al 1973; Winterkorn et al 1990). Even small doses of ergotamine tartrate, if taken regularly three or more times per week in some patients with migraine, can induce physical and psychological dependency. This condition is characterized by increasingly frequent migraine-like headaches and ergotamine tartrate usage leading to a vicious cycle of headache and medicament use.

Propranolol. This is a β-blocker used for the treatment of migraine but there are reports of aggravation of migraine on exposure to propranolol or after withdrawal (Robson 1977). This drug is also used for the treatment of hypertension and headache is reported as an adverse effect.

Sumatiptan. Sumatriptan is a potent and selective 5-HT$_{1D}$ receptor agonist, which can be administered orally and via the subcutaneous or intranasal route. The drug is well tolerated and is consistently highly effective in most patients. Significant limitations include the recurrence of headache within 24 h after initial successful treatment and in a minority of patients, abuse of sumatriptan with daily "sumatriptan-dependent headaches" (Ferrari and Haan 1995). As compared to older migraine therapies, there has been much less mention of sumatriptan's association with chronic daily headache. Five such cases were reported of patients on sumatriptan who developed daily headaches requiring the use of sumatriptan (Göbel et al 1996). Sumatriptan was withdrawn in all the cases and the frequency of migraine returned to that prior to institution of sumatriptan therapy.

Epidemiology of Drug-Induced Headache

Prevalence and incidence rates of drug-induced headache in the general population are not available. About 0.5% of the population has severe daily headaches the most common cause of which is primary headache disorders aggravated by analgesics. Approximately 40% of patients seen at major headache clinics suffer from chronic daily headache (Mathew 1993) and 73% of these patients use excessive amounts of analgesics, sedative-caffeine-analgesic combinations, or ergotamine on a daily basis. Analgesic rebound headaches were recognized as substantive components in more than 40% of 174 primary care practices surveyed (Rapoport et al 1996).

In Western Europe about a quarter of the population uses analgesics (75% to 90% of these are available over-the-counter without prescription) and 1% of the population abuses these medications. With this background, drug-induced headache would not be a rare phenomenon. Headache is the most frequently reported adverse effect of

drugs during clinical trials and the prevalence figures for some drugs are quoted in this chapter. Analgesic abuse headache is not confined to the adult population as several cases have been reported in children as well (Symon 1998).

Headaches Induced by Other Drugs and Substances

Antidepressants. Although antidepressants improve the headache due to depression, they have also been reported to cause headaches. In long term trials of moclobemide, headache along with insomnia was one of the most frequent events reported (Moll et al 1994).

Reports of headache with selective serotonin reuptake inhibitors (SSRIs) are rare. Headaches constituted 3% of 1202 reports describing 1861 adverse reactions to SSRIs submitted to the Swedish Adverse Drug Reactions Advisory Committee (Spigset 1999). Fluoxetine (Larson 1993) and paroxetine (Currie et al 1995) have been reported to be associated with headaches. Serotonin (5-hydroxytryptamine, 5-HT) is implicated in the pathogenesis of migraine. Cerebral vessels, whose constriction and dilatation are involved in migraine mechanisms, are innervated by serotonin fibers from the raphe nucleus and this is postulated to be the basis of antimigraine effect of serotonin antagonists such as methysergide. Trazodone has been reported to provoke migraine attack in a patient with genetic predisposition (Workman et al 1992). The explanation of this is that m-chlorophenylpiperazine, the major metabolite of trazodone can itself induce migraine.

Aspartame. There are only several controlled studies in the literature which deal with the relationship between aspartame and headache but the results are conflicting. One study found no difference between placebo and aspartame (Schiffman et al 1987), while the other found a significant increase of frequency of migraine attacks (Koehler and Glaros 1988; Van Den Eeden et al 1994). No definite opinion can be given on this topic.

Bromocriptine. Bromocriptine, also an ergot derivative used for suppression of lactation has been reported to induce headache Bromocriptine has been reported to induce headaches in postpartum women without previous history of migraine (Kulig et al 1991). Some of the headaches can be attributed to hypertension and stroke which have also been reported as adverse reactions to bromocriptine. Concomitant use of sympathomimetic drugs can produce cerebral vasospasm and intracerebral hemorrhage.

Cyclosporine. This is an immunosuppressive drug used widely in organ transplant and its use in non-transplant indications is increasing. Headache is the most frequent side effect of cyclosporine in patients receiving 2.5 mg/kg/day but not in those receiving half of this dose (Reitamo et al 1993). Cyclosporine-induced migraine with severe vomiting was reported in three cases and two of these lost the renal graft (Magrabi and Bohlega 1998). The exact pathomechanism of cyclosponine-induced headache is not known but cyclosporine has vasoactive properties or headache may be a manifestation of cyclosporine-induced encephalopathy. Propranolol has been used as treatment for these headaches (Gryn et al 1992). Switching of the patients to another immunosuppressive agent FK506 also relieves the headache although the mechanism of action of FK506 is unknown (Rozen et al 1996).

Glutamate. Vasospasm induced by glutamate and its metabolite glutamine is an explanation of monosodium glutamate-induced headache (Merritt and Williams 1990).

Intravenous Immune Globulins. Headache is commonly reported after intravenous infusion of immune globulins. Constantinescu and Chang (1993) reported a patient who developed migraine following first injection of gamma globulin and had a recurrence following the second injection. Further recurrences were prevented by prophylactic use of propranolol. The incidence of headache in patients receiving IVIG infusion has been reported to be 48% (Bertaroni et al 1995).

Nicotine. Transdermal nicotine is used as an aid to smoking cessation. Headache is reported in 10% of the patients using this therapy. This may be due to vasoconstrictive effect of nicotine.

Ondansetron. This is a 5-HT antagonist which is used to control the emesis associated with cancer chemotherapy. Headache has been reported as a common ADR of this drug in clinical trials (Siderov et al 1993, Markham and Sorkin 1993). Patients with history of migraine should be advised of this potential side effect.

Oral Contraceptives (OCs) and Migraine. Headache is one of the common complaints in women using oral contraceptives (OCs). Data on the relationship of migraine to OC use is conflicting. Most reports indicate increasing severity and/or frequency of attacks of migraine in OC users (Phillips 1968; Dalton 1976; Herzberg et al 1971; Ryan 1978). Four double-blind placebo-controlled studies showed no difference in headache among OC and placebo users (Nilsson and Solvell 1967; Goldzieher et al 1971; Silbergeld et al 1971; Cullberg 1972). A study conducted in Mexico showed that women receiving placebo who believed they were receiving OCs had a headache frequency of 15.6% (Aznar-Ramos et al 1969). Atypical patterns may appear in women suffering from migraine when they begin taking OCs, or migraine may appear for the first time in women with a family history of migraine. In a few cases migraine may even improve.

Risk Factors for Aggravation of Migraine in Women on OC

The following risk factors have been described by Dalton (1976):
- Age more than 30 years.
- Menstrual pattern of migraine.
- Length of menstrual cycle outside the conventional 27–30 days.
- Relief of migraine during the last trimester of pregnancy.
- Onset of migraine after pregnancy.

Pathomechanism. One pathomechanism that might cause worsening of migraine by OC use is increased platelet aggregation with small vessel occlusion by platelet thrombi (Linet and Stewart 1984). Patients with complicated migraine have increase in epinephrine-induced platelet aggregation (Mazal 1978).

Migraine headaches develop during the period of adaptation to oral contraception and attacks occur in the premenstrual period which indicates an estrogen-withdrawal. Vasoconstriction, which may have existed previously due to use of OC, may change over to relative vasodilatation during this period. The extent of this change may develop on the estrogen content of the pill and it has been shown that pills with low-estrogen content are less likely to provoke migraine than those with high-estrogen content (Karsay 1990).

Estrogen and progestin have potent effects on serotonergic and opioid neurons modulating both neuronal activity and receptor density. Headache associated with OC in menopausal hormone replacement may be related in part to periodic discontinuation of estrogens (Silberstein and Merriam 1991). An increase in frequency of headaches occurs in association with a fall in the estrogen content of the medication (Dennerstein et al 1978). Deterioration of migraine or first attack of migraine has been reported in menopausal women on transdermal estradiol therapy (Kaiser and Meienberg 1993).

Sildenafil (Pfizer's Viagra). Sildenafil, an oral therapy for erectile dysfunction, is a selective inhibitor of cyclic guanosine monophosphate (cGMP)-specific phosphodiesterase type 5 (PDE5), the predominant isozyme metabolizing cGMP in the corpus cavernosum. Headache as an adverse reaction has been reported in > 2% of cases in clinical trials (Goldenberg 1998). In another clinical trial, headaches were reported in 16% of the treated patients versus 4% of the patients on placebo (Morales et al 1998). One case has been reported of recurrence of cluster headache after starting treatment with sildenafil and these continued even after discontinuation of the drug (Stein 1999).

Vasodilators. Vasodilator drugs frequently cause headache. Drugs commonly implicated include antiangina agents (amyl nitrite, nitroglycerin), peripheral vasodilators (oxpentifylline, cyclandelate), and antihypertensives (prazosin, hydralazine). Bronchodilators like theophylline and nicotinic acid derivatives used in the treatment of hypercholesterolemia also possess vasodilator activity.

Nitroglycerin. Headache is the most frequent side effect of nitroglycerin and is sometimes so severe that its use in cardiac patients is limited. Migraineurs usually develop a headache after sublingual nitroglycerin (delayed nitroglycerin-induced headache) which is similar to their migraine attacks (Sicuteri et al 1987). A double-blind controlled study demonstrated that intravenous infusions of nitroglycerin produced a more severe and prolonged headache in migraine subjects as compared with normal controls (Oleson et al 1993). The fact that nitroglycerin, a nitric oxide donor, triggers genuine migraine attacks indicates that activation of nitric oxide cGMP pathway may cause migraine attacks (Thomsen et al 1994).

Pathomechanism. The exact mechanism of nitrate-induced headache is not known. The following explanations have been offered:

– In experimental models, intravenous nitroglycerin provokes a dose-dependent headache (Iversen et al 1992). In a study in human volunteers using 5-isosorbide mononitrate (5-ISM, an active metabolite of isosorbide dinitrate), the diameter of superficial temporal arteries was measured with high frequency ultrasound and correlated with headache. The authors concluded that headache after 5-ISM is caused by arterial dilatation or the mechanisms responsible for it.

– It has been suggested that nitric oxide, which is produced by the metabolism of both exogenous nitrates and endogenous L-arginine can play a key role in mediating vascular headaches (Oleson et al 1994).

– Recent studies of patients with chronic renal failure have shown that accumulation of asymmetrical dimethylarginine which is an analog of L-arginine, can impair endogenous nitric oxide synthesis through a competitive inhibition of nitric oxide synthase. Such patients are less likely to show vasodilating effect of nitrates. Serum creatinine and age have been independently and inversely associated with headache caused by nitrates (Pahor et al 1995).

Vitamin A Abuse. Excess intake of vitamin A can cause hypervitaminosis A and benign intracranial hypertension (see Chapter 17). However, isolated headache may occur as a symptom after overdose of vitamin A. A case was reported of patient who reported headache with occasional nausea and vomiting after taking 20,000 IU of vitamin A daily for two years (Friedland and Burde 1996). The patient experienced a significant relief of headache with 3 weeks of discontinuation of vitamin A.

Withdrawal Headaches

Withdrawal headaches can occur after discontinuation of several drugs whether used for the treatment of headache or other conditions. Headaches are also a part of the withdrawal syndromes following discontinuation of drugs of abuse. Examples are given of caffeine, valproic acid and octreotide.

- *Caffeine.* Headache is one of the symptoms in patients with caffeine withdrawal (discontinuation of caffeine intake). This may occur in persons who consume small to moderate amounts (median intake 2.5 cups of coffee per day) of caffeine (Silverman et al 1992). Caffeine withdrawal has been reported to precipitate migraine (Couturier et al 1992).

- *Valproic acid.* Onset of migraine after withdrawal of valproic acid treatment of epilepsy has been described in a young girl with family history of migraine (Pavese et al 1994).

- *Octreotide.* Rebound tension type headache has been reported after use of octreotide (somatostatin octapeptide analog) for acromegaly (May et al 1994). Headaches occur in about 50% of patients with pituitary tumors and subside with the use of octreotide. In the case reported they improved dramatically after administration of octreotide but recurred 6–8 hours later. The authors theorized that increasing octreotide doses cause up-regulation of substance P receptors, accounting for analgesic effect of this somatostatin analog and recurrence of headache on its withdrawal.

Headache Due to Non-CNS Adverse Effects of Drugs

Headache may be secondary to adverse effects involving systems other than the CNS. Two examples of these would be presented here: drug-induced hypertension and drug-induced myositis of head and neck muscles

Hypertension. Headache is one of the symptoms of severe hypertension. Several drugs produce hypertension. Hypertensive reactions between monoamine oxidase inhibitors (MAOI) and certain foods are well known (Blackwell et al 1967). Although postural hypotension is a frequent adverse reaction of MAOIs, spontaneous hypertensive reactions have also been reported (Fallon et al 1988). This reaction may present initially as a pounding occipital headache which radiates frontally and becomes generalized. These reactions occur within minutes to a few hours after ingestion of incompatible food or medication. The headache usually improves within an hour but dull ache may persist for some days. The most frequently recommended treatment of this reaction is intravenous phentolamine, or diazoxide, or nitroprusside. Golwyn and Sevlie (1993) have recommended the use of nifedipine to treat hypertensive headaches due to MAOIs.

When a patient who is taking a MAOI complains of headache, it is important to exclude other causes. MAOI drugs can also produce histamine headache particularly when taken with foods containing histamine whose degradation is impaired by MAOI. This is usually associated with hypotension and the logical treatment of this condition would be an antihistaminic (Davidson 1992).

Headache Due to Myositis of Head and Neck Muscles

Several drugs produce muscle pain and myositis. Patients complain of headache when head and neck muscles are involved. One example is filgrastim (Granulocyte colony stimulating factor) which is well known to produce muscle pain and headache.

References

Andersson PG: Ergotamine headache. Headache 1975; 15: 118–121.

Rasmussen BK: Epidemiology of headache. Cephalalgia 1995; 15: 45–68.

Aznar-Ramos R, Giner-Velazquez J, Lara-Ricalde R, et al: Incidence of side effects with contraceptive placebo. Am J Obstet Gynecol 1969; 105: 1144–1149.

Barnes TRE, Greenwood DT: Viloxazine and migraine. Lancet 1979; ii: 1368.

Bertaroni TE, Nance AM, Horner LH, et al: Complications of intravenous gamma globulin infusion in neuromuscular diseases (abstract). Neurology 1995; 45 (suppl 4): A236.

Blackwell B, Marley E, Taylor D: Hypertensive reactions between monoamine oxidase inhibitors and foodstuffs. Br J Psychiatry 1967; 113: 345–365.

Bonuccelli U, Nuti A, Lucetti C, et al: Amitriptyline and dexamethasone combined treatment in drug-induced headache. Cephalalgia 1996; 16: 198–200.

Bowdler I, Kilian J, Ganslenn-Blumberg S: The association between analgesic abuse and headache— coincidental or causal? Headache 1988; 28: 494.

Constantinescu CS, Chang AP: Recurrent migraine and intravenous immune globulin therapy. NEJM 1993; 329: 583–584.

Couturier EGM, Hering R, Steiner TJ: Weekend attacks in migraine patients: caused by caffeine withdrawal? Cephalalgia 1992; 12: 99–100.

Cullberg J: Mood changes and menstrual symptoms with different gestagen/estrogen combinations: a double-blind comparison with placebo. Acta Psychiatr Scand 1972; 236(suppl): 259–276.

Currie A, Ryman A, McAllister-Williams RH: Exacerbation of migraine with paroxetine: case report. Human Psychopharmacology: Clinical and Experimental 1995; 10: 349–350.

Dalton K: Migraine and oral contraceptives. Headache 1976; 15: 247–251.

Davidson JRT: Monoamine oxidase inhibitors. In Paykel ES (Ed.): Handbook of affective disorders, 2nd ed, New York, Guilford Press, 1992, pp 345–358.

Dennerstein L, Laby B, Burrows GD, et al: Headache and sex hormone therapy. Headache 1978; 18: 146–153.

Diener HC, Tfelt-Hansen P: Headache associated with chronic use of substance. In Oleson J, et al (Eds.): The headaches, New York, Raven Press, 1993, pp 721–727.

Diener HC, Dichgans J, Scholz E, et al: Analgesic-induced chronic headache: long-term results of withdrawal therapy. J Neurol 1989; 236: 9–14.

Diener HC, Gerber WD, Geiselhart D, et al: Short and long term effects of withdrawal therapy in drug-induced headache. In Diener HC, Wilkinson M (Eds.): Drug-induced headache, New York, Springer, 1988, pp 133–142.

Diener HC, Haab J, Peters C, et al: Subcutaneous sumatriptan in the treatment of headache during withdrawal from drug-induced headache. Headache 1991; 31: 205–209.

Edmeads J: Analgesic-induced headache: an unrecognized epidemic. Headache 1990; 30: 614–615.

Edmeads JG, Gawel MJ, Vickers J: Strategies for diagnosing and managing medication-induced headache. Canadian Family Physician 1997; 43: 1249–1254.

Elkind AH: Drug abuse and headache. Med Clin North Am 1991; 75: 717–732.

Elkind AH: Drug abuse in headache patients. Clin J Pain 1989; 5: 111–120.

Fallon B, Foote B, Walsh BT, et al: "Spontaneous" hypertensive episodes with monoamine oxidase inhibitors. J Clin Psychiatry 1988; 49: 163–165.

Ferrari MD, Haan J: Acute treatment of migraine attacks. Curr Opin Neurol 1995; 8: 237–42.

Friedland S, Burde RM: Chronic headache due to vitamin A abuse. Journal of Neuro-Ophthalmology 1996; 16: 72.

Garcia-Albea E, Cabrera F, Tejeiro J, et al: Jaqueca tipica y talidomida. Med Clin (Madrid) 1993; 100: 557.

Göbel H, Stolze H, Heinze A, et al: Easy therapeutical management of sumatriptan-induced headache. Neurology 1996; 47: 297–298.

Goldenberg MM: Safety and efficacy of sildenafil citrate in the treatment of male erectile dysfunction. Clin Ther 1998; 20: 1033–48.

Goldzieher JW, Moses LE, Averkin E, et al: A placebo-controlled, double-blind, crossover investigation of the side effects attributed to oral contraceptives. Fertil Steril 1971; 22: 609–623.

Golwyn DH, Sevlie CP: Monoamine oxidase inhibitor hypertensive crisis headache and orthostatic hypotension. J Clin Psychopharmacol 1993; 13: 77–78.

Gora ML: Nicotine transdermal systems. Ann Pharmacother 1993; 27: 742–750.

Granella F, Farina S, Malferrari G, et al: Drug abuse in chronic headache: a clinico-epidemiologic study. Cephalalgia 1987; 7: 15–19.

Gryn J, Goldberg J, Viner E: Propranolol for the treatment of cyclosporine-induced headaches. Bone Marrow Transplantation 1992; 9: 211–212.

Harinasuta T, Bunnag D, Lasserre R, et al: Trials of mefloquine in vivax and mefloquine plus "Fansidar" in symptomatic falciparum malaria. Bull WHO 1983; 61: 713.

Hering R, Steiner TJ: Abrupt outpatient withdrawal of medication in analgesic-abusing migraineurs. Lancet 1991; 337: 1442–1443.

Herzberg BN, Draper KC, Johnson AL, et al: Oral contraceptives, depression, and libido. BMJ 1971; 3: 495–500.

International Headache Society (Headache Classification Committee): Classification and diagnostic criteria for headache disorders, cranial neuralgias and facial pain. Cephalalgia 1988; 7(suppl): 1–96.

Isler H: Headache drugs provoking chronic headache: historical aspects and common misunderstandings. In Diener HC, Wilkinson M (Eds.): Drug-induced headache, Berlin, Springer-Verlag, 1988, pp 87–94.

Iversen HK, Nielsen TH, Garre K, et al: Dose-dependent headache response and dilatation of limb and extracranial arteries after three doses of 5-isosorbide mononitrate. Eur J Clin Pharmacol 1992; 42: 31–35.

Kaiser HJ, Meienberg O: Deterioration or onset of migraine under oestrogen replacement therapy. J Neurol 1993; 240: 195–197.

Karsay K: The relationship between vascular headaches and low-dose oral contraceptives. Ther Hung 1990; 38: 181–185.

Koehler SM, Glaros A: The effect of aspartame on headache. Headache 1988; 28: 10–14.

Kudrow L: Paradoxical effects of frequent analgesic abuse. In Critchley M, et al (Eds.): Advances in neurology, vol 33, Raven Press, New York, 1982, pp 335–341.

Kulig K, Moore LL, Kirk M, et al: Bromocriptine-associated headache: possible life-threatening sympathetic interaction. Obstet Gynecol 1991; 78: 941–943.

Lance E, Parkes C, Wilkinson M: Does analgesic abuse cause headache de novo? Headache 1988; 28: 61–62.

Larson EW: Migraine with typical aura associated with fluoxetine therapy: case report. J Clin Psychiatry 1993; 54: 235–236.

Linet MS, Stewart WF: Migraine headache: epidemiologic perspectives. Epidemiol Rev 1984; 6: 107–139.

Lippman CW: Characteristic headache resulting from prolonged use of ergot derivatives. J Nerv Ment Dis 1955; 121: 270–273.

Magrabi K, Bohlega S: Cyclosporine-induced migraine with severe vomiting causing loss of renal graft. Clin Neurol Neurosurg 1998; 100: 224–227.

Markham A, Sorkin EM: Ondasentron. An update of its therapeutic use in chemotherapy-induced and postoperative nausea and vomiting. Drugs 1993; 45: 931–952.

Mathew N: Chronic refractory headache. Neurology 1993; 43(suppl 3): S26–33.

Mathew NT, Kurman R, Perez F: Drug-induced refractory headache—clinical features and management. Headache 1990; 30: 634–638.

Mathew NT, Reuveni U, Perez F: Transformed or evolutive migraine. Headache 1987; 27: 102–106.

Mathew NT: Transformed migraine, analgesic rebound, and other chronic daily headaches. Neurol Clin 1997; 15: 167–86.

Mathew NT: Drug-induced headache. Neurologic Clinics 1990; 8: 903–912.

May A, Lederbogen S, Diener HC: Octreotide dependency and headache: a case report. Cephalalgia 1994; 14: 303–304.

Mazal S: Migraine attacks and increased platelet aggregability induced by oral contraceptives. Aust NZ J Med 1978; 8: 646–648.

McGregor EA, Vohrah C, Wilkinson M: Analgesic use: a study of treatments used by patients for migraine prior to attending City of London Migraine Clinic. Headache 1990; 30: 571–574.

Merritt JE, Williams PB: Vasospasm contributes to monosodium glutamate-induced headache. Headache 1990; 30: 575–580.

Moll E, Newmann N, Schmid-Burgk W, et al: Safety and efficacy during long-term treatment with moclobemide. Clin Neuropharmacol 1994; 17(suppl 1): S74–S87.

Morales A, Gingell C, Collins M, et al: Clinical safety of oral sildenafil citrate (VIAGRA) in the treatment of erectile dysfunction. Int J Impot Res 1998; 10: 69–74.

Nilsson L, Solvell L: Clinical studies on oral contraceptives—a randomized, double-blind, crossover study of four different preparations. Acta Obstet Gynecol Scand 1967; 46(suppl 8): 3–31.

Oleson J, Iversen HK, Thomsen LL: Nitric oxide supersensitivity. A possible molecular mechanism of migraine pain. NeuroReport 1993; 4: 1027–1030.

Oleson J, Thomsen LL, Iversen H: Nitric oxide is a key molecule in migraine and other vascular headaches. Trends Pharmacol Sci 1994; 15: 149–153.

Pahor M, Cecchi E, Fumagalli S, et al: Association of serum creatinine and age with headache caused by nitrates. Clin Pharmacol Ther 1995; 58: 470–481.

Pavese N, Baracchini G, Bonuccelli U: Valproate-withdrawal induced migraine. Headache 1994; 34: 445.

Phillips BM: Oral contraceptive drugs and migraine. BMJ 1968; 2: 99.

Polleri A, Murialdo G, Martignoni E, et al: Benserazide induces migraine attacks. Irrelevance of concomitant hyperprolactinemia. Farmaco (Sci) 1979; 34: 465–468.

Post RM, Silberstein SD: Shared mechanisms in affective illness, epilepsy and migraine. Neurology 1994; 44: S37–S47.

Rapoport A, Stang P, Gutterman DL, et al: Analgesic rebound headache in clinical practice: data from a physician survey. Headache 1996;36:14–9.

Rapoport AM, Weeks RE, Sheftel FD, et al: Analgesic rebound headache: theoretical and practical implications. Cephalalgia 1985; 5(suppl 3): 448.

Rapoport AM: Analgesic rebound headache. Headache 1988; 28: 662–665.

Raskin N: Repetitive intravenous dihydroergotamine as therapy for intractable migraine. Neurology 1986; 36: 995–997.

Reitamo S, Erkko P, Remitz A, et al: Cyclosporine in the treatment of palmoplantar pustulosis. A randomiized, double-blind, placebo-controlled study. Arch Dermatol 1993; 129: 1273–1279.

Robson RH: Recurrent migraine after propranolol. Br Heart J 1977; 39: 1157.

Rohr L, Floch J: Chronic headaches caused by drug abuse: danger for patients with migraine. Schweiz Rundsch Med Prax 1992; 81: 1417–1419.

Rowell AR, Neylan C, Wilkinson M: Ergotamine-induced headaches in migranous patients. Headache 1973; 13: 65–67.

Rozen TD, Wijdicks EFM, Hay JE: Treatment-refractory cyclosporine-associated headache: relief with conversion to FK-506. Neurology 1996; 47: 1347.

Ryan RE: A controlled study of the effect of oral contraceptives on migraine. 1978; 17: 250–251.

Schiffman S, Buckley CE, Sampson HA, et al: Aspartame and susceptibility to headache. NEJM 1987; 317: 1181–1185.

Shimomura T, Kowa H, Takahashi K: Analgesic-induced headaches: successful treatment with ibudilast. Headache 1991; 31: 483.

Shimomura T, Takahashi K: Alteration of platelet serotonin in patients with chronic tension type headache during cold pressor test. Headache 1990; 30: 581–583.

Sicuteri F, Del Bene E, Poggioni M, et al: Unmasking latent dysnociception in healthy subjects. Headache 1987; 27: 180–185.

Siderov J, Zalcberg J, Chambers B, et al: Migraine following the use of 5-hydroxytryptamine antagonist. Aust NZ J Med 1993; 23: 527–528.

Silbergeld S, Brast N, Noble EP: The menstrual cycle: a double-blind study of symptoms, mood, and behavior, and biochemical variables using Enovid and placebo. Psychosom Med 1971; 33: 411–428.

Silberstein SD, Young WB: Safety and efficacy of ergotamine tartarate and dihydroergotamine in the treatment of migraine and status migrainosus. Neurology 1995; 45: 577–584.

Silberstein SD, Lipton RB: Chronic daily headache. In Goadsby PJ, Silberstein SD (Eds.): Headache. Blue books of practical neurology, vol. 17, Boston, Butterworth-Heinemann, 1997, pp 201–25.

Silberstein SD, Merriam GR: Estrogens, progestins, and headache. Neurology 1991; 41: 786–793.

Silverman K, Evans SM, Strain EC, et al: Withdrawal syndrome after the double-blind cessation of caffeine consumption. NEJM 1992; 327: 109–114.

Spigset O: Adverse reactions of selective serotonin reuptake inhibitors: reports from a spontaneous reporting system. Drug Safety 1999; 20: 277–87.

Stein M: Viagra and cluster headaches. Headache 1999; 39: 58–59.

Stewart WF, Lipton RB, Celentano DD, et al: Prevalence

of migraine headache in the United States. JAMA 1992; 267: 64–69.

Symon DNK: Twelve cases of analgesic headache. Archives of Disease in Childhood 1998; 78: 555–556.

Tester-Dalderup CBM: Antifungal drugs. In Dukes MNG (Ed.): Meyler's side effects of drugs, 12th ed, Amsterdam, Elsevier, 1992, pp. 672–686.

Therasse DG: The safety profile of loracarbef. Am J Med 1992; 92: 20S–25S.

Thomsen LL, Kruuse C, Iversen HK, et al: A nitric oxide donor (nitroglycerin) triggers genuine migraine attacks. Eur J Neurol 1994; 1: 73–80.

Van Den Eeden SK, Koepsell TD, Longstreth WT, et al: Aspartame ingestion and headaches: a randomized crossover trial. Neurology 1994; 44: 1787–1793.

Wainscott G, Volans G, Wilkinson M: Ergotamine induced headaches. BMJ 1974; ii: 724.

Wallasch TM: Medikamentös induzierter Kopfschmerz. Fortschr Neurol Psychiatr 1992; 60: 114–118.

Welch KMA, Darnley D, Simkins RT: The role of estrogen in migraine: a review and hypothesis. Cephalalgia 1984; 4: 227–236.

Winterkorn JMS, Odel JG, Behrens MM: ergotamine headache mistaken for temporal arteritis. Ann Neurol 1990; 28: 396.

Wolfson W, Graham J: Development of tolerance to ergot alkaloids in patients with unusually severe migraine. NEJM 1949; 241: 296–298.

Workman EA, Tellian F, Short D: Trazodone induction of migraine headache through mCPP. Am J Psychiatry 1992; 149: 712–713.

Chapter 7
Drug-Induced Seizures

Introduction

Several drugs have been reported to cause seizures. Seizures may be defined as a "paroxysmal clinical event characterized by an altered state of consciousness with or without presence of motor activity or abnormal motor activity accompanied by epileptic EEG activity." An abnormal discharge may arise from neurons in either cortical or subcortical regions. The term epilepsy is not used for this adverse reaction except in rare circumstances when brain damage caused by a drug acts as an epileptic focus. This problem is difficult to evaluate because every human being can have a seizure under certain circumstances. About 10% of the population has a tendency to have seizures which can be triggered by such stimuli such as fever in infancy, drugs, biochemical disturbances.

Most of drug-induced seizures were described as complications of therapy with psychotropic drugs. After the introduction of antidepressants, the earliest reports of seizures were in 1950s and were particularly associated with imipramine therapy (Lehmann et al 1958). Epileptogenic effects of neuroleptic therapy were recognized in the 1960s. Penicillin, introduced in clinical use in 1939, was known to be epileptogenic when applied to cerebral cortex of experimental animals. Clinical reports of seizures due to penicillin started to appear in the 1960s (Weinstein et al 1964).

Clinical Features and Diagnosis

There are no characteristic clinical features of drug-induced seizures to differentiate them from idiopathic epileptic seizures. Generalized seizures with focal features are common and simple partial seizures are rare. Generalized seizures usually present with loss of consciousness, convulsions, tongue biting, and incontinence of urine. There is usually no preceding aura or focal disturbances and no residual neurological deficit. Severe attacks may lead to status epilepticus. Some of the conditions to be considered in the differential diagnosis of a drug-induced seizure are shown in Table 7.1.

Table 7.1. Differential diagnosis of drug-induced seizures.

Multiorgan failure
Renal failure and dialysis
Metabolic disorders secondary to organ failure
Raised levels of proconvulsant medications due to
  impaired clearance

Metabolic disorders
Hypoglycemia
Hyponatremia

Organic diseases of the brain
Post-traumatic epilepsy
Brain tumors
CNS infections

Cerebrovascular disorders
Stroke
Syncope
Drop attacks due to basilar insufficiency or migraine

In drug safety surveillance reports, information is often sketchy and there is no possibility of questioning the patients or the observers. Indication for the use of the drug is an important consideration in evaluating drug-induced seizures. Patients with acute CNS conditions are predisposed to seizures. Approximately 20 to 30% of children with meningitis with meningitis experience convulsions prior to presentation. It is difficult to evaluate the causal relationship of seizures to medication in these patients when they occur after start of antibiotic therapy. In this chapter, known pathomechanisms of seizures are described as well as hypotheses to explain seizures with drugs. Prevention and treatment of drug-induced seizures will be discussed according to the drugs involved.

Pharmacoepidemiology

Figures for the prevalence of epilepsy vary. Most studies show incidence rates varying from 20–70/100,000 per year and a point prevalence rate of 4–10/1000 in the general population. According to the World Health Organization, the life time prevalence, which is the measure of the number of people in general population who ever had epilepsy, is 5%. There are few studies of the prevalence of drug-induced convulsions. In series of 32,812 patients studied in the Boston Collaborative Drug Surveillance Program (Porter and Jick 1977), drug-associated convulsions occurred in 26 (0.08%). Messing et al (1984) evaluated 3,155 patients with seizures during a ten-year period in a neurology clinic and of these 45 (1.7%) had drug-induced seizures. Forty-five percent of these patients had single seizures, 40% suffered multiple convulsions, and 15% had status epilepticus. Most common drugs that caused seizures in this study were isoniazid, insulin, lidocaine, and psychotropic medications. Olson et al (1993) carried out a retrospective survey of seizures associated with poisoning and drug intoxication in San Francisco Bay area over a two year period. They found that the leading causes of seizures were cyclic antidepressants (29%), psychostimulant drugs (29%), antihistaminics (14%), theophylline (5%) and isoniazid (5%).

It is impossible to determine the incidence of drug-induced seizures in post-marketing spontaneous reports of adverse effects because the denominator is not known. It is also difficult to determine the incidence from clinical trials because most trials are carried out on relatively small number of patients. To detect one case of drug-induced seizure with an incidence of 1:1000 per year, about 3000 patients would have to be studied for this period.

Pathomechanism of Drug-Induced Seizures

Drugs may produce seizures by several mechanisms as shown in Table 7.2.

Table 7.2. Pathomechanisms of drug-induced seizures.

Direct effects on the CNS
  – disturbances of cerebral energy metabolism
  – stimulation of the CNS
  – neurotransmitter disturbances
  – chronic changes in α-2 receptors
  – cerebral cortical irritation
  – toxic effects on neurons
Indirect effects
  – cerebral blood flow disturbances
  – cerebral hypoxia
  – secondary to non-neurological drug reactions:
    • cardiac rhythm disturbances
    • electrolyte disturbances, e. g., hyponatremia, hypomagnesemia
    • metabolic disturbances, e. g., hypoglycemia
    • fever
Overdose of drugs affecting CNS
Sedative drug withdrawal
Drug interactions
  – interference with effect of antiepileptic drugs
  – concomitant use of two drugs where one drug raises the concentration of other drug known to induce epileptic seizures

Risk Factors for Drug-Induced Seizures

Risk factors which predispose to drug-induced seizures are shown in Table 7.3.

Drugs Associated with Seizures

The information on this topic is drawn from publications most of which are case reports and some are reviews of drug-induced seizures (Zaccara et al 1990; Garcia and Alldredge 1994). In some cases the causal relationship of the drug to the seizures is suspected but not proven. Various categories of drugs which have been reported to be associated with seizures are shown in Table 7.4.

Table 7.3. Risk factors for drug-induced seizures.

Patient related
- Family history of epilepsy or previous seizures
- Patients with CNS disorders without history of previous seizures: brain tumors, stroke, AIDS encephalopathy
- Breach of blood brain barrier such as occurs in head injury and meningitis
- Psychiatric disorders
- Patients at extremes of age: the elderly and the infants
- Systemic diseases affecting drug metabolism and excretion, particularly those affecting renal and hepatic functions
- High fever

Medication related
- Multiple medications: drug interactions
- Use of drugs known to induce seizures
- Factors affecting CNS levels of drugs: lipid solubility, protein binding transport by endogenous systems
- Serum levels of drugs: dose, frequency and route of administration
- Overdose
- Withdrawal

Table 7.4. Drugs associated with seizures.

Table 7.4. continued

Therapeutic categories	Radiological contrast agents*
Anesthesia	– intravascular
– local anesthetics	– intrathecal
– general anesthetics	Vaccines*
Antidepressants*	*Miscellaneous Drugs*
– tricyclics	Acyclovir
– monoamine oxidase inhibitors	Alcohol
– serotonin reuptake inhibitors	Allopurinol*
Antipsychotics	Aminophylline*
– butyrophenones	Aspartame
– phenothiazines*	Atropine sulfate
– clozapine*	Baclofen
– lithium	Beta-blockers
– zotepine	Bromocriptine
Antiepileptics	Camphor
Antihistaminics	Chloral hydrate
Antimalarial drugs	Desmopressin
Antimicrobial agents*	Digoxin
Antineoplastic agents	Domperidone
– alkylating agents	Drug abuse
– antimetabolites	Erythropoietin
– vinca alkaloids*	Famotidine
CNS stimulants theophylline*	Flumazenil*
– caffeine	Fluorescein
– cocaine	Ganciclovir
– amphetamine	Insulin*
– methylphenidate	Interferon-α
Immunosuppressive drugs	Iodine
– glucocorticoids	Isoretinoin
– cyclosporine	Levodopa
– azathioprine	Melatonin
– OKT3	Methyldopa
Non-steroidal anti-inflammatory drugs	Naftidrofuryl
– aspirin	Ondansetron
– indomethacin	Sulproston
– mefenamic acid	Terbutaline
Opioids and other narcotic analgesics	Thyroxine
– morphine	Ziperol
– meperidine*	

* Frequently reported.

Anesthesia

Neurological adverse effects of anesthesia are well known and are dealt with in more detail elsewhere (Jain 1999a, 1999b). For purposes of describing seizures as adverse effects, the following classification of anesthesia will be used:

– General anesthesia: Various types with the commonly used agents are as follows:

Inhalation: N_2OWN_2O;Nitrous oxide (most widely used), halothane, enflurane, isoflurane, sevoflurane

Intravenous: Barbiturates, benzodiazepines, propofol, ketamine

Narcotics: opioids, fentanyl

Muscle relaxants: polarizing and depolarizing

– Local anesthetics: lidocaine, ropivacaine, bupivacaine, mepivacaine, tetracaine, prilacaine, procaine, procainamide, and benzocaine

– Epidural anesthesia

Seizures following anesthesia are difficult to evaluate because of the complicating factors such as other medications and surgery. The emphasis here will be on the use of anesthetic agents rather than the procedures of anesthesia.

General Anesthetics. Seizures are uncommon during general anesthesia but have been observed following inhalation anesthesia with enflurane and isoflurane as well as with intravenous anesthetics.

Pathomechanism. Anesthetics produce both proconvulsant as well as anticonvulsant effects. The reasons for these contrasting effects are poorly understood at present. Biologic variability plays an important role in determining an individual patient's response to anesthetics. Variations in the responsiveness of inhibitory and excitatory neurons to the central depressant effects of these drugs could also explain these apparently conflicting data (Modica et al 1990). Predisposing factors include a history of epilepsy, hyperventilation syndrome, and oxygen toxicity.

Nitrous oxide has a cerebral excitatory effect and increases motor activity. An infant was reported to develop seizures on three occasions while receiving nitrous oxide (N_2O) anesthesia (Lannes et al 1997). EEG abnormalities were demonstrated under N_2O administration.

Enflurane is well known to produce generalized seizures (Quail 1989; Allan 1984) and has been used to activate epileptogenic foci during epilepsy surgery (Ito et al 1988). Electroencephalographic abnormalities following enflurane anesthesia can persist for several days following exposure (Kruczek et al 1980) and delayed convulsions may occur. No definite recommendations are available to prevent this complication. Concomitant use of nitrous oxide may have an anticonvulsant effect but rebound excitability can occur after nitrous oxide is withdrawn. Seizures are less likely to occur if low concentrations of enflurane are used and normocapnia is maintained.

Isoflurane has been reported to be associated with myoclonus and seizure activity in patients with no previous history of seizures (Harrison 1986; Hymes 1985).

Sevoflurane has been reported to be associated with clonic and tonic seizure-like movements of the extremities in a case report but no EEG was done and the possibility of this being myoclonus of the extremities was considered (Adachi et al 1992). Electroencephalographic evidence has been presented of seizure activity under deep sevoflurane anesthesia in a nonepileptic patient (Woodforth et al 1997).

Intravenous Anesthesia. *Ketamine* may initiate seizures in epileptic patients (Bennett et al 1973; Ferrer-Allado 1973). Convulsions have also been reported in non-epileptic patients (Elliot et al 1976; Page et al 1972). Two cases of tonic-clonic convulsions were reported following intramuscular injection of ketamine and atropine (Burmeister-Rother et al 1993). There is no clear statement regarding the effect of ketamine on convulsant neuronal activity but epilepsy remains a relative contraindication for its use.

Epileptogenic activity is enhanced with short-acting intravenous anesthetics *etomidate* (Krieger et al 1985) and *methohexital* (Musella et al 1971). The latter has been to be safe and reliable for activating epileptogenic foci during epilepsy surgery (Wyler 1987).

Fentanyl is an opioid used for induction of general anesthesia. There is considerable controversy regarding its seizure-inducing potential. Fentanyl produces subcortical seizures in rats associated with a hypermetabolic state in limbic structures and reduction of glucose utilization in the remainder of the brain (Tommasino et al 1984). In humans seizure-like movements have been observed following fentanyl infusion without signs of cortical seizure activity on EEG (Scott and Sarnquist 1985). A retrospective study of 127 patients undergoing anesthesia with high-dose opioid technique failed to demonstrate any evidence of true epileptiform EEG activity. Sprung and Schedewie (1992) described a case where focal motor activity resembling Jacksonian march developed during fentanyl induction of general anesthesia but EEG failed to show any evidence of an epileptic focus. The following three explanations have been proposed to explain the nature of opioid-induced muscle activity:

- The abnormal motor activity resembling convulsions actually represents myoclonus or clonus due to blocking of cortical inhibitory pathways allowing the lower CNS structures to express unrepressed excitability resulting in clonus.
- Opioid-induced motor activity represents a form of exaggerated muscle rigidity which may sometimes resemble seizures.
- Opioid-induced abnormal motor activity represents subcortical seizures which are unlikely to be detected by surface electrodes.

Electrodes placed in the epidural space have shown electrical seizure activity during induction with fentanyl for temporal lobe epilepsy surgery (Tempelhoff et al 1992). Factors which predispose to perioperative seizures are:

- Use of concomitant drugs known to predispose to seizures (see Neurobase article on this topic).
- Oxygen toxicity
- Discontinuation of antiepileptic medications in epileptic patients in the perioperative period.
- Metabolic abnormalities such as hyponatremia, hypocalcemia and hypoglycemia are associated with seizures.
- Hypothermic circulatory arrest for more than one hours increases the incidence of seizures to 15% (Miller et al 1995).

Fentanyl withdrawal seizures have been reported in a neonate following prolonged intrauterine exposure to fentanyl and rapid withdrawal of the agent after administration of naloxone 5 minutes after birth (Anwar et al 1995).

Propofol is a new intravenous short-acting anesthetic. Propofol infusion has been used for control of status epilepticus but use of this substance for induction of anesthesia has been reported to be followed by "convulsive movements" (de Lima et al 1992). DeFriez and Wong (1992) have reported two cases of seizure-like activity with opisthotonic posturing that occurred after propofol anesthesia. Mäkela et al (1993) presented five patients where seizures were associated with propofol anesthesia and recommended that its use should be avoided in epileptic patients. Seizures have been reported after re-exposure to propofol in a patient who had an uneventful induction of anesthesia using propofol on a previous occasion (Harrigan et al 1996). The seizures were controlled with clonazepam. Unilateral seizures occurred in another case following propofol-induced anesthesia and an previously asymptomatic infarct of the contralateral hemisphere was demonstrated by CT (Cochran et al 1996). There was no further recurrence of seizures. Propofol should be avoided in patients with cerebral lesions which are likely to be the focus of an epileptic discharge.

Management of anesthesia-associated seizures. The following measures have been suggested to reduce the possibilities of seizures:

- Avoidance of drugs known to cause seizures
- Monitoring to detect and to correct metabolic abnormalities such as hyponatremia and hypoglycemia.
- Maintenance of antiepileptic drug levels in epileptic patients. The drug may be given on the morning of surgery and as soon as the patient wakes up after surgery. If unable to take orally, it may be supplemented parenterally.
- In non-epileptic patients who are suspected to be at high risk of developing perioperative seizures, consideration should be given to starting prophylactic antiepileptic therapy preoperatively.

Most of the seizures associated with anesthesia are usually self-limiting and do not result in any sequelae. However, in patients who have undergone surgery, it is not desirable to have a convulsive movement. The management of perioperative seizures is similar to that of seizures due to other causes. Seizures due to an overdose of anticholinergic agent respond to physostigmine if standard anticonvulsants are not effective.

Local Anesthetics. Initial symptoms of CNS toxicity of local anesthetics are those of excitation which may be manifested by restlessness and dizziness. Other manifestations are tremors, slurring of speech and irrational conversation. This may proceed on to a seizure or CNS depression.

Cumulative toxicity of local anesthetics depends directly on the concentration achieved in plasma whereas CNS toxicity depends largely upon the membrane-stabilizing effect of the drug. Factors affecting plasma concentration and thus toxicity include the site and rate of injection, concentration and total dose administered, absorption, degree of tissue binding and rate of metabolism and excretion. The extent of absorption depends on tissue vascularity, sites and techniques of application, patient's disease state, and the dose/unit body weight. Lidocaine is eliminated mainly by the liver and both the drug as well as its toxic metabolite can accumulate in congestive heart failure and liver disorders, producing neurotoxicity at low drug concentrations.

Seizures are an adverse effect of overdose of local anesthetics and are likely to occur if the injection is made inadvertently into a blood vessel. A direct correlation exists between clinical symptoms and blood Seizures are an adverse effect of overdose of local anesthetics and are likely to occur if the injection is made inadvertently into a blood vessel. Cumulative toxicity of local anesthetics depends directly on the concentration achieved in plasma whereas CNS toxicity depends largely upon the membrane-stabilizing effect of the drug. Factors affecting plasma concentration and thus toxicity include the site and rate of injection, concentration and total dose administered, degree of plasma and tissue binding and rate of metabolism and excretion (Reynolds 1987).

Lidocaine. It has an anticonvulsant effect in subtoxic doses (below 4 mg/L) and has been used for the treatment of seizures (Taverner and Baine 1958; Michenfelder 1988). In patients with temporal lobe epilepsy and implanted depth electrodes, lidocaine was found to produce psychomotor seizures without other excitatory manifestations (De Jong and Watts 1966). Convulsant activity has been thought to be due to an imbalance in brain activity because excitatory pathways are considered to be more resistant than inhibitory pathways (Modica et al 1990). Lidocaine seems to exert its convulsant effect at the synaptic junctions rather than the neuronal membrane (Stone and Javid 1988). Lidocaine closes the chloride channels at the synaptic cleft; the resultant chloride ion flow hyperpolarizes the membrane and inhibits synaptic transmission. Cumulative toxicity during continuous extradural blockade with lidocaine may produce seizures. Lidocaine is eliminated mainly by the liver and both the drug as well as its toxic metabolite can accumulate in congestive heart failure and produce neurotoxicity at low drug concentrations. Acidosis increases the amount of unbound drug thus increasing its toxicity. Hypoxia and hypercapnia increase cerebral blood flow thus carrying more lidocaine to the brain. Correcting the acidosis and hypoxia in cases of lidocaine overdose is important for seizure control (Edgren et al 1986). Treatment with intravascular suxamethonium (succinylcholine) 80 mg to 100 mg and simultaneous ventilation by bag and mask using 100% oxygen is the immediate treatment of choice to stop convulsions rapidly; this treatment should be preferred to diazepam or barbiturates (Moore and Bonica 1985).

Although seizures are mostly associated with intravenous lidocaine, they have also been reported after topical administration, as for example, for airway anesthesia for bronchoscopy (Wu et al 1993). The extent of absorption depends on tissue vascularity, sites and techniques of application, patient's disease state, and the dose/unit body weight. Absorption from mucous membranes is usually more rapid than from subcutaneous tissues. A direct correlation exists between clinical symptoms and blood levels of lidocaine; as the level increases to 8–12 mg/L the probability of seizure increases. Seizures has been reported following local application of lidocaine to the oropharyngeal region (Kotaki et al 1996) and following ureteral stone manipulation with lido-caine (Pantuck et al 1997).

Bupivacaine. Local infusion of bupivacaine has been used for controlling postoperative pain. Patients receiving such infusions are at risk for developing systemic toxicity because of the pharmacokinetics of bupivacaine. Plasma level of bupivacaine associated with central nervous system toxicity in adults is estimated to be 4 µg/mL. Seizures along with hypotension and cardiac arrhythmias have been reported in children following continual caudal epidural infusions (McCloskey et al 1992). Seizures may also be a manifestation of bupivacaine toxicity in children in the absence of cardiovascular symptoms (Agarwal et al 1992). Pharmacodynamic interaction with flumazenil may increase convulsive activity of bupivacaine (Bruguerolle and Emperaire 1991). Animal experimental studies show that seizure-inducing effect of bupivacaine is reduced by encapsulating it in multilaminar liposomes when infused intravenously (Boogaerts et al 1993).

General management of seizures due to local anesthetics. Control of seizures is the most important part of neurological management of adverse reactions to local anesthetics. The patient should receive 100% oxygen. Diazepam or barbiturates should be used for control of seizures (Naguib et al 1998). Intravenous suxamethonium (succinylcholine) 2 mg/kg is used to facilitate intubation. Acidosis increases the amount of unbound drug thus increasing its toxicity. Hypoxia and hypercapnia increase cerebral blood flow thus carrying more lidocaine to the brain. Correcting the acidosis and hypoxia in cases of lidocaine overdose is important for seizure control.

Epidural Anesthesia. Inadvertent intravascular injection of anesthetics during attempted epidural anesthesia is a known complication. Intravascular injection of high doses of anesthetic has been reported and can cause seizures (Kenepp and Gutsche 1981). It can be prevented by aspiration of the catheter for blood.

Antiarrhythmic Drugs

Seizures have frequently been reported with the use of antiarrhythmic agents (Editorial 1989; Ol-son et al 1987; Schwartz et al 1981). *Lidocaine* is also an antiarrhythmic agent and its effect in producing seizures has already been discussed in the section on local anesthetics. *Mexiletine* and *tocainide* possess electrophysiological properties similar to those of lidocaine and both can induce central toxicity and convulsions. Severe hypoglycemia produced by *disopyramide* may cause seizures (Nappi et al 1983). Overdose with *quinine* can produce convulsions which can be controlled with intravenous diazepam (Bateman and Dyson 1986).

β-*blockers*, when administered in therapeutic doses, have an anticonvulsant effect but seizures have been reported in 58% of patients with β-blockers overdose, the majority of which involved propranolol (Weinstein 1984). It is unclear how propranolol can induce seizures at high dosages, but a non-specific effect on centrally located neurons, related to its membrane stabilizing effects, is probably involved, as well as the high lipophilicity of the drug and its ability to penetrate into the tissues (Buiumsohn et al 1979). Generalized convulsions have been reported in an elderly patient receiving an ultra-short-acting β-blocker (esmolol hydrochloride) infusion (Das and Ferris 1988).

Antidepressants

Antidepressants can have both anticonvulsive and convulsive properties. The former predominate at lower doses and the latter at higher doses or higher blood levels (Dailey and Naritoku 1996). Seizures are uncommon but serious adverse effects of antidepressants. The reported frequency of antidepressant-induced seizures is 0.1% (Jick et al 1983). Tricyclic antidepressants such as clomipramine maprolitine have a higher risk of seizures than selective serotonin reuptake inhibitors such as fluoxetine and monoamine oxidase inhibitors. Available publication, however, fails to provide reliable estimates of either the absolute or relative risk involved. Time interval to which the risk applies is an important consideration in calculating the risk estimate (Leber 1985). Animal data do not represent predictable outcome for humans. The risk of such

seizures depends on three critical factors (Skowron and Stimmel 1992):
- An individual's predisposing factors
- Pathomechanism of seizures and the relative epileptogenic potential of a particular drug.
- Amount and rate of dosage titration.

Rosenstein et al (1993) who have reviewed this subject emphasize that risk assessment of seizures in an individual should take into consideration the antidepressant involved, bioavailability of the drug, and the duration of the treatment.

Risk Factors. The following risk factors are considered to predispose a person to antidepressant-induced seizures:
- Long-term administration causes down-regulation of β-adrenergic receptor response and the resultant decrease in nor-adrenergic function may enhance seizure response. Seizures have been reported after extended use (more than 4 months) of maprotiline and fluoxetine
- Personal or family history of seizure disorder
- Mental retardation
- Degenerative diseases of the brain
- Advanced age
- EEG abnormalities
- Electroconvulsive therapy
- Multiple comedications
- Sedative and alcohol withdrawal
- Seizure risk for most antidepressants increases with dose (or blood levels).

Pathomechanism. The following mechanisms have been considered according to the class of antidepressant:
- Monoamine oxidase inhibitors decrease the reuptake of monoamines, increase the brain monoamine levels, and decrease the threshold for seizures.
- Seizure threshold increases with dopaminergic agents whereas dopamine-blocking drugs (antipsychotics and antidepressants) enhance seizures.
- The noradrenergic system can suppress or induce seizures. At low doses imipramine acts as an anticonvulsant but at high doses it can be epileptogenic by inhibiting the presynaptic reuptake of norepinephrine.
- Chronic changes in α-adrenoreceptors downregulate with chronic tricyclic administration

and may be a mechanism for seizure exacerbation (Karnaze 1992).
- The role of serotonin in the etiology of antidepressant-induced seizures is not clear. Enhancement of serotonin activity both increases the risk and protects against it in different animal models. Although serotonin is thought to be involved in a number of myoclonic seizure states, the relationship of these to other forms of epilepsy is still unclear (Deahl and Trimble 1991).
- Antidepressants also block the seizure-inhibiting effects of γ-aminobutyric acid (GABA) by antagonizing the GABA A receptor.
- Antidepressants are potent inhibitors of chloride influx into the neurons whereas anticonvulsant agents such as diazepam enhance it.
- Drugs can produce EEG changes without the occurrence of a seizure. Increase of slow waves and increase of fast activity such as following use of imipramine is considered more epileptogenic.
- Seizures are part of neurological picture following tricyclic antidepressant overdose.
- Seizures can occur in neonates following withdrawal from maternal clomipramine (Cowe et al 1982).

Drugs can produce EEG changes without the occurrence of a seizure. Increase of slow waves and increase of fast activity such as following use of imipramine is considered more epileptogenic. Non-convulsive status epilepticus has also been reported during antidepressant therapy (Yoshino et al 1997). Seizures are part of neurological picture following tricyclic antidepressant overdose. Seizures can occur in neonates following withdrawal from maternal clomipramine (Cowe et al 1982).

In evaluating seizures in association with antidepressants, the peculiar antagonism between epilepsy and depression should be taken into consideration. Seizures in patients with depression improve the depression and electroconvulsive therapy is still being used as a treatment for depression.

Tricyclic Antidepressants. Drugs reported to have epileptic potential in increasing order are desipramine, nortriptyline, trimipramine, imipramine, clomipramine, and amitriptyline. For imipramine, the most frequently studies of the drugs of this group, the reported seizure rate varies between 0.3% and 0.6% (Rosenstein et al 1993).

Convulsions are one of the main symptoms of tricyclic antidepressant poisoning but the reported incidence is only 4% (Starkey and Lawson 1980) but it is 13% in fatal cases (Crome and Newman 1979). Paraldehyde, phenobarbital, phenytoin and diazepam have all proven to be effective in the management of these convulsions when administered either alone or in combination.

Monoamine Oxidase Inhibitors. At therapeutic doses seizures do not seem to occur with monoamine oxidase (MAO) inhibitors. MAO inhibitors may even have an anticonvulsant effect. Interaction of MAO inhibitors with tricyclic antidepressants may, however, produce serotonin syndrome which may be accompanied by seizures in most serious cases (White and Simpson 1981).

Other Antidepressant Drugs. Incidence of convulsions with mianserin is reported to be no greater than that associated with tricyclic antidepressants (Edwards and Glen-Bott 1984). The occurrence of seizures with nomifensine is similar to that with tricyclic antidepressants (Edwards and Glen-Bott 1987).

Bupropion overdose has been reported to produce seizures (Storrow 1994). Davidson (1989) reported an overall crude incidence of seizures of 0.87% in patients on bupropion therapy. For patients taking doses of 450 mg or less per day, the seizure incidence dropped to 0.35%. This low incidence (0.36%) was confirmed by a later 102-center prospective study (Johnston et al 1991). At low doses the frequency of seizures is low (0.1%) with either bupropion or imipramine (Peck et al 1983). A seizure rate of 15.6% has been reported with maprotiline as compared to 2.2% for tricyclic antidepressants (Jabbari et al 1985). A seizure rate of 2.1% has been found in clinical trials of clomipramine (Peters et al 1990).

Fluoxetine was reported to be associated with low seizure activity (0.2%) in premarketing trials (Skowron and Stimmel 1992). Several case reports indicate association of fluoxetine with seizures (Murthy et al 1994; Madi et al 1994; Levine et al 1994). Concomitant use of fluoxetine with tricyclic antidepressants may cause the plasma levels of the latter to rise by more than 100% and lead to seizures. Seizures have been reported in patients on fluoxetine and adjuvant buspirone therapy (Grady et al 1992).

Antipsychotics

Almost all the antipsychotics in use are known to induce seizures in some predisposed patients. Seizures associated with antipsychotic medications occur in about 1% of the patients. In addition, approximately 7% of epileptic patients develop chronic psychosis requiring antipsychotic treatment (Cold et al 1990). Risk factors for antipsychotic-induced seizures are shown in Table 7.5.

Table 7.5. Risk factors for antipsychotic-induced seizures

History of epilepsy
Electroconvulsive therapy
Abnormal EEG
History of drug-induced seizures
Organic brain pathology
Head injury
Previous psychosurgery
Insulin shock therapy
Large doses of antipsychotics
Antipsychotics with sedative effects
Polypharmacy: two or more antipsychotics
Sudden changes in doses of antipsychotic medications

The potential of antipsychotic drugs to induce seizures may be related to effects on various neurotransmitter systems. Those agents with greater histaminic, adrenergic, and serotonergic affinity are associated with more reports of seizures than those with less affinity (Marks and Luchins 1991).

Butyrophenones. Haloperidol has been reported to be associated with seizures. EEG changes induced by haloperidol are similar to those observed after chlorpromazine but less marked (Small et al 1987).

Clozapine. Clozapine is an atypical antipsychotic drug used for treatment-resistant schizophrenia. Seizures have been shown to occur more commonly with clozapine than with conventional antipsychotics. Devinsky et al (1991) reviewed information on 1418 patients treated with clozapine in the United States between 1972 and 1988 and found that 41 (2.8%) had generalized tonic-clonic seizures during treatment with clozapine. These seizures appear to be dose-related; high-dose therapy was associated with a greater risk of seizures (4.4%) than medium (2.7%) or low doses (1.0%). Most of the patients were able to continue clozapine treatment despite seizure occurrence, either with reduction of dosage or addition of an antiepileptic medication.

EEG changes have been reported in adolescent schizophrenic patients on clozapine therapy (Braun-Scharm and Martinius 1991). Paroxysmal EEG patterns and generalized myoclonic seizures without alteration in consciousness have also been reported in adult schizophrenic patients (Gouzoulis et al 1991). Absence status seizures, accompanied by 3 Hz spiking wave abnormality on EEG, have also been reported in an adolescent after increase of dose of clozapine (Freedman et al 1994). Prolonged post-ictal encephalopathy following clozapine-induced seizures has also been reported (Karper et al 1992). Liukkonen et al (1992) reported 12 schizophrenic patients each of whom had one to six clozapine-associated convulsions. EEG showed irritative changes in one-third of the patients and paroxysmal slow wave activity in two-thirds. Seizure activity was self-limiting in 5 of the patients, and in the rest of the cases it was controlled with anticonvulsive therapy and clozapine treatment could be continued. In a retrospective study of EEG in 283 patients before, during, and after clozapine treatment, Gunther et al (1993) found slight to moderate abnormalities in 61.5% of the patients. However, seizures occurred only in three patients and no predictive information was available from the EEG records of these patients.

Pathomechanism. Clozapine lowers the seizure threshold in patients and propensity to cause seizures is dose-related. Concomitant use of clozapine and electroconvulsive therapy produced a seizure which went on for 6 minutes before it was terminated by intravenous diazepam (Bloch et al 1996).

Management. The following measures have been recommended for prevention and management of clozapine-induced seizures (Toth and Frankenburg 1994; Safferman et al 1991; Haller and Binder 1990):

- Clozapine should be administered with caution to patients with history of seizures or head injury.
- Pretreatment EEG may be obtained if there is history of seizures and if dose is increased. Guidelines for use of EEG have not been established as yet.
- On initiation of clozapine therapy, the dose should be raised slowly along with monitoring of blood levels.
- The use of comedications that increase the risk of seizures when combined with clozapine should be avoided.
- Valproic acid is the anticonvulsant of choice for prevention (add to clozapine in high risk situations) as well as for treatment of seizures. Other antiepileptic drugs such as phenytoin, carbamazepine, and phenobarbital, which cause hepatic enzyme induction and lower the blood levels of clozapine, should be avoided.

Lithium. The role of lithium in the causation of seizures is controversial. Although seizures have been reported in non-epileptic patients with plasma lithium in therapeutic range, lithium has also been noted to exert an anticonvulsant effect in some patients. Lithium poisoning is accompanied by EEG abnormalities and convulsions have been observed (Sansone and Ziegler 1985; Aronson and Reynolds 1992; Schindler and Ramchandani 1993).

Phenothiazines. Phenothiazines are known to produce seizures even in patients with no previous history of epilepsy. The aliphatic phenothiazines (e. g., chlorpromazine, promazine, and triflupromazine) are considered carry a higher risk for this adverse effect than the phenothiazines bearing a piperazine or piperidine moiety (Itil and Soldatos 1980). An incidence of 1.2% spontaneous seizures was reported in hospitalized psychiatric patients on phenothiazine therapy;

this increased to 9% in patients receiving large doses and dropped to 0.5% in those receiving low or moderate doses (Logothetis 1967). This observation conflicts with the studies of effects of these drugs in animal models of epilepsy; phenothiazines act as convulsant agents at lower doses but at higher doses they have an anticonvulsant effect (Lipka and Lathers 1987).

Pathomechanism. The biochemical basis of the seizures induced by phenothiazines is inhibition of GABAergic neural transmission. Enhancement of various EEG abnormalities has been noted during antipsychotic therapy. Chlorpromazine and thioridazine have been found to produce inverted U-shaped dose-response curves with a maximum epileptogenic effect at concentrations lower than therapeutic levels. Such patients are at increased risk of seizures at beginning of therapy and upon withdrawal. Seizures can also occur with overdose of these drugs.

Zotepine. This is a dibenzothiepin derivative which has been used to treat impulsive behavior and psychomotor retardation in schizophrenic patients. Hori et al (1992) have reported a prevalence of seizures in 17.1% of patients on this drug. Zotepine has a high affinity for the 5-HT$_1$ binding sites in the cerebral cortex and this property is considered to induce seizures.

Antiepileptics

Antiepileptic drugs (AEDs) can aggravate seizures (Guerrini et al 1998; Perucca et al 1998). Seizures may also be caused by AEDs. Various explanations of this paradoxical effect are:
- An incorrect choice of drugs in the treatment of epilepsy.
- A decrease in blood level of a previously effective AED.
- "Paradoxical intoxication" has been described in patients treated with phenytoin or carbamazepine in whom the seizure frequency increases as the blood levels of AED rise to supratherapeutic range.
- A progressive neurological condition in which there is increase in the frequency of seizures.

- Loss of efficacy of a previously effective AED (Jain 1993).
- Overdose effect of AED leading to neurotoxicity.
- Interactions of other drugs with AED leading to rise or fall of AED serum levels.
- Adverse effect caused specifically by the AED.
- Seizures due to electrolyte disturbances produced by AED. For example, hyponatremia produced by carbamazepine.
- Drug-induced IgA deficiency precipitates systemic lupus erythematosus (SLE) which has a 10% incidence of seizures associated with it (Aarli 1993). Association of carbamazepine with SLE-like syndromes has been described by Jain (1991).
- Reduced bioavailability of the AED. Use of moisture-exposed carbamazepine (CBZ) resulted in status epilepticus in a patient who was well controlled with CBZ previously. CBZ blood levels in this case decreased to 3.8:g/ml from the previous random CBZ levels of 9–13:g/ml (Bell et al 1993).
- Withdrawal of AEDs. Increase in seizure frequency in epileptics during withdrawal from barbiturate therapy is well known. In patients with complex partial seizures, increase in seizure frequency is seen when the blood phenobarbital levels fall below 20 mg/L (Theodore et al 1987). Epilepsy patients withdrawn from CBZ over a period of 4 days have been reported to experience significantly more seizures than those withdrawn over a period of 10 days (Malow et al 1993). Seizure exacerbation has been reported in 17 patients after rapid or abrupt discontinuation of clonazepam or replacement with nitrazepam (Sugai 1993). Seizures improved on restitution of the drug and did not occur in 54 other patients where clonazepam was discontinued gradually.

Examples of seizures caused by AEDs are:
- *Benzodiazepines* have been reported to produce status epilepticus when injected intravenously in children with Lennox-Gestaut syndrome. Another explanation of these seizures is the vehicle propylene glycol in the injection (Cronin 1992; McDonald et al 1987).
- *Carbamazepine.* Children with mixed seizure

disorders, particularly those with generalized slow spike-and-wave discharges on EEG become worse on carbamazepine. Carbamazepine has also been reported to cause myoclonic, atonic, and absence seizures (Sachdeo and Chakroverty 1985; Shields and Saslow 1983; Dhuna et al 1991). High doses of carbamazepine can lead to exacerbation of seizures without any other evidence of neurotoxicity. One such case has been described where lowering of carbamazepine dose led to improved seizure control (Neufeld 1993).

– *Lamotrigine.* Recent evidence indicates that lamotrigine is inappropriate in severe myoclonic epilepsy and may aggravate it.

– *Phenytoin* can aggravate absence seizures (Lerman 1986). Photosensitive complex partial seizures have also been reported to be aggravated by phenytoin (Shuper and Vining 1991). Seizures are an occasional manifestation of phenytoin toxicity (Stilman and Masdeu 1985).

– *Valproic acid* (VPA) occasionally induces status epilepticus. A case of non-convulsive status-epilepticus, with generalized sharp and slow wave activity on EEG, has been reported in a patient with complex partial seizures on VPA therapy (Steinhoff and Stodiek 1993). In animal experimental studies, chronic treatment with VPA has been shown to enhance seizures in gerbils (Cutler and Horton 1988). In a model nervous system (buccal ganglia of Helix pomata), the epileptogenic effect of VPA is believed to be exerted from the extracellular side of the cell membrane (Altrup et al 1992).

– *Vigabatrin* is rarely associated with aggravation of seizures, mostly in patients with therapy-resistant generalized seizures (Lortie et al 1993). Three cases have been reported of status epilepticus occurring during vigabatrin treatment (De Krom et al 1994).

Antihistaminics

Antihistaminics exert both a depressant as well as a stimulant effect on the CNS. Overdose of diphenhydramine can be characterized by jittery movement, tremors, and seizures (Krenzelok et al 1982). Children are particularly susceptible to the convulsive properties of these drugs (Magera et al 1981). Ethylenediamines and ethanolamines have the most tendency to produce seizures. Terfenadine, an antihistaminics structurally unrelated to older products, has also been reported to be associated with seizures (Tidswell and D'Assis-Fonesca 1993).

Pathomechnism. Evidence that histamine is involved in the termination of seizures and has a role as an endogenous anticonvulsant has been obtained in animal models of epilepsy (Tuomisto and Tacke 1986). Iinuma et al (1993) have found increased histamine H_1 receptor binding in the cortex of patients with epilepsy and have provided neurochemical evidence supporting the clinical observation that antihistamines exacerbate seizures in some cases of epilepsy.

Antimalarials

Prophylactic antimalarial drugs at standard doses can induce convulsions in healthy subjects and more frequently in those with a history of epilepsy. Fish and Espir (1988) have reported four cases who presented with tonic-clonic seizures while taking antimalarial drugs (chloroquine sulfate, dapsone, and pyrimethamine) prophylactically. Only one of the patients had a history of epilepsy. None of them had any recurrence of seizures after discontinuation of antimalarial drugs. Seizures have also been reported following mefloquine prophylactic treatment in non-epileptic subjects (Singh et al 1991; Bem et al 1992) and in an epileptic patient whose seizures were previously well controlled with valproic acid (Besser and Krämer 1991). Tonic-clonic seizures have been reported in a patient after quinine therapy of a mefloquine-resistant *Plasmodium falciparum* malaria (Miyashita et al 1994).

Pathomechanism. The mechanism of seizures induced by antimalarial drugs is uncertain. Chloroquine inhibits glutamate dehydrogenase activity and could reduce the concentration of inhibitory neurotransmitter gamma-aminobutyric acid.

Antimicrobial Agents

β-Lactam Antibiotics. These antibiotics are well known to have potent convulsant activity in humans but the frequency of this adverse effect is reported to be less than 1% (Norrby 1986; Perry 1984).

Penicillin. The incidence of penicillin-induced seizures was calculated to be 0.3% in the Boston Collaborative Study (1972). Because of a variety of statistical problems unavoidable in these epidemiological studies, the true incidence may differ from the values reported so far (Norrby 1986).

Pathomechanism. Penicillin produces focal seizures by topical application in vitro and in vivo and has been used to produce models for epilepsy research. The postulated mechanism of epileptogenic effect is by blocking of the effect of GABA when β-lactam ring binds to GABA receptors. Although penicillin does not readily cross the BBB, parenteral administration of large doses can cause neural hyperexcitability. This involves particularly the somatosensory cortex in the rat, a site where topical application produces similar effect.

Risk factors for penicillin-induced seizures are as follows (Barrons et al 1992):
- Patients with impaired renal function either as a primary condition or secondary to infection.
- Infants
- Aged persons
- Patients with meningitis
- Patients undergoing intraventricular antibiotic therapy
- Patients with history of seizures
- Intraoperative and early postoperative use in patients undergoing craniotomy for supratentorial pathology (Michenfelder et al 1990)

Ampicillin. Other penicillin analogues, including ampicillin, also have the β-lactam bond and are known to be epileptogenic when applied topically to the cerebral cortex in experimental animals. Ampicillin threshold concentration in epileptogenesis is seven times higher than that of penicillin. Seizures have been reported with ampicillin (Serdaru et al 1982; Hodgman et al 1984) and carbenicillin (Whelton et al 1971).

Cephalosporins. These have a potential to induce seizures as reported by Norrby (1987) in patients with impaired renal function who had been given high doses. Shah et al (1988) found no case of cefotaxime-induced seizures in a series of 602 consecutive patients treated with this drug. Ceftazidime has also been reported to induce non-convulsive status epilepticus in a patient (Klion et al 1994). Intraventricular cefazolin is a potent epileptogenic agent and should not be used by this route (Martin et al 1992).

Pathomechanism. Cephalosporins and carbapenems might also induce convulsions through the inhibition of GABA receptor binding when they accumulated in the CNS (Shimada et al 1992). CNS toxicity in patients treated with imipenem/cilastatin is considered to be caused by the accumulation of an open lactam metabolite of imipenem whereas cilastain appears to have no role. Observations on 1754 patients treated with imipenem/cilastin in phase III dose ranging studies in the United states revealed an incidence of seizures of 0.9% related to this therapy. Central nervous system lesions, seizure disorders, high doses and elderly patients with renal insufficiency are considered to be strong risk factors but seizures have been reported with other risk factors such as multi-organ failure (Leo and Ballow 1991) and history of head injury and stroke (Job and Dretler 1990).

Carbapenems. There is one case report of seizures in an elderly patient who received panipenem and later died because of renal failure (Katsuki et al 1998). The Japanese Ministry of Health has received over 20 reports of seizures following penepenem therapy. Caution is recommended in administering carbapenems to elderly patients who are likely to have renal or cerebrovascular disturbances which are risk factors for carbapenem-induced seizures.

Imipenem has been reported to cause CNS toxicity including seizures in 1.5–10% of patients. Imipenem-cilastatin is a broad spectrum antibiotic that is generally used for antibiotic-resistant hospital-acquired infections. Imipenem, inappropriately utilized for surgical prophylaxis in excessive doses (1 gram every six hours) and for a prolonged period of time (24 days), induced a tonic-clonic generalized seizure in a patient with no history of seizure activity (Hunter 1993).

Other Antibiotics. The aminoglycosides are usually not implicated in cases of drug-induced seizures even though they are known to produce ototoxicity and neuromuscular blockade. Convulsions can occur after treatment with enoxacin, pefloxacin, ciprofloxacin, or norfloxacin (Paton and Reeves 1992). Seizures have occurred in epileptic patients receiving a combination of ciprofloxacin and phenytoin where the possibility of reduction of phenytoin levels from drug interaction was considered to be a contributing factor (Langlois 1998).

Gentamicin has been rarely reported to induce seizures as a result of hypomagnesemia. Vancomycin and teicoplanin are not considered to be associated with seizures and have been occasionally administered intraventricularly. Convulsions have been observed following intraventricular use of teicoplanin in rats in a dose-related manner and caution should be exercised in human use of these drugs in this manner (Park and Christ 1992). Tetracyclines and macrolide antibiotics also have virtually no seizure potential. Quinolones may block receptors for antiepileptic agents in the brain or be directly neurotoxic.

Antitubercular Drugs. Neurotoxicity of antitubercular drugs has been reviewed by Holdiness (1987). Convulsions have been observed in 1 to 3% of patients on isoniazid therapy (Devadatta 1965).

Pathomechanism. The epileptogenic effect of isoniazid seems to result from its inhibitory effect on glutamic acid decarboxylase, the enzyme responsible for synthesis of GABA.

Management. Convulsions due to isoniazid intoxication are unresponsive to anticonvulsant therapy but respond to pyridoxine (Martin and DePadua 1983). Seizures are likely to occur as a result of isoniazid overdose (Tai et al 1996).

Antifungal Agents. Grand mal seizures have been rarely reported in patients treated with amphotericin B or miconazole.

Antihelminthic Agents. *Piperazine* has been used for the treatment of ascaris lumbricoides and enterobius vermicularis since the early 1950s. It has been associated with a variety of neurotoxic effects including seizures (Yohai and Barnett 1989). Seizures have also been observed with piperazine compounds used as antitussives. The pathomechanism of these seizures is not known, although inhibition of GABA system has been postulated.

Metronidazole, a 5-nitroimidazole, is widely used for the treatment of trichomoniasis, giardiasis, amoebiasis, and anaerobic infections. It produces a variety of adverse reactions on the nervous system including encephalopathy and seizures (Ahmed et al 1995; Halloran 1982).

Antineoplastic Agents

Antineoplastic agents can occasionally cause convulsions but the etiology and frequency of this adverse effect is not well known. Seizures may be a manifestation of encephalopathy due to neurotoxicity of antineoplastic agents. Because most of the patients are treated with combinations of antineoplastic agents, it is difficult to determine the role of any particular agent in the causation of seizures.

Alkylating Agents. High dose busulfan (HD-BU) therapy has been reported to be associated with seizures (Murphy et al 1992). Prophylactic phenytoin has been recommended and this should be started before HD-BU to allow for achieving adequate serum levels (Tiberghien et al 1992). Chlorambucil has epileptogenic properties and has been used to produce EEG patterns of petit mal epilepsy in rats (Mirsky et al 1966). Chlorambucil has been reported to cause seizures in children with history of myoclonic epilepsy (Williams et al 1978) and after overdose (Byrne et al 1981). Seizures have been reported following administration of mechlorethamine (Sullivan et al 1982).

Antimetabolites. Encephalopathy has been observed after high doses of methotrexate and some of these patients develop seizures (Kay et al 1972). Children with acute lymphoblastic leukemia treated with parenterally administered methotrexate have increased susceptibility to seizure development (Ochs et al 1984). Seizures in patients on multiple chemotherapy including methotrexate and cytarabine have been reported to be diminished by use of folate (Winick et al 1992).

Vinca Alkaloids. Vincristine is neurotoxic but mostly manifests as peripheral neuropathy. Lack of serious CNS toxicity is poor penetration across the BBB. However, it can cause hyponatremia by an excessive release of antidiuretic hormone. Seizures have, however, been observed in children treated with vincristine even in the absence of hyponatremia. Seizures occur with vincristine overdose (Kaufman et al 1976) and its inadvertent administration intrathecally (Legha 1986).

Other Antineoplastic Drugs. Seizures have been reported during cisplatin therapy (Whitshaw et al 1979; Berman and Mann 1980; Mead et al 1982). Cisplatin given by injection to frogs has been shown to produce tonic-clonic seizures (Blisard and Harrington 1989). A case has been reported of non-convulsive status epilepticus as a complication of therapy with ifosfamide, a nitrogen mustard derivative, which resolved after treatment with intravenous diazepam (Wengs et al 1993).

Central Nervous System Stimulants

This group contains drugs which share the ability to produce dose-related excitation of the central nervous system (CNS) leading to convulsions. The stimulation may be at cortical, brainstem, or spinal levels. Examples of cortical stimulants are: theophylline, caffeine, cocaine, amphetamine, ephedrine, methylphenidate. Brainstem stimulants such as picrotoxin and pentetrazol were used at one time to induce convulsions in psychotic patients but their use is obsolete now. Strychnine is a stimulant at spinal level and is not used therapeutically.

Amphetamine. Convulsions can occur in high dose "binge" users and in amphetamine poisoning but are rare among uses of low doses. Amphetamine increases dopaminergic transmission, decreases seizure activity, and improves EEG (Kobayashi and Mori 1977).

Caffeine. Caffeine has an intrinsic convulsant activity because of its adenosine receptor antagonizing properties. Animal studies have shown changes in the activity of norepinephrine, dopamine, and serotonin. The drug also acts directly on the cerebral arterial musculature to cause vasoconstriction and decrease in cerebral blood flow. Davis et al (1986) described seizure activity in two infants treated with intravenous and orally administered caffeine (20 mg/kg loading dose) to prevent a recurrence of apnea. Intravenous caffeine given before electroconvulsive therapy can prolong seizure duration but does not reduce the seizure threshold. Grandmal seizure has been reported in postpartum patient following intravenous infusion of caffeine sodium benzoate to treat persistent headache (Cohen et al 1992).

Cocaine. Cocaine was the first local anesthetic and convulsions are among its earliest known adverse effects. Cocaine augments the effects of catecholamine neurotransmitters, probably by blocking reuptake of these transmitters that restimulate receptors. Repeated high doses of cocaine produce a convulsive response in animal studies and seizure-kindled paradigms have shown that effects of cocaine on the electrical activity of the brain are similar to those of lidocaine (Russell and Stripling 1985).

In a retrospective review of 989 patients with complications related to cocaine abuse, seizures occurred in 29 of a total of 150 patients who experienced predominant neurological problems (Lowenstein et al 1988). Focal or generalized tonic-clonic seizures have been reported in 1.4 to 2.8% of cocaine users (Choy-Kwong and Lipton 1989). Cocaine-related seizures in adults may occur as acute provoked convulsions in patients known to have epilepsy, or spontaneously in otherwise normal individuals after snorting, or agonally with massive ingestion (Kramer et al 1990). Cocaine-induced seizures are usually generalized and tonic-clonic but complex partial status epilepticus has also been reported (Ogunyemi et al 1989).

Management. Use of propranolol is recommended for the management of adrenergic cocaine crisis (Ramoska and Sacchetti 1985). An alternative is labetalol which possesses both α-blocking (counter the cocaine-induced vasoconstriction and hypertension) and β-blocking capabilities which decrease the tachyarrhythmias (Gay and Luperka 1988). Diazepam can be administered to control the seizures and phenobarbital loading is used if status epilepticus develops (Lowenstein et al 1988).

Methylphenidate (Ritalin). This is an amphetamine-like compound and is used widely for the treatment of attention deficit hyperactivity disorder (ADHD) in children. The manufacturer, Novartis Pharmaceutical Corporation, lists the following warning in the Physicians' Desk Reference (1998):

There is some clinical evidence that Ritalin may lower the convulsive threshold in patients with prior history of seizures, with prior EEG abnormalities in the absence of seizures, and, very rarely, in the absence of history of seizures. Safe concomitant use of anticonvulsants and Ritalin has not been established. In the presence of seizures, the drug should be discontinued.

No evidence has been provided to support this statement. It has been shown that methylphenidate can be used safely in brain-injured patients, even those at high risk of seizures, as it is associated with a trend towards reduction rather than increase in seizure frequency in this population (Wroblewski et al 1992). Gross-Tsur et al (1997) carried out a double-blind/crossover study to evaluate the safety and efficacy of methylphenidate in children with dual diagnosis of epilepsy and ADHD. None of the 25 children of this sample who were seizure free had attacks while taking methylphenidate. Of the 5 children with seizures, 3 had an increase in attacks, whereas the other 2 showed no change or a reduction. There were no significant changes in antiepileptic drug (AED) levels or electroencephalographic findings. Methylphenidate benefited 70% of children and was found to be safe in children with no history of seizure. Caution is warranted for those still having seizures while receiving AED therapy.

Theophylline. Like other xanthines, theophylline is a powerful CNS stimulant. Seizures are a known complication of theophylline toxicity. Earlier reports suggested that theophylline levels in the high toxic range were required to produce seizures but later reports indicate that seizures in both children and adults may occur with therapeutic levels. Status epilepticus has been reported in asthmatic children with serum theophylline levels within therapeutic range (Dunn and Parekh 1991).

Pathomechanism. The precise mechanism of theophylline-induced seizures is not known, but may involve its action on adenosine and 5'-nucleotidase. There is usually clinical or EEG evidence of focal seizure activity in the absence of focal CNS disease (Nakada et al 1983). When the seizures are prolonged, the outcome is poor (Bahls et al 1991).

Various risk factors for serious outcome in theophylline-induced seizures are:
– Elderly patients
– History of previous seizures
– Neurological disease: encephalitis, cerebrovascular insufficiency
– Low serum albumin levels allow an increase in the absolute free theophylline concentration because theophylline is 55 to 65% protein bound
– Severe chronic obstructive pulmonary disease

Management. In patients with these risk factors, serum theophylline levels should be maintained below 10–15 mg/L. The seizures should be stopped as rapidly as possible to reduce the morbidity and mortality. Phenobarbital 10 mg/kg has been shown to possess the highest anticonvulsant activity against theophylline-induced seizures in animal studies while diazepam and phenytoin were less effective (Stone and Javid 1980). In humans theophylline-induced seizures are more refractory to treatment with diazepam (alone or in combination with phenobarbital or phenytoin. Treatment recommendations proposed by Gaudreault and Guay (1986):
– Give diazepam 5 to 20 mg intravenously at a low infusion rate within 5 to 20 minutes.
– If convulsions do not stop or recur, phenobarbital 15 mg/kg should be given intravenously.
– If seizures do not stop within 20 minutes, a loading dose of thiopental 3 to 5 mg/kg should be followed by an infusion of 2 to 4 mg/kg/h.

A study on healthy young volunteers has shown that vitamin B-6 supplementation reduces the

CNS stimulant effect of theophylline as demonstrated by reduction of tremor (Bartel et al 1994). Its use as a prophylactic against theophylline-induced seizures has not been tested as yet.

Immunosuppressive Drugs

Various immunosuppressant drugs used to prevent organ transplant rejection include cyclosporine, azathioprine, glucocorticoids, and monoclonal antibody OKT3. Leukoencephalopathy is a known complication of immunosuppressant drugs used to counteract transplant rejection. Seizures are a manifestation of this (Idilman et al 1998).

Azathioprine. This drug can also induce seizures although the incidence of this side effect is low. One such case has been reported by Lockskin and Kagen (1972).

Cyclosporine. Cyclosporine encephalopathy has been described elsewhere in this book (Chapter 3) and its manifestations include seizures. Convulsions are rare in the renal transplant patients (Beaman et al 1985), occur in less than 1% of heart transplant patients, and in approximately 3% of bone marrow transplant patients (Scott and Higenbottam 1988). It is difficult to evaluate seizures in patients with organ transplants because of various infections, rejection, or metabolic disturbances. However, cases have been described where other factors were excluded and seizures were attributed to cyclosporine (Shah et al 1989).

Cyclosporin-induced seizures are presumed to be caused by direct tissue damage. Both the brain and the kidney contain high concentrations of cytosolic-binding protein cyclophillin, suggesting that the drug can be taken up more readily into the cells of these tissues (Scott and Higenbottam 1988). High levels of metabolites of cyclosporine have been found in the serum of patients prior to seizures suggesting a toxic effect (Cilio et al 1993).

Glucocorticoids. These have been implicated occasionally in cases of drug-induced seizures. Seizures have been reported following intravenous pulse methylprednisolone in a renal transplant patient (El-Dahr et al 1987). The occurrence of seizures is more frequent in patients treated with a combination of cyclosporin and high dose methylprednisone (Durrant et al 1982; Boogaerts et al 1982).

OKT3 (an Anti-Pan-t-Cell Monoclonal Antibody). This substance has demonstrated usefulness as an effective immunosuppressive agent in acute allograft rejection and in graft-versus-host disease. Aseptic meningitis is known complication of this therapy (see Chapter 16) but a case of seizures with cerebritis has been reported by Capone and Cohen (1991).

Non-Steroidal Anti-Inflammatory Drugs

Aspirin. This is the most commonly ingested drug in overdoses in children. The toxic effects of aspirin are almost entirely mediated by salicylic acid which is formed by hydrolysis of the drug. Salicylate uncouples oxidative phosphorylation from electron transport and leads to depletion of body stores of glucose. Seizures are a part of the clinical picture of patients with salicylate intoxication and are believed to be due to depletion of brain glucose. Intravenous diazepam is considered to be the drug of choice for the management of salicylate-induced convulsions and short-acting barbiturates are the second-line agents.

Diclofenac. Seizures have been reported after the use of diclofenac (Heim et al 1990). The incidence is less than 1:100,000.

Indomethacin. This drug seems to be devoid of any significant seizure potential in clinical use. However, it has been shown to lower the threshold to pentetrazole-induced convulsions in mouse presumably by inhibition of cerebral prostaglandin and/or thromboxane synthesis (Steinhauer and Hertting 1981). Convulsions have been reported in a breast-fed infant after maternal use of indomethacin (Eag-Olofsson and Carl-Eric 1978).

Mefenamic Acid. Therapeutic doses of this drug are unlikely to cause seizures but an overdose can cause convulsions which are extremely resistant to intravenous diazepam.

Opioid Analgesics

High doses of intravenous opiates are an important method of treatment of severe pain in patients with cancer. Endogenous opioid peptides can evoke epileptiform activity on EEG in experimental animals and there is evidence that these epileptiform discharges are mediated by specific opioid receptors and that this activity can be antagonized by opioid antagonists such as naloxone (Gulya 1990; Ramabadran and Bansinath 1990).

Morphine. Cortical topical application of 24–400µg/kg of morphine in rats produces spiking of EEG and ultimately seizures at higher doses (Frenk et al 1984). These effects are unaltered by pretreatment with naloxone. Morphine can induce seizures in high doses in neonates and infants (Koren et al 1985). This may be due to an immature blood-brain barrier allowing a greater penetration of the drug into the CNS. In adults, seizures are a rare occurrence after intraspinal administration of morphine or other opioids (Cousins and Mather 1984). Seizures following intravenous morphine have been attributed to sodium bisulfite preservative contained in the morphine (Gregory et al 1992; Meisel and Welford 1992). Smith et al (1989) have reviewed EEGs of patients anesthetized with large doses of opioids and observed that the rigidity manifested by some of the patients was not accompanied by any evidence of epileptiform activity on EEG. These authors found no evidence to support the existence of opioid-induced seizures in the clinical setting.

Meperidine (Pethidine). Pethidine is metabolized to norpethidine which has half the analgesic potency of the parent compound but is twice as active as a convulsant. There are several reports of seizures associated with its use either intramuscularly or intravenously (Armstrong and Bersten 1986). The risk of seizures increases when meperidine is administered via patient-controlled analgesia pump (Hagmeyer et al

1993). Other risk factors for meperidine-induced seizures include:

– History of seizures
– Renal impairment leading to prolongation of elimination of norpethidine and greater accumulation. Patients with sickle cell crisis are more prone to develop seizures after intramuscular pethidine because of renal function impairment (Pryle et al 1992).
– Renal impairment leading to prolongation of elimination of norpethidine and greater accumulation. Patients with sickle cell crisis are more prone to develop seizures after intramuscular pethidine because of renal function impairment (Marinella 1997).
– High meperidine doses, i. e., daily doses exceeding 25 mg/kg.
– Coadministration of hepatic enzyme-inducing medications.
– Concomitant use of monoamine oxidase inhibitors which interact with pethidine giving an idiosyncratic reaction involving CNS excitation and seizures (Duthie and Nimmo 1987).

Naloxone does not reverse norpethidine toxicity and can, on the contrary, exacerbate the seizures by antagonizing the anticonvulsant effect of pethidine (Armstrong and Bersten 1986).

Radiologic Contrast Agents

Administration of radiologic contrast agents is associated with a variety of neurologic adverse effects and seizures are one of the most common complications. Their effect varies according to the agent used and the route of administration.

Intravascular Contrast Agents. The agents employed intravenously for studies such as angiography, urography, and computer tomography are usually sodium or methylglucamine salts of triiodinated derivatives of benzoic acid. The incidence of seizures following arteriography has been reported to be about 0.2 to 0.4% (Junck and Marshall 1983). Nelson et al (1989) reviewed contrast-induced seizures retrospectively in a consecutive series of 15,226 contrast-enhanced head examinations. An incidence of 0.19% was found. There was a strong association with history of spontaneous seizures and with the presence of structural intracranial abnormalities. These seizures were short-lived and self-limiting or easily controlled with small doses of intravenous diazepam. The epileptogenic effect of radiological contrast media seems to result from direct action of these substances on the cerebral cortex. High serum iodine content has been alleged to cause seizures and example has been quoted of a patient who developed seizures after mediastinal povidone-iodine irrigation and in whom the serum iodine levels were four times the normal range (Zec et al 1992). Hauben (1993) does not consider that the iodine content has a role in the neurotoxicity of radiological contrast agents. Large volume of contrast material during coronary angiography can led to retention of contrast material in the cerebral cortex and deep nuclei. In such a case described by May et al (1993), the patient suffered from prolonged seizures but survived and developed parkinsonian tremor. Aggressive medical management with gradual clearance of contrast material resulted in recovery.

Pathomechanism. The neurotoxicity of the contrast agents is probably related to disruption of the blood-brain barrier, disturbances in neuronal membranes or both. Because these agents can cross the intact blood-brain barrier only in very small quantities, they are safe in most of the cases. However, disruption of blood-brain barrier by brain pathology makes the patients more susceptible to seizures. Non-convulsive status epilepticus verified by EEG has been reported following intravenous contrast injection in a patient undergoing CT scan for glioblastoma multiforme (Lukovits et al 1996).

Agents for Intrathecal Administration. Metrizamide and iopamidol are non-ionic water-soluble agents used for myelography, cisternography, and ventriculography. A variety of seizures have been reported following metrizamide myelography. Metrizamide competitively inhibits brain hexokinase and may cause seizures by this means (Bertoni et al 1981). The incidence of seizures estimated from a large series of patients ranges from 0.6% (Amundsen 1977) to 0.02% (Dugstad and Eldevik 1977).

Iopamidol can also induce convulsions (Levey et al 1988; Vossler and Wright 1994). Seizures have also been reported after inadvertent administration of ionic water soluble contrast media for myelography.

Management. In patients who are at high risk for seizures, such as those with brain metastases, use of intravenous diazepam (5 mg) has been suggested as a prophylactic measure prior to injection of contrast agent for computer tomography. Oral phenytoin is more effective than diazepam against seizures induced by administration of contrast agents in the subarachnoid space and should be given prophylactically starting the day before the procedure to achieve therapeutic blood levels (de Vane et al 1986).

Vaccines

Postvaccinial encephalomyelitis has been discussed in more details in Chapter 3. Seizures are one of the manifestations. From a review of the yellow cards in UK, vaccines were shown to be the commonest reported cause of convulsions induced by drugs (Bem et al 1988). Pertussis vaccine, which is commonly administered with diphtheria and tetanus vaccine (DPT), is probably the most often implicated among those recommended and routinely used. The risk of seizure within 48 hours of DPT vaccination is 1 in 1750. It has been recommended that children who have had a major reaction to a previous vaccination, or children with progressive neurological disorders or a history of convulsions should not be given pertussis vaccination (Zimmerman et al 1987). Children at risk of febrile convulsions should not be given vaccines known to produce fever. Treatment of vaccine-induced seizures is the same as that of febrile convulsions.

Recently Farrington et al (1995) have reported the results of a new epidemiological and statistical methods based on record linkage to assess the risk of convulsions after DPT vaccine. They found an increased relative incidence for convulsions 0–3 days after DPT vaccine. The effect was limited to the third dose of the vaccine for which the attributable risk was 1 in 12,500 doses. The estimated absolute risk of 1 in 24,000 doses was

5 times that calculated from cases passively reported by the clinicians.

Miscellaneous Drugs

Drugs not belonging to the categories discussed above have been implicated as a cause of seizures. They are as follows:

Allopurinol. Seizures have been reported in a patient with hypoxanthine-guanine phosphoribosyl transferase deficiency who developed cerebral vasculitis following received allopurinol therapy (Weiss et al 1978). Allopurinol has anticonvulsant properties also and a case of status epilepticus has been reported following withdrawal of this drug (Kramer et al 1990).

Aminophylline. It is a methyxanthine and its effect is similar to that of theophylline and caffeine. In adults convulsions have occurred following intravenous administration (Schwartz and Scott 1974) whereas in children it has been reported following aminophylline suppositories (Parfrey and Davies 1979).

Aspartame. It is an artificial sweetener which can cause significant elevations in plasma and brain levels of phenylalanine. Anecdotal reports suggest that some persons suffer neurologic or behavioral reactions in association with aspartame consumption. There is controversy regarding aspartame's proconvulsant activity. Phenylalanine can be neurotoxic and can inhibit the synthesis of inhibitory monoamine neurotransmitters. In mice, pretreatment with 1000 mg/kg aspartame has been shown to potentiate pentylenetetrazol-induced seizures (Pinto and Maher 1988). Camfield et al (1992) have shown that aspartame appears to exacerbate the amount of EEG spike wave in children with absence seizures. These results have been disputed by Shaywitz and Novotny (1993) and further studies are needed to resolve this issue.

Atropine Sulfate. CNS toxicity of systemically ingested atropine is well known. Atropine sulfate eye drops can produce convulsions in children and exacerbation of akinetic seizures (Wright 1992).

Baclofen. Intrathecal baclofen is used to treat spasticity secondary to brain and spinal cord injuries. A case of status epilepticus after intrathecal baclofen has been described by Saltuari et al (1992). Three cases of encephalopathy with periodic generalized EEG sharp waves were been report previously (Hormes et al 1988; Abarbanel et al 1985). Zak et al (1994) presented a fourth similar cases and reviewed the previous cases. In their opinion all the four cases had generalized non-convulsive status epilepticus and not metabolic encephalopathies.

Pathomechanism. Baclofen is a $GABA_B$-antagonist with actions at pre- and post-synaptic sites in the CNS. Both proconvulsant and anticonvulsant effects of oral baclofen administered to humans have been described. A possible explanation of these seemingly contradictory effects may be the delicate balance between the suppression of recurrent inhibition by a presynaptic effect relative to the activation of receptors mediating postsynaptic inhibition. A greater suppression of inhibition than activation can lead to initiation of a seizure from a focus of damaged brain. Structural brain disease seems to be a prerequisite for the baclofen-induced seizures because they have not been reported to occur in patients receiving intrathecal baclofen for spasticity of solely spinal origin (Kofler et al 1994). Abrupt cessation of long term baclofen therapy has been associated with various forms of seizure activity (Terrance and Fromm 1981; Barker and Grant 1982).

Management. Intravenous diazepam and/or phenobarbital is suggested for control of these seizures. Caution should be exercised with major reductions in dosage or discontinuation of baclofen therapy.

β-Blockers. Generalized seizures due to therapy with these agents are rare. Most of the reported cases are due to overdose. Generalized seizure has been reported in a patient receiving infusion of an ultrashort-acting β-blocker esmolol hydrochloride. Possible mechanisms of seizures induced by β-blockers are:
- Marked bradycardia which may be induced by these agents
- Severe hypoglycemia is a known adverse effect of β-blockers.

– Membrane stabilizing property of β-blockers. This is comparable to seizures which occur with intravenous lidocaine infusions.

Bromocriptine. It is an ergot alkaloid-2Br-α-ergocriptine which is used for treatment of hyperprolactinemia and Parkinson's disease. In the past it was used for suppression of lactation by non-hormonal inhibition of prolactin release. Several cases have been reported in literature where the patient developed seizures after use of bromocriptine (Katz et al 1985; Kulig et al 1991; Gittelman 1991). In these cases the seizures were associated with other intracranial pathology such as cerebral vasospasm and stroke etc. These isolated reports are difficult to assess. Rothman et al (1990) conducted a record-based case control study of postpartum seizures to evaluate this relationship. They found that women taking bromocriptine had a 22% lower risk for seizures, i. e., relative risk estimate was 0.78 with a 90% confidence interval of 0.29 to 1.87. A reduction in seizure risk is consistent with the reports of antiseizure activity of bromocriptine in various species including humans.

Camphor. Camphor is present in several over-the-counter compounds of questionable use and may be ingested by children and cause convulsions (Siegel and Wason 1986).

Cimetidine. Seizures have reported as an adverse effect of cimetidine (Edmonds et al 1979; Schentag 1980). This drug does not normally cross the blood brain barrier but in various debilitating conditions, it may do so and produce neurotoxicity.

Desmopressin. This is a synthetic analogue of the endogenous peptide of arginine vasopressin, the antidiuretic hormone. Seizures have been reported with use of intranasal desmopressin for control of nocturnal enuresis in children (Yaouyanc et al 1992; Beach et al 1992; Hamed et al 1993). The pathomechanism is water intoxication with hyponatremia induced by desmopressin and excessive water intake. A preventive measure is limitation of fluid intake.

Digoxin. One of the extracardiac toxic effects of digitalis glycosides in humans is reported to be convulsions. In the patient reported by Kerr et al (1982), EEG disturbance was maximal when the plasma digoxin concentration exceeded 5.0 µg/L, and the gradual improvement in EEG coincided with the fall in plasma digoxin concentration as did the frequency of observed epileptiform episodes.

Pathomechanism. Digoxin, when given by intraventricular route in rats, induces a "popcorn type" of convulsion, though analogous to opioid seizures, is not mediated by opioid receptors or GABAergic systems (Kulkarni and Mehta 1983). The authors have suggested the involvement of Na/K-ATPase system in digoxin-induced convulsions.

Management. Clonidine and diazepam provide protection against digoxin-induced convulsions through an unknown mechanism.

Domperidone. This is a benzimidazole derivative which is effective for the control of chemotherapy-induced nausea and vomiting. The drug is supposed to exert its antiemetic effect at the level of dopamine receptors in the chemoreceptor trigger zone. Seizures have been reported in four patients after high dose intravenous domperidone as prophylaxis against chemotherapy-induced emesis (Weaving et al 1984).

Erythropoietin. The hormone erythropoietin which is produced mainly by the kidneys is the primary regulator of red cell production. Its deficiency in chronic renal failure leads to anemia which is treated with recombinant human erythropoietin (rHuEPO). Adverse effects of this therapy have been reviewed by Wong et al (1990). Seizures were observed in nearly all of the earlier studies of rHuEPO therapy. The risk of seizure with rHuEPO treatment is estimated to be 1 per 13 patient years. There is no evidence to support a pro-epileptic action of rHuEPO itself and many of the patients had seizures due to hypertensive encephalopathy which is known as an adverse effect of rHuEPO.

Famotidine. This is a H_2-receptor antagonist which is rarely observed to be neurotoxic. Yoshimoto et al (1994) observed two hemodialized neurosurgical patients who developed convulsions after intravenous famotidine therapy. The CSF concentrations of famotidine were four times that previously reported in non-neurosurgical patients with normal renal function.

Flumazenil. This is a new drug indicated for the reversal of sedative effects of benzodiazepines mediated at the benzodiazepine receptor site. Worldwide 43 cases of seizures associated with this drug have been reported some of which were probably unmasking of the anticonvulsant effect of the previously used benzodiazepines for a seizure disorder (Spivey 1992; Hoffman and Warren 1993). To minimize the likelihood of a seizure, it is recommended that flumazenil not be administered to patients who have used benzodiazepines for the treatment of a seizure disorder or who has ingested drugs that place them at risk for the development of seizures.

Fluorescein. Fluorescein sulfate is given intravenously for fundus fluorescein angiography. Estimated tonic-clonic seizures occur in 1:13900 angiograms (Yannuzi et al 1986). Topical fluorescein eye drops have also caused generalized tonic-clonic seizures (Cohen and Jocson 1981). Kelly et al (1989) have reported a case where convulsion following fluorescein angiography recurred on re-exposure in spite of prophylactic anticonvulsant medication.

Ganciclovir. This drug is used in the treatment of patients with AIDS. Seizures have been reported in association with this therapy (Barton et al 1992). The exact mechanism for the development of seizure activity is not clear. It can be difficult to differentiate between the disease and an adverse drug reaction in a patient with AIDS.

Insulin. Hypoglycemia is a well known complication of insulin therapy and can lead to seizures.

Iodine. Iodine content of the radiographic contrast media is one explanation for seizures as a complication of intravenous injection of such media. Systemic absorption of iodine may occur from topical applications. Zec et al (1992) described a case where seizures developed after mediastinal irrigation with povidone-iodine solution. This patient's serum iodine levels was four times the normal.

Isoretinoin. This may rarely induce epileptic attacks by mechanisms which are not well understood (Masson and Sztern 1991). Hull and Cunliffe (1989) reported that only one of the six epileptic patients on isoretinoin therapy had seizures while on this medication and consider it to be reasonably safe. Another case of seizures following isoretinoin therapy has been reported by Marroni et al (1993).

Levodopa. Only one case of myoclonus and seizures induced by levodopa has been found in the literature. Yoshida et al (1993) reported an elderly patient with Parkinson's disease who developed myoclonus and seizures after one year of levodopa therapy. These could be controlled with antiepileptic drugs. Rechallenge with levodopa resulted in recurrence of myoclonic jerks and generalized seizures. Sensory evoked potential studies showed that levodopa increased the amplitude indicating that cortical excitement was enhanced by the drug.

Melatonin. Melatonin was found to increase seizure activity in six children with multiple neurological deficits in a study in the United States (Sheldon 1998). The indication for use was chronic sleep disorders. Study was suspended when seizure activity was seen on EEG following melatonin therapy which returned to baseline levels when the drug was discontinued. After rechallenge with melatonin, the EEG abnormality recurred.

Methyldopa. This is an antihypertensive drug and its effect is thought to be due to its interference with transmission of impulses in the adrenergic nervous system. This effect is due to displacement of norepinephrine from nerve endings and its replacement by the weak pseudotransmitter metabolites alpha-methyldopamine and alpha-methylnorepinephrine. It is possible that a sudden release in large quantities after an intravenous injection of methyldopa may produce hypertension and seizures as reported by (Feldman et al 1967).

Naftidrofuryl. This is a vasodilator which is used for a wide variety of vascular disturbances. Convulsions have been recorded as a complication of high dose intravenous naftidrofuryl administration (Pohlmann-Eden et al 1991; Maier and Lohle 1993).

Ondansetron. During initial clinical trials of this drug to control vomiting associated with cancer chemotherapy, less than 1% of the patients were reported to have seizures. Most of these patients had risk factors for seizures but a case reported by Sargent et al (1993) did not have any risk factors.

Sulproston (Prostaglandin E₂ Derivative). Prostaglandins are widely used for termination of pregnancy in the second trimester. Convulsions have been reported in three out of four patients following intramuscular injection of the prostaglandin E₂ derivative sulproston (Brandenburgh et al 1990).

Terbutaline. This is a β-adrenergic agonist used in the treatment of asthma. Terbutaline can cause CNS irritability and seizures in certain predisposed individuals. Friedman et al (1982) have described a patient in whom seizures developed after high dose terbutaline therapy.

Thyrotropin-Releasing Hormone (TRH). TRH can cause EEG arousal and desynchronization in animals (Kruse 1975). TRH has been reported to cause recurrence of seizures in an epileptic patient previously controlled by phenobarbital and phenytoin (Maeda and Tanimoto 1981).

Ziperol. This is an antitussive agent considered to be less toxic than codeine and its derivatives. High doses of this drug are abused and cases of convulsions with cerebral edema have been reported (Perraro and Beorchia 1984).

Drug Withdrawal Seizures

Seizures due to withdrawal from antiepileptic drugs are discussed in section dealing with these drugs in this chapter. Seizures are also known to occur during withdrawal from benzodiazepines (Malcolm 1972; Tien and Gujavarty 1985; Ashton 1986). Diazepam withdrawal has been stressed as a cause of seizures because of the ubiquitous use of this drug (Vyas and Carney 1975). In a double-blind study where the patients were withdrawn from diazepam or lorazepam with substitution by propranolol, only 2.5% manifested epileptic seizures although other withdrawal symptoms were frequent (Tyrer et al 1981).

Pathomechanism. Many anxiolytic drugs produce their effect by enhancing brain gamma amino butyric acid (GABA) transmission. During long-term exposure to anxiolytics, the effectiveness is reduced as brain GABA synapses show adaptive changes. Abrupt cessation of anxiolytic treatment may, therefore, lead to an acute reduction in GABA function leading to seizures (Cowen and Nutt 1982).

Management. The use of a gradual withdrawal schedule of benzodiazepines may reduce the probability of a seizure but no controlled studies have been done to verify this. Substitution of another benzodiazepine does not necessarily control the seizures. Carbamazepine has been used successfully for the treatment of benzodiazepine withdrawal (Garcia-Borreguero et al 1991). In addition to controlling seizures, it reduces other withdrawal symptoms such as hypersensitivity to sensory stimuli and depersonalization.

Prevention of Drug-Induced Seizures

A knowledge of the drugs known to induce seizures is important and these drugs should be avoided or given cautiously to epileptic patients or those with risk factors for seizures such as infants with high fever (Galland et al 1992).

Appropriate dose monitoring should be done in patients receiving imipenem/cilastain combination which is associated with seizures in 2–4% of patients. Limitation of dose of 50 mg/kg/day in patients with normal renal function and to 20 mg/kg/day to those with impairment of renal function has been shown to reduce the frequency of seizures to below 1% (Guglielmo and Jacobs 1996).

Management of Drug-Induced Seizures

Most of the drug-induced seizures are self-limiting and do not result in severe sequelae. About

15% may present as status epilepticus which has potential for morbidity (Messing et al 1984). The treatment of drug-induced seizures is usually similar to that of seizures due to other causes, although they are more difficult to control. Special problems according to the drug involved are mentioned in this chapter. The problems of seizures due to overdose of drugs have been reviewed by Kulig (1992) and some of the special points to be noted are:

- In the case of overdose of tricyclic antidepressants, acidemia due to seizures makes the cardiotoxicity more severe.
- Theophylline seizures are usually refractory to usual anticonvulsant agents, and may require general anesthesia to control. Hemodialysis may be required to lower blood levels of the drug.
- If paralyzing agents are used, EEG monitoring should be used to monitor ongoing electrical seizure activity.
- Seizures due to drug-induced hypoglycemia should be recognized and treated quickly to avoid neurologic sequelae.
- Seizures induced by isoniazid usually respond quickly to the administration of pyridoxine.
- Seizures related to the overdose of anticholinergic agents may respond to physostigmine, if standard anticonvulsants are ineffective.
- Seizures in patients taking lithium or salicylates may indicate toxic concentrations of these drugs in the brain, which may require hemodialysis.

Intravenous diazepam is the most frequently used drug for the control of drug-induced seizures and it can be given rectally if intravenous access is not available.

References

Aarli JA: Immunological aspects of epilepsy. Brain Dev 1993; 15: 41–49.

Abarbanel J, Herishanu Y, Frisher S: Encephalopathy associated with baclofen. Ann Neurol 1985; 17(6): 617–618.

Adachi M, Ikemoto Y, Kubo K, et al: Seizure-like movements during induction of anesthesia with sevoflurane. Br J Anesthesia 1992; 68: 214–215.

Agarwal R, Gutlove DP, Lockhart CH: Seizures in pedi-

atric patients receiving continuous infusion of bupivacine. Anesth Analg 1992; 75: 284–286.

Ahmed A, Loes DJ, Bressler EL: Reversible magnetic resonance imaging finding in metronidazole-induced encephalopathy. Neurology 1995; 45: 588–589.

Allan MW: Convulsions after enflurane. Anesthesia 1984; 39: 605–606.

Altrup U, Reith H, Speckman EJ: Effects of valproate in a model nervous system (buccal ganglia of helix pomata): epileptic actions. Epilepsia 1992; 33: 753–759.

Amundsen P: Metrizamide in cervical myelography: survey and present state. Acta Radiologica 1977; 355: 85–97.

Anwar M, Garretson M, Huddleston K, et al: Withdrawal seizures in a neonate following prolonged fentanyl use. J Toxicol 1995; 33: 493.

Armstrong PJ, Bersten A: Norperidone toxicity. Anesthesia and Analgesia 1986; 65: 536–538.

Aronson JK, Reynolds DJM: Lithium. BMJ 1992; 305: 1273–1276.

Ashton CH: Adverse effects of prolonged benzodiazepine use. Adverse Drug Reactions Bulletin 1986; No. 118: 440.

Bahls FH, Ma KK, Bird TD: Theophylline associated seizures with "therapeutic" or low toxic serum concentrations: risk factors for serious outcome in adults. Neurology 1991; 41: 1309–1312.

Barker I, Grant IS: Convulsions after abrupt withdrawal of baclofen. Lancet 1982; 2: 556.

Barrons RW, Murray KM, Richey RM: Populations at risk for penicillin-induced seizures. Ann Pharmacother 1992; 26: 26–29.

Bartel PR, Ubbink JB, Delport R, et al: Vitamin B-6 supplementation and theophylline-related effects in humans. Am J Clin Nutrition 1994; 60: 93–99.

Barton TL, Rousch MK, Dever LL: Seizures associated with ganciclovir therapy. Pharmacotherapy 1992; 12: 413–415.

Bateman DN, Dyson EH: Quinine toxicity. Adverse Drug Reactions and Acute Poisoning Reviews 1986; 4: 215–233.

Beach PS, Beach RE, Smith LR: Hyponatremic seizures in a child treated with desmopressin to control enuresis. Clin Paediatr 1992; 31: 566–569.

Beaman M, Parvin S, Veitch PS, et al: Convulsions associated with cyclosporin A in renal transplant recipients. BMJ 1985; 290: 139–140.

Bell WL, Crawford IL, Shiu GK: Reduced bioavailability of moisture-exposed carbamazepine resulting in status epilepticus. Epilepsia 1993; 34: 1102–1104.

Bem JL, Breckenridge AM, Mann RD, et al: Review of yellow cards (1986): report to the Committee on Safety of Medicines. Brit J Clin Pharmacol 1988; 26: 679–689.

Bem JL, Kerr L, Stuerchler D: Mefloquine prophylaxis: an overview of spontaneous reports of severe psychiatric reactions and convulsions. J Tropical Medicine and Hygiene 1992; 95: 167–179.

Bennett DR, Madsen JA, Jordan WS, et al: Ketamine anesthesia in brain damaged epileptics. Neurology (New York) 1973; 23: 449.

Berman IJ, Mann MP: Seizures and transient cortical

blindness associated with cis-platinum (II) diamminedichloride (PDD) therapy in a thirty-year old man. Cancer 1980; 45: 764–766.

Bertoni JM, Schwartman RJ, Van Horn G, et al: Asterixis and encephalopathy following metrizamide myelography: investigation into possible mechanisms and review of literature. Ann Neurol 1981; 9: 366–370.

Besser R, Krämer G: Verdacht auf anfallfördernde Wirkung von Mefloquin (Lariam7). Nervenarzt 1991; 62: 760–761.

Blisard KS, Harrington DA: Cisplatin-induced neurotoxicity with seizures in frogs. Ann Neurol 1989; 26: 336–341.

Bloch Y, Pollack M, Mor I: Should the administration of ECT during clozapine therapy be contraindicated? Br J Psychiatry 1996; 169: 253–4.

Boogaerts J, Declerq A, Lafont N, et al: Toxicity of bupivacine encapsulated into liposomes and injected intravenously: comparison with plain solutions. Anesth Analg 1993; 76: 553–555.

Boogaerts MA, Zache P, Verwilghen RL: Cyclosporin, methylprednisolone, and convulsions. Lancet 1982; 2: 1216–1217.

Boston Collaborative Drug Surveillance Program: Drug-induced convulsions. Lancet 1972; 2: 677–679.

Brandenburgh H, Jahoda MGJ, Wladimiroff JW, et al: Convulsions in epileptic women after administration of prostaglandin E_2 derivative. Lancet 1990; 336: 1138.

Braun-Scharm H, Martinius J: EEG-Veränderungen und Unfälle unter Clozapin-Medikation bei schizophrenen Jugendlichen. Z Kinder-/Jugendpsychiat 1991; 19: 164–169.

Bruguerolle B, Emperaire N: Flumazenil and bupivacaine-induced toxicity: inverse against type activity. Life Sci 1991; 49: 185–188.

Buiumsohn A, Eisenberg ES, Jacob H, et al: Seizures and intraventricular conduction defect in propranolol poisoning. Ann of Int Med 1979; 91: 860–862.

Burmeister-Rother R, Streatfield KA, Yoo MC: Convulsions following ketamine and atropine. Anesthesia 1993; 43: 82.

Byrne TN, Moseley TA, Finer MA: Myoclonic seizures following chlorambucil overdose. Ann Neurol 1981; 191: 191–194.

Calandra G, Lydick E, Carrigan J, et al: Factors predisposing to seizures in seriously ill infected patients receiving antibiotics: experience with imipenem/cilastatin. Am J Med 1988; 84: 911–918.

Camfield PR, Camfield CS, Dooley JM, et al: Aspartame exacerbates EEG spike-wave discharge in children with generalized absence epilepsy. Neurology 1992; 42: 1000–1003.

Capone PM, Cohen ME: Seizures and cerebritis associated with administration of OKT3. Pediatr Neurol 1991; 7: 299–301.

Choy-Kwong M, Lipton RB: Seizures in hospitalized cocaine users. Neurology 1989; 39: 425–7.

Cilio MR, Danhaive D, Gadisseux JF, et al: Unusual cyclosporin related neurological complications in recipients of liver transplants. Arch Dis Child 1993; 68: 405–407.

Cochran D, Price W, Gwinnutt CL: Unilateral convulsion after induction of anesthesia with propofol. Brit J Anesthaesia 1996; 76: 570–572.

Cohen SM, Laurito CE, Curran MJ: Grand mal seizures in a postpartum patient following intravenous infusion of caffeine sodium benzoate to treat persistent headache. J Clin Anesth 1992; 4: 48–51.

Cohen HC, Jocson VL: A unique case of grandmal seizure after Fluress. Ann Ophthalmol 1981; 13: 1379–1380.

Cold JA, Wells BG, Froemming JH: Seizure activity associated with antipsychotic therapy. DICP Ann Pharmacother 1990; 24: 601–606.

Cousins MJ, Mather LE: Intrathecal and epidural administration of opioids. Anesthesiology 1984; 61: 276–310.

Cowe LA, Lloyd DJ, Dawling S: Neonatal convulsions caused by withdrawal from maternal clomipramine. BMJ 1982; 284: 1837–1838.

Cowen PJ, Nutt DJ: Abstinence symptoms after withdrawal of tranquillizing drugs: is there a common neurochemical mechanism? Lancet 1982; 2: 360–362.

Crome P, Newman B: The problem of tricyclic antidepressant poisoning. Postgrad Med J 1979; 55: 528–532.

Cronin CMG: Neurotoxicity of lorazepam in a premature infant. Paediatrics 1992; 89: 1129–1130.

Cutler MG, Horton RW: Paradoxical enhancement of seizures in the gerbil after chronic treatment with sodium valproate. Neuropharmacology 1988; 27: 617–21.

Dailey JW, Naritaku DK: Antidepressants and seizures. Biochemical Pharmacology 1996; 52: 1323–1329.

Das G, Ferris JC: Generalized convulsions in a patient receiving ultrashort-acting β-blocker infusion. Drug Intell Clin Pharm 1988; 22: 484–485.

Davidson J: Seizures and bupropion: a review. J Clin Psychiatry 1989; 50: 256–261.

Davis JM, Metrakos K, Aranda JV: Apnoea and seizures. Arch Dis Child 1986; 61: 791–3.

De Jongh RH, Walt LF: Lidocaine-induced psychomotor seizures in man. Acta Anesthesiol Scan 1966; suppl 23: 598.

de Lima JC, Scarf MG, Cooper MG: Propofol convulsions again? Anesthesia and Intensive Care 1992; 20: 397–398.

de Vane PJ, MacPherson P, Teasdale E, et al: The prophylactic use of phenytoin during iopamidol contrast studies of the subarachnoid space. Europ J Clin Pharmacol 1986; 29: 747–749.

Deahl M, Trimble M: Serotonin reuptake inhibitors, epilepsy and myoclonus. Br J Psychiatry 1991; 159: 433–435.

DeFriez CB, Wong HC: Seizures and opisthotonus after propofol anesthesia. Anesth Analg 1992; 75: 630–632.

De Krom MCTFM, Verduin N, Visser E, et al: Three cases with status epilepticus during vigabatrin treatment. JNNP 1994; 57: 1294–1295.

Devadatta S: Isoniazid-induced encephalopathy. Lancet 1965; 2: 440–441.

Devinsky O, Honigfeld G, Patin J: Clozapine-related seizures. Neurology 1991; 41: 369–371.

Dhuna A, Pascal-Leone A, Talwar D: Exacerbation of

partial seizures and onset of non-epileptic myoclonus with carbamazepine. Epilepsia 1991; 32: 275–278.

Dugstad G, Eldevik P: Lumbar myelography. Acta Radiologica 1977; 355: 17–30.

Dunn DW, Parekh HU: Theophylline and status epilepticus in children. Neuropediatrics 1991; 22: 24–26.

Durrant S, Chiping PM, Palmer s, et al: Cyclosporin A, methylprednisolone, and convulsions. Lancet 1982; 2: 829–830.

Duthie DJ, Nimmo WS: Adverse effects of opioid analgesic drugs. Br J Anaesth 1987; 59: 61–77.

Eag-Olofsson O, Carl-Eric E: Convulsions in a breast-fed infant after maternal indomethacin. Lancet 1978; 2: 215.

Edgren B, Tilleli J, Gehrz R: Intravenous lidocaine overdosage in a child. Clin Toxicol 1986; 24: 51–58.

Editorial: Drugs for cardiac arrhythmias. Medical Letter 1989 (April 21); 790

Edmonds ME, Ashford RFU, Brenneer MK, et al: Cimetidine; does neurotoxicity occur? Report of three cases. J Roy Soc Med 1979; 72: 172–175.

Edwards JG, Glen-Bott M: Mianserin and convulsive seizures. Br J Clin Pharmac 1984; 15(suppl 2): 299S–311S.

Edwards JG, Glen-Bott M: Nomifensine and convulsive seizures. Human Toxicol 1987; 6: 247–249.

Edwards JG, Long SK, Sedgwick EM, et al: Antidepressants and convulsive seizures: clinical, electroencephalographic, and pharmacological aspects. Clin Neuropharmacol 1986; 9: 329–360.

El-Dahr S, Chevalier RL, Gomez RA, et al: Seizures and blindness following intravenous pulse methylprednisolone in a renal transplant patient. Int J Ped Nephrology 1987; 8: 87–90.

Elliott E, Hamid TK, Arthur LJ, et al: Ketamine anesthesia for medical procedures in children. Arch Dis Child 1976; 51: 56.

Förstl H, Pohlman-Eden, Rothenberger A: Veränderungen somatosensibel evozierter Potentiale bei pharmakogener Myoklonie. Nervenarzt 1992; 63: 359–362.

Farrington P, Pugh S, Colville A, et al: A new method for active surveillance of adverse events from diptheria /tetanus/pertussis and measles/mumps/rubella vaccines. Lancet 1995; 345: 567–569.

Feldman W, Hilman D, Baliah T: Hypertension and seizures following methydopa infusion. Pediatrics 1967; 39: 780–782.

Ferrer-Allado T, Breckner VL, Dymond A, et al: Ketamine-induced electroconvulsive phenomenon in the human limbic and thalamic regions. Anesthesiology 1973; 38: 333.

Fish DR, Espir MLE: Convulsions associated with prophylactic antimalarilal drugs: implications for people with epilepsy. BMJ 1988; 297: 526–527.

Freedman JF, Wirshing WC, Russell AT, et al: Absence status seizures during successful long-term clozapine treatment of an adolescent with schizophrenia. J Child & Adolescent Psychopharmacology 1994; 4: 53–62.

Frenk H, Watkins LR, Miller J, et al: Non-specific convulsions are induced by morphine but not D-Ala2-methionine-enkephalinamide at cortical sites. Brain Res 1984; 299: 51–9.

Friedman R, Zitelli B, Jardine B, et al: Seizures in a patient receiving terbutaline. AJDC 1982; 136: 1091.

Galland MC, Griguer S, Morange-Sala S, et al: Convulsions fJbriles: faut-il contre-indiquer certains medicaments? Therapie 1992; 47: 409–414.

Garcia PA, Alldredge BK: Drug-induced seizures. Neurologic Clinics 1994; 12: 85–99.

Garcia-Borreguero D, Bronisch T, Apelt S, et al: Treatment of benzodiazepine withdrawal symptoms with carbamazepine. Eur Arch Psychiatry Clin Neurosci 1991; 241: 145–150

Gaudreult P, Guay J: Theophylline poisoning: pharmacological considerations and clinical management. Medical toxicology 1986; 1: 169–191.

Gay GR, Luperka KA: Control of cocaine-induced hypertension with labetolol. Anesthesia and Analgesia 1988; 67: 92.

Gittelman DK: Bromocriptine associated with postpartum hypertension, seizures, and pituitary hemorrhage. Gen Hosp Psychiatry 1991; 13: 278–280.

Gouzoulis E, Grunze H, Bardeleben UV: Myoclonic epileptic seizures during clozapine treatment: report of three cases. Eur Arch Psychiatry Clin Neurosci 1991; 240: 370–372.

Grady TA, Pigott TA, L'Heureux F, et al: Seizures associated with fluoxetine and adjuvant busipirone therapy. J Clin Psychopharmacol 1992; 12: 70–71.

Gregory RE, Grossman S, Sheidler VR: Grand mal seizures associated with high-dose intravenous morphine infusions: incidence and possible etiology. Pain 1992; 51: 255–258.

Gross-Tsur V, Manor O, van der Meere J, et al: Epilepsy and attention deficit hyperactivity disorder: is methylphenidate safe and effective? J Pediatr 1997; 130: 670–674.

Guerrini R, Belmonte A, Genton P: Antiepileptic drug-induced worsening of seizures in children. Epilepsia 1998; 39(suppl 3): S2–S10.

Guglielmo BJ, Jacobs RA: Impact of dosage-monitoring system on frequency of seizures associated with imipenem-cilastin. American Journal of Health-System Pharmacy 1996; 53: 2097–2098.

Gulya K: The opioid system in neurologic and psychiatric disorders and in their experimental models. Pharmac Ther 1990; 46: 395–428.

Gunther W, Baghai T, Naber D, et al: EEG alterations and seizures during treatment with clozapine. Pharmacopsychiatry 1993; 26: 69–74.

Hagmeyer KO, Mauro LS, Mauro VF: Mepederine-related seizures associated with patient-controlled analgesia pumps. Ann Pharmacotherapy 1993; 27: 29–32.

Haller E, Binder RL: Clozapine and seizures. Am J Psychiatry 1990; 147: 1471–1475.

Halloran TJ: Convulsions associated with high cumulative doses of metronidazole. Drug Intell Clin Pharmacy 1982; 16: 409.

Hamed M, Mitchel H, Clow J: Hyponatremic convulsions associated with desmopressin and imipramine treatment. BMJ 1993; 306: 1169.

Hargrave R, Martinez D, Bernstein AJ: Fluoxetine-induced seizures. Psychosomatics 1992; 33: 236–237.

Harrigan PW, Browne SM, Quail AW: Multiple seizures

following re-exposure to propofol. Anaesth Intensive Care 1996; 24: 261–4.

Harrison JL: Postoperative seizures after isofluorane anesthesia. Anesthesia and Analgesia 1986; 65: 1235–1236.

Hauben M: Seizures after povidone-iodine mediastinal irrigation. N Engl J Med 1993; 328: 355–356.

Heim M, Nadvorna H, Azaria M: Grand mal seizures following treatment with diclofenac and pentazocine. South African Medical Journal 1990; 78: 700–701.

Hodgman T, Dasta JF, Armstrong DK, et al: Ampicillin induced seizures. Southern Medical Journal 1984; 77: 1323–1325.

Hoffman EJ, Warren EW: Flumzenil: A benzodiazepine antagonist. Clin Pharm 1993; 12: 641–656.

Holdiness MR: Neurological manifestations and toxicities of antituberculous drugs: a review. Medical Toxicology 1987; 2: 33–51.

Holliday W, Brasfield KH, Powers B: Grand mal seizures induced by maprotiline. Am J Psychiatry 1982; 139: 673–674.

Hori M, Suzuki T, Sasaki M, et al: Convulsive seizures in schizophrenic patients induced by zotepine administration. Jpn J Psychiatr Neurol 1992; 46: 161–167.

Hormes JT, Benarroch EE, Rodriguez M, et al: Periodic sharp waves in baclofen-induced encephalopathy. Arch Neurol 1988; 45: 814–5.

Hull SM, Cunliffe WJ: The safety of isoretinoin in patients with acne and systemic diseases. J Dermatological Treatment 1989; 1: 35–37.

Hunter WJ: Imipenem-induced seizure: a case of inappropriate, excessive, and prolonged surgical prophylaxis. Hosp Pharm 1993; 28: 986–8.

Hymes JA: Seizure activity during isoflurane anesthesia. Anesthesia and Analgesia 1985; 64: 367–368.

Idilman R, De Maria N, Kugelmas M, et al: Immunosuppressive drug-induced leukoencephalopathy in patients with liver transplant. Eur J Gastroenterol Hepatol 1998; 10: 433–436.

Iinuma K, Yokoyama H, Otsuki T, et al: Histamine H$_1$ receptors in complex partial seizures. Lancet 1993; 341: 238.

Insel TR, Cohen RM, Murphy DL: Possible development of seerotonin syndrome in man. Am J Psychiatry 1982; 7: 954–955.

Itil TM, Soldatos C: Epileptogenic side effects of psychotropic drugs. JAMA 1980; 244: 1460–1463.

Ito BM, Sato S, Kufta CV, et al: Effect of isoflurane and enflurane on the electrocorticogram of epileptic patients. Neurology 1988; 38: 924–928.

Jabbari B, Bryan GE, Marsh EE, et al: Incidence of seizures with tricyclic and tetracyclic antidepressants. Arch Neurol 1985; 42: 480–481.

Jain KK: Investigation and management of loss of efficacy of an antiepileptic medication using carbamazepine as an example. J Roy Soc Med 1993; 86: 133–136.

Jain KK: Lupus erythematosus like syndromes associated with carbamazepine therapy. Drug Safety 1991; 6: 350–360.

Jain KK: Neurological complications of general anesthesia, Neurobase, Arbor Publiction Corporation, San Diego, California, 1999a.

Jain KK: Neurological complications of local anesthesia. Neurobase, Arbor Publiction Corporation, San Diego, California, 1999b.

Jick H, Dinan RN, Hunter JR, et al: Tricyclic antidepressants and convulsions. J Clin Psychopharmacol 1983; 3: 182–185.

Job ML, Dretler RH: Seizure activity with imipenem therapy: incidence and risk factors. DICP Ann Pharmacother 1990; 24: 467–469.

Johnston JA, Lineberry CG, Ascher JA, et al: A 102-center prospective study of seizure in association with bupropion. J Clin Psychiatry 1991; 52: 450–456.

Junck L, Marshall WH: Neurotoxicity of radiological contrast agents. Ann Neurol 1983; 13: 469–484.

Kando JC, Tohen M, Castillo J, et al: Concurrent use of clozapine and valproate in affective and psychotic disorders. J Clin Psychiatry 1994; 55: 255–257.

Karnaze DS: The low incidence of seizure exacerbation in epileptic patients treated with tricyclic antidepressants and "atypical" antidepressants: postulated mechanisms. Epilepsia 1992; 33(suppl 3): 112.

Karper LP, Salloway SP, Seibyl JP, et al: Prolonged postictal encephalopathy in two patients with clozapine-induced seizures. J Neuropsychiat Clin Neurosci 1992; 4: 454–457.

Katsuki K, Shinohara K, Yamada T: A case of fatal seizure and unconsciousness caused by panipenem/betamipron. Kansenshogaku Zasshi 1998; 72: 651–3.

Katz M, Kroll D, Pak I, et al: Puerperal hypertension, stroke, and seizures after suppression of lactation with bromocriptine. Obstet Gynecol 1985; 66: 822–824.

Kaufman IA, Kung FH, Koenig HM, et al: Overdosage with vincristine. J Pediatrics 1976; 89: 671–674.

Kay HE, Knapton PJ, O'Sullivan JP: Encephalopathy in acute leukemia associated with methotrexate therapy. Arch Dis Child 1972; 47: 344–354.

Kelly SP, MacDermott NJG, Saunders DC, et al: Convulsions following intravenous fluorescein angiography. Br J Ophthalmol 1989; 73: 655–656.

Kenepp NB, Gutsche BB: Inadvertent intravascular injections during lumbar epidural anesthesia. Anesthesiology 1981; 54(2): 172–3.

Kerr DJ, Elliott HL, Hills WS: Epileptiform seizures and electroencephalographic abnormalities as manifestations of drug toxicity. BMJ 1982; 284: 162–163.

Klion AD, Kallsen J, Cowl CT, et al: Ceftazidime-related non-convulsive status epilepticus. Arch Int Med 1994; 154: 586–589.

Kobayashi K, Mori A: Brain monoamine in seizure mechanism. Folia Psychiatrica et Neurologica Japonica 1977; 31: 483–489.

Kofler M, Kronenberg MF, Rifici C, et al: Epileptic seizures associated with intrathecal baclofen application. Neurology 1994; 44: 25–27.

Koren G, Butt W, Chinyanga H, et al: Postoperative morphine infusion in newborn ilnfants: assessment of disposition characteristics and safety. J Pediatrics 1985; 107: 963–967.

Kotaki H, Tayama N, Ito K, et al: Safe and effective application dose of lidocaine for surgery with laryn-goscopy. Clin Pharmacol Ther 1996; 60: 229–235.

Kramer LD, Locke GE, Ogunyemi A, et al: Cocaine-related seizures in adults. Am J Drug Alcohol Abuse 1990; 16: 309–317.

Krenzelok M, Anderson GM, Mirick M: Diphenhydramine overdose resulting in death. J Emerg Med 1982; 11: 212–213.

Krieger W, Copperman J, Laxer KD: Seizure with etomidate anesthesia. Anesthesia and Analgesia 1985; 64: 1226–1227.

Kruczek M, Albin MF, Wolf S, et al: Postoperative seizure activity following enflurane anesthesia. Anesthesiology 1980; 53: 175–176.

Kruse H: Thyrotropin-releasing hormone: interaction with chlorpromazine in mice, rats, and rabbits. J Pharmacol (Paris) 1975; 6: 249–268.

Kulig K, Morre LL, Kirk M, et al: Bromocriptine-associated headache: possible life-threatening sympathomimetic interaction. Obstet Gynecol 1991; 78: 941–943.

Kulig K: Initial management of ingestions of toxic substances. NEJM 1992; 326: 1677–1680.

Kulkarni SK, Mehta AK: Possible mechanism of digitoxin-induced convulsions. Psychopharmacology 1983; 79: 287–289.

Langlois C: Risk of seizures from concomitant use of ciprofloxacin and phenytoin in patients with epilepsy. CMAJ 1998; 158: 104–105.

Lannes M, Desparmet JF, Zifkin BG: Generalized seizures associated with nitrous oxide in an infant. Anesthesiology 1997; 87: 705–8.

Leber P: "Time-less" risks (a hazard of risk assessment: the example of seizure and antidepressants). Psychopharmacology Bulletin 1985; 21: 334–338.

Legha SS: Vincristine neurotoxicity: pathophysiology and management. Med Toxicol 1986; 1: 421–427.

Lehmann HE, Cahn CH, de Verteuil RL: The treatment of depressive conditions with imipramine. Can J Psychiat 1958; 3: 155–163.

Leo RJ, Ballow CH: Seizure activity associated with imipenem use: clinical reports and review of literature. DICP Ann Pharmacother 1991; 25: 351–354.

Levey AI, Weiss H, Yu R, et al: Seizures following myelography with iopamidol. Ann Neurol 1988; 23: 397–399.

Levine R, Kenin M, Hoffman JS, et al: Grandmal seizures associated with the use of fluoxetine. J Clin Psychopharmacol 1994; 14: 145–146.

Lipka LJ, Lathers CM: Psychoactive agents, seizure production, and sudden death in epilepsy. J Clin Pharmacol 1987; 27: 169–183.

Liukkonen J, Koponen HJ, Nousiainen U: Clinical picture and long-term course of epileptic seizures that ocur following clozapine treatment. Psychiatry Research 1992; 44: 107–112.

Lockskin MD, Kagen LJ: Meningitic reactions after azothioprine. NEJM 1972; 286: 1321–1322.

Lockton JW, Holmes O: Site of initiation of penicillin-induced epilepsy in the cortex cerebri of the rat. Brain Res 1980; 190: 301–304.

Logothetis J: Spontaneous epileptic seizures and elec-troencephalographic changes in the course of phenothiazine therapy. Neurology 1967; 17: 869–877.

Lortie A, Chiron C, Mumford J, et al: The potential for increasing seizure frequency, relapse, and appearance of new seizure types with vigabatrin. Neurology 1993; 43(suppl 5): S24–S27.

Lowenstein D, Aminoff M, Simon R: Barbiturate anesthesia in the treatment of status epilepticus: clinical experience with 14 patients. Neurology 1988; 38: 395–400.

Lukovits TG, Fadul CE, Pipas JM, et al: Non-convulsive status epilepticus after intravenous contrast medium administration. Epilepsia 1996; 37: 1117–1120.

McDonald MG, Getson PR, Glasgow AM, et al: Propylene glycol: increased incidence of seizures in low birth weight infants. Pediatrics 1987; 79: 622–625.

Madi L, O'Brien AAJ, Fennel J: Status epilepticus secondary to fluoxetine. Postgraduate Medical Journal 1994; 70: 383–384.

Maeda K, Tanimoto K: Epileptic seizures induced by thyrotropic releasing hormone. Lancet 1981; 1: 1058–1059.

Magera BE, Betlach CJ, Sweatt AP: Hydroxyzine intoxication in 13- month old child. Pediatrics 1981; 67: 280–283.

Maier W, Lohle E: Convulsive state during intravenous infusion of naftidrofuryl. HNO 1993; 41: 539–541.

Mäkela JP, Iivanainen M, Pieninkeroinen IP, et al: Seizures associated with propofol anesthesia. Epilepsia 1993; 34: 832–835.

Malcolm MT: Temporal lobe epilepsy due to drug withdrawal. Br J Addict 1972; 67: 309–312.

Malow BA, Blaxton TA, Stertz B, et al: Carbamazepine withdrawal: effects of taper rate on seizure frequency. Neurology 1993; 43: 2280–2284.

Marinella MA: Mperidine-induced generalized seizure with normal renal function. Southern Medical Journal 1997; 90: 556–558.

Marks RC, Luchins DJ: Antipsychotic medications and seizures. Psychiatric Medicine 1991; 9: 37–52.

Marroni M, Bellomo G, Bucaneve G, et al: Isoretinoin: possible cause of acute seizure and confusion. Ann Pharmacother 1993; 27: 793.

Martin DR, DePadua L: Recognition of INH-toxicity seizures. Phillipine J Int MLed 1983; 21: 190.

Martin ES, Bagwell T, Bush-Veith S, et al: Seizures after intraventricular cefazolin administration. Clin Pharm 1992; 11: 104–105.

Masson C, Sztern A: IsotrJtinoine, cause possible de crise d'Jpilepsie. Presse MJdicale 1991; 20: 2264–2265.

May EF, Ling GSF, Geyer CA, et al: Contrast agent overdose causing brain retention of contrast, seizures, and parkinsonism. Neurology 1993; 43: 836–838.

McCloskey JJ, Haun SE, Deshpande JK: Bupivacaine toxicity secondary to continuous caudal epidural infusion in children. Anesth Analg 1992; 75: 287–290.

Mead GM, Arnold AM, Green JA, et al: Epileptic seizures associated with cisplatin administration. Cancer Treat Rep 1982; 66: 1719–1722.

Meisel SB, Welford PK: Seizures associated with high-dose intravenous morphine containing sodium bisulfite preservative. Ann Pharmacotherapy 1992; 26: 1515–1517.

Messing RO, Closson RG, Simon RP: Drug-induced seizures: a 10-year experience. Neurology 1984; 34: 1582–1586.

Michenfelder JD, Cucchiara RF, Sundt TM: Influence of intraoperative antibiotic choice on the incidence of early postcraniotomy seizures. J Neurosurg 1990; 72: 703–705.

Michenfelder JD: Local anesthetics. In Michenfelder JD: Anesthesia and the brain, New York, Churchill Livingstone, 1988, pp 135–143.

Miller G, Eggli KD, Contant C, et al: Postoperative neurological complications after open heart surgery on young infants. Arch Pediatr Adolesc Med 1995; 149: 764–768.

Mirsky AF, Bloch S, Rojas S: Experimental petit mal epilepsy produced by chlorambucil. Acta Biologica Experimenta 1966; 26: 55–68.

Miyashita T, Tokumura Y, Nishiya H, et al: A case of mefloquine-resistant Plasmodium falciparum malaria with convulsions after antimalarial treatment. Kansenshogaku Zasshi 1994; 68: 152–156.

Modica PA, Templehof R, White PF: Pro- and anticonvulsant effects of anesthetics. Anesthesia Analgesia 1990; 70: 305–315.

Moore DC, Bonica JJ: Convulsions and ventricular tachycardia from bupivacaine with epinephrine: successful resuscitation. Anesthesia Analgesia 1985; 64: 844–845.

Murphy CP, Harden EA, Thompson JM: Generalized seizures secondary to high-dose busulfan therapy. Ann Pharmacother 1992; 26: 26–30.

Murthy R, Newton K, Qureshi J: The association of fluoxetine with seizures. J Psychopharmacol 1994; 8: 187–188.

Musella L, Wilder BJ, Schmidt RP: EEG activation with intravenous methohexital in psychomotor epilepsy. Neurology 1971; 21: 594–601.

Naguib M, Magboul MMA, Samarkandi AH: Adverse effects and drug interactions associated with local and regional anaesthesia. Drug Safety 1998; 18: 221–250.

Nappi JM, Dhanani S, Lovejoy J, et al: Severe hypoglycemia associated with dysopyramide. West J Med 1983; 138: 95–97.

Nelson M, Bartlett RJV, Lamb JT: Seizures after intravenous contrast media for cranial computed tomography. JNNP 1989; 52: 1170–1175.

Neufeld MY: Exacerbation of focal seizures due to carbamazepine treatment in an adult patient. Clin Neuropharmacol 1993; 16: 359–361.

Norrby SR: Problems in evaluation of adverse reactions of lactam antibiotics. Med Toxicol 1986; 1: 358–370.

Norrby SR: Side effects of cyclosporins. Drugs 1987; 34(suppl 2): 105–120.

Ochs JJ, Bowman WP, Pui C-H, et al: Seizures in childhood lymphoblastic leukemia patients. Lancet 1984; 2: 1422.

Ogunyemi A, Locke GE, Kramer LD, et al: Complex partial status epilepticus provoked by "crack" cocaine. Ann Neurol 1989; 26: 785–786.

Olson KR, Kearney TE, Dyer JE, et al: Seizures associated with poisoning and drug overdose. Am J Emerg Med 1993; 11: 565–568.

Olson KR, Pental PR, Kelley MT: Physical assessment and diagnosis of the poisoned patient. Med toxicol 1987; 2: 52–81.

Page P, Morgan M, Loh L: Ketamine anesthesia in pediatric procedures. Acta Anesthesiol Scand 1972; 16: 155.

Pantuck AJ, Goldsmith JW, Kuriyan JB, et al: Seizures after ureteral stone manipulation with lidocaine. Journal of Urology 1997; 157: 2248.

Parfrey P, Davies SJ: Seizures after aminophylline suppository. BMJ 1979; 3: 497–498.

Park HH, Christ W: Teicoplanin produces convulsions in rats, when administered intraventricularly. Europ J Clin Res 1992; 3: 151–156.

Paton JH, Reeves DS: Adverse reactions to the fluoroquinolones. Adverse Drug Reactions Bulletin 1992; No.153: 575–578.

Peck AW, Stern WC, Watkinson C: Incidence of seizures during treatment with tricyclic antidepressant drugs and bupropion. J Clin Psychiatry 1983; 44: 197–201.

Perraro F, Beorchia A: Convulsions and cerebral oedema associated with ziperol abuse. Lancet 1984; 1: 45–46.

Perry MF: Toxic and adverse reactions encountered with a new β-lactam antibiotic. Bull NY Acad Med 1984; 60: 358–368.

Perucca E, Gram L, Avanzini G, et al: Antiepileptic drugs as a cause of worsening seizures. Epilepsia 1998; 39: 5–17.

Peters MD, Davis SK, Austin LS: Clomipramine: an antiobsessional tricyclic antidepressant. Clin Pharm 1990; 9: 165–78.

Physicians' Desk Reference, Montvale, NJ, Medical Economics Company, 1998, p 1897.

Pinto JM, Maher TJ: Administration of aspartame potentiates pentylenetetrazole- and fluorothyl-induced seizures in mice. Neuropharmacology 1988; 27: 51–5.

Pohlmann-Eden B, Linden D, Bergler W: Konvulsive Krisen und kardiovaskuläre Komplikationen nach hochdosierter parenteraler Naftidrofuryl-Gabe. DMW 1991; 116: 1453.

Porter J, Jick H: Drug-induced anaphylaxis, convulsions, deafness, and extrapyramidal symptoms. Lancet 1977; 1: 587–588.

Pryle BJ, Grech H, Stoddart PA, et al: Toxicity of norpethidine in sickle cell crisis. BMJ 1992; 304: 1478–1479.

Quail AW: Modern inhalational anesthetic agents. A review of halothane, isoflurane and enflurane. Med J Australia 1989; 150: 95–102.

Ramabadran K, Bansinath M: Endogenous opioid peptides and epilepsy. Int J Clin Pharmcol Ther Toxicol 1990; 28: 47–62.

Ramoska E, Sacchetti A: Propranolol-induced hypertension in treatment of cocaine intoxication. Ann Emergency Med 1985; 14: 12–13.

Ratcliffe SG, Axworthy DG: Mefenic acid poisoning and epilepsy. BMJ 1979; 3: 672.

Reynolds F: Adverse effects of local anesthetics. Br J Anesth 1987, 59: 78–95.

Rosenstein DL, Nelson JC, Jacobs SC: Seizures associated with antidepressants: a review. J Clin Psychiatry 1993; 54: 289–299.

Rothman KJ, Funch DP, Dreyer NA: Bromocriptine and puerperal seizures. Epidemiology 1990; 1: 232–238.

Russell RD, Stripling J: Monoaminergic and local anesthetic components of cocaine's effect on kindled seizure expression. Pharmacology Biochem Behav 1985; 22: 427–434.

Sachdeo R, Chakroverty S: Enhancement of absences with CBZ. Epilepsia 1985; 26: 534.

Safferman AZ, Lieberman JA, Kane JM, et al: Update on the clinical efficacy and side effects of clozapine. Schizophrenia Bulletin 1991; 17: 247–258.

Saltuari L, Marosi MJ, Kofler M, et al: Status epilepticus complicating intrathecal baclofen overdose. Lancet 1992; 339: 373–374.

Sansone ME, Ziegler DK: Lithium toxicity: a review of neurologic complications. Clin Neuropharmacol 1985; 8: 142–248.

Sargent AI, Deppe SA, Chan FA: Seizures associated with ondansetron. Clin Pharm 1993; 12: 613–615.

Schentag JJ: Cimetidine-associated mental confusion. Further studies in 36 severely ill patients. Therapeutic Drug Monitoring 1980; 2: 133–142.

Schindler BA, Ramchandani D: Partial complex status epilepticus in a lithium toxic patient. Psychosomatics 1993; 34: 521–522.

Schwartz JB, Keefe D, Harrison DC: Adverse effects of antiarrhythmic drugs. Drugs 1981; 21: 23–45.

Schwartz MS, Scott DF: Aminophylline-induced seizures. Epilepsia 1974; 15: 501–505.

Scott JC, Sarnquist FH: Seizure-like movements during fentanyl infusion with absence of seizure activity in simultaneous EEG recording. Anesthesiology 1985; 62: 812–814.

Scott JP, Higenbottam TW: Adverse reaction and interactions of cyclosporin. Med Toxicol 1988; 3: 107–127.

Serdaru M, Diquet B, Lhermitte F: Generalized seizures and ampicillin. Lancet 1982; 2: 617–618.

Shah D, Rylance PB, Rogerson ME, et al: Generalized epileptic fits in renal transplant recipients given cyclosporin A. BMJ 1989; 289: 1347–1348.

Shah PM, Wiesel M, Stille W: Clinical experience with cefotaxime in internal medicine between 1981 and 1984. Drugs 1988; 35(suppl 2): 190–194.

Shaywitz BA, Novotny EJ: Aspartame and seizures. Neurology 1993; 43: 630.

Sheldon SH: Pro-convulsant effects of oral melatonin in neurologically disabled children. Lancet 1998; 351: 1254.

Shields WD, Saslow E: myoclonic, atonic, and absence seizures following institution of carbamazepine therapy. Neurology 1983; 33: 1487–1489.

Shimada J, Hori S, Kanemitsu K, et al: A comparative study on the convulsant activity of carbapenems and β-lactams. Drug Exptl Clin Res 1992; 18: 377–381.

Shuper A, Vining EPG: Photosensitive complex partial seizures aggravated by phenytoin. Pediatr Neurol 1991; 7: 471–472.

Siegel E, Wason S: Camphor toxicity. Pediatr Clin North Am 1986; 33: 375–379.

Singh K, Shanks GD, Wilde H: Seizures after mefloquine. Ann Int Med 1991; 114: 994.

Skowron DM, Stimmel GL: Antidepressants and risk of seizures. Pharmacotherapy 1992; 12: 18–22.

Small JG, Milstein V, Small IF, et al: Computerized EEG profile of haloperidol, chlorpromazine, clozapine, and placebo in the treatment of resistant schizophrenia. Clinical Electroencephalography 1987; 18: 124–134.

Smith NT, Benthuysen JI, Bickford RG, et al: Seizures during opioid anesthesia induction—are they opioid-induced rigidity? Anesthesiology 1989; 71: 852–862.

Spivey WH: Flumazil and seizures: analysis of 43 cases. Clin Ther 1992; 14: 292–305.

Sprung J, Schedewie HK: Apparent focal motor seizure with a jacksonian march induced by fentanyl: a case report and review of literature. J Clin Anesth 1992; 4: 139–143.

Starkey IR, Lawson AA: Psychiatric aspects of acute poisoning with with tricyclic and related antidepressants: a ten year review. Scottish Med J 1980; 25: 303–308.

Steinhauer HB, Hertting G: Lowering of the convulsive threshold by non-steroidal anti-inflammatory drugs. Europ J Pharmacol 1981; 69: 199–203.

Steinhoff BJ, Stodiek SR: Temporary abolition of seizure activity by flumazenil in a case of valproate-induced non-convulsive status epilepticus. Seizure 1993; 2: 261–265.

Stilman N, Masdeu JC: Incidence of seizures with phenytoin toxicity. Neurology 1985; 35: 1769–1772.

Stone WE, Javid MJ: anticonvulsive and convulsive effects of lidocaine: comparison with those of phenytoin, and implications for mechanism of action concepts. Neurological Research 1988; 10: 161–168.

Stone WE, Javid MJ: Aminophylline and imidazole as convulsants. Archives Internationales de Pharmacodynamie et de Therapie 1980; 248: 121–131.

Storrow AB: Bupropion overdose and seizure. Am J Emergency Med 1994; 12: 183–184.

Sugai K: Seizures with clonazepam: discontinuation and suggestions for safe discontinuation rates in children. Epilepsia 1993; 34: 1089–1097.

Sullivan KM, Storb R, Shulman HM: Immediate and delayed neurotoxicity after mechlorethamine preparation for bone marrow transplantation. Ann Int Med 1982; 97: 182–189.

Tai DYH, Yeo JKS, Eng PCT, et al: Intentional overdose with isoniazid: case report and review of literature. Singapore Medical Journal 1996; 37: 222–225.

Taverner D, Baine DAC: Intravenous lidocaine as anticonvulsant. Lancet 1958; 2: 1145–1147.

Tempelhoff R, Modica PA, Bernardo KL, et al: Fentanyl-induced electrocorticographic seizures in patients with complex partial epilepsy. J Neurosurg 1992; 77: 201–208.

Terrence CG, Fromm GH: Complications of baclofen wilthdrawal. Arch Neurol 1981; 38: 588.

Theodore WH, Porter RJ, Raubertas RF: Seizures during barbiturate withdrawal: relation to blood level. Ann Neurol 1987; 22: 644–647.

Tiberghien P, Flesch M, Paitaud G, et al: More on high-dose busulfan and seizure prophylaxis. Bone Marrow Transplantation 1992; 9: 147.

Tidswell P, D'Assis-Fonesca A: Generalized seizure due to terfenadine. BMJ 1993; 307: 241.

Tien AY, Gujavarty KS: Seizure following withdrawal from triazolam. Am J Psychiatry 1985; 142: 1516–1517.

Tommasino C, Maekawa T, Shapiro HM: Fentanyl-induced seizures activate subcortical brain metabolism. Anesthesiology 1984; 60: 283–290.

Toth P, Frankenburg FR: Clozapine and seizures: a review. Can J Psychiatry 1994; 39: 236–238.

Tuomisto L, Tacke U: Is histamine an anticonvulsive inhibitory transmitter? Neuropharmacology 1986; 25: 955–958.

Tyrer P, Rutherford D, Huggett T: Benzodiazepine withdrawal symptoms and propranolol. Lancet 1981; 1: 520–522.

Vossler DG, Wright SJ: Convulsive status epilepticus following intrathecial iopamidol adminsitration. J Epilepsy 1994; 7: 18–20.

Vyas I, Carney MWP: Diazepam and withdrawal fits. BMJ 1975; 2: 44.

Weaving A, Bezwoda WR, Derman DP: Seizures after antiemetic treatment with high dose domperidone: report of four cases. BMJ 1984; 288: 1728.

Weinstein L, Lerner PI, Chew WR: Clinical and bacteriological studies of the effect of "massive" doses of penicillin G on infections caused by gram negative bacilli. NEJM 1964; 271: 525–533.

Weinstein RS: Recognition and management of poisoning with β-adrenergic blocking agents. Ann Emerg Med 1984; 13: 1123–1131.

Weiss FB, Forman P, Rosenthal IM: Allopurinol-induced arteritis in partial HGPRTase deficiency: atypical seizure manifestation. Arch Int Med 1978; 138: 1743–1744.

Wengs WJ, Talwar D, Bernard J: Ifosfamide-induced non-convulsive status epilepticus. Arch Neurol 1993; 50: 1104–1105.

Whelton A, Carter GG, Garth MA, et al: Carbenicillin-induced acidosis and seizures. JAMA 1971; 218: 1942–1943.

White K, Simpson G: Combined MAOI-tricyclic antidepressant therapy: a re-evaluation. J Clin Psychopharmacol 1981; 1: 264–282.

Whitshaw E, Subramanian S, Alexopoulos C: Cancer of the ovary: a summary of experience with cis-dichlorodiammineplatinum at the Royal Marsden Hospital. Cancer Treatment Reports 1979; 63: 1545–1548.

Williams SA, Makker SP, Grupe WE: Seizures: a significant side effect of chlorambucil therapy in children. J Pediat 1978; 93: 516–518.

Wilson AJ, Evill CA, Sage MR: Effects of non-ionic contrast media on the blood-brain barrier: osmolality versus chemotoxicity. Invest Radiol 1984; 19: 329–332.

Winick NJ, Bowman WP, Kamen BA, et al: Unexpected neurologic toxicity in the treatment of children wit h acute leukemia. J Ntl Cancer Inst 1992; 84: 252–256.

Wong KC, Li PK, Liu SF, et al: The adverse effects of recombinant human erythropoietin therapy. Adverse Drug React Acute Poisoning Rev 1990; 9: 183–206.

Woodforth IJ, Hicks RG, Crawford MR, et al: Electroencephalographic evidence of seizure activity under deep sevoflurane anesthesia in a nonepileptic patient. Anesthesiology 1997; 87: 1579–1582.

Wright BD: Exacerbation of kinetic seizures by atropine eye drops. Br J Ophthalmol 1992; 76: 179–180.

Wroblewski MS, Leary JM, Phelan AM, et al: Methylphenidate and seizure frequency in brain injured patients with seizure disorders. J Clin Psychiatry 1992; 53: 86–89.

Wu F, Razzaghi A, Souney PF: Seizure after lidocaine for bronchoscopy: case report and review of use of lidocaine in airway anesthesia. Pharmacotherapy 1993; 13: 72–78.

Wyler AR, Richey ET, Atkinson RA, et al: Methohexital activation of epileptogenic foci during acute electrocorticography. Epilepsia 1987; 28: 490–494.

Yannuzi LA, Rohrer KT, Tindel LJ, et al; Fluorescein angiography complication survey (FACS). Ophthalmology 1986; 93: 611–617.

Yaouyanc G, Jonville AP, Yaouyanc-Lapalle H, et al: Seizure with hyponatremia in a child prescribed desmopressin for nocturnal enuresis. Clin Toxicol 1992; 30: 637–641.

Yohai D, Barnett SH: Absence and atonic seizures induced by piperazine. Pediatr Neurol 1989; 5: 393–394.

Yoshida K, Moriwaka F, Matsuura T, et al: Myoclonus and seizures in a patient with Parkinson's disease: induction by levodopa and its confirmation on SEPs. Jpn J Psychiat Neurol 1993; 47: 621–625.

Yoshimoto K, Saima S, Echizen H, et al: Famotidine-associated central nervous system reactions and plasma and cerebrospinal drug concentrations in neurosurgical patients with renal failure. Clin Pharmacol Ther 1994; 55: 693–700.

Yoshino A, Watanabe M, Shimizu K, et al: Nonconvulsive status epilepticus during antidepressant treatment. Neuropsychobiology. 1997; 35: 91–94.

Zaccara G, Muscas GC, Messori A: Clinical features, pathogenesis, and management of drug-induced seizures. Drug Safety 1990; 5: 109–151.

Zak R, Solomen G, Petito F, et al: Baclofen-induced generalized non-convulsive status epilepticus. Ann Neurol 1994; 36: 113–114.

Zec N, Donovan W, Aufiero TX, et al: Seizures in a patient treated with continuous povidone-iodine mediastinal irrigation. NEJM 1992; 326: 1784.

Zimmerman B, Gold R, Lavi S: Adverse effects of immunization. Is prevention possible? Postgraduate Med 1987; 82: 225–232.

Chapter 8
Drug-Induced Movement Disorders

Introduction

Movement disorders are common and an important part of neurological practice. Drugs, particularly those used for the treatment of psychiatric disorders, contribute significantly to the pathogenesis of movement disorders. These are often referred to as neuroleptics (literal meaning "one that grips the nerve") and include all antipsychotic drugs: classical antipsychotic drugs (Table 8.1) and atypical antipsychotics (Table 8.2). Antipsychotics belong to the category of dopamine receptor blocking agents which also includes drugs such as metoclopramide which are not used for psychiatric disorders but have the potential of antipsychotic activity if given in

Table 8.1. Classical antipsychotic (neuroleptic) drugs.

Butyrophenones: e. g., haloperidol
Dibenzoxazepines: e. g., loxapine
Diphenylbutylpiperidines: e. g., pimozide
Phenothiazines: e. g., chlorpromazine
Piperidine subgroup: e. g., thioridazine, mesoridazine
Piperazine subgroup: e. g., trifluoperazine,
    fluphenazine, Perphenazine
Thioxanthenes: e. g., chlorprothixene

high doses. Movement disorders can also be the adverse reactions to non-antipsychotic drugs. There is a vast amount of literature on this subject. The current state of knowledge on this topic will be summarized in this chapter and only selected references will be quoted.

Terminology and Classification of Movement Disorders

There is considerable confusion and misunderstanding regarding the terminology of movement disorders. This is reflected in spontaneous reports of adverse drug reactions submitted to the manufacturers as well as in publications. The term extrapyramidal disorders is very non-specific. It usually refers to acute effects such as rigidity with abnormal posturing etc. Extrapyramidal motor disturbances may mean parkinsonism. The use of the term "extrapyramidal" in describing the movement disorders is discouraged because it refers to the anatomical location of the presumed site of action of the drug rather than the clinical description. The term "extrapyramidal syndromes" is often used because the

Table 8.2. Newer atypical antipsychotics.

Drug	Mechanism of action/comments
Clozapine	This was the first atypical antipsychotic. It show the greater affinity for 5-HT$_{1C}$ and 5-HT$_2$ receptors than other receptors. It is associated with agranulocytosis in about 1% of the patients.
Olanzapine	The receptor affinity of this drug is similar to that of clozapine but it has more potent anticholinergic effects.
Risperidone	This is a dual 5-HT$_2$ and dopamine receptor antagonist.
Sertindole	It has a$_1$ adrenergic blocking activity which may cause hypotension.
Quetiapine	This is considered to be more selective for 5-HT$_2$ receptors than D$_2$ receptors.
Ziprasidone	This blocks 5-HT$_{2A}$, 5-HT$_{2C}$ and 5-HT$_{1D}$ receptors as well as D$_2$ receptors. It causes less hypotension and sedation than the traditional antipsychotics.

manifestations usually involve more than one symptom. A list with brief definition of various terms used in this chapter follows:

- *Dyskinesia* is the overall term for drug-induced movement disorders. It can be further specified as hypokinesia or hyperkinesia.
- *Hypokinesia* is reduction of spontaneous activity.
  - *Akinesia* is poverty or lack of movement.
  - *Bradykinesia* is reduction of speed of movement.
- *Hyperkinesia* is abnormal or involuntary movement of striated muscles, which are recurring and uncontrolled, and result in movement of the affected parts. This term includes various types of movements (see Table 8.3) with some mixed types such as choreoathetosis.
- *Parkinsonian* syndrome is an akinetic rigid syndrome. The tremor component of it, however, is a hyperkinesia.
- *Tardive dyskinesia*. This term is used for movement disorders associated with chronic antipsychotic therapy. It includes choreoathetosis which, as an acute effect, is classified under hyperkinesias. Other variants of tardive dyskinesia are: tardive dystonia, tardive akathisia, and tardive tics or Tourette-like syndrome.
- *Akinetic mutism*. This is a condition characterized by loss of spontaneous movement and apathy but with preserved consciousness.

Antipsychotic-Induced Deficit Syndrome (NIDS)

This term has been coined by to distinguish between the negative symptoms of schizophrenia and the adverse effects of psychotropic drugs (Lader 1993). This describes the counter-therapeutic effect of antipsychotic medication in impairing the patient's overall well-being. Adverse effects grouped together in this syndrome include sedation, extrapyramidal symptoms (dystonias, tremor, parkinsonism, and akathisia), hypotension, a subjective feeling of dysphoria, and impaired cognitive dysfunction. Antipsychotics are not unique in their association with such symptoms. Many other psychotropics, used as adjuncts in the treatment of schizophrenia have effects similar to those of antipsychotics and can produce this syndrome.

Assessment of Neurological Status of Schizophrenic Patients

For evaluating neurological adverse effects of antipsychotics, one should know the baseline neurological status of these patients. This information is usually not available in older patients but it would be important to establish the clinical neurological status of new patients prior to institution of antipsychotic therapy.

Presence of neurological signs (disorders of equilibrium, tremor, and adiadochokinesia) in schizophrenic patients in the publications of pioneers who described this disease in the pre-antipsychotic era (Bleuler 1908; Kraepelin 1919). Neurological soft signs have been reported to be more frequently present in schizophrenic patients than in other psychiatric patients and normal subjects but it is possible that antipsychotics contribute to the prevalence of these abnormali-

Table 8.3. Types of hyperkinesias (modified from Jeste and Wyatt 1982).

Type	Rhythmicity	Speed	Localization
Akathesia	Absent	Variable	Limbs, axial muscles
Athetosis	Present	Slow	Distal parts of limbs
Asterixis	Absent	Variable	Neck, arms, trunk
Ballism	Absent	Variable	Limbs, uni- or bilateral
Chorea	Absent	Rapid	Proximal limbs, orofacial
Dystonia	Absent	Slow	Axial muscles
Myoclonus	Absent	Rapid	Limbs
Tic	Variable	Variable	Limbs, orofacial
Tremor	Present	3–20/sec	Fingers, toes, head, tongue

ties (Gupta et al 1995). Modern neuroimaging techniques and neuropathologic techniques have shown structural abnormalities in schizophrenic patients. These abnormalities have been reviewed by Nasrallah (1993) include the following:

- Dilated cerebral ventricles as shown on CT scan
- Widening of sulci and fissures
- Decreased cerebral volume as measured by MRI. On postmortem, brains of schizophrenics weigh 5% less than the controls
- Cerebellar dysplasia
- Medial temporal lobe hypoplasia. Reduction of white matter in the parahippocampal gyrus. Reduction of the granule layer of dentate gyrus of the hippocampal formation
- Reduction of the volume of globus pallidus
- An excess of congenital neuroanatomic abnormalities

Factors that Influence Onset of Drug-Induced Movement Disorders

Some of the factors which influence the onset of drug-induced neurological disorders are some diseases and methods of drug administration. Some examples are:

- *HIV infection.* Patients with AIDS are more susceptible to DIND (Chapter 2). The use of antipsychotic agents in patients with HIV infection frequently results in the development of extrapyramidal symptoms. An example of this is a case report of a patient with AIDs psychosis who developed treatment-resistant tardive dyskinesia after only 6 months of oral fluphenazine therapy (Shedlack et al 1994).
- *Degenerative CNS disorders.* Patients with cerebral atrophy and Parkinson's disease are more susceptible to neurological adverse effects of drugs including aggravation of movement disorders.
- *Hypoglycemia.* Choreoathetosis can be seen in drug-induced hypoglycemia (Newman and Kinkel 1984). A case of hypoglycemic choreoathetosis and ballismus complicating pentamidine therapy of *Pneucystitis carinii* pneu-

monia has been described (Sweeney et al 1994).

- *Method of drug administration.* Considerable discussion centers around the effect of depot preparations for antipsychotic agents on the frequency of extrapyramidal movement disorders. This subject has been reviewed by Barnes and Curson (1994). Although no significant relationship has been demonstrated, depot medications have the disadvantage that they cannot be withdrawn quickly in case of adverse reactions.

Akathisia

This term means an inability to remain seated (Greek kathisia—"the act of sitting" and a—"negative prefix"). This is also called motor restlessness or the feeling of a need to move. Haskovec (1902) identified the syndrome of spontaneously occurring restless long before the introduction of antipsychotics and felt that it was secondary to psychological disorders. It was later linked to extrapyramidal disorders, and finally with the introduction of antipsychotics, akathisia has become the most frequently reported movement disorder resulting from these medications. The prevalence figures vary between 12.5% to 75% of the patients treated with antipsychotics. The newer atypical antipsychotics have also been reported to be associated with akathisia although the frequency of this occurrence is less. These include clozapine (Safferman et al 1993), olanzapine (Kurzthaler et al 1997) and risperidone withdrawal (Rosebush et al 1997). Prochlorperazine, an antipsychotic which is used as an antiemetic in chemotherapy for cancer, has also been reported to be associated with akathisia (Dukoff et al 1996).

Although akathisia is considered to be mostly related to antipsychotic use, non-antipsychotic drugs have also been reported to cause it (Table 8.4). Akathisia has also been described in head-injured patients not receiving any antipsychotic medications.

Akathisia with Antidepressant Treatment. This was first described by Zubenko et al (1987) in 5 of 1000 patients who were antipsychotic-

Table 8.4. Non-antipsychotic drugs causing akathisia.

Antianxiety agent: buspirone (Patterson 1988)
Antidepressants:
  Tricyclic
  – desipramine
  – imipramine
  – nortriptyline
  Selective serotonin reuptake inhibitors (Gerber and
  Lynd 1998)
  – fluoxetine (Bauer 1996; Arya 1997)
  – fluvoxamine
  – sertraline
  – paroxetine (Olivera 1996)
  5-HT$_2$ receptor inhibitors trazodone, nefazodone
  (Eberstein et al 1996)
  MAO inhibitor: tranylcypromine
Benzodiazepines (Joseph and Wroblewski 1993)
Carbamazepine (Schwarzc et al 1986)
Dopamine storage and transport inhibitors*
  α-methyltyrosine
  Reserpine
  Tetrabenazine
Droperidol (Foster et al 1996)
Levodopa* (Riley and Lang 1994)
Lithium (Channabasavanna & Goswami 1987; Price
  & Zimmer 1987; Patterson 1988)
Metachlopramide* (Miller and Jankovic 1989; Robin-
  son et al 1994; Weimer 1995; Hamilton 1987)
Sumatriptan (Lopez-Alemany et al 1997)

* Well documented.

free and receiving antidepressant agents: imipramine, desipramine, trazodone and tranylcypromine. Akathisia has also been described with
the use fluoxetine (Coulter and Pillans 1995),
nortriptyline (Sabaawi et al 1993), and sertraline
(Shihabuddin et al 1994).

Drug-induced akathisia was considered to be
a factor in intense suicidal ideation during fluoxetine treatment. In the most convincing study
implicating drug-induced akathisia in fluoxetine-associated suicidality, three depressed patients were re-exposed to fluoxetine after having
made suicidal attempts and monitored closely
(Rothschild and Locke 1991). All the three developed akathisia and stated that akathisia had
precipitated the suicide attempt.

Epidemiology. The prevalence rate varies widely. Some of the published figures are:
– 21% in patients treated with high as well as
  low potency antipsychotics for 3–6 m (Ayd
  1961).

– 75% of patients treated with haloperidol within one week (Van Putten et al 1984).
– 18% of patients treated with fluphenazine
  (Chakos et al 1992)
– 24% of 120 schizophrenic patients receiving
  antipsychotics. Another 18% had pseudoakathisia (Halstead et al 1994).
– 9.8 to 25% of patients receiving antidepressant fluoxetine (Lipinski et al 1989).

Clinical Features. Motor disturbances associated with akathisia are repeated leg crossings,
swinging of one leg, lateral knee movements,
sliding of feet and rapid walking (Gibb and Lees
1986). It is also described a "jitteriness syndrome." Pre-requisites for the diagnosis of drug-
induced akathisia (DIA) are:
– Drug exposure
– Presence of characteristic clinical features
– Exclusion of non-drug causes.

Classification. Akathisia has been divided into
the following categories (Sachdev 1994):
– *Acute.* Starts within hours or days but not
  more than 6 weeks after initiation or increase
  in dose of the drug.
– *Tardive.* Onset after 3 months of continuous
  use of the drug.
– *Withdrawal.* Onset within 6 weeks after discontinuation of the drug.
– *Chronic.* DIA which persists beyond 3 months
  after discontinuation of the drug. It overlaps
  categories 1–3.

Further subcategories of chronic akathisia have
been proposed by Lang (1994) which include va-
rieties such as *pseudoakathisia*. Patients with
pseudoakathisia have objective motor movements of akathisia without subjective complaints
of restlessness. Patients with akathisia are at
greater risk for developing tardive dyskinesia.
All these forms of akathisia may be a point in
continuum. The term "cognitive akathisia" is
used for describing the inner feeling of restlessness without motor disturbances (Melvin and
Arana 1992).

Pathogenesis. This has not been established but
some of the hypotheses are:
– Association of akathisia with dopamine antagonists (antipsychotics) suggests that dopamin-

ergic systems are involved. According to a hypothesis based on animal experimental studies, postsynaptic dopamine receptor blockade in the mesocortical dopamine system may be responsible (Marsden and Jenner (1980).

- Therapeutic benefit of β-adrenergic antagonists (Adler et al 1991) points to a mechanism that involves an altered balance of central dopaminergic and noradrenergic transmission. The possible mechanism entails an overactive noradrenergic system in relation to increased dopamine transmission in the ventral tegmental area.

- The antidopaminergic hypothesis of akathisia implicates either receptor blockade by antipsychotics or antidepressant-induced serotonergic and/or noradrenergic inhibition of dopamine neurotransmission. The precise mechanism and significance of inverse balance between dopaminergic and noradrenergic activity are yet to be defined (Sabaawi et al 1994).

- Role of serotonin. Serotonin reuptake inhibitors potentiate an inhibitory effect of serotonin on the metabolic production or release of dopamine by neurons of the basal ganglia (Bouchard et al 1989). Fluoxetine inhibits levodopa storage in the striatum. Serotonin reuptake inhibitors may induce extrapyramidal side effects.

- Withdrawal akathisia. Akathisia has been reported in a manic depressive patient following withdrawal of pimozide which had controlled the psychiatric symptoms (Lang 1994). Akathisia resolved after pimozide was reinstated and recurred after a second withdrawal.

Measurement. Several attempts have been made to quantify the motor restlessness of akathisia by using electronic movement meters but the specificity and sensitivity of these methods remains undetermined. The best instrument for assessment is Barnes' four-item akathisia scale (Barnes 1989; Adler et al 1992). This scale provides rating points for the subjective awareness of restlessness, observable restlessness, and a global severity item. Akathisia is rated in both sitting and standing positions. This scale has been found to have a high inter-rater reliability.

Treatment. Various strategies for the treatment of drug-induced akathisia are:
- *Lowering the dose of antipsychotics*. This has been found to be the only consistently effective treatment (Braude et al 1983). If this is not possible, switching to a lower potency antipsychotic or use of one of the following drugs is recommended:
- *Anti-parkinsonian drugs*. These are useful if other extrapyramidal symptoms are present: anticholinergics and amantadine. Trihexiphenidyl (anticholinergic) and propranolol combination has been found to be useful for the treatment of fluvoxamine-induced akathisia (Chong and Tan 1996).
- *Benzodiazepines*. The following drugs of this category have been used for akathisia: diazepam, lorazepam, and clonazepam (Kutcher et al 1989). In a recent study in France, antipsychotic-induced akathisia was reduced significantly more with clonazepam than with placebo (Pujalte et al 1994). The optimal daily dose was found to be 10–40 mg/kg/day.
- *β-blockers*. Propranolol, a lipophilic non selective β-blocker has been used most frequently for the treatment of akathisia. Selective β-antagonist betaxolol appears to be the most promising. Propranolol has been reported to resolve akathisia induced by triptyline in the treatment of depression in two patients (Sabaawi et al 1993).
- *Clonidine*. This is a central α_2 agonist that has been reported to be effective for treating akathisia but its use is limited by development of hypotension and sedation (Adler et al 1987).
- *Bupropion*. Antipsychotic-induced akathisia responds dramatically to bupropion (Tanquary et al 1993).
- *Nicotine*. In a prospective study, nicotine patch was shown to significantly reduce antipsychotic-induced akathisia in non-smoker patients (Anfung and Pope 1997).

Akinetic Mutism

Although this condition is characterized by lack of movement, it is usually not discussed under movement disorders in textbooks of neurology.

The patient is usually alert but apathetic. In some cases associated with leukoencephalopathy, cognitive function may be impaired. This condition is usually seen in bilateral medial frontal lobe lesions and communicating hydrocephalus. It should be distinguished from locked-in syndrome where the patient is quadriplegic but awake. Locked-in syndrome is due to bilateral destruction of the medulla or the anterior pons with sparing of the tegmentum and thus preservation of consciousness. Akinetic mutism has been reported as an adverse reaction to various drugs listed in Table 8.5.

Table 8.5. Drugs associated with akinetic mutism.

5-fluorouracil
Baclofen
Cyclosporine A
Diphenylhydantoin (phenytoin) toxicity
Methylphenidate test dose
Antipsychotics

Aoki (1986) reported two cancer patients are who presented with altered consciousness 2 and 3 months, respectively, after the administration of 5-fluorouracil derivatives, and progressed to a state of akinetic mutism. CT scanning revealed diffuse decreased attenuation of the cerebral white matter, indicative of leukoencephalopathy, without association of mass lesion. Upon discontinuing the drugs, both patients made significant recovery and the decreased attenuation on the CT also disappeared.

Akinetic mutism have been reported in patients with renal insufficiency who are on baclofen therapy (Parmar 1991). Rubin and So (1999) reported a patient with normal renal function who developed akinetic mutism after 3 days of receiving low-dosage baclofen. Electroencephalography showed a diffusely slow background with intermittent generalized sharp wave discharges. The condition resolved after discontinuing baclofen. The pathomechanism of this condition is unknown, but it may result from selective binding of the drug to the $GABA_B$ receptors located in the frontal lobes or thalamic nuclei, interrupting the thalamocortical limbic pathways.

Three patients were reported to have developed akinetic mutism on the third day after the introduction of intravenous cyclosporin A, given for immunosuppression after liver transplantation (Bird et al 1990). One patient recovered completely after withdrawal of cyclosporin. The other two patients showed abnormalities in the pons on MRI scanning, suggesting central pontine myelinolysis. None of the patients had experienced significant fluctuations in serum sodium or other risk factors for central pontine myelinolysis. In these patients the time course of the akinetic mutism and extrapyramidal syndrome, which developed in the absence of any other identifiable cause, suggests cyclosporin A was the precipitating factor.

Akinetic mutism has been reported as a complication of diphenylhydantoin (DPH) toxicity with DPH level greater than 40 µg/mL (Tutuncuoglu et al 1997). MRI showed mild cerebellar atrophy and the patient regained motor and mental activity within two months after carbamazepine was substituted for DPH.

A case of akinetic mutism was described in a menopausal, depressed woman with onset following a mood challenge with 40 mg of methylphenidate taken orally over a 3-hour period (Wiener and Kennedy 1985). This was considered to be a conversion disorder precipitated by drug-induced dysphoria. It is suggested that increased susceptibility to dysphoria may have been related to prior clomipramine administration and hypoestrogenism.

Asterixis

This consists of arrhythmic lapses of sustained posture, in which the sudden interruptions in muscular contraction allow gravity or the inherent elasticity of muscles to produce a movement, which the patient then corrects, sometimes with overshoot. Asterixis differs physiologically from both tremor and myoclonus and is incorrectly described as "flapping tremor." It is elicited by asking the patient to hold the arms outstretched with hands dorsiflexed, or to dorsiflex the hands and extend the fingers while resting the forearms on the arms of a chair; flexion movements of the hands may occur several times a minute. As-

Table 8.6. Drugs associated with asterixis.

Antiepileptic drugs:
- Carbamazepine (Rivelli et al 1988; Rittmannsberger et al 1991)
- Phenobarbitone
- Primidone (Chadwick et al 1976)
- Valproic acid

Ceftazidime (Hillsley and Massey 1991)
Levodopa (Glantz et al 1982)
Methyldopa (Yamadori and Albert 1972)
Metrizamide used for myelography (Vincent 1980)
Antipsychotic drugs

terixis was first observed in patients with hepatic encephalopathy. It is also observed in hepatic encephalopathy induced by drugs (see Chapter 3). Drugs reported to be associated with asterixis are shown in Table 8.6.

Rittmannsberger (1996) has observed 10 cases of asterixis in psychiatric inpatients, most with affective spectrum disorders being treated with combination therapy. The drugs most often used were clozapine (eight cases), lithium (seven cases), and carbamazepine (seven cases). There were neither metabolic disorders nor structural brain lesions that might explain the occurrence of asterixis. Because dosage in general was moderate and serum levels were within therapeutic boundaries in most cases, the symptom seemed to have been caused by an interaction of drugs rather than by a single agent. Therefore, it is recommended that clozapine, carbamazepine, and lithium should be combined with each other only with great care.

Athetosis

This is characterized by inability to sustain the fingers and toes, or any other part of the body in one position. The maintained posture is interrupted by a relatively slow, sinuous, purposeless movements which have a tendency to flow into one another. The basic pattern of the movements is alteration between extension-pronation, and flexion-supination of the arm, and between flexion and extension of the fingers, the flexed and adducted thumb being trapped by the flexed fingers as the hand closes. the movements appear to be slower than those of chorea, but all grada-

tions between the two are seen, and in some cases, it is impossible to distinguish between them, hence the term choreoathetosis. Athetosis may involve all the limbs or may be restricted to certain groups of muscles.

Drug-induced athetosis may occur with antipsychotic medications such as phenothiazines and haloperidol. Among the non-antipsychotic drugs, choreoathetosis has also been reported with phenytoin and carbamazepine.

Ballism

This is wide amplitude flinging movements usually involving the proximal muscles and one side of the body (hemiballismus). Bilateral movements are called biballismus or paraballismus. This movement disorder is closely related to chorea. Besides the antipsychotic drugs such as phenothiazines and haloperidol, ballismus has been reported as an adverse effect of levodopa, phenytoin (Lazaro 1982), and carbamazepine.

Chorea

Chorea refers to involuntary arrhythmic movements of a forcible, rapid, jerky type. These movements may be simple or quite elaborate and of variable distribution. Although the movements are purposeless, the patient may incorporate them into a deliberate movement, as if to make them less noticeable. When superimposed on voluntary movements, they may assume an exaggerated and grotesque character. Usually the movements are discrete, but if they are very numerous, they become confluent and resemble athetosis or the patient may develop a mixed form called choreoathetosis. The chronic form of it due to antipsychotics is referred to as tardive dyskinesia. In addition to antipsychotics, other drugs which may produce chorea are listed in Table 8.7. A few are discussed in detail in the following text.

Phenytoin-Induced Chorea. Since the first report in 1962, 73 patients were documented to have developed this complication in a review in 1993 (Harrison et al 1993). Several more cases

Table 8.7. Non-antipsychotic drugs that may produce chorea.

Aminophylline (Ferreyros and Alfonso 1992)
Amoxapine
Anabolic steroids: oxymetholone (Tilzey et al 1981)
Anticholinergics: benzhexol (Warne and Gubbay 1979)
Anticonvulsants (Chadwick et al 1976; Lazaro 1982)
   – Carbamazepine (Bimpong-Buta and Froescher 1982)
   – Ethosuximide (Kirschberg 1975)
   – Gabapentin in neurologically impaired patients
     (Chudnow et al 1997)
   – Phenobarbital (Lightman 1978)
   – Phenytoin (see text)
   – Valproic acid (Lancman et al 1994a)
Antihistaminics: H_1 and H_2
Baclofen therapy in Alzheimer's disease (Crystal 1990)
Benzodiazepines
Cimetidine (Kushner 1982)
CNS stimulants*
   – Amphetamines (Lundh and Turving 1981)
   – Cocaine (Daras et al 1994)
   – Methylphenidate
   – Pemoline
Cyclosporine (Cambarros et al 1993)
Dopamine agonists*: levodopa (see section on
levodopa-induced dyskinesias)
Interferon-α-2a (Neu et al 1996)
Lithium (Peters 1949; Podskalny and Factor 1996)
Methadone (Wasserman and Yahr 1980)
Oral contraceptives (Bickerstaff 1975; Riddoch et al
   1971)
Propofol (Diltoer et al 1996)
Selective serotonin reuptake inhibitors
   – Fluoxetine in a patient with CYP2D6 deficiency
     (Marchioni et al 1996)
   – Paroxetine (Fox et al 1997)
Sulfasalazine (Quinn et al 1991)
Theophylline (Stuart et al 1992; Pranzatelli et al 1991)
Tricyclic antidepressants

* Well documented.

have been reported since then (Shulman et al 1996; Koukkari et al 1996). Patients with brain damage are more likely to show this adverse reaction. Considering the extensive use of this drug, chorea is considered to be rare complication.

Pathomechanism. Although the exact mechanism is not known, the following explanations are offered:
– Direct toxic effect of phenytoin on the dopaminergic system to produce a dyskinesia-like event
– A disturbance in the functional equilibrium of the basal ganglia output system

– A differential effect on the dopamine receptor subtypes or their second messenger systems
– An idiosyncratic reaction

Dystonia

Dystonia or torsion spasm is a persistent attitude or posture in one or the other of the extremes of athetoid movements. It may take the form of an overextension or overflexion of the hand, inversion of the foot, rotation and lateral flexion of the head, torsion of the spine, with arching and twisting of the back, or forceful closure of the eyes and a fixed grimace. Defined this way it is closely allied to athetosis, differing only in the duration and persistence of the postural abnormality and the disproportionate involvement of the larger axial muscles. The pathophysiology of dystonia is poorly understood. Some primary dystonias are caused by specific genetic mutations. However, the focus of this section is drug-induced dystonias which may be acute or tardive.

Acute Dystonia. The reported prevalence of acute dystonic reactions in patients treated with antipsychotics varies from 2.5 to 50%. Higher prevalence rates are found in studies where patients are treated with high doses of potent antipsychotics and in patients under the age of 35 years. Acute dystonic reactions are the earliest extrapyramidal reactions to appear after initiating antipsychotic treatment. Approximately 90% of these occur within 3 days of starting therapy. Acute dystonic reactions last from seconds to a few hours and occur more frequently in the afternoon and the evening. These are usually localized to the face, neck and upper part of the body whereas the involvement of the lower part of the body is rare. The symptoms remit on discontinuing the antipsychotics or starting anticholinergic treatment.

There is a correlation between the potency of the drug used to control schizophrenia and its propensity to induce dystonia. Piperazine compounds have the highest potential to induce dystonia and patients without concomitant anticholinergic therapy have a higher frequency of dystonia than those on anticholinergic therapy (Spina et al 1993).

Table 8.8. Dystonia as a result of drug interactions.

Drugs	Comments
Sertraline and trazodone	Both drugs augment serotonergic neurotransmission and impair nigrostriatal dopamine activity (Lewis et al 1997)
Sertraline and metoclopramide	Combination of serotonergic effect of sertraline (SSRI) with dopamine-blocking properties of metoclopramide (Christensen and Byerly 1996)
Fluvoxamine and spiramycin	Dystonia resolved on discontinuation of spiramycin but the facilitating role of fluvoxamine (SSRI) could not be excluded (Benazzi 1997)
Fluoxetine and chlorpromazine overdose	Laryngeal dystonia due to overdose of an antipsychotic was facilitated by SSRI fluoxetine (Murray 1995)
Haloperidol and metachlorophenylpiperazine (mCPP)	mCPP is a non-selective 5-HT-receptor agonist/antagonist that is used in psychiatry to assess central serotonergic function (Adityanjee and Lindenmeyer 1993)
Risperidone and phenytoin	Dystonia occurred after addition of phenytoin to risperidone and resolved when phenytoin was discontinued (Sanderson 1996)

Clozapine, an atypical antipsychotic, is less likely to produce movement disorders. Adverse reaction profile of this clozapine has been reviewed by Dev and Krupp (1995).

Tardive Dystonia. The term "tardive dystonia" is used if dystonia persists after discontinuation of antipsychotics and usually do not respond to anticholinergic treatment. It is often considered a subtype of dystonia but justifies recognition as a separate syndrome. It should be differentiated from tardive dyskinesia (see the following section on dyskinesia) but both forms can coexist in some patients. Criteria for the diagnosis of tardive dystonia are:
- Presence of dystonic movements or postures
- Development of symptoms during treatment with dopamine receptor blocking agents for within two months of their discontinuation
- Exclusion of other causes of secondary dystonia
- No family history of dystonia.

Drugs Producing Dystonia. Antipsychotics are well recognized as a cause of dystonia and various antipsychotics will not be listed here. Dystonia may result from drug interactions of antipsychotic and well as non antipsychotic medications (Table 8.8) and non-antipsychotic drugs can also induce dystonia (Table 8.9). Serotonergic drugs are involved in several of the drug interactions producing dystonia.

Pathomechanism. The pathomechanism of antipsychotic-induced dystonia is not known. It has been hypothesized to be due to either a hypo- or hyperdopaminergic state associated with dopamine receptor blockade in the caudate, putamen or the globus pallidus. Acute dystonic reactions after administration of a single dose of an antipsychotic medication tend to occur when plasma antipsychotic level is decreasing, indicating the transient effect of increased dopamine output. Such reactions are less frequent in the elderly because striatal dopamine receptors decrease with age and older patients may have a striatal hypodopaminergic status protecting them from acute dystonic reactions.

Some clues have emerged from the animal studies reviewed by Rupniak and Marsden (1986). All studies agreed that antipsychotics induce increase of striatal acetylcholine and that cholinergic agents induce dystonia in antipsychotic-primed monkeys which were reversed by anticholinergic agents. Dopaminergic agents like levodopa can induce dystonia by systemic administration as well as by direct intrastriatal application of dopamine in monkeys. An imbalance in a critical relationship between dopamine receptor antagonists and possibly other neurotransmitters may be important in accounting for the mechanisms underlying dystonia. Dystonia with relapse of schizophrenia has been reported in a patient after withdrawal of clozapine therapy

Table 8.9. Non-antipsychotic drugs reported to induce dystonia.

Anesthetics
  – ketamine
  – fentanyl
Anticholinergic agents: benzotropine
Antiepileptic drugs
  – Phenytoin (Chadwick et al 1976; Moss et al 1994)
  – Carbamazepine (Crosley and Swender 1979; Bradbury et al 1982; Soman et al 1994)
Antihistaminics: diphenhydramine (Joseph and King 1995)
Antimalarials: chloroquine (Singhi et al 1977)
Benzodiazepines
  – Diazepam
  – Midazolam (Stolarek and Ford 1990)
Calcium antagonists
  – Cinnarizine
  – Flunarizine
  – Nifedipine
Cholinomimetic agents: bethanecol
Dextromethorphan (Graudins and Fern 1996)
Disulfiram (de Mari et al 1993)
Dopamine agonists*: levodopa (see section on levodopa-induced dyskinesias)
Metoclopramide withdrawal *(Lauterbach 1992)
Monoamine oxidase inhibitors (Pande and Max 1989; Jarecke and Reid 1990)
Ondansetron (Halpern and Murphy 1991; Garcia-del-Muro et al 1993)
Ranitidine overdose (Maack and Spiller 1993)
Selective serotonin reuptake inhibitors (Gerber and Lynd 1998)
  – Fluvoxamine (Chong 1995; Bronner and Vanneste 1998)
  – Fluoxetine (Dave 1994; Coulter & Pillans 1994; Black and Uhde 1992; Recoppa et al 1990)
Sumatriptan (Garcia 1994; Jones-Fearing 1996; Oterino and Pasqual 1998)
Tricyclic antidepressants: amitriptyline

*Well documented.

(Dickson et al 1994). Dystonia appearing in patients being switched from clozapine to risperidone is attributed to a "cholinergic rebound phenomenon" (Radford et al 1995).

The role of GABA and serotonin in acute dystonia is much less studied. GABA antagonists such as picrotoxin aggravate dystonia. There is some evidence of the role of haloperidol-sensitive sigma receptors in the induction of acute dystonias (Walker et al 1988).

Treatment. The treatment of acute dystonia differs from that of tardive dystonia and the two will be described separately.

– *Acute dystonia.* Reduction of antipsychotic dosage or total withdrawal leads to disappearance of dystonia within 24–48 hours. If this is not possible any of the following drugs may be used:

• Anticholinergics. This is the most practical approach for concomitant medication. Intravenous agents such as benzotropine can lead to disappearance of dystonia within minutes but such treatments should not be carried out regularly because they increase the risk of developing tardive dyskinesia.

• Dopamine agonists. The reaction can also be reversed by low doses of dopamine agonists such as apomorphine. Its effect is possibly related to the presynaptic action which would be expected to reduce the compensatory decrease in dopamine turnover following antipsychotic-induced postsynaptic dopamine receptor blockade. Terguride, a partial dopamine agonist has been shown to mitigate the undesirable extrapyramidal effects of antipsychotics while potentiating the antipsychotic effect (Filip et al 1992).

• Mianserin. This is a serotonin antagonist that may have a beneficial effect on SSRI-induced dystonia (Poyurovsky et al 1997).

• Benzodiazepines. Diazepam have been reported to relieve muscle spasm but midazolam can induce dystonia.

• Diphenylhadramine. This drug has been used to treat phenytoin-induced dystonia (Moss et al 1994).

– *Tardive dystonia.* The treatment is individualized and an algorithm for the management of tardive dystonia is shown in Figure 8.1. If ongoing antipsychotic therapy is required, atypical antipsychotics are used in stead of classical antipsychotics as they are less likely to induce dystonic reactions. Other methods that are used include the following:

• Combination of clozapine and clonazepam. This has been recommended for the tardive dystonia as both movement disorder and the psychiatric symptoms are managed (Blake et al 1991).

• Tetrabenazine. In contrast to typical antipsychotics, tetrabenazine is a monoamine depleting and dopamine receptor blocking

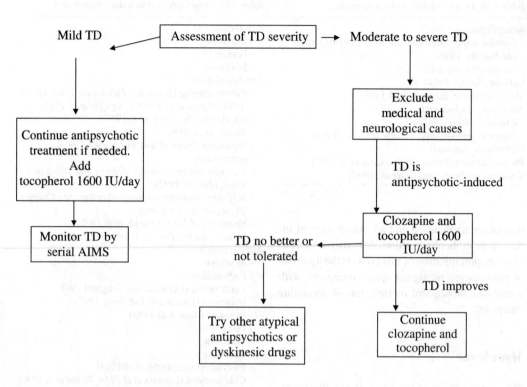

Figure 8.1. Algorithm for the management of tardive dystonia (TD). AIMS = abnormal involuntary movement scale, IU = international unit (modified from Gardos 1999).

drug which has not been associated with tardive dystonia.

- Tocopherol (vitamin E). Tardive dystonia secondary to antipsychotic therapy has been treated with high dose vitamin E (titrated to 1200 mg daily) resulting in significant improvement (Dannon et al 1997). The rationale is antioxidant effect of vitamin E based on the hypothesis that tardive dystonia is mediated by free radical damage of neurons.
- Botulinum toxin injections are shown to be effective for the treatment of focal dystonias
- Baclofen has been used for the treatment of idiopathic dystonias and its use has been extended to tardive dystonia.
- Surgery. Local denervation, myectomy, thalamotomy, pallidotomy and deep brain stimulation are considered only for patients with disabling dystonia where medical therapies have failed.

Oculogyric Crisis (OCG)

This is a variant of acute dystonia and is involuntary ocular deviation following administration of dopamine receptor blocking agents. It was originally described in association with epidemic encephalitis lethargica but it has been reported to occur as an adverse effect of the drugs listed in Table 8.10.

OGC has been reported in 4% schizrenic patients treated with antipsychotics (Sachdev 1993). Clonazepam has been reported to be useful in the management of antipsychotic-induced oculo-gyric crises (Horiguchi and Inami 1989). A case of OGC has been reported in an epileptic patient on gabapentin therapy (Reeves et al 1996). Discontinuation of the drug and a single dose of lorazepam led to rapid resolution of the pentazocine for pain relief (Burstein and Fullerton 1993). The crisis resolved after discontinua-

Table 8.10. Drugs causing oculogyric crisis.

Antiepileptics
  Carbamazepine (Berchou and Rodin 1979: Gorman
  and Barkley 1995)
  Gabapentin (see text)
Lithium (Sandyk 1984)
Metaclopramide (Edwards et al 1989)
Antipsychotics (see text)
  Classical antipsychotics
  Atypical antipsychotic: clozapine (Dave 1994)
Pentozocine (see text)
Phenothiazines (Harries 1967; Skorin et al 1987)
Tensilon test (Nucci and Brancato 1990)

tion of the medication and administration of intravenous diphenhydramine. A plausible mechanism for precipitation of this crisis is the agonism
of pentazocine on sigma opiate receptors, with
postulated subsequent modulation of dopamine
receptors.

Myoclonus

This is defined as sudden, brief, shock-like involuntary movement that may be caused by both active muscle contraction (positive myoclonus) or
inhibition of ongoing muscle activity (negative
myoclonus). Such contractions occur once or re-
peatedly for a few times and are localized to a
group of muscles such as those of the arm or the
leg or may be generalized. It is usually arrhythmic and irregular. Myoclonus can be physiologic
such as "sleep jerks," epileptic, drug-induced, or
idiopathic. Drugs which have been reported to induce myoclonus are shown in Table 8.11.

Treatment. Treatment of myoclonus usually involves withdrawal of the suspected drug causing
it. Valproic acid has been used for treatment of
clozapine-induced myoclonus (Meltzer and
Ranjan 1994). Dantrolene has been used successfully for treating myoclonus associated with
morphine.

Restless Legs Syndrome (RLS)

In this disorder the movement occurs secondary
to a subjective need to move. The patient may

Table 8.11. Drugs reported to induce myoclonus.

Anesthetics
  – Enflurane
  – Fentanyl
  – Isoflurane
Anticonvulsants
  – Carbamazepine (Joyce and Gunderson 1980; Jacome
    1979; Martinon et al 1980; Aguglia et al 1987)
  – Phenytoin (Chadwick et al 1976;
    Duarte et al 1996)
  – Vigabatrin (Neufeld and Vishnevska 1995)
Antidepressants
  – Tricyclic antidepressants* (Garvey and Tollefson
    1987; Masand 1992)
  – Selective serotonin reuptake inhibitors (see Chapter
    21, serotonin syndrome)
  – Fluoxetine (Ghika-Schmidt et al 1997)
  – Monoamine oxidase inhibitors (White 1987)
Antimicrobials
  – Acyclovir
  – Carbencillin
  – Cefmetazole (Uchihara and Tsugoshi 1988)
  – Imipenem (Frucht and Eidelberg 1997)
  – Isoniazid (Yagi et al 1989)
  – Pefloxacin
  – Penicillin
Antineoplastics
  – Prednimustine (Martin et al 1993)
  – Chlorambucil (LaDelfa et al 1985; Wyllie et al 1996)
Antipsychotics*
  – Typical (Fukuzako et al 1990; Brogmus and Lesch
    1995)
  – Atypical: clozapine (Berman et al 1992; Meltzer and
    Ranjan 1994; Barak et al 1996)
Benzodiazepines
  – Midazolam (Magny et al 1994)
  – Lorazepam (Lee et al 1994)
  – Diazepam withdrawal
Bismuth salts* (Buge and Rancurel 1977)
Bromocriptine (Buchman et al 1987)
Cardiovascular drugs
  – Diltiazem (Jeret et al 1992)
  – Flecainide (Ghika et al 1994)
  – Nifedipine (Pedro-Botet et al 1989)
  – Propafenone (Chua et al 1994; Devoize et al 1986)
Dopamine agonists
  – Amantadine (Pfeiffer 1996)
  – Levodopa* (Klawans et al 1975)
Lithium (Rosen and Stevens 1983)
Metoclopramide (Lu and Chu 1988)
Opioids: intrathecal, intravenous and epidural–
  – Morphine (Galvina and Robertshaw 1988)
  – Diamorphine (Turner 1992; Jayawardena and Hill
    1991)
Miscellaneous drugs
  – Norpethidine (Reutens et al 1989)
  – Physostigmine (Mayeux et al 1987)
  – Propofol (Hughes and Lyon 1995)

*Well documented.

complain of uncomfortable creeping sensation in muscles, usually in the legs and thighs. The trouble is more pronounced when an affected person lies in a resting position for prolonged periods or tries to sleep. This may lead to insomnia or nocturnal myoclonus. RLS has been known for centuries but diagnostic criteria has emerged only in recent years. Four clinical characteristics are minimal for the diagnosis of RLS.

1. Desire to move the limbs usually associated with paresthesias
2. Motor restlessness
3. Symptoms are worse or exclusively present at rest
4. Symptoms must be worse in the evening or at night

Family history is positive in most of the cases of RLS and a genetic linkage is suggested (Montplaisir et al 1997). RLS can also be a symptom of such systemic disorders as cancer, diabetes mellitus, uremia, primary amyloidosis, and vitamin deficiencies. Neurological examination is usually normal. EMG, nerve conduction studies, and sural nerve biopsies in these patients have shown a peripheral axonal neuropathy (Iannaccone et al 1995). These patients had no systemic diseases and no family history of peripheral neuropathy. The authors stated that all of the eight patients had used benzodiazepines and one of these had used carbamazepine as well but did not point out the recognized role of these drugs in causing peripheral neuropathy.

Antipsychotic-induced akathisia might change its feature as RLS during night sleep as shown by polysomnographic studies (Nishimatsu et al 1997). RLS has been reported with the drugs shown in Table 8.12.

Table 8.12. Drugs associated with restless legs syndrome.

Benzodiazepines
Carbamazepine (Milne 1992; Schwarcz et al 1986).
Cimetidine (O'Sullivan and Greenberg 1993)
Droperidol to counteract vomiting with epidural morphine (Athanassiadis and Karamis 1992).
Levodopa
Mianserin (Markkula and Lauerma 1997)
Antipsychotics
Psychotropic drugs (Terao et al 1992)

Tics

Tics are abrupt, transient, stereotyped, coordinated movements that vary in intensity and are repeated at irregular intervals. The movements are often brief and jerky (clonic tics) but slower and more prolonged movements (dystonic tics) may also occur. These can be voluntarily suppressed for short periods. Tics may be motor or phonic (making sounds) and each may be simple or complex. Gilles de la Tourette syndrome is a neuropsychiatric disorder consisting of multiple vocal and motor tics often accompanied by echolalia, echopraxia, coprolalia, mutilations, and obsessive compulsive symptoms. The cause is not known. Long-term antipsychotic therapy may be associated with "tardive Tourette syndrome" and will be described with tardive dyskinesia. Although they can occur with antipsychotic therapy, drug-induced tics are usually associated with non-antipsychotic drugs, mostly CNS stimulants (Lowe et al 1982). Various drugs are listed in Table 8.13.

Motor tics are associated with methylphenidate (Golden 1977) and have been observed in 1.3% of children receiving this drug (Deckla et al 1976). Tics usually disappear when the therapy is discontinued. Other CNS stimulants such

Table 8.13. Drugs that can induce tics.

Antidepressants
Antipsychotics
  – Clozapine (Lindenmeyer et al 1995)
Anticonvulsants
  – Carbamazepine (Robertson et al 1993)
  – Clonazepam (Gilman and Sandyk 1987)
  – Phenobarbital (Sandyk 1986b)
CNS stimulating agents
  – Cocaine (Attig et al 1994)
  – Dextroamphetamine
  – Methylphenidate
  – Pemoline
Corticosteroids (Dietl et al 1998)
Dopamine receptor blocking agents other than antipsychotics
Levodopa (Shale et al 1986)
Opioids (Bruun and Kurlan 1991)
  – Opioid antagonist (naloxone) withdrawal (Sandyk 1986a)
Selective serotonin reuptake inhibitors
  – Fluoxetine (Eisenhauer and Germain 1993)
  – Sertraline (Hauser and Zesiewicz 1995)

as dextroamphetamine and pemoline can induce tics (Mitchell and Matthews 1980). The adverse effect of CNS stimulants on Tourette's syndrome supports the hypothesis that this condition results from relative excess of catecholaminergic activity in the CNS (Pollack et al 1977). Tics following antipsychotic therapy have been reviewed by Bharucha and Sethi (1995). From the few reports available, one cannot be certain of the causal relationship.

The pathomechanism of tics is not known. Exacerbation of Tourette's syndrome following antidepressant therapy points to the involvement of dopaminergic system as well (Müller 1992). Tics are usually managed by administration of haloperidol.

Tremor

Tremor may be defined as rhythmical involuntary oscillations of a part of body around a fixed point, usually in one plane. The rhythmic quality distinguishes tremor from other involuntary movements; its biphasic character distinguishes it from clonus. Clinically tremor may be of three types (Lane 1984):

1. *Resting (static) tremor* occurs in a part that is supported and relaxed. It is typically found in Parkinson's disease and is rare as an adverse effect of drugs which are antipsychotics and amiodarone (Lustman and Moncu 1974).
2. *Action tremor* is one that develops only during movement. The intention tremor of cerebellar disease is an action tremor that shows progressive exaggeration in goal-directed movements, as in finger-nose test. This type of tremor indicates cerebellar dysfunction and is rare with drugs except anticonvulsants and lithium (see Chapter 15).
3. *Postural tremor* is the type of tremor which appears when the position of the body is actively maintained against the force of gravity —physiological tremor and benign familial (essential) tremor being the commonest examples.

Physiological tremor is present in all muscle groups and can rarely be seen by the naked eye. It is present throughout the waking state and in some phases of sleep as well. It ranges in frequency between 8–13 Hz. The amplitude of this type of tremor can be increased directly, or indirectly, by drugs.

Benign Familial Essential Tremor. This is an idiopathic, dominantly inherited, postural tremor of variable amplitude with frequency range similar to that of physiological tremor. Cardioselective β-blockers, such as metoprolol and atenolol, may relieve essential tremor whereas non-selective β-blocker pindolol exacerbates it (Hod et al 1980).

Drug-Induced Tremor. Characteristically the drug-induced tremors are postural although they can produce a typical resting parkinsonian tremor. Antipsychotic drugs produce a low frequency postural tremor whereas anticonvulsant drugs produce a high frequency, low-amplitude tremor. Other drugs may enhance physiological tremor when it is referred to as drug-induced tremor. Drug-induced tremor may be a part of other syndromes such as serotonin syndrome and drug-induced parkinsonism. Various drugs which induce or enhance tremor are listed Table 8.14.

Tardive tremor. This term is used for antipsychotic-induced tremor which persists after discontinuation of the offending drug and is usually accompanies by tardive dyskinesia and tardive dystonia. Tardive tremor is predominantly postural with a frequency range of 3 to 5 Hz (Stacy and Jancovic 1992).

Pathomechanism. Pathomechanism of tremor is not well understood. Several other drugs exacerbate physiological and essential tremors by different mechanisms. While the parkinsonism and tardive dyskinesia of antipsychotics is related to dopamine receptor blocking properties, the tremor-inducing effect may result from other properties. Physiological tremor may be exacerbated through the increase in catecholamines. Cimetidine is postulated to increase tremor by blockade of central H_2 receptors. The mechanism underlying the genesis of slower and more complex and disabling drug-induced tremor is even less clear.

Treatment. Propranolol is frequently used for treatment of tremor but it is not always effective.

Table 8.14. Drugs that induce or enhance physiological tremor.

Anticonvulsants*
 – Lamotrigine (Reutens et al 1993)
 – Valproic acid (Karas et al 1982; Hyman et al 1979)
Antidepressants*
 – Monoamine oxidase inhibitors
 – Selective serotonin reuptake inhibitors (see Chapter 21, serotonin syndrome)
 – Tricyclic antidepressants
Antihyperglycemic drugs*
β-adrenergic agonists* (Larsen and Schmekel 1993)
Calcium channel blockers*
 – Cinnarizine
 – Flunarizine (Jimenez-Jimenez and Garcia-Ruiz 1993)
Cardiac antiarrhythmics
 – Amiodarone
 – Procainamide
Cimetidine (Bateman 1981)
CNS stimulants*
 – Amphetamines
 – Caffeine
 – Cocaine
 – Ephedrine
Corticosteroids*
Cotrimoxozole (Aboulafia 1996)
Cyclosporine
Dopamine receptor blocking agents
 – Antipsychotics*
 – Domperidone
 – Droperidol
 – Metoclopramide
Histamine H$_1$-antagonists (Soto et al 1993)
Levodopa* (see section on levodopa-related movement disorders)
Lithium * (Stacy and Jankovic 1992)
Methyldopa
Metoclopramide (Ahronheim 1982)
Nicotine
Pindolol
Reserpine
Theophylline*
Thyroxine*
Tumor necrosis factor (Ferbert et al 1993)
Vidarabine
Withdrawal*
 – Alcohol
 – Barbiturates
 – Benzodiazepines
 – Beta Blockers
 – Opiates

*Well documented.

Valproate-induced tremor has been managed successfully by adding acetazolamide to the therapy (Lancman et al 1984b).

Drug-Induced Parkinsonism (DIP)

Historically, it has been noted that reserpine, when used for treating psychiatric disorders, often induced a syndrome identical to idiopathic Parkinson's disease (IPD). This led to the discovery that catecholamine stores were depleted in parkinsonism and that dopamine was reduced. This was a key factor in the development of levodopa for use in treating IPD. Initially it was debated whether DIP was an untoward effect or whether DIP was required for antipsychotic effect of drugs. Now it is known that DIP is not necessary for the antipsychotic effect of drugs and that IPD and schizophrenia do not preclude each other (Friedman et al 1987).

Epidemiology. The epidemiology of drug-induced parkinsonism reflects the epidemiology of the disorder being treated, the doses required, and the sensitivity of the population. The vast majority of patients who develop drug-induced parkinsonism have psychiatric disorders, generally schizophrenia which affects about 1% of the population. Depending on the risk factors, the prevalence of DIP in psychiatric patients has ranged from 50% to 75% in older literature. The prevalence is expected to be lower with the use of newer atypical antipsychotics.

Several studies in Spain have reported that drug-induced parkinsonism accounts for 24% to 35% of all parkinsonian syndromes (Jiménéz-Jiménéz et al 1996). The prevalence of drug-induced parkinsonism is estimated to be 32.7 per 100,000 persons in Italy (Morgante et al 1992). In Germany, the prevalence of drug-induced parkinsonism is 410 per 100,000 individuals over the age of 65 years compared to 710 cases of Parkinson's disease in a similar population (Trenkwalder et al 1995).

Clinical Features. Clinically DIP is difficult to differentiate from IPD as it has the same features: rigidity, bradykinesia, and tremor at rest. DIP is usually bilateral but may be unilateral. Tremor is less frequent (35%) in DIP than in IPD (80%). The history of drug exposure is the most important factor in establishing the diagnosis of DIP. Other causes of parkinsonism such as degenerative diseases of the CNS, environmental toxins, and brain disorders such as tumors and hydrocephalus can also produce parkinsonism. DIP is a temporary phenomenon and ameliorates after discontinuation of the offending drug or treatment with antiparkinsonian drugs.

Pathomechanism. Various pathomechanisms of DIP are shown in Table 8.15.

Antipsychotic-Induced DIP

This has also been termed antipsychotic-induced pseudoparkinsonism (Osser 1992). It is the commonest adverse effect of antipsychotics, especially with the use of high potency oral preparations and depot injections. At any given time it is estimated that 20% of those given depot injection with be affected by parkinsonism and as many as 89% in a 6-month period (Bristow and Hirsch 1993). DIP and tardive dyskinesia can coexist and this topic has been reviewed by Gardos and Cole (1992). The available data provide no clear support either for the notion that DIP and tardive dyskinesia are opposites, or for the view of their coexistence. Parkinsonism develops later than akathisia and dystonia and in 90% of the cases develops within the first 72 hours (Ayd 1961). Epidemiologic data suggest that parkinsonism observed early in the course of treatment with antipsychotics can lead to subsequent development of tardive dyskinesia. Antiparkinsonian drugs, when used for treatment of DIP may aggravate orofacial type of tardive dyskinesia. The explanation of coexistence of DIP and tardive dyskinesia may be the biochemical altera-

tions occurring simultaneously in different regions of the brain. Risk factors related to the drug are use of high potency antipsychotics and increased drug dosage (Casey 1991). Risk factors related to the patients are as follows:

– *Age*. The elderly are at a greater risk for DIP due to antipsychotics. This may be due to diminished number of nigral dopaminergic neurons with aging. In a prospective study, 9% of all new cases referred to a geriatric clinic were of parkinsonism and half of these were drug-induced (Stephen and Williamson 1984).
– *Sex*. Females are twice as liable to suffer from DIP due to antipsychotics than men (Ayd 1961).
– *Cerebral atrophy*. This has been implicated as a predisposing factor for DIP due to antipsychotics (Hoffman et al 1987).
– *AIDS*. Patient with psychosis due to AIDS are 2.4 times more likely to develop parkinsonian adverse effects if treated with antipsychotics than psychotic patients without AIDS (Hriso et al 1991).
– *Genetic factors* may predispose to the development of DIP. Six patients with family history of IPD were reported to have developed DIP on antipsychotic regimes that did not produce any extrapyramidal reactions in other patients (Gartmann et al 1993).

Pathomechanism of Antipsychotic-Induced DIP. All antipsychotics except clozapine induce similar biochemical, physiological, and behavioral changes in animals and presumably in humans. The blocking of dopamine type 2 receptors (D_2) by antipsychotics over prolonged peri-

Table 8.15. Pathomechanisms of drug-induced parkinsonism.

Mechanism	Examples of drugs
Inhibition of mitochondrial complex	Calcium channel blockers Antipsychotics
Presynaptic dopamine depletion	Reserpine
Blocking of dopamine synthesis	Methyldopa
Blocking of dopamine receptors	Antipsychotics
Increase of serotonin has an inhibitory effect on the metabolic production or release of dopamine by neurons of the basal ganglia	Selective serotonin reuptake inhibitors
Cholinomimetic action with disturbance of motor circuitry	Tacrine
GABAergic over activity	Valproic acid

ods leads to two further effects: an increase in dopamine synthesis and an increase in the number of D_2 receptors (denervation supersensitivity). Over the course of several weeks following initial D_2 receptor blockade, typical antipsychotics gradually suppress the formation of striatal and ventral tegmental presynaptic dopamine neurons in rat the brain (Chiado and Bunney 1983). This "depolarization block" could be the neurophysiologic correlate of DIP and the antipsychotic effect of the antipsychotics, with both occurring simultaneously. In contrast to classical antipsychotics, clozapine, has a greater affinity for other dopamine receptor subtypes (D_1 and D_4 relative to its affinity for the D_2 receptor. In addition, clozapine exerts its effects on other neurotransmitter systems as well. The explanation, however, for marked antipsychotic activity with paucity of extrapyramidal effects is the preferential effect of clozapine on the mesolimbic and amygdaloid rather than the neostriatal dopaminergic system.

Antipsychotics also affect the non-dopamine systems. Most of them have a certain degree of anticholinergic activity. The antipsychotics may also act as H_1 receptor antagonists and may also antagonize serotonin binding in the brain which would further inhibit the generation of serotonin-sensitive cAMP.

Course and Prognosis. The clinical course of antipsychotic-induced parkinsonism may be characterized by rapid remission of symptoms with a few days to a few months. In some cases, the symptoms may persist while in others, they may deteriorate. Persistence of symptoms is associated with MRI abnormalities such as putaminal hyperintensities in younger patients and striatal hyperintensities in older patient (Bocola et al 1996).

Management. Management of antipsychotic-induced parkinsonism has been reviewed by Mamo et al (1999). Various methods that have been used include the following:
- Reduction of dose (Levinson 1991).
- Discontinuation of antipsychotics.
- Substitution of classical antipsychotics by atypical antipsychotics with low potential for inducing parkinsonism such as clozapine.

- Substitution by antipsychotic with increased cholinergic effects such as chlorpromazine.
- Addition of anticholinergic drugs such as benzatropine or trihexyphenidyl to the antipsychotic.
- Dopaminergic agents. The only such agent that has been found to be useful is amantadine. Levodopa is usually not recommended as it may increase psychotic symptoms. Selegeline has also been found to be useful for treatment of parkinsonism due to antipsychotics.
- Electroconvulsive has been used successfully in a case of antipsychotic-induced parkinsonism which persisted after discontinuation of antipsychotics (Hermesh et al 1992).
- No experience with surgical procedures has been reported in such cases.

Non-Antipsychotic Drugs that Induce Parkinsonism

Drugs other than antipsychotics have been reported to be associated with DIP as an adverse effect are shown in Table 8.16. These include some antipsychotics used for non-psychiatric indications as well as non-antipsychotics used for psychiatric indications.

Tardive Dyskinesia (TD)

Tardive dyskinesia (TD) is an abnormal involuntary movement disorder resulting from the chronic (< 3 months) use of antipsychotics. The word "tardive" is of French origin indicating late onset. There are some exceptions to this definition as TD has been reported in some patients with less than 3 months' treatment and also in association with non-antipsychotic medications.

Historical records suggest dyskinesia was observed in severely ill institutionalized patients with schizophrenia in the pre-neuroleptic era. The first report of TD was by Schonecker (1957) who described a lip-smacking dyskinetic movement disorder following chlorpromazine treatment. The term "tardive dyskinesia" was first used by Faurbye et al (1964) to describe abnormal movements that developed during or follow-

Table 8.16. Non-antipsychotic drugs associated with induction or aggravation of parkinsonism.

Antidepressants
  Selective serotonin reuptake inhibitors
    Fluoxetine (Bouchard et al 1989; Chouinard and Sultan 1992; Touw et al 1992; Steur 1993)
    Fluvoxamine (Meco et al 1994)
    Paroxetine
    Sertraline (Cano and Roquer 1995)
  Monoamine oxidase inhibitors
    Phenelzine (Teusink et al 1984)
    Trazodone
    Bupropion
Antiepileptics
  Lamotrigine (Ho et al 1997)
  Phenytoin
  Valproic acid (Alvarez-Gomez et al 1993; Sasso et al 1994; Sassod et al 1993; Armon et al 1996)
Antimicrobials
  Amphotericin B (Manley et al 1998)
  Cephaloridine (Mintz et al 1971)
Antineoplastic agents (Boranic & Raci 1979; Howell & Sager 1994)
  Paclitaxel (Bauer and Munter 1995)
  Carboplatin/cyclophosphamide(Linn et al 1998)
  Cyclophosphamide/etoposide (Fleming and Mangino 1997)
  Cytarabine (Sirvent et al 1998)
Calcium antagonists (Gracia-Ruiz et al 1992; Malaterre et al 1992; Negrotti et al 1992)
  Amlodipine (Sempere et al 1995)
  Cinnarizine* (Micheli et al 1989)
  Diltiazem (Dick and Barold 1989)
  Flunarizine*
  Manidipine hydrochloride (Nakashima et al 1994)
  Verapamil (Garcia-Albia et al 1993)
Dopamine depleting drugs
  Reserpine (Ross 1990)
  Tetrabenazine
Dopamine synthesis blockers
  α-methylpara-tyrosine
  Methyldopa (Gillman and Sandyk 1984; Rosenblum and Montgomery 1980)
Dopamine receptor blocking agents
  Metaclopramide*
  Droperidol
  Domperidone
  Prochlorperazine
Miscellaneous agents
  Amiadarone (Werner & Olanow 1989)
  Clebopride (Marti-Masso et al 1993; Montagna et al 1992; Martinez-Martin 1993; Sempere et al 1996)
  Cyclosporine (Wasserstein and Honig 1996)
  Diazepam
  Disulfiram (Laplane et al 1992; de Mari et al 1993)
  Donepezil (Bourke and Druckenbrod 1998)
  Lithium (Lecamwasam et al 1994)
  Lovastatin (Müller et al 1995)
  Manganese for parenteral nutrition (Ejima et al 1992)
  Meperidine (Lieberman and Goldstein 1985a; Olive et al 1994)
  Methyphenidate (Ross 1990)
  Naproxen (Shaunak et al 1995)
  Procaine (Gjerris 1971)
  Tacrine (Ott and Lanon 1992)
  Vaccines (Alves et al 1992)
  Tetanus vaccine (Reijneveld et al 1997)

* Well documented.

ing long-term treatment with antipsychotic. General acceptance of TD as an adverse effect of long-term antipsychotic therapy occurred in 1970s.

TD is a choreic disorder. Choreic movements are usually non-patterned but in the setting of TD, they may be patterned. The most common clinical presentation is orofacial dyskinesias but it may involve the trunk and extremity muscles also.

Epidemiology. Abnormal movements in psychiatric patients may be a manifestation of subtle brain damage rather than antipsychotic exposure. The prevalence of TD in never medicated elderly schizophrenic patients is 41% (similar figure to those who are treated with antipsychotics) and is higher than the 15% incidence of TD in the first degree relatives of these patients (McCreadie et al 1996). However, most epidemiological studies support the association between antipsychotics and TD and have uncovered risk factors. Klawans et al (1988) have reviewed the problems of evaluating epidemiological studies because of the variability of diagnostic criteria for TD, variations in dose of antipsychotics, and modification of symptoms by treatment. Estimates for the prevalence of TD in patients receiving antipsychotics range from 0.5% to 70%. The average prevalence is about 20% against a background prevalence of spontaneous dyskinesia of about 6% (Kane and Smith 1982; Casey and Gerlach 1988). The incidence rate or the risk of a schizophrenic patient to develop TD after one year of continuous antipsychotic therapy is 4% to 5% (Gardos and Cole 1980). Integration of incidence and prevalence rates requires knowledge of risk factors for the development of TD and persistence afterwards (Kane et al 1986).

Risk Factors. Factors related to the patient characteristics are:

- *Age*. There is low prevalence with nearly complete reversibility in pediatric patients. It increases with advancing age until the seventh decade when it reaches a plateau (Koshino et al 1992). The elderly are more susceptible to TD (Yassa et al 1992).
- *Sex*. TD occurs more often in women than in men with an approximate ratio of 1.7 to 1.

- *Prior electroconvulsive therapy (ECT)*. There is lack of correlation between ECT and TD. ECT may unmask a latent TD or even improve it some cases.
- *Nature of psychiatric disorder*. Patients with schizoaffective disorders appear to be at greater risk than those with schizophrenia.
- *Brain damage*. This would be expected to predispose to development of TD but empirical studies do not support this hypothesis.
- *Drug-induced parkinsonism (DIP)*. Patients who develop DIP are more likely to develop TD.
- *Genetic predisposition*. Steen et al (1997) have found a high frequency (22–24%) of homozygosity for the Ser9Gly variant (allele 2) of the DRD_3 gene among subjects with TD as compared with the relative under-representation (4–6%) of this genotype in patients with no or fluctuating TD. Their results indicate that autosomal inheritance of two polymorphic Ser9Gly alleles (2–2 genotype), but not homozygosity for the wild-type allele (1–1 genotype), is a susceptibility factor for the development of TD.
- *Diabetes mellitus*. Patients with diabetes mellitus are at greater risk for developing TD (Ganzini et al 1992).
- *Antipsychotic drug dose and duration of treatment*. Higher doses and longer durations of treatment are suspected to be risk factors but no studies so far have settled this issue. The only risk factor related to drug exposure is in older patients where is a significant correlation between TD and length as well as total dose of antipsychotics only during the first 2 to 3 years of therapy.
- *Neuroleptic drug type*. The newer atypical antipsychotics such as clozapine are less likely to produce TD than the classical antipsychotics. Controlled clinical trials have indicated a significantly lower risk of tardive dyskinesia with olanzapine than with haloperidol (Beasley et al 1999).

Course of TD. It is difficult to study the natural course of TD after discontinuation of antipsychotics because of relapses of the psychiatric illness and resumption of antipsychotic therapy before an adequate follow-up period is over. Various rating scales are used so that data from several studies from different centers can be compared. One of the frequently used scales in the studies quoted here is AIMS (abnormal involuntary movement scale) devised by Guy (1976).

Several authors have observed that continuous antipsychotic therapy is preferable to interrupted therapy as TD is more likely to persist in the latter group (Bergen et al 1992; Jeste et al 1979). Risk factors for poor outcome and persistence are the same as for the initial occurrence of TD. TD which does not recover beyond 1–2 years should be considered persistent rather than permanent (Klawans et al 1984). Cavallaro et al (1993) reported that 28% of the patients recovered completely and 30% improved. Prognostic factors for favorable outcome are:

1. Young female patients. This may be due to the protective effect of estrogens.
2. Less severe forms of TD

Intellectual Impairment in TD. Intellectual impairment is seen in some patients with TD. Ueyama et al (1993) have observed that schizophrenic patients with TD tend to suffer more brain damage than those without TD. Intellectual impairment in these patients was related to cerebral atrophy shown in CT.

Pathomechanism. Various hypotheses to explain TD are:

– *Dopamine supersensitivity.* This is based on similarity between levodopa-induced dyskinesia and TD. Chronic antipsychotic treatment produces a hypersensitivity of striatal dopamine receptors, similar to denervation-induced hypersensitivity seen in peripheral muscles. Chronic antipsychotic treatment produces an increase in dopamine receptor density in the striatum as well as behavioral supersensitivity to dopamine. Dopamine agonists such as levodopa and amphetamine can exacerbate TD. Dopamine antagonists suppress TD while anticholinergics tend to enhance it. Mechanism by which dopamine receptor blockade leads to dopaminergic supersensitivity is not known. Observations from several animal experimental studies and human patients are difficult to reconcile with this hypothesis.

Lee et al (1997) have transfected a bovine dopamine transporter (bDAT) cDNA was into CV-1 cells, a cell line that lacks vesicular storage and release mechanisms. Using this cell line, the effects of neuroleptic drugs on DAT-mediated uptake and release of dopamine (DA) were examined. All of the neuroleptic drugs tested, inhibited DA uptakes in DAT expressing cells, and most of them were shown to promote spontaneous release of DA at the same time. These results imply that neuroleptic drugs would cause an overflow of DA in the synaptic cleft of extrapyramidal dopaminergic neurons, which could be one of the possible mechanisms of drug-induced tardive dyskinesia.

– *GABA depletion.* Animal studies suggest GABAergic hypofunction in TD (Fibiger and Lloyd 1984) and human studies support the hypothesis that a dysfunction of GABA-mediated neurotransmission may be the basis of TD (Cassady et al 1992).

– *Norepinephrine overactivity.* Central noradrenergic neurons innervate the striatum and appear to influence movement and to modulate dopamine-induced hyperactivity. There is no convincing evidence to support this hypothesis.

– *Serotonergic mechanisms.* These may be involved in regulating abnormal movements perhaps by modulating dopamine release. Serotonin (5-HT) may play a role in basal ganglia dysfunction underlying TD, but this role remains to be proven.

– *Neurotoxicity.* Excitotoxic mechanisms may be involved in the pathogenesis of TD (De Keyser 1991). Movement disorders induced by chronic antipsychotic treatment may result, at least in part, from a hypersensitivity of the presynaptic D_2 receptor regulating the release of glutamate. Gunne and Andren (1993) have developed an animal model and hypothesized that TD is due to an excitotoxic lesion of the inhibitory GABAergic afferents. This may open the possibility of preventing TD by addition of a glutamate antagonist or NMDA receptor antagonist to chronic antipsychotic treatment. Increase in dopamine turnover produced by antipsychotics may increase oxygen free radical formation (Cadet and Lohr 1987; Shriqui and Jones 1990). According to this hypothesis concomitant use of free radical scavengers should be helpful in preventing TD.

- *Structural abnormalities in the striatum.* In vivo studies done by MRI in TD patients have shown that volume of the caudate nuclei of patients with TD are significantly smaller as compared to that in patients without TD and normal controls (Mion et al 1991). This abnormality may be related to some previous condition which may prove to be a substrate that is necessary for TD to evolve. Further studies are required to determine the pathophysiologic nature of these alterations.
- *Inhibition of Complex I of the Electron Transport Chain.* Antipsychotics have been shown to alter mitochondrial electron transport chain function in the rat brain both in vivo and in vitro (Jackson-Lewis and Przedborski (1994). Complex I is particularly sensitive to free radical attack and these authors have shown that

free radical scavengers compounds such as ascorbic acid, glutathione, and superoxide dismutase attenuate the fluphenazine-induced inhibitory effect on complex I activity. Therefore, the use of antioxidant therapy as cotreatment to the antipsychotic therapy may prevent or reduce the severity of TD.

Differential Diagnosis of TD. All patients with TD should have a thorough physical examination and laboratory tests but the diagnosis is mostly clinical and not based on the results of laboratory tests. TD should be differentiated from the conditions shown in Table 8.17. The most frequently encountered dyskinesia which needs to be differentiated from TD is that due to levodopa. A comparison of the dyskinesias induced by levodopa and antipsychotic is given in the section on levodopa-induced dyskinesias.

Drug-Induced TD

Antipsychotics are the best known among drugs associated with TD but several non-antipsychotic drugs can also produce dyskinesias (Table 8.18).

Some of the drugs listed in Table 8.18, such as anxiolytics and antidepressants, are also used in the treatment of TD but they can also induce or aggravate TD. Antidepressants have been reported to induce TD when given to patients with Creutzfeldt-Jakob disease (Clark et al 1992). TD has been reported with use of tricyclic antidepressants for treatment for depression (Clark et al 1992; Gersten 1993; Clayton 1996; Vandel et al 1997). TD has been reported following use of buspirone in a patient with dementia (Strauss 1988) and also in a patient without previous neurological disorder (LeWitt et al 1993).

Selective serotonin reuptake inhibitors have been associated with TD (Gerber and Lynd 1998). Fluoxetine can induce TD in patients with schizoaffective disorders (Budman and Bruun 1991), with fluvoxamine (Arya and Szabaldi 1993) and with paroxetine (Botsaris and Sypek 1996).

Tardive dyskinesia-like syndrome has also been associated with the use of lithium and carbamazepine in an epileptic patient with bipolar disorder (Lazarus 1994).

Table 8.17. Conditions to be considered in the differential diagnosis of tardive dyskinesia (TD).

Drug-induced tardive dyskinesia (see Table 8.18)
TD-like syndromes in patients with schizophrenia who have never been treated with antipsychotics
Abnormal movements with neurological disorders
  – Brain tumor involving basal ganglia
  – CNS infections: meningitis, encephalitis
  – Focal dystonia
  – Huntington's disease
  – Hypoxic encephalopathies
  – Idiopathic torsion dystonia
  – Oral dyskinesia associated with dementia
  – Status epilepticus
  – Sydenham's chorea
  – Tourettte's syndrome
  – Wilson's disease
Drug-induced parkinsonism
Serotonin syndrome
Neuroleptic malignant syndrome
Metabolic and endocrine disorders
  – Diabetic ketoacidosis
  – Hartnup disease
  – Hepatic encepahalopathy
  – Hepatocerebral degeneration
  – Hyper- and hypo-natremia
  – Hyperglycemia
  – Hyperparathyroidism
  – Hyperthyroidism
  – Hypomagnesemia
  – Pyruvate decarboxylase deficiency

Table 8.18. Drugs associated with the development of tardive dyskinesia.

Anticholinergic drugs (see text)
Antidepressants (see text)
  Tricyclic antidepressants
  Selective serotonin reuptake inhibitors
  Fluoxetine
  Fluvoxamine
  Paroxetine
Antiepileptic drugs
  Carbamazepine (see text)
  Methusuximide
Antihistaminic drugs (Hale and Heins 1978)
Antipsychotics*
Anxiolytics
  Buspirone (see text)
  Lorazepam (Sandyk 1986)
Dopamine receptor blocking drugs* (used for indications other than schizophrenia)
  Clebopride (Sempere et al 1994)
  Metachlopramide (Ganzini et al 1993; Putnam et al 1992; Orme and Tallis 1984)
  Sulpiride (Harraiz et al 1991)
Fentanyl (Petzinger et al 1995)
Lithium (Lazarus 1994; Meyer-Lindenberg and Krausnick 1997)
Norpseudoephedrine (see text)
Withdrawal of therapy
  Benzatropine/clozapine treatment (Songer and Schulte 1996)
  Prochlorperazine withdrawal (Alberts et al 1996)

---

* Well documented.

The prevalent theory of tardive dyskinesia indicates that this condition may result from an imbalance of the cholinergic-dopaminergic system. Thus, claims have been made that anticholinergic drugs may increase the incidence of tardive dyskinesia and the severity of the established form of this syndrome. Yassa (1988) found evidence to indicate that anticholinergic drugs may increase the severity of established tardive dyskinesia. Thus, it is recommended that anticholinergic drugs should be discontinued when a patient develops tardive dyskinesia

Thiel and Dressler (1993) described two patients who developed dyskinesias after use of norpseudoephedrine as appetite suppressant. These cleared up after discontinuation of the drug. There are isolated case reports of TD in patients treated with anticholinergic and antihistaminic drugs but no causal relationship can be established.

Variants of TD. The following variants of TD will be considered:
- Tardive dystonia
- Tardive akathisia
- Tardive Tourette-like syndrome
- Tardive myoclonus
- Withdrawal dyskinesia

Tardive dystonia. This is rare with a prevalence of 2% in chronically medicated schizophrenic patients (Yassa et al 1989). This subject has been reviewed by Burke and Kang (1988). It is distinguished from the chronic oral-buccal form of TD, not only by the dystonic nature of the involuntary movements, but also by the frequency with which it causes significant neurological disability. Acute antipsychotic-induced dystonia usually resolves when antipsychotics are discontinued whereas tardive dyskinesia does not. There is past history of acute dystonia in 40% of patients who later present with tardive dystonia (Sachdev 1993). Bruxism (grinding movements of the jaws) has been reported as a form of focal tardive dystonia (Micheli et al 1993).

Tardive dystonia should be differentiated from idiopathic dystonia because the clinical pharmacological approach is different. Tardive dystonia responds to treatment with dopamine depleting drugs or antagonists which are usually ineffective in idiopathic dystonia.

Tardive akathisia. This is akathisia which develops during long-term antipsychotic treatment or within three months of cessation and is present for at least one month. Akathisia may be a precursor or concomitant feature of some cases of TD. Akathisia may be difficult to differentiate from chronic psychiatric conditions. It differs from acute akathisia from a clinical pharmacological point of view. It does not respond to β-blockers and the response to dopamine antagonists is opposite to that of acute dystonia. It shares the pharmacological characteristics of TD in that it is exacerbated or provoked by drug reduction or withdrawal and improves temporarily when the dose is increased.

Tardive Tourette-like syndrome. Tourette's syndrome has been reported following antipsychotic treatment in schizophrenic patients without previous history of tic disorder (Klawans et al

1982). Dopamine receptor supersensitivity may play a part in the pathophysiology of Tourette-like syndrome in some cases. Tardive Tourette-like syndrome is more closely related to TD than to idiopathic Tourette's syndrome and responds to antidopaminergic drugs (Fog et al 1982).

Tardive myoclonus. Several of the patients with tardive dystonia also have myoclonus. Pure tardive myoclonus has also been described as a complication of antipsychotic therapy. Clonazepam has been considered to be effective in the management of tardive myoclonus.

Withdrawal tardive dyskinesia. The terms "withdrawal dyskinesia" and "withdrawal emergent dyskinesia" are used for movement disorders that are associated with discontinuation or reduction of dosage of antipsychotics (Gerhard 1992). The term "covert dyskinesia" describes existing TD which is unmasked after antipsychotic therapy is reduced or discontinued, leading to withdrawal TD. The exact frequency of occurrence of withdrawal dyskinesias is not known but up to 40% of previously asymptomatic patients develop dyskinesias when antipsychotics are discontinued. These dyskinesias usually manifest within a few days after discontinuation of therapy. Dyskinesias which appear during antipsychotic therapy may be aggravated on discontinuation and may become irreversible. Schooler and Kane (1982) use the term "withdrawal tardive dyskinesia" for abnormal movements that persist for at least three months after discontinuation of antipsychotics.

The pathomechanism of withdrawal dyskinesia is not known. It is probably similar to that of TD. A similar phenomenon has been reported with amoxapine and is considered to be due to its dopamine receptor blocking activity.

The prognosis of withdrawal dyskinesia is uncertain. The disorder is usually self-limited. Patients with withdrawal dyskinesias are considered to be more likely to develop TD when antipsychotics are readministered but there are no studies to prove this.

Management. Acute extrapyramidal syndromes including dystonia are associated with the use of virtually all antipsychotic agents. Various strategies have been reviewed by Gardos

(1999). A careful assessment of TD is the basis of effective management. Of the numerous published rating scales, the Abnormal Involuntary Movements Scale (AIMS) is the most widely used and is considered to be the gold standard (Guy 1976).

Adjunctive agent used in the treatment are anticholinergic agents, amantadine, benzodiazepine, or β-blockers. In patients on long-term antipsychotic therapy, the prophylactic use of agents to control movement disorders is controversial. An algorithm outlining the clinical strategies for managing tardive dyskinesia (TD) is shown in Figure 8.2.

Prevention. This is the treatment of choice for TD. Various approaches are (Tanner and Klawans 1986):
– Conservative use of antipsychotics with reduction of long-term use. Use should be reserved for major psychiatric disorders.
– Use of lowest effective dose.
– Preferential use of antipsychotics with low risk of inducing TD.
– Caution in using antipsychotics in patients with risk factors.
– Early detection of TD.

Antipsychotic withdrawal is the usual recommended course and complete remission was reported in five out of six patients after 2–4 years of abstinence (Fahn 1985). Risks and benefits of discontinuation of antipsychotics should be weighed carefully before making this decision.

Pharmacotherapy. Various approaches are as follows:
– Suppressive therapy with antipsychotics is successful in 75% of the patients but the long-term safety has not been demonstrated.
– Newer atypical antipsychotics such as clozapine. Early clinical trials of clozapine demonstrated its efficacy with few extrapyramidal side effects (Casey 1989). A prospective study was unable to conclude whether clozapine causes tardive dyskinesia but it was considered to be less likely to do so than other antipsychotics (Kane et al 1993). Clozapine has also been used in the treatment of TD and has been shown to improve symptoms in 44% of the pa-

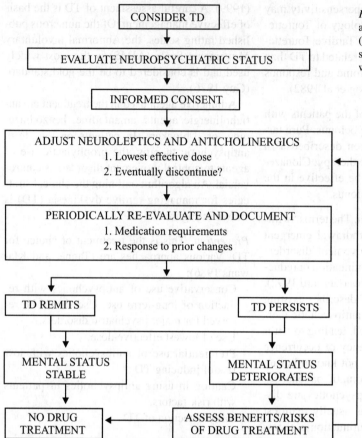

Figure 8.2. An algorithm for managing tardive dyskinesia (TD) (from Casey DE: Tardive dyskinesia. West J Med 153: 538, 1990, with permission)

CONSIDER TD

EVALUATE NEUROPSYCHIATRIC STATUS

INFORMED CONSENT

ADJUST NEUROLEPTICS AND ANTICHOLINERGICS
1. Lowest effective dose
2. Eventually discontinue?

PERIODICALLY RE-EVALUATE AND DOCUMENT
1. Medication requirements
2. Response to prior changes

TD REMITS

TD PERSISTS

MENTAL STATUS STABLE

MENTAL STATUS DETERIORATES

NO DRUG TREATMENT

ASSESS BENEFITS/RISKS OF DRUG TREATMENT

tients (Lamberti and Bellnier 1993; Bajulaiye and Addonizio 1992; Friedman 1994). Risperidone is also considered to be associated with less extrapyramidal reactions than classical antipsychotics (Curtis and Kerwin 1995).

- Dopamine antagonists. Of these, the dopamine depleters such as reserpine, tetrabenazine, and α-methyldopa relieve symptoms in 50% of the patients (Huang and Wang 1981).
- Sulpride, D₂ receptor antagonist, has been reported to be effective in TD (Schwartz et al 1990). Direct dopamine agonists (e. g., apomorphine), and indirect dopamine agonists (e. g., amantadine and bromocriptine) are somewhat effective.
- Noradrenergic antagonists such as β-blocker propranolol may suppress TD in up to 73% of the patients (Schrodt et al 1982). Clonidine, an α₂-antagonist has been shown to be effective (Nishikawa et al 1984).
- Anticholinergics. Dopamine and acetylcho-

line appear to have opposite effects on striate-mediated behavior. Anticholinergic, in the presence of dopamine supersensitivity, would be expected to make TD worse but intravenous benztropine has been found useful for treatment of dyskinesias. However, long-term use of anticholinergics worsens TD. Cholinergic agents, though theoretically expected to improve TD, have not been found to useful for the treatment with the exception of meclofenoxate which is an acetylcholine-releasing agent (Izumi et al 1986).

- GABA agonists such as baclofen, valproic acid, diazepam and clonazepam have not proven to be useful. Some studies show that progabide, a mixed GABA_A and GABA_B agonist, may have significant therapeutic effect in TD but further studies are needed. The effectiveness of this agent may support the GABA deficiency hypothesis of the pathogenesis of TD.

- Antioxidants. Vitamin E, an antioxidant and free radical scavenger, has been reported to be effective for the treatment of TD (Elkashef et al 1990; Lohr et al 1988). In a randomized cross-over study, vitamin E showed no difference from placebo in the treatment of TD. In a review of this topic, Schneiderhan (1993) concluded that the efficacy of vitamin E in TD is questionable and that further studies are needed.
- Calcium channel blockers. Verapamil has been reported to be useful in the treatment of TD in a pilot study (Dinan 1989). In a review, Cates et al (1993) consider calcium channel blockers to be potentially useful and worthy of further trials in the treatment of TD.
- Serotonergic agents. Buspirone and fluoxetine have been reported to be useful but further studies are needed. Risperidone (selective 5-HT_2 and 5-HT_{1C} antagonist) reduces TD when given concomitantly with haloperidol and further investigations are needed to evaluate this therapeutic approach.
- Branched chain amino acids (BCAA). A clinical trial has shown that BCAA decreases TD symptoms (Richardson et al 1999). This is based on the lessened ability of TD patients to clear phenylalanine (Phe)—the ingested form of the large neutral amino acid (LNAA). Greater availability of a group of LNAA, BCAA, concomitant with the lower availability of Phe to the brain are associated with a decrease in TD symptoms.
- Miscellaneous agents. Lithium, cerulitide (a CKK antagonist), and prednisone have been reported to be effective but no adequate evidence is available.

Dyskinesias Associated with Antiparkinsonian Drugs

Among antiparkinsonian drug, levodopa is the one which is frequently associated with dyskinesias. Other drugs used in the treatment of Parkinson's disease which have rarely been reported to be associated with dyskinesia are: Apomorphine (Cotzias et al 1976), bromocriptine (Lieberman

and Goldstein 1985b) and propofol (Krauss et al 1996).

Levodopa-Induced Dyskinesias

The original report of Cotzias et al (1967) which stated that levodopa ameliorated the signs and symptoms of Parkinson's disease included the observation that athetoid movements were induced in some patients by the drug. Subsequent reports indicated that the occurrence of dyskinesias in Parkinson's disease treated with levodopa was as high as 50% (Cotzias et al 1969) and more recently quoted figures are as high as 80% (Nutt 1990).

Clinical Features. Patients with Parkinson' disease may suffer from one or more of the following movement disorders during chronic treatment with levodopa.
- *Choreoathetosis.* This is the most common pattern.
- *Dystonia.* Occurs in 20% to 30% patients.
- *Akathisia.* Occurs in 26% of patients. May precede treatment.
- *Ballism.* This can be very severe.
- *Stereotyped movements.* Stepping or kicking movements of legs.
- *Myoclonus.* Rare. Usually in association with dementia.
- *Tremor.* Present before treatment. Difficult to evaluate.

Clinical pharmacological classification of levodopa-induced dyskinesia has been reviewed by Luquin et al (1992). Three types are recognized: Peak-dose dyskinesia, off-dose dystonia, and diphasic dyskinesia.
- *Peak dose dyskinesia.* This is also called on-dyskinesia. This occurs at the peak dose and is the most frequent type. The movements are mostly choreoathetotic. It usually occurs in patients with good therapeutic response to levodopa and is present during the time that the patient is experiencing a reduction in symptoms of parkinsonism.
- *Off-dose (end-of-dose) dystonia.* This occurs when levodopa levels are low and affects mainly the legs. Crampy pain is almost always

present. It manifests in the morning in patients who switch to a single daily dose and is also called "early morning dystonia." Dystonia occurs when the drug is not working and parkinsonism is more apparent. It also occurs after levodopa withdrawal but disappears within a day. Dystonia may also occur spontaneously in Parkinson's disease. Differentiation of various other types of dystonia from that occurring during levodopa therapy has been discussed by Carella et al (1993). Parkinsonism and levodopa-induced dystonia may be present simultaneously but in different parts of the body. Dystonia reflects the degree rather than the rate of reduction in dopaminergic stimulation and may involve the interaction of dopamine with a receptor subpopulation that does not mediate antiparkinsonian efficacy (Bravi et al 1993).

– *Diphasic dyskinesia.* This occurs when levodopa begins to take effect and as the drug effect wanes with minimal manifestations during the peak dose. These can be very severe with ballistic movements. Clinical and EMG analysis of dyskinesias after administration of levodopa has shown that their timing, distribution and severity is not chaotic but follows a certain pattern (Marconi et al 1994). In this continuum-oscillator model of pathophysiology of levodopa-induced dyskinesias, one type of abnormal movement (onset-of-dose) evolves into another (peak-dose). Levodopa-induced dyskinesias (LID) wax and wane with emotional state of the patient and with activity and disappear when the patient is asleep. LID start in the foot in patients who respond well to levodopa initially. This is consistent with the observation that loss of dopaminergic function is more marked in dorsolateral striatum that corresponds somatotopically to the foot area (Vidailhet et al 1994). There is worsening of the tremor before emergence of dyskinesia indicating that dyskinesia and postural tremor may stem from a common pathophysiological mechanism (Caliguiri and Lohr 1993). There is a broad spectrum of levodopa-related fluctuations in Parkinson's disease, which, in addition to movement disorders, induce psychiatric disturbances as well (Riley and Lang 1993). Dyskinesias occurs in patients with an adequate response to levodopa and those with no therapeutic benefit have little or no dyskinesia. A retrospective study has shown that there is no relation between the dose or duration of levodopa therapy and onset of dyskinesias (Peppe et al 1993).

Table 8.19. Comparison of tardive dyskinesias induced by levodopa and antipsychotics.

Variable	Levodopa	Antipsychotics
Prevalence	50%–80%	20%
Clinical Manifestations		
– orofacial involvement	Less common	More common
– limb dyskinesia	Common	Less common
– unilateral dyskinesias	Frequent	Rare
Etiologic factors		
– primary illness	Parkinson's	Psychiatric
– dose and length of treatment	Unimportant	Important
– aging as a risk factor	Less important	Important
Course		
– "On" and "off" phenomena	Present	Not reported
– drug withdrawal dyskinesias	Rare	Frequent
– persistence on drug withdrawal	Not reported	Frequent
Treatment		
– dose reduction	Effective	Less effective
– dose increase	Worsens	May be masked
– surgery (e. g., thalamotomy)	Available	Not done

Movement disorders associated with chronic levodopa therapy are also referred to as tardive dyskinesias (TD) and need to be differentiated from the TD due to antipsychotics. This comparison is shown in Table 8.19.

Risk Factors. Patients with young age of onset of Parkinson's disease have a higher prevalence of levodopa-induced dystonia (Wu et al 1993). This may be due to higher doses given for longer periods to younger patients who tolerate higher doses better than the elderly. Patients with severe Parkinson's disease are more likely to develop dyskinesias with levodopa therapy. High carbohydrate with low protein diet may trigger dyskinesias by decreasing the plasma large neutral amino acids and raising levodopa level relative to this (Wurtman et al 1988).

Pathophysiology. The pharmacological mechanisms of levodopa-induced dyskinesia are:

- Dopaminergic denervation is required. Dyskinesias occur exclusively in patients with Parkinson's disease and not in healthy volunteers (Arts et al 1991).
- Intact striatal outflow is required for the emergence of dyskinesias which appear in patients with good response to levodopa. Patients with variants of Parkinson's disease who do not respond to levodopa, rarely experience these complications.
- Dyskinesias are induced by levodopa therapy. They are rare at onset of therapy but appear after weeks months or years of therapy. Recent clinical and preclinical pharmacological findings suggest that the pathogenesis of this complication reflects factors related both to the natural progression of Parkinson's disease and levodopa toxicity. Degeneration of nigrostriatal dopaminergic projections can alter function in the downstream neuronal systems and increase their susceptibility to change as a result of subsequent exposure to dopaminergic drugs (Chase et al 1993).
- Chronic administration of levodopa can cause alterations in mitochondrial and respiratory chain activity in rats that is likely related to an oxidative stress imposed by increased dopamine turnover (Przedborski et al 1993). This mechanism may exaggerate a mitochondrial

defect already present in the brains of patients with Parkinson's disease and may play a role in the progression of the disease.
- Role of pharmacologic variables such as dosing schedules, magnitude of individual and cumulative dose of the drug, the balance of D_1 and D_2 receptor stimulation are being explored as critical determinants of development of dyskinesias.
- Conversion of exogenously applied levodopa to dopamine and its storage might cause dopaminergic neurons in the disease state to be exposed to excessive load of dopamine which may exert toxic effect by generation of free radicals (Kuno 1994).
- Free radicals have been implicated in the pathogenesis of Parkinson's disease. Levodopa oxidation produces free radicals which may accelerate neuronal degeneration (Ogawa 1994).

A model of basis ganglia function producing levodopa-induced dyskinesia in a patient with Parkinson's disease is shown in Figure 8.3.

Management

Treatment of dyskinesias is unsatisfactory. There is no specific antidyskinesic drug. Strategies for preventing and treating levodopa-induced dyskinesias have been reviewed by Durif (1999).

- The most common strategy is to adjust the dose of levodopa, i. e., to give smaller doses of levodopa more frequently.
- Change of method of administration to provide a steady concentration of levodopa at the basal ganglia and prevent the "off effect" (Florence and Jani 1994):
  · by carbidopa-levodopa preparations
  · controlled release preparations
  · polymeric implants
- Partial dopamine agonist terguride, both as a monotherapy and in combination with levodopa, can reduce dyskinesias in 53% of the patients.
- Initial bromocriptine therapy before levodopa delays the onset of dyskinesias (Montastruc et al 1993). Bromocriptine, a dopamine agonist, has a neuroprotective effect by its free-radical

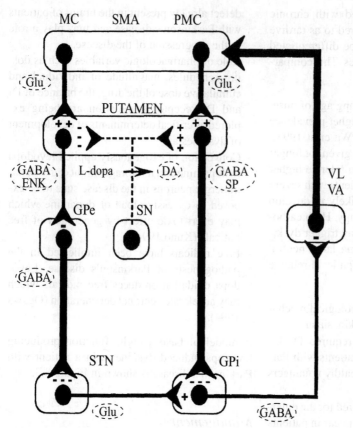

Figure 8.3. Model of basal ganglia function producing levodopa-induced dyskinesia in a parkinsonian subject. Levodopa, converted to dopamine in the putamen, reverses the balance of excitation and inhibition in GPi by augmenting the direct inhibitory input while reducing the indirect excitatory input. This reduces or abolishes the parkinsonism but concomitantly induces dyskinesia.

Abbrev. GPi and GPe = globus pallidus internal and external, SMA = supplementary motor area, STN = subthalamic nucleus, VL and VA = ventrolateral an anterior nuclei of thalamus, SN = substania nigra, PMC = premotor cortex, SMA = supplementary motor area, MC = primary motor cortex.

Reproduced from Nutt JG: Dyskinesia induced by levodopa and dopamine agonists in patients with Parkinson's disease. In Lang AE and Weiner WJ (Eds.) Drug-induced Movement Disorders, Mt. Kisco, Futura Publishing Company, 1992, pp. 281–314.

Table 8.20. Named syndromes of drug-induced movement disorders.

Syndromes	Feature	Drug(s) involved	Comment
Pisa syndrome (pleurothotonus)	Unilateral dystonia with bending to one side	Clozapine (Kurtz et al 1993); Sertindole (Padberg et al 1998); Antidepressants (Suzuki et al 1997)	27 cases reported in literature. Some are unrelated to drugs
Metronome or alternating Pisa syndrome	Alternating dystonia from one side to the other	Clozapine (Bruneau & Stip 1998)	Considered to be a form of tardive dystonia
Rabbit syndrome	An atypical form of drug-induced parkinsonism in which perioral muscular movements strikingly imitate the movements of a rabbit's mouth. The tongue is spared	Antipsychotics (Villaneuve 1972); Risperidone (Schwartz et al 1998); Antidepressants (Fornazzari et al 1991); Sulpiride (Kakigi et al 1982)	20 cases reported in literature. One denovo case deteriorated with levodopa and improved with neuroleptic treatment (Nishiyama et al 1993)
Serotonin syndrome	Includes tremor as one of the features	See Chapter 21	
Neuroleptic malignant syndrome	Includes muscular rigidity as one of the features	See Chapter 23	

scavenging activity. Combination of levodopa and bromocriptine appears to create a better balance between post-synaptic D_2 and D_1 receptors and to maintain normal dopaminergic transmission for longer periods than does high dose levodopa alone (Ogawa 1994).

- Apomorphine (a dopaminergic drug) injection or continuous subcutaneous infusion may be tried for diphasic dyskinesia (de Saint Victor et al 1992).

- Antioxidants. Vitamin E has been shown to be beneficial (Ford and Fahn 1993). Vitamin C and deprenyl prevent levodopa toxicity by unrelated mechanisms in catecholamine-rich human neuroblastoma cell lines (Pardo et al 1993).

- Fluoxetine. It has been suggested that increasing brain serotonergic transmission with fluoxetine may reduce levodopa- or dopamine agonist-induced dyskinesias without aggravating parkinsonian motor disability.

- Clozapine has been shown to suppress dyskinesias in advanced Parkinson's disease (Bennett et al 1993)

- Riluzole. This drug is an inhibitor of glutamatergic transmission in the CNS and is used for the treatment of amyotrophic lateral sclerosis. Riluzole has been reported to attenuate levodopa-induced dyskinesias without deterioration of the basic disease or suppression of clinical benefits of levodopa (Merims et al 1999).

- Buspirone have been reported to be useful (Kleedorfer et al 1991).

- Thalamic stimulation (Caparros-Lefebre et al 1993) and thalamotomy (Hillier et al 1999) have been reported to be successful for the management of persistent dyskinesias due to levodopa.

- Magnetic fields. Sandyk et al (1992) have reported one case of levodopa-induced dyskinesia which was treated successfully by application of weak magnetic fields to the head.

- Gene therapy. Grafts of dopamine-producing fibroblasts or myoblasts, genetically modified *in vitro* to express tyrosine hydroxylase can be used for the treatment of Parkinson's disease. These cells produce and secrete dopamine and provide it in high concentrations only to the damaged part of the brain and thus avoid the "on" and "off" phenomenon (Jain 1998).

Drug-Induced Extrapyramidal Syndromes

Various drug-induced movement disorders already described in this chapter are also reported as extrapyramidal syndromes. Special syndromes of drug-induced movement disorders are shown in Table 8.20. Some of these have multiple neurological features ad are dealt with in other chapters.

References

Abouafia DM: Tremors associated with trimethoprim-sulfamethoxazole therapy in a patient with AIDs: case report and review. Clinical Infectious Diseases 1996; 22: 598–600.

Adityanjee, Lindenmeyer JP: Precipitation of dystonia by m-CPP in a schizophrenic patient treated with haloperidol. Am J Psychiatry 1993; 150: 737–738.

Adler LA, Angrist B, Rotrosen J: Acute neuroleptic-induced akathisia. In Lang AE, Weiner WJ (Eds.): Drug-induced movement disorders, Mt. Kisco, Futura Publishing Co, 1992, pp 85–119.

Adler LA, Angrist B, Rotrosen J: Efficacy of betaxolol in neuroleptic-induced akathisia. Psychiatry Research 1991; 39: 193–198.

Alberts VA, Catalano G, Poole MA: Tardive dyskinesia as a result of long-term prochlorperazine use. Southern Medical Journal 1996; 89: 989–991.

Alvarez-Gomez MJ, Vaamonde J, Narbona J, et al: Parkinsonian syndrome in childhood after sodium valproate administration. Clin Neuropharmacology 1993; 16: 451–455.

Alves RSC, Barbosa ER, Scaff M: Postvaccinal parkinsonism. Mov Dis 1992; 7: 178–180.

Anfung MK, Pope HG: Treatment of neuroleptic-induced akathisia with nicotine patches. Psychopharmacology 1997; 134: 153–156.

Aoki N: Reversible leukoencephalopathy caused by 5-fluorouracil derivatives, presenting as akinetic mutism. Surg Neurol 1986; 25(3): 279–82.

Arblaster LA, Lakie M, Murch WJ, et al: A study of the early signs of drug induced parkinsonism. JNNP 1993; 56: 301–303.

Armon C, Shin C, Miller P, et al: Reversible parkinsonism and cognitive impairment with chronic valproate use. Neurology 1996; 47: 626–635.

Aronheim JC: Metoclopramide and tremor. Ann Int Med 1982; 97: 621.

Arts N, van de Vlasakker, Tacke T, et al: Is levodopa harmful? Lancet 1991; 338: 1210–1211.

Arya DK, Szabadi E: Dyskinesia associated with fluvoxamine. J Clin Psychopharmacology 1993; 13: 365–366.

Arya DK: Existing brain condition may predispose to SSRI-induced extrapyramidal symptoms. Austr and NZ J of Psychiatry 1997; 31: 773–774.

Athanassiadis C, Karamanis A: Akathisia after long-term epidural use of droperidol: a case report. Pain 1992; 50: 203–204.

Attig E, Amyot R, Botez T: Cocaine-induced chronic tics. JNNP 1994; 57: 1143–1144.

Ayd F: A survey of drug-induced extrapyramidal reactions. JAMA 1961; 175: 1054–1060.

Bajulaiye R, Addonizio G: Clozapine in the treatment of psychosis in an 82-year old woman with tardive dyskinesia. J Clin Psychopharmacol 1992; 12: 364–365.

Barak Y, Levine J, Weisz R: Clozapine-induced myoclonus: two case reports. J Clin Psychopharmacol 1996 Aug; 16(4): 339–40.

Barnes TR: A rating scale for drug-induced akathisia. Br J Psychiatry 1989; 154: 672–6.

Barnes TRE, Curson DA: Long-term depot antipsychotics: a risk-benefit assessment. Drug Safety 1994; 10: 464–479.

Baronti F, Mouradian MM, Conant KE, et al: Partial dopamine agonist therapy of levodopa-induced dyskinesias. Neurology 1992; 42: 1241–1243.

Bateman DN, Bevan P, Langley BP, et al: Cimetidine-induced postural and action tremor. JNNP 1981; 44: 9.

Bauer M, Hellweg R, Baumgartner A: Fluoxetine-induced akathisia does not reappear after switch to paroxetine. J Clin Psychiatry 1996; 57: 593–594.

Beasley CM, Dellva MA, Tamura RN, et al: Randomised double-blind comparison of the incidence of tardive dyskinesia in patients with schizophrenia during long-term treatment with olanzapine or haloperidol. Br J Psychiatry 1999; 174: 23–30.

Benazzi F: Spiramycin-associated acute dystonia during neuroleptic treatment. Canad J Psychiat 1997; 42: 665–666.

Bennett JP, Landow ER, Schuh LA: Suppression of dyskinesias in advanced Parkinson's disease. neurology 1993; 43: 1551–1555.

Bergen J, Kitchin R, Berry G: Predictors of the course of tardive dyskinesia n patients receiving neuroleptics. Biol Psychiatry 1992; 32: 580–594.

Berman I, Zalma A, DuRand CJ, et al: Clozapine-induced myoclonic jerks and drop attacks. J Clin Psychiatry 1992; 53: 329–330.

Bharucha KJ and Sethi KD: Tardive Tourettism after exposure to neuroleptic therapy. Mov Dis 1995; 10: 791–793.

Bickerstaff ER: Neurological complications of oral contraceptives, Oxford, Clarendon Press, 1975.

Bird GL, Meadows J, Goka J, et al: Cyclosporin-associated akinetic mutism and extrapyramidal syndrome after liver transplantation. J Neurol Neurosurg Psychiatry 1990; 53(12): 1068–1071.

Black B, Uhde TW: Acute dystonia and fluoxetine. J Clin Psychiatry 1992; 53: 327.

Blake LM, Marks RC, Nierman P, et al: Clozapine and clonazepam in tardive dystonia. J Clin Psychopharmacol 1991; 11: 268.

Bleuler E (1908): Dementia praecox or the group of schizophrenias. Translated by Zinkin J, New York, International Universities Press, 1950, pp170–180.

Bocola V, Fabbrini G, Sollecito A, et al: Neuroleptic-induced parkinsonism: MRI findings in relation to clinical course after withdrawal of neuroleptic drugs. JNNP 1996; 60: 213–216.

Boranic M, Raci F: A Parkinson-like syndrome as side effect of chemotherapy with vincristine and adriamycin in a child with acute leukemia. Biomedicine 1979; 31: 124–125.

Botsaris SD, Sypek JM: Paroxetine and tardive dyskinesia. J Clin Psychopharmacol 1996; 16: 258–259.

Bouchard RH, Pourcher E, Vincent P: Fluoxetine and extrapyramidal side effects. Am J Psychiatry 1989; 146: 1352–1353.

Bourke D, Druckenbrod RW: Possible association between donepezil and worsening Parkinson's disease. Ann Pharmacother 1998; 32: 610–611.

Bower JH, Muenter MD: Temporary worsening of parkinsonism in a patient with Parkinson's disease after treatment with paclitaxel for a metastatic grade IV adenocarcinoma. Mov Disord 1995; 10(5): 681–2.

Braude WM, Barnes TRE, Gore SM: Clinical characteristics of akathisia. Brit J Psychiatry 1983; 143: 139–1150.

Bravi D, Mouradian MM, Roberts JW, et al: End-of-dose dystonia in Parkinson's disease. Neurology 1993; 43: 2130–2131.

Bristow MLF, Hirsch SR: Pitfalls and problems of long-term use of neuroleptic drugs in schizophrenia. Drug Safety 1993; 8: 136–148.

Brogmus KE, Lesch A: Psychotropic drug-induced myoclonus. Psychiatr Prax 1995; 22(2): 77–79.

Bronner IM, Vanneste JAL: Complex movement disorder associated with fluvoxamine. Mov Dis 1998; 13: 848–850.

Bruneau MA, Stip E: Metronome or alternating Pisa syndrome: a form of tardive dystonia under clozapine treatment. Int Clin Psychopharmacol 1998; 13: 229–232.

Bruun R, Kurlan R: Opiate therapy and self-harming behavior in Tourette's syndrome. Mov Dis 1991; 6: 184–185.

Buchman AS, Bennett DA, Goetz CG: Bromocriptine-induced myoclonus. Neurology 1987; 37: 885.

Budman CL, Bruun RD: Persistent dyskinesia in a patient receiving fluoxetine. Am J Psychiatry 1991; 148: 1403.

Buge A, Rancurel G, Dechy H: Encéphalopathies myocloniques bismuthiques. Formes évolutives, complications tardives, durables ou dèfinitives. A propos de 41 cases. Rev Neurol (Paris) 1977; 133: 401–415.

Burke RE, Kang UJ: Tardive dystonia: clinical aspects and treatment. Adv Neurol 1988; 49: 199–210.

Burstein AH, Fullerton T: Oculogyric crisis possibly related to pentazocine. Ann Pharmacother 1993; 27(7–8): 874–876

Cadet JL, Lohr JB: Free radicals and developmental

pathobiology of schizophrenic burnout. Intergr Psychiatry 19887; 5: 40–48.

Calabresi P, De Murtas M, Mercuri NB, et al: Chronic neuroleptic treatment: D₂ dopamine receptor supersensitivity and striatal glutamatergic transmission. Ann Neurol 1992; 31: 366–373.

Caliguiri M, Lohr JB: Worsening of postural tremor in patients with levodopa-induced dyskinesia: a quantitative analysis. Clin Neuropharmacol 1993; 16: 244–250.

Cano A, Roquer J: Parkinsonism secondary to use of sertraline. Medicinia Clinica 1995; 105: 797–798.

Caparros-Lefebvre D, Blond S, Vermesch P, et al: Chronic thalamic stimulation improves tremor and levodopa induced dyskinesias in Parkinson's disease. JNNP 1993; 56: 268–273.

Carella F, Giovannini P, Girotti F, et al: Dystonia and Parkinson's disease. Adv Neurol 1993; 60: 558–561.

Case Q, McAndrew JB: Dexedrine dyskinesia. Clin Pediatrics 1974; 13: 69–72.

Casey DE: Clozapine: neuroleptic-induced EPS and tardive dyskinesia. Psychopharmacology 1989; 45: 789–796.

Casey DE, Gerlach J: Tardive dyskinesia. Acta Psychiatr Scand 1988; 77: 369–378.

Casey DE: Neuroleptic drug-induced extrapyramidal syndromes and tardive dyskinesia. Schizophrenia Research 1991; 4: 109–120.

Cassady SL, Thaker GK, Moran M, et al: GABA agonist-induced changes in motor, oculomotor, and attention measures correlate in schizophrenics with tardive dyskinesia. Biol Psychiatry 1992; 32: 302–311.

Cates M, Lusk K, Wells BBG: Are calcium channel blockers effective in the treatment of tardive dyskinesia? Ann Pharmacother 1993; 27: 191–196.

Cavallaro R, Regazzetti MG, Mundo E, et al: Tardive dyskinesia outcomes: clinical and pharmacologic correlates of remission and persistence. Neuropsychopharmacology 1993; 8: 233–239.

Chakos MH, Meyerhoff DI, Loebel AD, et al: Incidence and correlates of acute extrapyramidal symptoms in first episodes of schizophrenia. Psychopharmacology Bulletin 1992; 28: 81–86.

Chase TN, Engber TN, Mouradian MM: Striatal dopaminoceptive system changes and motor response complications in L-dopa-treated patients with advanced Parkinson's disease. Adv Neurol 1993; 60: 181–185.

Chiado IA, Bunney BI: Typical and atypical neuroleptics: differential effects of chronic administration on the activity of A9 and A10 midbrain dopaminergic neurons. J Neuroscience 1983; 3: 1607–1610.

Chong SA, Tan CH: Fluvoxamine and akathisia. J Clin Psychopharmacology 1996; 16: 334–335.

Chong SA: Fluvoxamine and mandibular dystonia. Canad J Psychiat 1995; 40: 430–431.

Chouinard G, Sultan S: A case of Parkinson's disease exacerbated by fluoxetine. Human Psychopharmacology 1992; 7: 63–66.

Chua TP, Farrel T, Lipkin DP: Myoclonus associated with propafenone. BMJ 1994; 308: 113.

Chudnow RS, Dewey RB, Lawson CP: Choreoathetosis as a side effect of gabapentin therapy in severely neu-

rologically impaired patients. Arch neurol 1997; 54: 910–912.

Clarke CE, Bamford JM, House A: Dyskinesia in Creutzfeldt-Jakob disease precipitated by antidepressant therapy. Mov Dis 1992; 7: 86–87.

Clayton AH: Antidepressant-induced tardive dyskinesia: a review and case report. Psychopharmacology Bulletin 1995; 31: 259–264.

Combarros O, Fabrega E, Polo JM, et al: Cyclosporine-induced chorea after liver transplantation for Wilson's disease. Ann Neurol 1993; 33: 108.

Cotzias GC, Papavasiliou PS, Gellene R: Modification of parkinsonism chronic treatment with levodopa. NEJM; 1969; 280: 337–345.

Cotzias GC, Papavasiliou PS, Tolosaes Mendez JS, et al: Treatment of Parkinson's disease with aporphines: possible role of growth hormone. NEJM 1976; 294: 567–572.

Cotzias GC, Van Woert MH, Schiffer LM: Aromatic amino acids and modification of parkinsonism. NEJM 1967; 276: 374–379.

Coulter DM, Pillans PI: Fluoxetine and extrapyramidal side effects. Am J Psychiatry 1995; 152: 122–125.

Crystal HA: Baclofen therapy may be associated with chorea in Alzheimer's disease. Ann Neurol 1990; 28: 839.

Curtis VA, Kerwin RW: A risk-benefit assessment of risperidone in schizophrenia. Drug Safety 1995; 12: 139–145.

Dannon PN, Grunhaus I, Iancu I, et al: Vitamin E treatment in tardive dyskinesia. Clin Neuropharmacology 1997; 20: 434–437.

Daras M, Koppel BS, Atos-Radzion E: Cocaine-induced choreoathetoid movements (crack dancing). Neurology 1994; 44: 751–752.

Dave M: Fluoxetine-associated dystonia. Am J Psychiatry 1994; 151: 149.

Dave M: tardive oculogyric crisis with clozapine. J Clin Psychiatry 1994; 55: 264–265.

De Keyser J: Excitotoxic mechanisms may be involved in the pathophysiology of tardive dyskinesia. Clin Neuropharmacol 1991; 14: 562–565.

De Mari M, De Blasi R, Lamberti P, et al: Unilateral pallidal lesion after acute disulfiram intoxication. A clinical and magnetic resonance imaging study. Mov Dis 1993; 8: 247.

de Mari M, De Blasi R, Lamberti P, et al: Unilateral pallidal lesions after acute disulfiram intoxication: A clinical and magnetic resonance study. Mov Dis 1993; 8: 247–249.

de Saint Victor JF, Pollak P, Gervason CL, et al: Levodopa-induced diphasic dyskinsias improved by subcutaneous apomorphine. Mov Dis 1992; 7: 283–287.

Deckla MB, Bemporad JR, MacKay MC: Tics following methylphenidate administration. JAMA 1976; 235: 1349–1351.

Dev V, Krupp P: Adverse event profile and safety of clozapine. Reviews in Contemporary Pharmacotherapy 1995; 6: 197–208.

Dick RS, Barold SS: Diltiazem-induced parkinsonism. Am J Med 1989; 87: 95–96.

Dickson R, Williams R, Dalby JT: Clozapine withdrawal. Canadian Journal of Psychiatry 1994; 39: 184.

Dietl T, Kumpfel T, Hinze-Selch D, et al: Exacerbation of tics by prednisolone. Nervenarzt 1998; 69: 1111–1114.

Diltoer MW, Rosseneu S, Ramet J, et al: Anticholinergic treatment for choreoathetosis in a child after induction with propofol. Anesthesia and Analgesia 1996; 82: 670.

Dinan TG: A pilot study of verapamil in the treatment of tardive dyskinesia. Hum Psychopharmacol 1989; 4: 55–58.

Duarte J, Sempere AP, Cabezas MC, et al: Postural myoclonus induced by phenytoin. Clin Neuropharmacol 1996; 19: 536–538.

Dukoff R, Horak ID, Hassan R, et al: Akathisia associated with prochlorperazine as an antiemetic: a case report. Annals of Oncology 1996; 7: 103.

Durif F: Treating and preventing levodopa-induced dyskinesias. Drugs & Aging 1999; 14: 337–345.

Eberstein S, Adler LA, Angrist B: Nefazodone and akathisia. Biol Psychiatry 1996; 40: 798–799.

Edwards M, Koo MW, Tse RK: Oculogyric crisis after metoclopramide therapy. Optom Vis Sci 1989; 66(3): 179–180.

Eisenhaueer G, Jermain DM: Fluoxetine and tics in an adolescent. Ann Pharmacother 1993; 27: 725–726.

Ejima A, Imamura T, Nakamura S, et al: Manganese intoxication during total parenteral nutrition. Lancet 1992; 339: 426.

Elkashef AM, Ruskin PE, Bacher N, et al: Vitamin E in the treatment of tardive dyskinesia. Am J Psychiatry 1990; 147: 505–506.

Fahn S: A therapeutic approach to tardive dyskinesia. J Clin Psychiatry 1985; 46: 19–24.

Fann WE, Sullivan JL, Richman BW: Dyskinesias associated with tricyclic antidepressants. Br J Psychiatry 1976; 128: 490–493.

Faurbye A, Rasch PJ, Petersen PB, et al: Neurological symptoms in pharmacotherapy in psychoses. Acta Psychiatr Scand 1964; 40: 10.

Ferbert A, Biniek R, Kindler J, et al: Myoclonus and tremor induced acutely by administration of tumor necrosis factor. Mov Dis 1993; 8: 232–233.

Ferreyos J, Alfonso I: Dyskinesia secondary to aminophylline. Pediatr Neurol 1992; 8: 157.

Fibiger HC, Lloyd KG: Neurobiological substrates of tardive dyskinesia: the GABA hypothesis. TINS 1984; 12: 462–464.

Filip V, Marsalak M, Halkova E, et al: Treatment of extrapyramidal side effects with terguride. Psychiatry Research 1992; 41: 9–16.

Fleming DR, Mangino PB: Parkinsonian syndrome in a dialysis-supported patient receiving high-dose chemotherapy for multiple myeloma. Southern Medical Journal 1997; 90: 364–365.

Florence A, Jani PU: Novel oral drug formulations. Drug Safety 1994; 10: 233–266.

Fog R, Pakkenberg H, Regeur L, et al: "Tardive" Tourette Syndrome in relation to long-term neuroleptic treatment of tics. In Friedhoff AJ, Chase TN (Eds.): Gilles de la Tourette syndrome, New York, Raven Press, 1982, pp 419–421.

Ford B, Fahn S: Effect of antioxidants on prevention of dopa-induced complications of Parkinson's disease. Neurology 1993; 43(suppl 2): A156–A157.

Fornazzari L, Ichise M, Remington G, et al: Rabbit syndrome, antidepressant use, and cerebral perfusion SPECT scan findings. J Psychiatry Neurosci 1991; 16(4): 227–9.

Foster PN, Stickle BR, Laurence AS: Akathisia following low-dose droperidol for antiemesis in day-case patients. Anesthesia 1996; 51: 491–494.

Fox GC, Ebeid S, Vincenti G: Paroxetine-induced chorea. Brit J Psychiatry 1997; 170: 193–194.

Freyhan FA: Psychomotility and parkinsonism in treatment with neuroleptic drugs. Arch Neurol Psychiatry 1957; 78: 465–472.

Friedman JH, Max J, Swift R: Idiopathic Parkinson's disease in a chronic schizophrenic patient: long-term treatment with clozapine and levodopa. Clin Neuropharmacol 1987; 10: 470–475.

Friedman JH: Clozapine treatment of psychosis in patients with tardive dystonia. Mov Dis 1994; 9: 321–324.

Froomes PR, Stewart MR: A reversible parkinsonism syndrome and hepatotoxicity following addition of carbamazepine to sodium valproate. Australian and New Zealand Journal of Medicine 1994; 24: 413–414.

Frucht S, Eidelberg D: Imipenem-induced myoclonus. Mov Dis 1997; 12: 621–622.

Fukuzako H, Tominaga H, Izumi K, et al: Postural myoclonus associated with long-term administration of neuroleptics in schizophrenic patients. Biol Psychiatry 1990 15; 27: 1116–26.

Ganzini L, Casey DE, Hoffman WF, et al: Tardive dyskinesia and diabetes mellitus. Psychopharmacol Bull 1992; 28: 281–286.

Ganzini L, Casey DE, Hoffman WF, et al: The prevalence of metoclopramide-induced tardive dyskinesia and acute extrapyramidal movement disorders. Arch Int Med 1993; 153: 1469–1475.

Garcia G: Dystonic reaction associated with sumatriptan. Ann Pharmcocther 1994; 28: 1199.

Garcia-Albia E, Jiménéz-Jiménéz FJ, Ayuso-Peralta L, et al: Parkinsonism unmasked by verapamil. Clin Neuropharmacol 1993; 16: 263–265.

Garcia-del-Muro X, Cardenal F, Ferrer P: Extrapyramidal reaction associated with ondansetron. Eur J Cancer 1993; 29A: 288.

Garcia-Ruiz P, Garcia de Yebenes J, Jiménéz-Jiménéz FJ, et al: Parkinsonism associated with calcium channel blockers: a prospective follow-up study. Clin Neuropharmacol 1992; 15: 19–26.

Garcia-Ruiz PJ, de Yebenes JG, Jiménéz-Jiménéz FJ, et al: Parkinsonism associated with calcium channel blockers: a prospective follow-up study. Clin Neuropharmacol 1992; 15: 19–26.

Gardos G, Cole JO: Drug-induced parkinsonism and concomitant dyskinesia. In Joseph AB, Young RR (Eds.): Movement disorders in neurology and neuropsychiatry, Boston, Blackwell Scienfic Publications, 1992, pp 60–66.

Gardos G, Cole JO: Overview of public health issues in tardive dyskinesia. Am J Psychiatry 1980; 137: 776–781.

Gardos G: Managing antipsychotic-induced tardive dyskinesia. Drug Safety 1999; 20: 167–193.

Gartmann J, Hartmann K, Kuhn M: Sanz-Streiflicht Nr. 14. Schweiz Ärzt Zeitung 1993; 29: 1163–1164.

Garvey MJ, Tollefson GD: Occurrence of myoclonus in patients treated with cyclic antidepressants. Arch Gen Psychiatry 1987; 44: 269–282.

Gelenberg AJ, Jefferson JW: Lithium tremor. J Clin Psychiatry 1995; 56: 283–287.

Gerber PE, Lynd LD: Selective serotonin-reuptake inhibitor-induced movement disorders. Ann Pharmacother 1998; 32: 692–698.

Gerhard AL: Withdrawal dyskinesia. In Joseph AB, Young RR (Eds.): Movement disorders in neurology and neuropsychiatry, Boston, Blackwell Scientific Publications, 1992, pp 81–87.

Gersten SP: Tardive dyskinesia-like syndrome with clomipramine. Am J Psychiatry 1993; 150: 165.

Ghika J, Goy JJ, Naegeli C, et al: Acute reversible ataxo-myoclonic encephalopathy with flecainide therapy Schweiz Arch Neurol Psychiatr 1994; 145: 4–6.

Ghika-Schmidt F, Ghika J, Vuadens P, et al: Acute reversible myoclonic encephalopathy associated with fluoxetine therapy. Mov Dis 1997; 12: 622–623.

Gibb WRG, Lees AJ: The clinical phenomenon of akathisia. JNNP 1986; 49: 861–866.

Gillman MA, Sandyk R: Clonazepam-induced Tourette's syndrome in a subject with hyperexplexia. Postgrad Med J 1987; 63: 311–312.

Gillman MA, Sandyk R: Parkinsonism induced by methyldopa. South Afr Med J 1984; 65: 194.

Gjerris F: Transitory procaine-induced parkinsonism. JNNP 1971; 34: 20–22.

Glantz R, Weiner WJ, Goetz CG, et al: Drug-induced asterixis in Parkinson disease. Neurology 1982; 32(5): 553–5.

Glavina MJ, Robertshaw R: Myoclonic spasms following intrathecal morphine. Anesthesia 1988; 43: 389–390.

Glazer WM, Morgenstern H, Schooler H, et al: Predictors of improvement in tardive dyskinesia following discontinuation of neuroleptic therapy. Br J Psychiatry 1990; 157: 585–592.

Golden GS: The effect of central nervous system stimulants on Tourette's syndrome. Ann Neurol 1977; 2: 69–70.

Gorman M, Barkley GL: Oculogyric crisis induced by carbamazepine. Epilepsia 1995; 36(11): 1158–60.

Graudins A, Fern RP: Acut edystonia in a child associated with therapeutic ingestion of a dextromethorphan containing cough and cold syrup. J Toxicol-Clin Toxicol 1996; 34: 351–352.

Gunne LM, Andren PE: An animal model for coexisting tardive dyskinesia and tardive parkinsonism: a glutamate hypothesis for tardive dyskinesia. Clin Neuropharmacol 1993; 16: 90–95.

Gupta S, Andreason NC, Arndt S, et al: Neurological soft signs in neuroleptic-naive and neuroleptic-treated schizophrenic patients in normal comparison subjects. Am J Psychiatry 1995; 152: 191–196.

Guy W: ECDEU assessment manual for psychopharmacology. Revised edition. Washington, DC: Department of Health, Education and Welfare, 1976.

Guy W: Assessment Manual for Psychopharmacology. Washington, DC, US Department of Health Education and Welfare, 1976: 534–537.

Hale C, Heins T: Tardive dyskinesia and antihistamines. Med J Aust 1978; 1: 112–3.

Halperin JR, Murphy B: Extrapyramidal reaction to ondansetron. Cancer 1992; 69: 1275.

Halstead SM, Barnes TRE, Speller JC: Akathisia: prevalence and associated dysphoria in an in-patient population with chronic schizophrenia. Brit J Psychiatry 1994; 164: 177–183.

Hamilton PA: Metaclopramide-induced akathisia. Military Medicine 1987; 152: 585–586.

Harries JR: Oculogyric crises due to phenothiazines. Br Med J 1967; 3(559): 241.

Harrison MLB, Lyons GR, Landow ER: Phenytoin and dyskinesias: a report of two cases and review of literature. Mov Dis 1993; 8: 19–27.

Haskovec L: Akathesie. Arch Bohemes Med Clin 1902; 3: 193–200.

Hauseer RA, Zesiewicz TA: Sertraline-induced exacerbation of tics in Tourette's syndrome. Mov Dis 1995; 10: 682–683.

Hermesh H, Aizenberg D, Friedberg G, et al: Electroconvulsive therapy for persistent neuroleptic-induced akathisia and parkinsonism: a case report. Biol Psychiatry 1992; 31: 407–411.

Herraiz J, Cano A, Roquer J: Tardive dyskinesia due to sulpiride. Med Clin (Barc) 1991; 97: 235–236.

Hillier CE, Wiles CM, Simpson BA: Thalamotomy for severe antipsychotic induced tardive dyskinesia and dystonia. J Neurol Neurosurg Psychiatry 1999; 66: 250–251.

Hillsley RE, Massey EW: Truncal asterixis associated with ceftazidime, a third generation cephalosporin. Neurology 1991; 41: 2008.

Ho GJ, Swartz BE, Kaplan LR: Lamotrigine-induced parkinsonism: report of three cases in non-Parkinson's patients. Ann Neurol 1997; 42: 446.

Hod H, Har-Zahar J, Kaplinsky N, et al: Pindolol-induced tremor. Postgrad Med J 1980; 56: 346.

Hoffman WF, Labs SM, Casey DE: Neuroleptic-induced parkinsonism in older schizophrenics. Biol Psychiatry 1987; 22: 427–439.

Horiguchi J, Inami Y: Effect of clonazepam on neuroleptic-induced oculogyric crisis. Acta Psychiatr Scand 1989; 80: 521–523.

Howell SJL, Sager SJ: A progressive parkinsonism syndrome developing after chemotherapy and radiotherapy for non-Hodgkin's lymphoma. Movement Disorders 1994; 9: 373–375.

Hriso E, Kuhn T, Masdeu JC, et al: Extrapyramidal symptoms due to dopamine blocking agents in patients with AIDS encephalopathy. Am J Psychiatry 1991; 148: 1558–1561.

Huang CC, Wang RH: Reserpine and alpha methyldopa in the treatment of tardive dyskinesia. Psychopharmacology 1981; 73: 359–362.

Hughes NJ, Lyons JB: Prolonged myoclonus and meningism following propofol. Can J Anaesth 1995; 42: 744–746.

Hyman NM, Dennis PD, Sinclair KGA: Tremor due to sodium valproate. Neurology 1983; 29: 1177–1188.

Iannaccone S, Zucconi M, Marchettini P, et al: Evidence of peripheral axonal neuropathy in primary restless legs syndrome. Movement Disorders 1995; 10: 2–9.

Izumi K, Tamminaga H, Koja T, et al: Meclofenoxate therapy in tardive dyskinesia. Biol Psychiatry 1986; 21: 151–160.

Jackson-Lewis V, Przedborski S: Neuroleptic medications inhibit complex I of the electron transport chain. Neurology 1994; 35: 244–245.

Jain KK: Textbook of hyperbaric medicine. Hogrefe & Huber, Göttingen, 1998.

Jarecke CR, Reid PJ: Acute dystonic reaction induced by a monoamine oxidase inhibitor. J Clin Psychopharmacol 1990; 10: 144–145.

Jayawardena B, Hill DJ: Myoclonic spasms after epidural diamorphine infusion. Anaesthesia 1991; 46: 473–474.

Jeret JS, Somasundaram M, Asaikar S: Diltiazem-induced myoclonus. NY State J Med 1992; 92: 447–478.

Jeste DV, Potkin SG, Sinha S, et al: Tardive dyskinsia —reversible and persistent. Arch Gen Psychiatry 1979; 36: 585–590.

Jeste DV, Wyatt RJ: Understanding and Treating Tardive Dyskinesias. New York, Guilford, 1982.

Jiménéz-Jiménéz FJ, Orti-Pareja M, Ayuso-Peralta L, et al: Drug-induced parkinsonism in a movement disorder unit. A four-year survey. Parkinsonism-Related Disord 1996; 2: 145–149.

Jiménéz-Jiménéz FJ, Garcia-ruiz PJ: Flunarizine and essential tremor. Neurology 1993; 43: 239.

Jones-Fearing K: SSRIs and EPS with fluoxetine. J Am Acad Child Adolesc Psychiat 1996; 35: 1107–1108.

Joseph AB, Wroblewski BA: Paradoxical akathisia caused by clonazepam, clorazepate and lorazepam in patients with traumatic encephalopathy and seizure disorders: a subtype of benzodiazepine-induced disinhibition. Behavioral Neurology 1993; 6: 221–223.

Joseph M, King WD: Dystonic reaction with antihistamine/decongestant cold syrup. Vet Hum Toxicol 1993; 35: 343.

Joseph MM, King WD: Dystonic reaction following recommended use of cold syrup. Ann Emerg Med 1995; 26: 749–751.

Joyce RP, Gunderson CH: Carbamazepine induced orofacial dyskinesia. Neurology 1980; 30: 1333.

Kakigi R, Kuroda Y, Shibasaki H: The rabbit syndrome induced by sulpiride: a case report. Rinsho Shinkeigaku 1982; 22(6): 557–562.

Kane JM, Smith JM: Tardive dyskinesia. Arch Gen Psychiatry 1982; 39: 473–481.

Kane JM, Woerner M, Borenstein M, et al: Integrating incidence and prevalence of tardive dyskinesia. Psychopharmacology Bulletin 1986; 22: 254–258.

Kane JM, Woerner MG, Pollack S, et al: Does clozapine cause tardive dyskinesia? J Clin Psychiatry 1993; 54: 327–330.

Karas BJ, Wilder BH, Hammond EJ, et al: Valproate tremors. Neurology 1982; 32: 428–432.

Kirschberg GJ: Dyskinesia—an unusual reaction to ethosuximide. Arch Neurol 1975; 32: 137–138.

Klawans HL, Nausieda PA, Goetz CC, et al: Tourette-like symptoms following chronic neuroleptic therapy. In Friedhoff AJ, Chase TN (Eds.): Gilles de la Tourette syndrome, New York, Raven Press, 1982, pp 415–418.

Klawans HL, Tanner CM, Barr A: The reversibility of "permanent" tardive dyskinesia. Clin Neuropharmacol 1984; 7: 153–159.

Klawans HL, Tanner CM, Goetz CG: Epidemiology and pathophysiology of tardive dyskinesias. Adv Neurol 1988; 49: 185–197.

Kleedorfer B, Lees AJ, Stern GM: Buspirone in the treatment of levodopa-induced dyskinesias. JNNP 1991; 54: 376–377.

Koshino Y, Madokaro S, Ito T, et al: A survey of tardive dyskinesia in psychiatric inpatients in Japan. Clin Neuropharmacol 1992; 15: 34–43.

Koukkari MW, Vanefsky MA, Steinberg GK, et al: Phenytoin-related chorea in children with deep hemispheric vascular malformations. J Child Neurol 1996; 11(6): 490–491

Kraepelin E: Dementia praecox and paraphrenia (1919). Translated by Barclay RM; edited by Robert GM, New York, Robert E Krieger, 197, pp 77–83.

Krauss JK, Akeyson EW, Giam P, et al: Propofol-induced dyskinesias in Parkinson's disease. Anesthesia and Analgesia 1996; 83: 420–422.

Kuno S: Dilemma in the treatment of Parkinson's disease with L-dopa. Eur Neurol 1994; 34(suppl 3): 17–19.

Kurtz G, Kapfhammer HP, Peuker B: Pisa-Syndrom unter Clozapintherapie. Nervenarzt 1993; 64: 742–746.

Kurzthaler I, Hummer M, Kohl C, et al: Propranolol treatment of olanzapine-induced akathisia. Am J Psychiatry 1997; 154: 1316.

Kushner MJ: Chorea and cimetidine. Ann Int Med 1982; 96: 126-.

Kutcher S, Williamson P, McKenzie S, et al: Successful clonazepam treatment of neuroleptic induced akathisia in older adolescents and young adults: a double-blind, placebo-controlled study. J Clin Psychopharmacol 1989; 9: 403–406.

LaDelfa I, Bayer N, Myers R, et al: Chlorambucil-induced myoclonic seizures in an adult. J Clin Oncol 1985; 3: 1691–1692.

Lader MH: Neuroleptic-induced deficit syndrome (NIDS). J Clin Psychiatry 1993; 54: 493–494.

Lamberti JS, Bellnier T: Clozapine and tardive dyskinesia. J Nerv Ment Dis 1993; 181: 137–138.

Lancman ME, Asconape JJ, Penry JK: Choreiform movements associated with the use of valproate. Arch Neurol 1994a; 51: 702–704.

Lancman ME; Asconape JJ, Walker F: Acetazolamide appears effective in the management of valproate-induced tremor. Mov Dis 1994b; 9: 369.

Lane RJM: Drugs and tremor. Adverse React Bull 1984; no.106: 392–395.

Lang AE: Withdrawal akathisia: case reports and a proposed classification of chronic akathisia. Movement Disorders 1994; 9: 188–192.

Laplane D, Attal N, Sauron B, et al: Lesions of basal ganglia due to disulfiram neurotoxicity. JNNP 1992; 55: 925–929.

Larsen K, Schmekel B: Tremor in healthy volunteers after bambuterol and terbutaline CR-tablets. Eur J Clin Pharmacol 1993; 45: 303–5.

Lauterbach EC: Haloperidol-induced dystonia and parkinsonism on discontinuing metoclopramide: implications for differential thalamocortical activity. J Clin Psychopharmacol 1992; 12: 442–443.

Lazaro RP: Involuntary movements induced by anticonvulsants. Mt Sinai J Med 1982; 49: 274–281.

Lazarus A: Tardive dyskinesia-like syndrome associated with lithium and carbamazepine. J Clin Psychopharmacol 1994; 14: 146–147.

Lecamwasam D, Synek B, Moyles K, et al: Chronic lithium neurotoxicity presenting as Parkinson's disease: a cross-sectional study of patients with 15 years or more on lithium. International Clinical Psychopharmacology 1994; 9: 127–129.

Lee DS, Wong HA, Knoppert DC: Myoclonus associated with lorazepam therapy in very-low-birth-weight infants. Biol Neonate 1994; 66: 311–315.

Lee SH, Oh DY, Jung SC, et al: Neuroleptic drugs alter the dopamine transporter-mediated uptake and release of dopamine: a possible mechanism for drug-induced tardive dyskinesia. Pharmacol Res 1997; 35: 447–450.

Levinson DF: Pharmacologic treatment of schizophrenia. Clin Therapeutics 1991; 13: 326–352.

Lewis CF, DeQuardo JR, Tandon R: Dystonia associated with trazodone and sertraline. J Clin Psychopharmacol 1997; 17: 64–65.

LeWitt PA, Walters A, Hening W, et al: Persistent movement disorders induced by buspirone. Mov Dis 1993; 8: 331–334.

Lieberman AN, Goldstein M: Bromocriptine in parkinson's disease. Pharmacol Rev 1985b; 37: 217–227.

Lieberman AN, Goldstein M: Reversible parkinsonism related to meperidine. NEJM 1985a; 312: 509.

Lieberman JA: Neuroleptic-induced movement disorders and experience with clozapine in tardive dyskinesia. J Clin Psychiatry 1990; 8: 3–8.

Lightman SL: Phenobarbital dyskinesia. Postgrad Med J 1978; 54: 114–115.

Lindenmayer JP, Da Silva D, Buenda A, et al: Tic-like syndrome after treatment with clozapine. Am J Psychiatry 1995; 152: 649.

Linn M, Brodt E, Gutschow K, et al: Progression of Parkinson's disease with impairment of vision under carboplatin/cyclophosphamide therapy for ovarian cancer. Cancer Chemotherapy and Pharmacology 1998; 41: 427–428.

Lohr JB: Vitamin E in the treatment of tardive dyskinesia. The possible involvement of free radical mechanisms. Schizophrenia Bull 1988; 14: 291–296.

Lopez-Alemy M, Ferrer-Tuset C, Bernacer-Alpera B: Akathisia and acute dystonia induced by sumatriptan. J Neurol 1997; 244: 131–133.

Lowe TL, Cohen DJ, Detlor J, et al: Stimulant medications precipitate Tourette's syndrome. JAMA 1982; 247: 1168–1169.

Lu C, Chu N: Acute dystonic reactions with asterixis and myoclonus following metoclopramide therapy. JNNP 1981; 551: 1002–1003.

Lundh H, Turving K: An extrapyramidal choreiform syndrome caused by amphetamine addiction. JNNP 1981; 44: 728–730.

Luquin MR, Scipioni O, Vaamonde J, et al: Levodopa-induced dyskinesias in Parkinson's disease: clinical and pharmacological classification. Mov Dis 1992; 7: 117–124.

Lustman F, Moncu G: Amiodarone and neurological side effects. Lancet 1974; i: 568.

Magny JF, d'Allest AM, Nedelcoux H, et al: Midazolam and myoclonus in neonate. Eur J Pediatr 1994; 153: 389–90.

Malaterre HR, Lauribe P, Paganelli F, et al: Syndrome parkinsonien, effet indésirable possible des inhibiteurs calciques. Arch Mal Coeur 1992; 85: 1335–1337.

Malhotra AK, Litman RE, Picker D: Adverse effects of antipsychotic drugs. Drug Safety 1993; 9: 429–436.

Mamo DC, Sweet RA, Keshavan MS: Managing antipsychotic-induced parkinsonism. Drug Saf 1999 Mar; 20(3): 269–75.

Manley TJ, Chusid MJ, Rand SD, et al: Reversible parkinsonism in a child after bone marrow transplantation and lipid-based amphotericin B therapy. Pediatric Infectious Diseases Journal 1998; 17: 433–434.

Marchioni E, Perucca E, Soragna D, et al: Choreiform syndrome associated with fluoxetine treatment in a patient with deficient CYP2D6 activity. Neurology 1996; 46: 853.

Marconi R, Lefebvre-Caparros D, Bonnet AM, et al: Levodopa-induced dyskinesias in Parkinson's disease phenomenology and pathophysiology. Movement Disorders 1994; 9: 2–12.

Markkula J, Lauerma H: Mianserin and restless legs. Int Clin Psychopharmacol 1997; 12(1): 53–58.

Marsden CD, Jenner P: The pathophysiology of extrapyramidal side-effects of neuroleptic drugs. Psychol Med 1980; 10: 55–72.

Marti Masso JF, Carrera N, Urtasun M, et al: Drug-induced parkinsonism: a growing list. Mov Dis 1993; 8: 125–126.

Martin M, Diaz-Rubio E, Valverde JJ, et al: Prednimustine-induced myoclonus—a report of three cases. Acta Oncologica 1994; 33: 81–82.

Martinez-Martin P: Transient dyskinesia induced by clebopride. Mov Dis 1993; 8: 125–126.

Masand P: Drug-induced oropharyngeal disturbances: stuttering and jaw myoclonus. J Clin Psychopharmacol 1992; 12: 444–445.

Mateos V, Caminal L, Colosia VP, et al: Parkinsonismo inducido por metoclopramida. Rev Clin Espanola 1993; 192: 200–201.

Mayeux R, Albert M, Jenike M: Physostigmine-induced myoclonus in Alzheimer's disease. Neurology 1987; 37: 345–6.

McCreadie RG, Thara R, Kamath S, et al: Abnormal movements in never-medicated Indian patients with schizophrenia. Br J Psychiatry 1996; 168(2): 221–226.

Meco G, Bonifati V, Fabrizio E, et al: Worsening of parkinsonism with fluvoxamine—two cases. Human Psychopharmacology: Clinical and Experimental 1994; 9: 439–441.

Meltzer HY, Ranjan R: Valproic acid in lthe treatmlent of clozapine-induced myoclonus. Am J Psychiatry 1994; 151: 1246–1247.

Melvin JA, Arana GW: Cognitive akathisia: Clinical and theoretical aspects. In Joseph AB, Young RR (Eds.): Movement disorders in neurology and psychiatry, Boston, Blackwell Scientific Publications, 1992, pp 100–105.

Merims D, Ziv I, Djaldetti R, et al: Riluzole for levodopa-induced dyskinesias in advanced Parkinson's disease. Lancet 1999; 353: 1764–5.

Meyer-Lindenberg A, Krausnick B: Tardive dyskinesia in a neuroleptic-naive patient with bipolar-1 disorder: persistent exacerbation after lithium intoxication. Mov Dis 1997; 12: 1108–1109.

Micheli EF, Fernandez Pardal M, Giannaula R, et al: Movement disorders and depression due to flunarizine and cinnarizine. Movement Disorders 1989; 4: 139–146.

Micheli F, Pardal MF, Gatto M, et al: Bruxism secondary to antidopaminergic drug exposure. Clin Neuropharmacol 1993; 16: 315–323.

Miller LG, Jankovic J: Metaclopramide-induced movement disorders. Clinical findings with a review of the literature. Arch Int Med 1989; 149: 2486–2492.

Milne IK: Akathisia associated with carbamazepine therapy. NZ Med J 1992; 105: 182.

Mintz U, Liberman UA: Parkinsonian syndrome due to cephaloridine. JAMA 1971; 216: 1200.

Mion CC, Andreason NC, Arndt S, et al: MRI abnormalities in tardive dyskinesia. Psychiatry Research Neuroimaging 1991; 40: 157–166.

Mitchell E, Matthews KL: Gilles de la Tourette's disorder associated with pemoline. Am J Psychiatry 1980; 137: 1618–1619.

Montagna P, Gabellini AS, Monari L, et al: Parkinsonian syndrome after along-term treatment with clebopride. Mov Dis 1992; 7: 89–90.

Montastruc JL, Rascol O, Senard JM, et al: Does initial bromocriptine treatment delay levodopa-induced motor complications in Parkinson's disease? A prospective randomized study. Neurology 1993; 43(suppl 2): S740.

Montplaisir J, Boucher S, Poirier G, et al: Clinical, polysomnographic, and genetic characteristics of restless legs syndrome: a study of 133 patients diagnosed with new standard criteria. Mov Dis 1997; 12: 61–65.

Morgante L, Rocca WA, De Rosa AE, et al: Prevalence of Parkinson's disease and other types of parkinsonism: a door-to-door survey in three Sicilian municipalities. The Sicilian Neuro-Epidemiology Study (SNES) Group. Neurology 1992; 42: 1901–1907.

Moss W, Ojukwu C, Chiriboga CA: Phenytoin-induced movement disorder. Clinical Pediatrics 1994; 33: 634–636.

Müller N: Exacerbation of tics following antidepressant therapy in a case of Gilles-de-la-Tourette syndrome. Pharmacopsychiatr 1992; 25: 243–244.

Müller T, Kuhn W, Pöhlau D, et al: Parkinsonism unmasked by lovastatin. Ann Neurol 1995; 37: 685–686.

Murray V: Laryngeal dystonia. Brit J Psychiatry 1995; 167: 698–699.

Nasrallah HA: Neurodevelopmental pathogenesis of schizophrenia. Psychiatr Clin North Am 1993; 16(2): 269–280.

Negrotti A, Calzetti S, Sasso E: Calcium entry blockers-induced parkinsonism: possible role of inherited susceptibitlity. Neurotoxicology 1992; 13: 261–264.

Neu J-P, Guilhot F, Boinot C, et al: Development of chorea with lupus anticoagulant after interferon therapy. Eur Neurol 1996; 235–236.

Neufeld MY, Vishnevska S: Vigabatrin and multifocal myoclonus in adults with partial seizures. Clin Neuropharmacol 1995; 18: 280–283.

Newman RP, Kinkel WR: Paroxysmal choreoathetosis related to hypoglycemia. Arch neurol 1984; 41: 341–342.

Nishikawa T, Tanaka M, Tsuda A, et al: Clonidine therapy for tardive dyskinesia and related syndromes. Clin Neuropharmacol 1984; 7: 239–245.

Nishimatsu O, Horiguchi J, Inami Y, et al: Periodic limb movement disorder in neuroleptic-induced akathisia. Kobe J Med Sci 1997; 43(5): 169–77.

Nishiyama K, Masuda N, Kurisaki H: A case of rabbit syndrome—its unique pharmacological feature. Rinsho Shinkeigaku 1993 Jun; 33(6): 663–5.

Nucci P, Brancato R: Oculogyric crisis after the Tensilon test. Graefes Arch Clin Exp Ophthalmol 1990; 228(4): 384–5.

Nutt JG: Levodopa-induced dyskinesia. Neurology 1990; 40: 340–345.

Ogawa N: Levodopa and dopamine agonists in the treatment of Parkinson's disease: advantages and disadvantages. Eur Neurol 1994; 34(suppl 3): 20–28.

Olive JM, Masana L, Gonzalez J: Meperidine and reversible parkinsonism. Movement Disorders 1994; 9: 115–116.

Olivera AA: A case of paroxetine-induced akathisia. Biological Psychiatry 1996; 39: 910.

Osser DN: Neuroleptic-induced pseudoparkinsonism. In Joseph AB, Young RR (Eds.): Movement disorders in neurology and psychiatry, Boston, Blackwell Scientific Publications, 1992, pp 70–80.

O'Sullivan RL, Greenberg DB: H_2 antagonists, restless leg syndrome, and movement disorders. Psychosomatics 1993; 34: 530–531.

Oterino A, Pascual J: Sumatriptan-induced axial dystonia in a patient with cluster headache. Cephalalgia 1998; 18: 360–361.

Ott BR, Lannon MC: Exacerbation of parkinsonism by tacrine. Clin Neuropharmacol 1992; 15: 322–325.

Padberg F, Stübner S, Buch K, et al: Pisa syndrome during treatment with sertindole. Brit J Psychiatry 1998; 173: 351–352.

Pande AC, Max P: A dystonic reaction occurring during treatment with tranylcypromine. J Clin Psychopharmacol 1989; 9: 229–230.

Pardo B, Mena MA, Fahn S, et al: Ascorbic acid protects against levodopa-induced neurotoxicity on a catecholamine-rich human neuroblastoma cell line. Mov Dis 1993; 8: 278–284.

Parmar MS: Akinetic mutism after baclofen. Ann Intern Med 1991 15; 115(6): 499–500.

Patterson JF: Amoxapine-induced chorea. South Med J 1983; 76: 1077-.

Pedro-Botet ML, Bonal J, Caralps A: Nifedipine and myoclonic disorders. Nephron 1989; 51: 281.

Peppe A, Dambrosia JM, Chase TN: Risk factors for motor response complications in L-dopa-treated parkinsonian patients. Adv Neurol 1993; 60: 698–702.

Peters HA: Lithium intoxication producing chorea athetosis with recovery. Wisconsin Medical Journal 1949; Dec: 1–2.

Petzinger G, Mayer SA, Przedborski S, et al: Fentanyl-induced dyskinesias. Mov Dis 1995; 10: 679–680.

Pfeiffer RF: Amantadine-induced vocal myoclonus. Mov Dis 1996; 11: 104–106.

Podskalny GD, Factor SA: Chorea caused by lithium intoxication: a case report and literature review. Mov Dis 1996; 11: 733–737.

Pollack MA, Cohen NL, Friedhoff AJ: Gilles de la Tourette's syndrome. Arch Neurol 1977; 34: 630–632.

Poyurovsky M, Schniedman M, Weizman A: Successful treatment of fluoxetine-induced dystonia with low-dose mianserin. Mov Dis 1997; 12: 1102–1105.

Pranzatelli MR, Albin RL, Cohen BH: Acute dyskinesias in young asthmatics treated with theophylline. Pediatr Neurol 1991; 7: 216–219.

Przedborski S, Jackson-Lewis V, Muthane U, et al: Chronic levodopa administration alters cerebral mitochondrial respiratory chain activity. Ann Neurol 1993; 34: 715–723.

Pujalte D, Bottai T, Hue B, et al: A double-blind comparison of clonazepam and placebo in treatment of neuroleptic-induced akathisia. Clinical Neuropharmacology 1994; 17: 236–242.

Putnam PE, Orenstein SR, Wessel HB, et al: Tardive dyskinesia associated with use of metoclopramide in a child. J Pediatr 1992; 121: 983–985.

Quinn AG, Ellis WR, Burn D, et al: Chorea precipitated by sulphasalazine. BMJ 1991; 302: 1025.

Radford JM, Brown TM, Borison RL: Unexpected dystonia while changing from clozapine to risperidone. J Clin Psychopharmacol 1995; 15: 225–226.

Reccoppa L, Welch WA, Ware MR: Acute dystonia and fluoxetine. J Clin Psychiatry 1990; 51: 487.

Reeves AL, So EL, Sharbrough FW, et al: Movement disorders associated with the use of gabapentin. Epilepsia 1996; 37(10): 988–990.

Reijneveld LB, Taphoorn MJB, Hoogenraad TU, et al: Severe but transient parkinsonism after tetanus vaccination. JNNP 1997; 63: 258.

Reutens DC, Stewart-Wynne EG: Norpethidine induced myoclonus in a patient with renal failure. J Neurol Neurosurg Psychiatry 1989; 52: 1450–1.

Richardson MA, Bevans ML, Weber JB, et al: Branched chain amino acids decrease tardive dyskinesia symptoms. Psychopharmacology (Berl) 1999; 143: 358–364.

Riddoch D, Jefferson M, Bickerstaff ER: Chorea and oral contraceptives. BMJ 1971; iv: 217.

Riley DE, Lang AE: The spectrum of levodopa-related fluctuations in Parkinson's disease. Neurology 1993; 43: 1459–1464.

Rittmannsberger H: Asterixis induced by psychotropic drug treatment. Clin Neuropharmacol 1996; 19(4): 349–355.

Robertson PL, Garofalo EA, Silverstein FS, et al: Carbamazepine-induced tics. Epilepsia 1993; 34: 965–968.

Robinson D, Omar SJ, Dangel C, et al: Metaclopramide-induced extrapyramidal symptoms in a diabetic patient. J Am Geriatr Soc 1994; 42: 1307–1308.

Rosebush PI, Kennedy K, Dalton B, et al: Protracted akathisia after risperidone withdrawal. Am J Psychiatry 1997; 154: 437–438.

Rosen PD, Stevens R: Action myoclonus in lithium toxicity. Ann Neurol 1983; 13: 221–222.

Rosenblum AM, Montgomery EB: Exacerbation of parkinsonism by methyldopa. JAMA 1989; 244: 2727–2728.

Ross RT: Drug-induced parkinsonism and other movement disorders. Can J Neurol Sci 1990; 17: 155–162.

Rothschild AJ, Locke CA: Reexposure to fluoxetine after serious suicide attempts by three patients: the role of akathisia. J Clin Psychiatry 1991; 52(12): 491–3.

Rubin DI, So EL: Reversible akinetic mutism possibly induced by baclofen. Pharmacotherapy 1999; 19(4): 468–470.

Rupniak NMJ, Marsden CD: Acute dystonia induced by neuroleptic drugs. Psychopharmacology 1986; 88: 403–419.

Sabaawi M, Fragala MR, Holmes TF: Drug-induced akathisia: subjective experience and objective findings. Military Medicine 1994; 159: 286–291.

Sabaawi M, Richmond DR, Fragala MR: Akathisia in association with nortriptyline therapy. Am Fam Phys 1993; 48: 1024–1026.

Sachdev P: Clinical characteristics of 15 patients with tardive dyskinesia. Am J Psychiatry 1993; 150: 498–500.

Sachdev P: Research diagnostic criteria for drug-induced akathisia: conceptualization, rationale and proposal. Psychopharmacology 1994; 114: 181–186.

Sachdev P: Tardive and chronically recurrent oculogyric crises. Mov Dis 1993; 8: 93–97.

Safferman AZ, Lieberman JA, Pollack S, et al: Akathisia and clozapine treatment. J Clin Psychopharmacol 1993; 13(4): 286–7.

Sanderson DR: Drug interaction between risperidone and phenytoin resulting in extrapyramidal symptoms. J Clin Psychiatry 1996; 57: 177.

Sandyk R, Anninos PA, Tsagas N: Magnetic fields in the treatment of Parkinson's disease. Intern J Neurosci 1992; 63: 141–150.

Sandyk R: Nalaxone withdrawal exacerbates Tourette's syndrome. J Clin Psychopharmacol 1986a; 6: 58–59.

Sandyk R: Oculogyric crisis induced by lithium carbonate. Eur Neurol 1984; 23(2): 92–94.

Sandyk R: Orofacial dyskinesias associated with lorazepam therapy. Clin Pharm 1986; 5: 419–421.

Sandyk R: Phenobarbital-induced Tourette-like symptoms. Pediatr Neurol 1996b; 2: 54–55.

Sasso E, Delsoldato S, Mancia D: Reversible parkinsonism induced by valproate (abstract). Epilepsia 1993; 34(suppl 2): 162.

Sasso E, Delsoldato S, Negrotti A, et al: Reversible valproate-induced extrapyramidal disorders. Epilepsia 1994; 35: 391–393.

Schneiderhan ME: Vitamin E in tardive dyskinesia. Ann Pharmacother 1993; 27: 311–313.

Schonecker M: Ein eigentümliches Syndrom im oralen Bereich bei megaphen Applikation. Nervenarzt 1957; 28: 35.

Schooler NR, Kane JM: Research diagnoses for tardive dyskinesia. Arch Gen Psychiatry 1982; 39(4): 486–7.

Schrodt GR, Wright JH, Simpson R, et al: Treatment of tardive dyskinesia with propranolol. J Clin Psychiatry 1982; 43: 328–331.

Schwartz M, Beny A, Sharf B: Risperidone-induced rabbit syndrome. Br J Psychiatry 1998; 173: 267–268.

Schwartz M, Moguillansky L, Lanyi G, et al: Sulpride in tardive dyskinesia. JNNP 1990; 53: 800–802.

Sempere AP, Duarte J, Garcia F, et al: An estimate of the risk of movement disorders associated with the chronic use of clebopride. Mov Disord 1996; 11(5): 582–583.

Sempere AP,Duarte J, Cabezas c, et al: Parkinsonism induced by Amlodipine. Movement Disorders 1995; 10: 115–116.

Shale H, Fahn S, Mayeux R: Tics in a patient with Parkinson's disease. Mov Dis 1986; 1: 79–83.

Shaunak S, Brown P, Morgan-Hughes JA: Exacerbation of idiopathic Parkinson's disease by naproxen. BMJ 1995; 422.

Shedlack KJ, Soldato-Couture C, Swanson CL: Rapidly progressive tardive dyskinesia in AIDS. Biol Psychiatry 1994; 35: 147–148.

Shihabuddin L, Rapport D: Sertraline and extrapyramidal side effects. Am J Psychiatry 1994; 151: 288.

Shriqui C, Jones B: Free radicals and tardive dyskinesia. Can J Psychiatry 1990; 35: 282–284.

Shriqui CL, Bradwejn J, Annable L, et al: Vitamin E in the treatment of tardive dyskinensia: a double-blind placebo-controlled study. Am J Psychiatry 1992; 1149: 391–393.

Shulman LM, Singer C, Weiner WJ: Phenytoin-induced focal chorea. Mov Disord 1996; 11(1): 111–114.

Singhi S, Singhi P, Singh I: Chloroquine-induced involuntary movements. BMJ 1977; no. 6085: 520.

Sirvent N, Monpoux F, Benet L, et al: Acute basal ganglia necrosis associated with cytarabine therapy. Medical and Pediatric Oncology 1998; 30: 308.

Skorin L Jr, Onofrey BE, DeWitt JD: Phenothiazine-induced oculogyric crisis. J Am Optom Assoc 1987; 58(4): 316–8.

Soman P, Jain S, Rajsekhar V, et al: Dystonia—a rare manifestation of carbamazepine toxicity. Postgrad Med J 1994; 70: 54–55.

Songer DA, Schulte HM: Withdrawal dyskinesia after abrupt cessation of clozapine and benztropine. J clin Psychiatry 1996; 57: 40.

Soto J, Sacristan JA, Alsar MJ, et al: Terfenadine-induced tremor. Ann Neurol 1993; 33: 226.

Spina E, Sturiale V, Valvo S, et al: Prevalence of acute dystonic reactions associated with neuroleptic treatment with and without anticholinergic prophylaxis. Int Clin Psychopharmacol 1993; 8: 21–24.

Stacy M, Jankovic J: Tardive tremor. Mov Disord 1992; 7: 53–57.

Steen VM, Lovlie R, MacEwan T, et al: Dopamine D_3-receptor gene variant and susceptibility to tardive dyskinesia in schizophrenic patients. Mol Psychiatry 1997; 2(2): 139–145.

Stephen PJ, Williamson J: Drug-induced parkinsonism in the elderly. Lancet 1984; ii: 1082–1083.

Steur EN: Increase of Parkinson disability after fluoxetine medication. Neurology 1993; 43: 211–213.

Stolarek IH, Ford MJ: Acute dystonia induced by midazolam and abolished by flumazenil. BMJ 1990; no. 6724: 614.

Strauss A: Oral dyskinesia associated with buspirone use in an elderly woman. J Clin Psychiatry 1988; 49: 322–323.

Stuart AM, Worley LM, Spillane J: Choreiform movements observed in an 8-year-old child following use of an oral theophylline preparation. Clin Pediatr 1992; 31: 692–694.

Suzuki T, Kurita H, Hori T, Sasaki M, et al: The Pisa syndrome (pleurothotonus) during antidepressant therapy. Biol Psychiatry 1997; 41(2): 234–236.

Sweeney BJ, Edgecombe J, Chrchill DR, et al: Choreoathetosis/ballismus associated with pentadimine-induced hypoglycemia in a patient with acquired immunodeficiency syndrome. Arch Neurol 1994; 51: 723–725.

Tanner CM, Klawans HL: Tardive dyskinesia: prevention and treatment. Clin Neuropharmacol 1986; 9(suppl 2): S76–S84.

Tanquary J: Case report: Akathisia responsive to bupropion. J Drug Dev 1993; 6: 69–70.

Terao T, Yoshimura R, Terao M, et al: Restless legs syndrome induced by psychotropics. Ann Clin Psychiatry 1992; 4: 127–130.

Teusink JP, Alexopoulos GS, Shamoian CA: Parkinsonian side effects induced by a monamine oxidase inhibitor. Am J Psychiatry 1984; 141: 118–119.

Thiel A, Dressler D: Dyskinesias possibly induced by norpseudoephedrine. J Neurol 1994; 241: 167–169.

Tilzey A, Heptonstall J, Hamblin T: Toxic confusional state and choreiform movements after treatment with anabolic steroids. BMJ 1981; 283: 349.

Touw DJ, Gernaat HBPE, Woude JVD: Parkinsonism after addition of fluoxetine to neuroleptic or carbamazepine medication. Ned Tidjschr Geneeskd 1992; 136: 332–334.

Trenkwalder C, Schwarz J, Gebhard J, et al: Starnberg trial on epidemiology of parkinsonism and hypertension in the elderly. Prevalence of Parkinson's disease and related disorders assessed by a door-to-door survey of inhabitants older than 65 years. Arch Neurol 1995; 52: 1017–1022.

Turner D: Diamorphine toxicity. Anesthesia 1992; 47: 168–169.

Tutuncuoglu S, Kantar M, Tekgul H, et al: Akinetic mutism due to diphenylhydantoin toxicity. Turk J Pediatr 1997; 39(3): 403–407.

Uchihara T, Tsukagoshi H: Myoclonic activity associated

with cefmetazole, with a review of neurotoxicity of cephalosporins. Clin Neurol Neurosurg 1988; 90: 369–371.

Ueyama K, Fukuzako H, Takeuchi K, et al: Brain atrophy and intellectual impairment in tardive dyskinesia. Jpn J Psychiat Neurol 1993; 47: 99–104.

Van Putten T, May PRA, Marder SR: Akathisia with haloperidol and thiothixene. Arch Gen Psychiatry 1984; 41: 1036–1039.

Vandel P, Bonin B, Leveque E, et al: Tricyclic antidepressant-induced extrapyramidal side effects. Eur Neuropsychopharmacol 1997; 7: 207–212.

Vidailhet M, Bonnet AM, Marconi R, et al: Do parkinsonian symptoms and levodopa-induced dyskinesias start in the foot. Neurology 1994; 44: 1613–1616.

Villeneuve A: The rabbit syndrome: a peculiar extrapyramidal reaction. Can Psychiatr Assoc J 1972; suppl 2: S669–S672.

Vincent FM: Asterixis after metrizamide myelography. JAMA 1980; 244: 2727.

Walker JM, Matsumoto MA, Bowen WD, et al: Evidence for the role of haloperidol-sensitive d-"opiate" receptors in the motor effects of antipsychotic drugs. Neurology 1988; 38: 961–965.

Warne RW, Gubbay SS: Choreiform movements induced by cholinergic therapy. Med J Austr 1979; i: 465.

Wasserstein PH, Honig LS: Parkinsonism during cyclosporine treatment. Bone Marrow Transplantation 1996; 18: 649–650.

Weimer S: Akathisia in a cancer patient treated with antiemetics. Am J Psychiatry 1995; 152: 960–961.

Werner EG, Olanow CW: Parkinsonism and amiodarone therapy. Ann Neurol 1989; 25: 630–632.

White PD: Myoclonus and episodal delirium associated with phenelzine: a case report (letter). J Clin Psychiatry 1987; 48: 340–341.

Wiener J, Kennedy S: Akinesia and mutism following a methylphenidate challenge test. J Clin Psychopharmacol 1985; 5(4): 231–3.

Wu RM, Chiu HC, Wang M, et al: Risk factors on the occurrence of response fluctuations and dyskinesias in Parkinson's disease. J Neural Transm 1993; 5: 127–133.

Wurtman R, Caballero B, Salzman E: Facilitation of levodopa-induced dyskinesias by dietary carbohydrates. NEJM 1988; 319: 1288–1289.

Wyllie ARJ, Bayliff CD, Kovacs MJ: Myoclonus due to chlorambucil in two adults with lymphoma. Ann Pharmacother 1997; 31: 171–174.

Yagi S, Moriya O, Nakajima M, et al: A case of tuberculous pleurisy associated with myoclonus and Quincke's edema due to isoniazid and isoniazid sodium methanesulfonate. Kekkaku 1989; 64: 407–412.

Yamadori A, Albert ML: Involuntary movement disorder caused by methyldopa. NEJM 1972; 285: 610.

Yassa R, Nair V, Iskander H: A comparison of severe tardive dystonia with severe tardive dyskinesia. Acta Psychiatr Scand 1989; 80: 155–189.

Yassa R, Nastase C, Dupont D, et al: Tardive dyskinesia in elderly psychiatric patients: a 5-year study. Am J Psychiatry 1992; 149: 1206–1211.

Yassa R: Tardive dyskinesia and anticholinergic drugs. A critical review of the literature. Encephale 1988; 14 Spec No: 233–9.

Zubenko GS, Cohen BM, Lipinski JFJr. Antidepressant-related akathisia. J Clin Psychopharmacol 1987; 7(4): 254–257.

Chapter 9
Drug-Induced Cerebrovascular Disorders

Introduction

The term "cerebrovascular disorders" (CVD) covers diseases of the brain resulting from pathological processes of the blood vessels and disturbances of cerebral blood flow (CBF). Intracerebral hemorrhage and subarachnoid hemorrhage due to rupture of cerebral arterial aneurysms are separate categories in addition to cerebral infarction which may be hemorrhagic or non-hemorrhagic. The term "stroke" is used to describe the sudden onset of neurological deficit due to disturbance of blood flow to the brain. The incidence of stroke varies from 50 to 200 cases per 1,000,000 population per year. There are numerous causes and risk factors for CVD. While stroke has a long history of documentation in medical literature, there are few reports of drug-induced stroke. One of the earlier reports was that of a 41-year old women who had an ischemic stroke while taking oral contraceptives (Lorentz 1962). Drugs are still among the rare causes of stroke but no figures are available for drug-induced CVD. The classification of drug-induced CVD is shown in Table 9.1. Various drugs that have been associated with CVD are shown in Table 9.2. Several of these are anecdotal case reports whereas others have an established association.

Table 9.1. Classification of drug-induced CVD.

Secondary to drug-induced cardiovascular disorders
 – Cardiac arrhythmias
 – Hypertension
 – Hypotension
Drug-induced reduction of cerebral blood flow
Drug-induced hemorrheological disturbances
Drug-induced cerebral vasculitis
Drug-induced vasoconstriction and vasospasm
Drug-induced thromboembolic disease
Drug-induced cerebral hemorrhage
Drug-induced intrauterine and perinatal cerebral hemorrhage
Drug-induced immunological disturbances

Table 9.2. Various drugs that have been associated with CVD.

Therapeutic substances
Allopurinol
Androgens
Anticoagulants*
Antineoplastic drugs*
β-blockers
Calcium channel blockers
Cytokines: interleukin-2 and interferons*
Decongestants containing pseudoephedrine
Epsilon-aminocaproic acid
Ergot derivatives*
Erythropoietin
Fenfluramine
Ginkgo biloba extract
Ginseng
Immunoglobulins
Isoretinoin (Amalfitano et al 1995)
Nicotine
Nitrates
Oral contraceptives*
Praziquantel for neurocysticercosis (Bang et al 1997)
Thrombolytics*

Diagnostics
Cerebral angiography
Radiologic contrast media
Pharmacologic stress-testing using adenosine perfusion
 imaging (Khan and Samual 1997)

Substance abuse
Alcohol
Drugs abuse*

* Indicates an established association.

Drug-Induced Cardiovascular Disturbances

It is beyond the scope of this book to cover various cardiovascular disturbances associated with drugs. This information can be obtained from standard texts on adverse drug reactions such that by Davies (1991). Only hypertension and hypotension will be mentioned here briefly.

Hypertension. Drug-induced hypertension is a major risk factor for stroke. A 5 to 6 mm Hg increase in diastolic blood pressure maintained over a few years may be associated with a 67% increase in total stroke risk (Johnson 1997). Several drugs can induce hypertension and those which are well known for this effect are: NSAIDs, erythropoietin, cyclosporin, corticosteroids, and sympathomimetic drugs (Thomas 1993). These may result in intracerebral hemorrhage. Subarachnoid hemorrhage and cardiac arrest occurred in a patient treated with subcutaneous epinephrine for an allergic reaction (Horowitz et al 1996). The patient had a blood pressure of 220/160 mm Hg and epinephrine is contraindicated at this level of blood pressure.

Hypotension. Drug-induced hypotension can be mediated by a fall in cardiac output or direct myocardial depression. It can be due to reduced venous return or decrease of peripheral resistance. Postural hypotension may occur due to effect of antihypertensive drugs or drug-induced polyneuropathy where there is impairment of neural control of peripheral vascular resistance and as fall in venous return due to muscle paralysis.

Postural hypotension may result in syncope (see Chapter 4) and the patient may recover consciousness promptly on lying down with no cerebrovascular sequelae. Sudden major fall of blood pressure may cause localized necrosis of the gray as well as the white matter at the boundary zones ("water sheds") between major arterial territories. Elderly subjects with atherosclerotic disease of cerebral arteries are liable to suffer a major stroke during a sustained hypotensive episode. Moderate but sustained hypotension may lead to diffuse neuronal loss in the cerebral cortex (Adams et al 1966).

In a Dutch study, 7% of the patients admitted to the hospital with strokes or transient ischemic attacks (TIA) had significant change in the antihypertensive or diuretic therapy over the previous three weeks (Jansen et al 1986). Symptoms of stroke have been noted after fall of BP on antihypertensive therapy. TIA has been reported with nitrates and nifedipine.

Although antihypertensive drugs protect the brain against harmful effects of prolonged hypertension, cerebral ischemia may occur during antihypertensive treatment under the following circumstances (Strandgaard 1987):

− Patients with malignant hypertension in the initial phase of treatment.

− Elderly hypertensive patients.

− Patients with acute stroke and high blood pressure.

− Patient with stenosis of functional cerebral arteries.

It is difficult to predict the risk of cerebral hypoperfusion due to antihypertensive medications in an individual patient (Fagan et al 1989). Because of the increasing evidence that patients with severe hypertension are particularly liable to ischemic brain damage due to regional or global reduction in cerebral perfusion pressure, attempts should be made to lower the pressure gradually in order to allow the cerebral circulation to recover its normal reactivity (Graham 1983).

Drug-Induced Reduction of Cerebral Blood Flow

Theophylline is known to reduce cerebral blood flow (CBF) in patients with chronic obstructive pulmonary disease (Bowton et al 1988). Aminophylline decreases CBF under hypoxic as well as normoxic conditions and, therefore, reduces oxygen delivery. Indomethacin has also been shown to decrease CBF and cognitive function (Hemler et al 1990).

Drug-Induced Hemorrheological Disturbances

Hemorrheological disturbances are an important cause of cerebrovascular disease. Several drug-induced hematological disturbances particularly those involving the elements of the blood can impair cerebral microcirculation. Of particular concern are drugs which produce proliferation of leucocytes or increase platelet aggregation. Increase in number of leucocytes in drug-induced leukemias may affect cerebral microcirculation or the leukemic blasts may compete for oxygen in the microcirculation and they may be invasive, damaging vessel wall (Lichtman and Rowe 1982). A critical factor is the deformability and size of the leucocytes. Total white blood counts in excess of 400,000/μL can be tolerated in chronic lymphoid leukemia if the cells are small and easily deformable (Ernst et al 1987). No adverse effects of leukocytosis on cerebral circulation are usually noted in total WBC of less than 100,000/μL. However, Prentice et al (1982) reported a two-fold increase in incidence of strokes if biannual leucocyte counts were > 10,000/μL.

Platelets can be affected by several drugs. The usual adverse effect of drugs is thrombocytopenia which would tend to lead to complications such as cerebral hemorrhage and thromboembolism. Heparin-induced thrombocytopenia occurs in approximately 1–2% of patients treated with heparin and leads to thromboembolic complications including stroke (Becker and Miller 1989). These are known complications in cancer patients on chemotherapy. Some of these patients are treated with granulocyte colony-stimulating factor (G-CSF) to counteract the neutropenia re-

sulting from chemotherapy. Strokes have been reported in these patients but the relationship to G-CSF is uncertain. However, it has been shown that G-CSF increases the serum levels of granulocyte elastase indicating highly activated leucocytes which can injure tissues (Iijima et al 1993). Thrombocytopenia is also known to occur in patients receiving G-CSF and platelet activation has been shown in human volunteers (Avenarius et al 1992). Platelets possess G-CSF receptors and G-CSF-augmented adenosine diphosphate induced platelet aggregation has been reported in vitro (Shimoda et al 1993a) as well as in human volunteers (Shimoda et al 1993b). This may occur in patients with severe chronic benign neutropenia who are on G-CSF therapy and do not have concomitant chemotherapy to produce thrombocytopenia.

Drug-Induced Cerebral Vasculitis

Central nervous system (CNS) may be involved secondary to systemic vasculitis. For example, subarachnoid hemorrhage and stroke have been reported in Henoch-Schönlein purpura (Lewis and Philpott 1956). Cerebral vasculitis may occur without any other systemic manifestations and it shares with other vasculitides the histologic features of inflammation and necrosis of blood vessels. Inflammatory process may be primary or secondary to other processes.

Pathomechanism. Vasculitis associated with drugs is usually "hypersensitivity vasculitis" but this is not an accurate description as immune mechanisms are involved in the pathogenesis of the condition. Hypersensitivity vas-

Table 9.3. Differentiation between primary and drug-induced vasculitis (Modified from Glick et al 1987).

Feature	Drug-induced	Primary
Vessels involved	Small arteries	Arteries and veins
Predominant cellular infiltrate	Polymorphonuclear leucocytes	Lymphocytes, monocytes
Giant cells	None	Characteristic
Granulomas	None	Characteristic
Necrosis	Marked	Moderate
Vessel wall involvement	Marked	Moderate
	Intimal	Adventitial

culopathy can be considered as an explanation of acute neurological deficits resulting from administration of drugs which normally do not affect the cerebral blood vessels. Two cases have been described of neurological deficits following carbamazepine therapy where lymphocyte proliferation test suggested a hypersensitivity reaction to carbamazepine (McIntyre et al 1994). A case of cerebral vasculitis with neurological deficits was described following treatment of metastatic renal cancer with interleukin (Michel et al 1995). This resolved following treatment with prednisolone. Asymptomatic cerebral vasculitis has been associated with allopurinol therapy. Only one case report describes a stroke associated with an immune-complex-mediated reaction to allopurinol (Rothwell and Grant 1996). It is possible to distinguish drug-induced vasculitis from primary CNS vasculitis (Table 9.3).

Cerebral Vasoconstriction and Vasospasm

- *Vasoconstriction.* Arterial hypertension has been considered as a factor in etiology of cerebral vasoconstriction due to ergot alkaloids but vasculitis appears to be a more likely mechanism.
- *Drug-induced vasospasm.* Vasospasm of the middle cerebral artery, verified by angiography, has been reported in a patient with Guillain-Barré syndrome following treatment with intravenous immunoglobulin (Voltz et al 1996). The spasm and neurological deficit resolved following treatment.

Clinical Manifestations. The clinical effects of tissue ischemia in cerebral vasculature vary but the symptoms may be transient or prolonged and strokes are a frequent complication (Moore and Cupps 1983). Vasculitis is a major pathology in patients who present with stroke due to drug abuse. This is dealt with in more detail in the section on drug abuse.

Cerebral vasculitis has been reported as an adverse effect of therapeutic drugs or drug abuse (Table 9.4).

Table 9.4. Drugs associated with cerebral vasculitis.

Therapeutic and diagnostic pharmaceuticals
Allopurinol
Amphetamine*
Ergot alkaloids
Ephedrine
Ginseng (Ryu and Chien 1995)
Iapamidol as contrast agent for myelography
Interleukin-2
Oxymetazole
Penicillin
Phenylpropanolamine
Pseudoephedrine
Sympathomimetic drugs
Tacrolismus (Pizzolato et al 1998)
Vaccine: hepatitis B (Le Hello et al 1999)

Drug abuse
Cocaine
Heroin
Methylphenidate
Pentozocine
Phencyclidine
Sympathomimetic drugs*

* Used therapeutically but also abused.

Cerebral Vasculitis Associated with Therapeutic Drugs. The following drugs have been reported to induce cerebral vasculitis and in some publications it is referred to as cerebral angiopathy.
- *Allopurinol.* This drug was reported to produced cerebral vasculitis and seizures in a case but the patient recovered following discontinuation of the drug (Weiss et al 1978).
- *Ergot Alkaloids.* Ergonovine is an ergot alkaloid derivative used for control of postpartum hemorrhage. Baringarrementeria et al (1992) reported a case of postpartum cerebral angiopathy due to ergonovine and have reviewed seven similar cases from literature. Two cases of stroke with seizures have been reported following the use of bromocriptine (another ergot derivative) for suppression of lactation (Katz et al 1985). A case of cerebral vasculitis was reported in a 20-year old woman 10 days after start of bromocriptine to suppress lactation (Janssens et al 1995). She presented with headaches and seizures but no hypertension. Cerebral angiography showed the typical beaded appearance of cerebral arteries. She was treated with heparin and steroids and re-

covered in 3 months. Three other cases of cerebral vasculitis (confirmed by angiography) due to bromocriptine therapy in the postpartum period have been reported and all the patients recovered after discontinuation of the drug (Lucas et al 1996).

– *Iapamidol.* May et al (1994) reported the case of a patient without previous cerebral problems who developed loss of consciousness and hemiplegia following iapamidol myelography. Vasculitis was identified on cerebral angiography and multiple cerebral infarcts were identified on MRI.

– *Penicillin* can produce allergic vasculitis (Popper et al 1978).

– *Phenylpropanolamine* (PPA) is a nasal vasoconstrictor. Le Coz et al (1988) reported two patients who developed cerebral vasculitis after daily use of this drug. Intracerebral hemorrhage developed in one of the patients but both recovered after discontinuation of the drug and radiographic evidence of vasculitis disappeared. Another case of cerebral hemorrhage has been reported but it is not known if it was associated with vasculitis (Thompson et al 1998).

Structurally and functionally PPA is similar to amphetamine. Adolescents are a particularly susceptible group influenced by its action as an anorexiant. Forman et al (1989) reviewed 10 cases in literature and presented an eleventh case of PPA-associated intracerebral hemorrhage with cerebral vasculitis following ingestion of an overdose of diet-aid pills.

The possible pathomechanisms of cerebrovascular accidents following PPA are as follows:

– Rise of blood pressure
– Arterial spasm
– Immuno-allergic vasculitis
– Direct toxic effect of PPA on arterial wall

Drug-Induced Thromboembolic Disease

Several drugs produce disturbances of blood coagulation and produce cerebral infarction by thromboembolism. The main categories of drugs are oral contraceptives and antineoplastic drugs

which will be discussed in separate sections. The same drugs may also produce other types of stroke as well.

Drug-Induced Cerebral Hemorrhage

The most important drugs in this categories are anticoagulants and thrombolytics which are discussed in separate sections. Cerebral hemorrhage may also occur due to thrombocytopenic effect of drugs as well as due to drug-induced hypertension. Cerebral hemorrhage associated with anticoagulant therapy is well documented.

Intrauterine Fetal Cerebral Hemorrhage

β-sympathomimetic agents are commonly used in an attempt to delay preterm delivery which is associated with periventricular hemorrhage as a complication. In a retrospective study of 2827 women in a multicenter pre-term birth prevention trial, β-sympathomimetic tocolysis was found to be associated with more than two-fold increase in the incidence of neonatal periventricular hemorrhage (Groome et al 1992).

β-sympathomimetic tocolysis may exert a number of effects on the fetal cardiovascular system which may predispose the premature infant to periventricular and intraventricular hemorrhages. The immature preterm brain is not well protected by autoregulation against the fluctuations in blood pressure. An increase in mean arterial blood pressure and a redistribution of the fetal cardiac output in favor of the upper body may place a premature infant at risk of periventricular-intraventricular hemorrhage after initiation of β-sympatholytic tocolysis.

Neonatal Intracranial Hemorrhage

Spontaneous hemorrhage into the cerebral ventricles is relatively common in premature infants. As many as 55% of infants with birth weight under 1500 g have periventricular-intraventricular hemorrhage detected by computerized tomography or echoencephalography. The exact cause of such hemorrhage is not known but it is multifactorial. The role of drugs in the causation of neonatal hemorrhages will be described by using examples from the maternal use of drugs as well as drugs given to the newborn.

Maternal Use of Drugs. The following drugs used during pregnancy have been reported to be associated with bleeding disorders in the neonate:

– *Anticoagulant therapy (coumarins).* Use of these drugs in pregnancy has been associated with cerebral hemorrhage and hydrocephalus in the infant (Pohl and Kornhuber 1966).

– *Aspirin.* Maternal use of aspirin has been reported to be associated with an increase in incidence of cerebral hemorrhage in the neonate (Rumack et al 1981). There is controversy about the methodology of this study and further studies are needed (Soller and Stander 1981; Corby 1981).

– *Antiepileptic drugs (AEDs).* Relation of maternal use of AED to neonatal hemorrhage has been examined by Moslet and Hansen (1992). These authors reviewed reported cases of neonatal cerebral hemorrhage where the mothers were treated by at least one AED of the hydantoin type or a derivative of barbituric acid which are hepatic enzyme inducers or by polytherapy. One case of neonatal subdural hematoma was reported as a result of in utero exposure to phenobarbital and the patient was treated successfully by drainage of the hematoma, fresh frozen plasma and an intravenous preparation of vitamin K (Renzulli et al 1998). The incidence of such hemorrhages was markedly reduced in those cases where oral vitamin K was given to the mother prior to delivery. The authors made the following recommendations:

  · Vitamin K tablets should be given to the epileptic mother on AED during the last month of pregnancy and phytomenadione should be given intravenously to the infant immediately after birth.

  · Cord blood specimens should be submitted for clotting studies and if diminished vita-

min K-dependent factors are found, fresh frozen plasma should be given to the infant.

  · Alternatively, the AED treatment of the pregnant epileptic women should be changed to non-enzyme inducing AED such as clonazepam.

Drugs Administered to the Infant. The following drugs have been reported to produce cerebral hemorrhage in the neonate.

– *Heparin.* This is often used to maintain the patency of catheters for vascular access placed in the umbilical arteries of premature infants. Routine use of heparin in neonatal intensive care units is associated with a fourfold increase in the risk of periventricular-intraventricular hemorrhage (Lesko et al 1986).

– *Benzyl alcohol.* This is a bacteriostatic agent, is used to flush intravascular catheters. The volume of alcohol is significantly related to the development of kernicterus and intraventricular hemorrhage and the use of this substance is not recommended (Jardine and Rogers 1989).

– *Sodium bicarbonate.* This substance, when administered in excess to neonates, with or without hypernatremia, may place them at greater risk of intracranial hemorrhage (Simmons et al 1974; Volpe 1974). Hypertonic loads of saline built up in the administration of sodium bicarbonate to correct acidosis in infants with respiratory distress syndrome can precipitate intraventricular hemorrhage (Reichert and Fuller 1980).

Drug-Induced Immunological Disturbances

Phenothiazines such as chlorpromazine can induce immunological disturbances such as lupus anticoagulant which can result in thromboembolic events such as stroke. Another neuroleptic, haloperidol has been reported to be associated with stroke in patient and the presence of lupus anticoagulant was confirmed (Laugharne et al 1994).

Drug Abuse

Drug abuse is recognized to be a cause of stroke but there is limited information of drug abuse in patients who present with stroke. Up to half of all strokes in patients younger than 45 years of age may be associated with the use of recreational drugs. History of drug abuse was obtained in 11 (19.5%) of 116 stroke patients entered in Maryland Stroke Data Bank during one year from 1988 to 1989 (Sloan et al 1991). Drugs usually implicated are heroin, amphetamines, methylphenidate, phencyclidine, and cocaine.

Pathomechanism of Stroke in Drug Abuse. The following mechanisms have been reviewed by Caplan et al (1982):

- *Endocarditis*, common in addicts, is a well known cause of stroke.
- *Direct toxic injury to blood vessels* is an uncommon mechanism of stroke in drug addicts. Rarely a drug is injected into the carotid artery instead of the jugular vein.
- *Embolization of foreign matter*. Most of the drug substances injected by the addicts contain contaminants in the form of particulate foreign matter. This produces a granulomatous reaction with obliteration of the pulmonary arterioles leading to pulmonary hypertension which opens functional arteriovenous shunts. When the lungs cease to be efficient filters, intravenously injected particulate matter can be released into the systemic circulation and may block the cerebral arteries. such particulate matter has been identified in the cerebral arteries but does not appear to be the cause of intracerebral and subarachnoid hemorrhages in drug abusers.
- *Pharmacologically mediated vascular changes*. Amphetamine, methylphenidate, and cocaine share the potential for altering vascular tone. By preventing the uptake of sympathomimetic neurotransmitter by nerve terminals, cocaine sensitizes the end organ response of vessels to epinephrine and norepinephrine. Although cocaine is postulated to produce peripheral vasoconstriction, it produces vasodilatation of cat cerebral arteries when applied locally. This appears to be mediated by mechanisms that depend on the stimulation of β-adrenergic receptors (Dohi et al 1990). The diagnosis of vasculitis produced by cocaine has been documented in a patient by biopsy (Fredericks et al 1991).
- *Immunological mechanism*. This is a more common and universal mechanism of vascular injury and according to Caplan et al (1982), the clinical evidence for this is delay in onset after injection and there is abstinence for a period before reintroduction of the drug. The laboratory evidence for it is as follows:
  - Eosinophilia
  - Elevated γ globulins and immune globulins
  - Angiographically documented polyarteritis-like lesions
  - Lymph node hypertrophy
  - Morphine binding to γ globulin fraction
  - Positive Coombs test
- *Intracerebral hemorrhage* may occur due to rupture of pre-existing intracranial cerebrovascular malformations (McEnvoy et al 1998).

Heroin. There are several case reports of cerebral infarction in addicts who use intravenous heroin (Brust and Richter 1976). This may follow the injection immediately or 6 to 24 hours later. Angiography has shown narrowing of the internal carotid arteries and beading of the small intracranial arteries in these cases.

Amphetamines. Amphetamine-associated stroke is heterogeneous clinically, pathologically and etiologically (Heye and Hankey 1996). In contrast to heroin, these drugs cause intracerebral and subarachnoid hemorrhages. Nearly half of the reported cases have followed oral use of the drug. Delaney and Estes (1980) described one case of cerebral vasculitis due to amphetamine and reviewed 14 others from the literature. In 4 of these cases vasculitis was demonstrated by cerebral angiography and in 2 cases at autopsy. Cerebral hemorrhage in these cases was considered to be due to either vasculitis or amphetamine-related hypertension. Pathology of amphetamine-related vasculitis has been well defined. There is fibrinoid necrosis of the media and intima of medium sized cerebral arteries with leucocytic infiltration. In late stages muscular and elastic tissue is replaced by collagen. Angiography shows beaded arteries and segmental changes in vessel caliber. In an experimental study by Rumbaugh et al (1971), rhesus monkeys were given intravenous amphetamine in the same dose range as in human addicts for two weeks and then they were sacrificed. In the acute phase angiography showed vasospasm of the cerebral arteries and at autopsy there was brain swelling and focal areas of ischemia and infarction.

Amphetamine-induced vasculitis has been reported to respond to prednisone in two cases with improvement in clinical and angiographic features (Salanova and Taubner 1984; Yu et al 1983).

Methylphenidate. Tablets of this substance are occasionally injected intravenously by drug abusers and strokes have been reported following this. Talc and corn starch content of the tablets is seen as emboli to the retinal vessels by ophthalmoscopy.

Phencyclidine (PCP, Angel dust). This substance can lead to hypertensive encephalopathy.

Ephedrine. Ephedrine is a direct α- and β-sympathetic agonist and an indirect adrenoreceptor agonist. It releases norepinephrine from synaptic as well as sympathetic neurons and acts as a CNS stimulant. Ischemic as well as hemorrhagic strokes has been reported after abuse of ephedrine with typical changes of vasculitis as seen on cerebral angiography (Wooten et al 1983; Conci et al 1988). Bruno et al (1993) reported ephedrine-related stroke in 3 patients. One had a thalamic infarct after ingesting a large amount of ephedrine for weight loss. Two patients had fatal intracerebral hemorrhage after ingestion of unknown amounts of ephedrine. Only one of these patients who had cerebral vasculitis, also had a history of drug abuse. The other patient who did not have a history of drug abuse was found to have hemorrhage from an arteriovenous malformation.

Pentazocine (Talwin) and Tripelenamine (Ts and Blues). Intravenous abusers of "Ts and blues" can have cerebral infarction independent of infective endocarditis. The ischemia can result from vasculitis or toxic effects of the drug (Caplan 1982).

Lysergic Acid Diethylamide (LSD). This is an amine derivative of the ergot alkaloids which are potent vasoconstricting agents. Lieberman et al (1974), reviewed previous reports and described a case of a young woman who developed hemiplegia after ingestion of LSD and angiography showed constriction and later occlusion of the carotid siphon.

Cocaine. This substance may be inhaled or injected subcutaneously, intramuscularly, or intravenously. Association of cocaine with vasculitis and cerebral infarction is well known (Levine and Welch 1988). Angiographic appearance is similar to that seen in vasculitis associated with amphetamine use (Fredericks et al 1991). Cases of biopsy-proven cerebral vasculitis associated with cocaine abuse have been reported (Krendel et al 1990; Fredericks et al 1991; Case Records of the Massachusetts General Hospital 1993). Cocaine administration induced dose-related cerebral vasoconstriction has been demonstrated by MRI angiography (Kaufman et al 1998). These changes occurred at low doses and in the absence of other risk factors such as polydrug abuse. Outcome stratification by previous drug users indicates that cocaine may have a cumulative residual effect on inducing cerebrovascular dysfunction. Cocaine-related cerebral hemorrhage is due to cocaine-induced hypertension rather than vasculitis as shown in autopsy studies (Nolte et al 1996).

Since the introduction of the free base cocaine known as "crack," the number of cocaine-related strokes (cerebral infarcts) has been increasing steadily. A 3-year prospective study of over 30,000 admissions to an inner city emergency hospital in Detroit revealed 33 patients (3% of total 979 cocaine related admissions) who had an acute stroke (infarct or hemorrhage) related to cocaine abuse (Peterson et al 1991). Klonoff et al (1989) reviewed 47 patients (mean age 32.5 years) with stroke related to cocaine. Intracranial aneurysms and arteriovenous malformations were present in 17 of the 32 patients studied angiographically or at autopsy. Cerebral vasculitis was present in two patients, intracranial hemorrhage occurred in 22 (49%), subarachnoid hemorrhage in 13 (29%), and cerebral infarction in 10 (22%). There is an unusually high incidence of intracranial aneurysms and vascular malformations in this series. Cocaine-related strokes occur primarily in the young adult. A thorough history of the use of cocaine and toxicological screening of urine and serum should be part of the evaluation of young patients with stroke (Levine et al 1990).

Marijuana. In contrast to other drugs mentioned above, stroke has been reported only rarely with the use of marijuana. Two cases of cerebral infarction in young men who smoke marijuana heavily were investigated and were postulated to be due to vasospasm associated with fluctuation in blood pressure caused by marijuana (Zachariah 1991).

Oral Contraceptives and Cerebrovascular Disorders

Since Lorentz (1962) described a 41-year old women who had an ischemic stroke while taking oral contraceptives (OC), considerable evidence has accumulated in the published literature of association between oral contraceptives and cerebrovascular diseases CVD). The following types of CVD have been reported:
- Cerebral arterial occlusive disease with hemorrhagic or non-hemorrhagic infarction.
- Subarachnoid hemorrhage
- Miscellaneous vascular lesions: Superior sagittal sinus thrombosis, bilateral carotid artery occlusion, vasculitis, dural arteriovenous fistula.

Epidemiological Studies on the Relation of OC to Stroke. A retrospective study by Inman and Vessey (1968) showed that OC are a cause of cerebral thrombosis and pulmonary thromboembolism in the absence of predisposing factors. Their data suggested an yearly incidence of stroke of 1:10,000 in women on OC. Around this time several other reports linked OC to stroke (Hutchinson and McCall 1968; Hunt and Sutherland 1968; Jennett 1969; Heyman et al 1969). McFarland (1970) reported regression of cerebral arterial lesions after cessation of OC.

The Collaborative Group for the Study of Stroke in Young Women (1973) estimated that the risk of thrombotic stroke is increased about two-fold in women using OC. In a study from UK, death rate from diseases of the circulatory system in women who had used oral contraceptives was five times that of controls who had never used them, and the death rate in those who had taken the pill continuously for five years was more than ten times that of controls (Royal College of General Practitioner's Oral Contraceptive Study 1977). In the Boston Collaborative Drug Surveillance Program (Jick et al 1978) the relative risk estimate for stroke among OC users compared with non-users was 26 (lower 90% one-sided confidence bound = 7.0). Conclusions of the Walnut Creek Contraceptive Drug Study (Ramachandaran et al 1980) about CVD were:
- Subarachnoid hemorrhage was positively associated with OC use both past and current. This risk was increased in smokers.
- The risk of cerebral thrombosis (stroke) or ischemic cerebrovascular disease was not increased in OC users who never smoked.

The reduced risk of stroke in more recent studies may be due to lowering of the estrogen content of the pills. Vessey et al (1984) observed no stroke among women using low estrogen ($< 50\,\mu g$) in the Oxford Family Planning Association Prospective Study.

Lidegaard (1998) analyzed the mortality of CVD in Denmark for men and women 15–44 years of age in a 14-year period before and after the appearance of OC in 1966. Women showed a 33% rise in deaths from cerebral thromboembolism while men showed a 14% fall.

A number of subsequent investigations failed to demonstrate a risk in former smokers or those who had ever used the pill (Stampfer et al 1988; Vessey et al 1969; Thorogood et al 1992). A nested case-control analysis of the data collected during the Royal College of General Practitioners Oral Contraception Study was performed by Hannaford et al (1994). A significant doubling of all stroke risk was observed in current users of OCs—both smokers as well as non-smokers. Former users had a small non-significant elevation in risk of all stroke but a stronger risk of fatal event. The effect in former smokers was restricted to women who smoked.

The risk estimates in more recent studies are lower. An international, multicenter, case control study about the ischemic stroke and combined oral contraceptives concluded that the risk of ischemic stroke is low in women of reproductive age and any risk attributable to OCs is small (WHO Collaborative Study of Cardiovascular Disease and Steroid Hormone Contraception 1996a). The risk can be further reduced, if users are younger than 35 years of age, do not smoke, and do not have a history of hypertension. The risk of hemorrhagic stroke attributable to OC use is not increased in younger women and is only slightly increased in older women (WHO Collaborative Study of Cardiovascular Disease and Steroid Hormone Contraception 1996b). The relative risk of thrombotic stroke among users of OCs compared with non-users is about 1.5 and does not change with increasing age (Lidegaard 1993). The absolute risk, on the other hand, increases near exponentially with increasing age. For a 20-year old healthy woman, the absolute risk of a cerebral thrombosis is about 2 per 100,000 individuals per year. In a study conducted in Washington State, USA, the odds ratios for hemorrhagic stroke was elevated to 3.28 (95% CI 1.27–8.57) compared with patients who were not current users of OCs (Schwartz et al 1997). According to a European matched case-control study, there is a small relative risk of occlusive stroke for women of reproductive age who currently use oral contraceptives and first generation oral contraceptives seem to be associated with a higher risk (Heinemann et al 1998).

With the conflicting reports from several well controlled studies, it is difficult to give a definite statement about the risk of stroke in a women on OCs. There is adequate evidence that there is no increased risk of stroke with low dose OCs. The hormonal content of estrogens and progesterone as well as the background diseases have a bearing on the risk for stroke.

Pathophysiology of Stroke in Relation to OC. Irey et al (1978) found vascular lesions in the form of intimal hyperplasia with and without associated thrombus in the cerebral arteries of young women who developed strokes while taking OC and died. Combined OCs increase the production of factor X, factor II, and plasminogen; decrease the production of antithrombin; and increase platelet aggregation by reducing the production of prostacyclin (Mammen 1982). Estrogens used in OC have effects on the laboratory measures of clotting such as fibrinogen, factor VII, and antithrombin III but the effect is difficult to translate into clinical risk of vascular events (Psaty et al 1993). It has been hypothesized that OCs, somehow, make cerebral vasculature more prone to aneurysm formation and rupture.

It is interesting compare the OC with the use of estrogen replacement therapy in postmenopausal women. Thompson et al (1989), in a case-controlled study of women with myocardial infarction or stroke, found no evidence that the use of hormone replacement therapy contributes a major cardiovascular risk or benefit. Hormone replacement therapy with potent estrogens alone or cyclically combined with progestins can, when started shortly after menopause, reduce the risk of stroke (Falkeborn et al 1993).

Risk Factors for Stroke in Women on OC. Risk factors for stroke in patients on OCs which been identified in various studies are shown in Table 9.5. Stroke in young women and it should not be ascribed to OC unless other possible causes are excluded.

– *Smoking*. This is clearly identified as increasing the risk in most of the studies.
– *Hypertension*. Combined OCs can cause hypertension in about 4–5% of normotensive women and increase blood pressure in about 9–16% of women with existing hypertension (Russell and Sullivan 1970). Malignant hypertension has been reported in two women secondary to the use of low dose oral contraceptives (Bortolotto et al 1994). Both improved after discontinuation of OCs. Start of OC in a previously hypertensive woman can increase the risk of hemorrhagic stroke.
– *Migraine*. It is generally accepted that migraine is aggravated by OCs (see Chapter 6). The Collaborative Group for the Study of

Table 9.5. Risk factors for stroke in women on OC.

Age over 35
Hypertension
Insulin dependent diabetes mellitus
Migraine
Previous history of thromboembolic disease
Smoking

Stroke in Young Women (1975) reported that "our data do not support previous reports suggesting that migraine may increase the risk of stroke in women using OCs." However, women with focal migraine (symptoms localized to one side of the head) and associated with a major "aura" or hemiparesis should not use the combined pill since there is a risk of localized cerebrovascular occlusion (Fraser 1993).

Subarachnoid Hemorrhage (SAH). Inman (1979) conducted a case control study of deaths from SAH in women aged 15–44 in UK. There was a small excess of deaths among those who used OCs as compared to healthy controls but this was not statistically significant. SAH was not considered to be a serious cause for concern in healthy non-hypertensive women using OCs.

A critical review of the literature by Auff et al (1986) indicates that the incidence of SAH is increased in women taking OCs and that the mortality is higher. In a 10-year follow-up study (1970–79) of middle-aged Swedes, Lidegaard et al (1987) found that the prevalence rate of SAH was 2.8 times higher in the females than in the males. This was considered to mainly due to an accumulation of non-hypertensive aneurysmal SAH in women born in the period 1932–40 who used high-estrogen content OC.

Miscellaneous Cerebrovascular Lesions in Women Taking OCs. The following have been reported:

- *Superior Sagittal Sinus Thrombosis.* This is a rare but well recognized clinical and pathological entity. The cause can be determined in most of the cases. The result is cerebral infarction, cerebral edema, and seizures. Sudden occlusion of the whole length of the sinus may be fatal. There are several reports of superior sagittal sinus thrombosis in women on OCs (Atkinson et al 1970; Buchanan and Brazinsky 1970; Sissons and Hall 1970; Dindar and Platts 1974; Piper and Mathias 1989). In contrast to the arterial thrombotic stroke, the risk of cerebral venous sinus thrombosis is in-

creased with the third generation OCs (de Bruijn et al 1998).
- *Bilateral internal carotid artery occlusion* has been described in a young woman (Mandel and Strimmel 1969). This is more rare than unilateral carotid occlusion in a young adult.
- *Carotid dural arteriovenous fistula* has been reported in a case and was postulated to be due to estrogen-induced vasodilatation of the arteries (Donaldson and Ramsey 1983).

Conclusions Regarding OC and Stroke. The combined relative risk of mortality from stroke in women using OC in three major studies (Royal College of General Practitioners, Walnut Creek, and Oxford Family Planning Association) was calculated to be 2.5 (Vecchia et al 1990). OCs were the main cause of 20% increase in mortality in users as compared with non-users. The knowledge gained from earlier epidemiological studies partly contributed to the reduction in the frequency of stroke with modern low estrogen-content OCs. There is paucity of data with newer pills due to this decreased incidence and there is difficulty in conducting studies with acceptable statistical power.

The evidence from these epidemiological studies supports the contention that oral contraceptives are *associated* with stroke but the question whether they *cause* stroke is less settled (Longstreth and Swanson 1984). These studies have identified other risk factors such as hypertension and smoking whose control could prevent more deaths due to vascular disease than could be prevented by limiting the use of oral contraceptives. Use of OC should be avoided in women over 35 with risk factors and those over 44 even without risk factors.

Strokes in women on OCs are sometimes preceded by transient neurological symptoms such as paresthesias or weakness of limbs and the preparation should be stopped at once under these circumstances (Kjaer et al 1971). Gschwend (1976) suggested the use of aspirin not exceeding 1 G/day to prevent the embolic complications of OCs but this hypothesis has never been tested.

Antineoplastic Agents and Cerebrovascular Disorders

Vascular complications associated with antineoplastic agents are being reported with increasing frequency Cerebrovascular events are most common after cisplatin based chemotherapy (Martinez et al 1992; Doll et al 1986a; Goldhirsch et al 1983). Strokes have been reported after use of combination of chemotherapeutics and some examples are:

– Vinblastine, bleomycin, and cisplatin (Samuels et al 1987; Kukla et al 1982)
– Cisplatin and 5-fluorouracil (El Amrani et al 1998)
– Carboplatin and cyclophosphamide (Ikeda et al 1999)
– Aspariginase, vincristine, daunorubicin and prednisolone (Lim et al 1998)

Patients with breast cancer receiving multiagent chemotherapy are at risk for developing stroke than expected in a general group of women not receiving chemotherapy (Wall et al 1989). Dural sinus thrombosis has been reported in two patients with breast cancer; one treated with L-asparaginase and the other with medroxyprogesterone acetate (Matsumo et al 1992). The pathophysiology of thrombosis in women with breast cancer treated with chemohormonal therapy is poorly understood.

Other chemotherapeutic agents have also been reported to be associated with CVD. A case of cerebral infarction has been reported following 5-FU therapy (Gandia et al 1992). A stroke-like syndrome with white matter hypodense lesions seen on MRI has also been reported in cancer patients treated with methotrexate (Borgna-Pignatti et al 1992; Follezou et al 1993). Pectasides et al (1992) reported eight patients who developed cerebrovascular accidents after various hormono-chemotherapeutic regimens. None of these patients had any other significant risk factor for stroke except malignancy.

Pathomechanism of CVD in Chemotherapy for Cancer. Possible mechanisms of cerebrovascular disturbances due to antineoplastic agents have been reviewed by Doll et al (1986b) and are shown in Table 9.6. More than one of these

Table 9.6. Possible mechanisms of cerebrovascular disorders due to antineoplastic agents

Drug-induced endovascular damage
Disturbances of clotting mechanism
Platelet activation
Abnormalities of thromboxane-prostacyclin homeostasis
Autonomic dysfunction
Vasculitis
Stimulation of fibroblasts

mechanisms may be operative in an individual patient.

Coagulation disorders are a common occurrence in patients with cancer and of cytotoxic drugs have a procoagulant potential (Walsh et al 1992). Pihko et al (1993) reported that 9 out of 90 children treated for acute lymphoblastic leukemia or non-Hodgkin's lymphoma had visual hallucinations and seizures following chemotherapy. Brain imaging studies revealed cortical and subcortical white matter lesions in watershed areas of major cerebral arteries suggesting ischemia as the cause. The lesions resolved after discontinuation of the chemotherapy.

Anticoagulants and Stroke

Both hemorrhagic and thromboembolic complications have been reported in patients on anticoagulant therapy for cardiac indications. A non-hemorrhagic cerebral infarct may convert to a hemorrhagic infant after anticoagulant therapy.

Intracerebral Hemorrhage. Bleeding complications are an inherent risk of anticoagulation (AC) treatment and most of the fatal bleedings are intracerebral (Landefeld and Goldman 1989). The incidence of spontaneous intracerebral hemorrhage in various reports varies from 9 to 23% (Wintzen et al 1984). Fogelholm et al (1992) reported that 14.2% of 288 stroke patients with primary intracerebral hemorrhage were on AC treatment at the onset of stroke. The estimated age-adjusted odds ratio of being on AC treatment at the time of intracerebral hemorrhage was 6.7%. The cause of fatality rate during the first week and mortality during the follow-up of 32 months were slightly higher, the functional outcome being slightly worse in the AC group. Anticoagulant therapy is used as a treatment for CVD and may increase the risk of hemorrhagic transformation (Cerebral Embolism Study Group 1987).

Babikian et al (1989) studied 10 stroke patients with intracerebral hemorrhage after anticoagulation with heparin and found that these hemorrhages, like in the 16 cases reported before, occur early after stroke onset with moderate sized or large infarcts, and with excessive anticoagulation in some patients. In a case-control analysis, 121 consecutive adult patients taking warfarin who developed intracranial hemorrhage were each matched to three contemporary controls randomly selected from among outpatients managed by anticoagulant therapy (Hylek and singer 1994). The hemorrhage was intracerebral in 77 patients (fatal in 46%) and subdural in 44 (20% fatal). The major risk factor was identified as prothrombin time ratio (PTR). For each 0.5% increase in PTR over the entire range, the risk for intracerebral hemorrhage doubled. The authors emphasized the importance of maintaining PTR under 2.00 to prevent intracerebral hemorrhage. The risk of hemorrhage varies according to the type of CVD. Hemorrhage occurred only in two of 85 patients (2.3%) with TIA who received intravenous heparin within 96 hours of onset in the study reported by Bogousslavsky and Regli (1985). A trial to test the hypothesis that streptokinase is better than placebo in severe ischemic stroke, was terminated prematurely because of excess mortality and intracranial hemorrhage in the intervention group (Shahar and McGovern 1995).

Patients with pre-existing vascular lesions such as intracranial aneurysms may rupture during anticoagulant therapy (Finney and Gholston 1967). An excess rate of major cerebral hemorrhages occurred in a clinical trial of oral anticoagulants in patients with a history of transient ischemic attacks during the preceding six months (SPIRIT Study Group 1997).

Extracerebral Intracranial Hemorrhages. In one series of 116 anticoagulation-related intracranial hemorrhages, 76 were extracerebral; 69 of these were in the subdural space and seven in the subarachnoid space (Mattle et al 1989). Trauma is a precipitating factor in subdural hematomas which are more likely to occur with long-term oral anticoagulation (Diamond et al 1988).

Intracerebral Hemorrhage as a Complication of Thrombolytic Therapy

Thrombolytic therapy, which acts by pharmacological dissolution of an established thrombus is used both for coronary artery occlusion and acute strokes due to cerebrovascular arterial occlusion. Complications of thrombolytic therapy in these indications will be considered separately.

Thrombolytic Therapy for Myocardial Infarction. This has been shown to reduce the mortality rate in patients with evolving myocardial infarcts. Six thrombolytic agents are either approved for clinical use or have undergone clinical trials (Collen 1993). These are streptokinase, two-chain urokinase (tcu-PA), plasminogen streptokinase activator complex, recombinant staphylokinase, recombinant single-chain urokinase-type plasminogen activator (rscu-PA, pro-urokinase), and recombinant tissue plasminogen activator (rt-PA, altepase). Of these streptokinase and rt-PA are widely used for thrombolysis. Intracerebral hemorrhage is one of the complications. The incidence rate has been reported to be 1% in a prospective multicenter study involving 2469 patients with acute myocardial infarction treated with thrombolytic agents (De Jaegere et al 1992). Elderly patients and those on oral anticoagulation prior to hospitalization were at a higher risk for intracerebral hemorrhage. The incidence of stroke in clinical trials of rt-PA was reported to be 1.8% in patients with acute myocardial infarction. Intracerebral hemorrhage was an unpredictable risk but cerebral infarction could be related to myocardial infarction and poor left ventricular function (O'Connor et al 1990). In a smaller series, the overall prevalence of intracerebral hemorrhage was 3.4% (Urban et al 1992). This rate is higher than that in the clinical trials but presents a more realistic view of the situation in clinical practice outside the constraints of clinical trials.

Maggioni et al (1992) have reported on the results of the GISSI-2 study in Italy and the International Study Group involving more than 20,000 patients with acute myocardial infarction. Those who receive thrombolytic therapy have a small risk of stroke. Treatment with t-PA as compared with streptokinase resulted in a small but significant excess of stroke. Subcutaneous heparin, given together with t-PA or streptokinase and aspirin did not result in an increased risk of stroke.

Simoons et al (1993) have developed a model for the assessment of an individual's risk of intracranial hemorrhage during thrombolysis. If the overall incidence of intracranial hemorrhage is assumed to be 0.75%, patients without risk factors who receive streptokinase have a 0.26% probability of having intracranial hemorrhage. The risk is 0.96%, 1.32%, and 2.1% in patients with one, two, or three risk factors respectively.

In the pilot phase of a randomized trial, recombinant hirudin (a direct thrombin inhibitor) in combination with altepase and aspirin was associated with an increase rate of intracranial hemorrhage in patients with myocardial infarction (Neuhaus et al 1994). The possibility of delayed intracranial hemorrhage after thrombolytic therapy should also be considered. Nathan et al (1994) reported the case of an elderly patient who presented with headache 3 months after altepase and heparin treatment for coronary artery occlusion and was found to have a chronic subdural hematoma. Clinical features and pathogenesis of intracerebral hemorrhage (ICH) after rt-PA and heparin therapy in Thrombolysis in Myocardial Infarction (TIMI) Phase II Clinical Trial have been published (Sloan et al 1995). ICH in these cases may be associated with cerebral amyloid angiopathy and other cerebrovascular lesions. Contributing factors in some of the cases were hypertension and ventricular arrhythmias. The time of occurrence and sites of ischemic infarction in these cases were similar to those reported for similar cases in prethrombolytic era (Sloan et al 1997).

Pathomechanism. The mechanism of hemorrhage with thrombolysis is not clear. Excessive prolongation of the activated partial thromboplastin time and elevated fibrin degradation products may contribute to intracranial hemorrhage in some patients (Kase et al 1992). Computer tomographic findings of multiple cerebral hematomas, fluid levels in the hematomas, and blood in multiple compartments serves to differentiate fibrin-

olysis-induced hemorrhage from hemorrhage due to other causes (Wijdicks and Jack 1993).

Transient ischemic attacks (TIA) have also been reported as a complication of thrombolytic therapy (Caramelli et al 1992). These can be explained by the release of small thrombi into the cerebral circulation (Sloan 1987). Usually there are no permanent sequelae because these small emboli are finally dissolved by the thrombolytic therapy. However, a case of severe persisting neurologic deficit has been reported in a patient following altepase therapy for thrombotic obstruction of a mitral prosthetic valve. Embolic occlusion of peripheral as well as cerebral arteries was found (Hirschl et al 1994).

Risk of Cerebral Hemorrhage and Edema After Altepase-(t-PA)Therapy for Stroke. The only approved thrombolytic agent for stroke currently is tissue plasminogen activator (t-PA). One of the complications is intracerebral hemorrhage. In the first 36 hours, symptomatic intracranial hemorrhage is reported in 6.4% of patients treated with t-PA as compared with 0.6% (p < 0.01) of those treated with placebo (NINDS-t-PA Stroke Study Group 1997).

Cerebral edema associated with stroke may also be aggravated by thrombolysis. Forced reperfusion of already irreversibly damaged tissue increases edema formation and enlarges developing infarcts with an increase of intracranial pressure (Rudolf et al 1998). Although the incidence of edema associated with thrombolytic therapy is lower than that associated with conventional treatments, it may assume a "malignant" form in patients who are treated beyond the therapeutic windows and do not respond to thrombolysis.

Miscellaneous Drugs Associated with CVD

Various types of cerebrovascular events have been reported as adverse effects of several drugs. The causal relationship is not proven in most of the cases. The following drug-related CVD has been reported in literature:

Androgens. Thromboembolic complications are

not generally recognized as side effects of androgen therapy. However, there is some experimental evidence that testosterone stimulates thrombus formation by suppressing prostacyclin production in arterial smooth muscles cells. Stroke has been reported in a 21-year old hypogonadal man who overzealously self-administered testosterone with blood testosterone levels 10 times the usual in similar patients on testosterone replacement therapy (Nagelberg et al 1986). Anabolic androgenic steroids have been reported to cause a stroke in a young athlete (Frankle et al 1988).

β-Blockers. Sabin et al (1993) have reported two cases and quoted three cases from publications where β-blockers administered to patients with migraine have been related to the onset of a cerebrovascular ischemic event. Another case has been reported where there was a temporal association between stroke and treatment with propranolol (Mendizabal et al 1997). Migraine itself is a risk factor for stroke. Non-selective β-blockers, in addition to their vasoconstrictive effect, cause an increase in platelet activity by stimulation of the platelet α_2 receptors.

Bromocriptine. This is an ergot derivative which has been reported to produce cerebral angiopathy. Cerebrovascular accidents have been reported in women who used bromocriptine for suppression of lactation during the postpartum period (This indication has been withdrawn now). A case of intracranial hemorrhage 4 days postpartum in a 31-year old woman who was placed on bromocriptine within hours of delivery (Iffy 1994). She had gestational hypertension which was considered to have gotten worse after bromocriptine therapy and produced vasospasm leading to cerebral infarction. CT scan showed an intracerebral hematoma in the left temporal lobe. Follow-up CT scan showed infarcted brain tissue at site of hemorrhage. Another ergot alkaloid derivative lisuride has been associated with post-partum intracerebral hemorrhage (Roh and Parks 1998).

Calcium Channel Entry Blockers. There are 2 case reports of stroke associated with verapamil overdose (Shah and Passalacqua 1992; Samniah and Schlaeffer 1988). Both these patients had hypotension, bradyarrhythmia, hyperglycemia, and mild acidosis. The authors hypothesized that during recovery from verapamil overdose, an increased number of convertible inactive calcium channels may have been available to the α-adrenoreceptor agonist effect of dopamine. Dopamine infusion given to these patients at a high rate acts as an agonist for α-adrenoreceptors producing vasospasm and aggravate cerebral hypoperfusion due to hypotension.

Epsilon-Aminocaproic Acid (EACA). This agent has been used for the management of the acute phase of subarachnoid hemorrhage due to ruptured intracranial aneurysm still vasospasm clears up and the patient can undergo surgical repair of the aneurysm. Sonntag and Stein (1974) treated seven patients with EACA and three of them developed arteriographic changes resembling arteritis (distinct from vasospasm) or intravascular thrombosis with clinical deterioration.

Fenfluramine. This is an anorectic drug used for weight control. Two women on this therapy have been reported to develop small infarctions of the cochlear, retinal, and brain tissue, termed SICRET syndrome by Schwitter et al (1992).

Immunoglobulin. Intravenous immunoglobulin (IVIG) therapy has been used for the treatment of Guillain-Barré syndrome and myasthenia gravis. One case of cerebral infarction has been reported following high dose IVIG therapy for polyneuritis cranialis in a 84-year old man (Silbert et al 1992). Old age with atherosclerosis, increased serum γ globulin level, and altered blood viscosity may be predisposing factors for thromboembolic events (Dalakas 1994). Another report concerns a case of a 4-year old boy who experienced a stroke after IV injection of immunoglobulin 400 mg/kg administered over a period of four hours (Morales and Chaudhary 1994). Hemiplegia and aphasia developed within 8 hours of receiving the injection. MRI showed left striatocapsular infarction. Risk factor in this case was protein S deficiency. A 27-year old woman with myasthenia gravis and history of migraine developed aseptic meningitis and bilateral cerebral thrombosis after a 5-day course of

IVIG (Steg and Lefkowitz 1994). The precise mechanism of cerebral thrombosis in this patient could not be determined but migraine may have been a risk factor. In view of these reports caution should be exercised when using IVIG in patients with risk factors for cerebrovascular disease such as high serum viscosity and pre-existing cerebrovascular disease.

Nicotine. Transdermal nicotine is used for management of smoking cessation. Adverse effects of nicotine are seen in some patients and stroke has been reported in a patient where the nicotine patch was considered to have precipitated cerebral vasospasm (Pierce 1994).

Nitrates. Various nitrates are used as vasodilators for treatment of angina pectoris. In patients with cerebral atherosclerosis, nitrates fail to dilate the diseased cerebral arteries and the blood is shunted to the dilated normal vessels may precipitate a TIA (Purvin and Dunn 1981). A case of intracranial hemorrhage has been reported following transdermal nitrate application (Boggild 1992).

Radiologic Contrast Media. Stroke is a known complication of cerebral angiography for investigation of cerebrovascular diseases. Most of the these complication are due to the procedure itself such as occlusion of the arteries with catheters, detaching of atherosclerotic plaques, etc. In some cases complications have been attributed to the effect of contrast material on the cerebral vessels (Maurer 1991). Vasospasm has been observed. Cerebral embolism has been reported after lymphography with oily contrast media (Rasmussen 1990).

Sumatriptan. Two cases of hemiparesis have been reported following subcutaneous injection of sumatriptan (Luman and Gray 1993). Sumatriptan is known to produce vasoconstriction of the middle cerebral and internal carotid arteries (Caekebeke et al 1992) but the pathomechanism of stroke is not clear. Cavazos et al (1994) have described the case of a young woman on oral contraceptives who was given sumatriptan for chronic bifrontal headache which was misdiagnosed as migraine. If fact she had pseudotumor cerebri. The first injection of sumatriptan was in-

effective and repeat injection was followed by right hemiplegia. MRI showed a cortical infarct in the left frontoparietal region and superior sagittal sinus thrombosis. She recovered after anticoagulation. The authors postulated that cerebral arterial vasoconstriction induced by sumatriptan decreased the mean cerebral arterial pressure in the setting of increased venous pressure due to superior sagittal sinus thrombosis and this resulted in the development of cerebral infarction. The case history of this patient was atypical of migraine and according to Sykes et al (1994), this patient should not have received sumatriptan. One case of intracerebral hemorrhage has been reported in a migraine patient who abused dihydroergotamine and sumatriptan (Nighoghossian et al 1998).

Adverse Effect of Drugs on Recovery from Stroke

The following drugs have an adverse effect on recovery from stroke and should be avoided in all stroke patients, particularly those with a drug-induced form (Jain 1998):

– Anticholinergics when given late after cerebral infarction
– Antihypertensives: clonidine and prazosin
– Anxiolytics acting through GABA/benzodiazepine receptor complex
– Barbiturates such as phenobarbital
– Dopamine receptor antagonists
– Haloperidol

Concluding Remarks

Cerebrovascular disease has diverse pathological lesions and clinical manifestations. Pathophysiology of most of these is not well understood. With this background, it is difficult to evaluate the role of drugs in producing cerebrovascular disturbances. Animals experimental studies are not helpful in resolving most of these issues. Further pharmaco-epidemiological studies are necessary.

References

Adams HP, Butler MJ, Biller J, et al: Nonhemorrhagic cerebral infarction in young adults. Arch Neurol 1986; 43: 793–796.

Adams JH, Brierley JB, Connor PCR, et al: The effect of systemic hypotension upon the human brain. Brain 1966; 89: 235–268.

Atkinson EA, Fairburn B, Heathfield KWG: Intracranial venous thrombosis as complication of oral contraception. Lancet 1970; 1: 914–918.

Auff A, Zeiler K, Holzner F, et al: Zum Stellenwert der oralen Kontrazeptiva als Risikofaktor zerebraler Gefässerkrankungen. Wien Klin Wochenschr 1986; 98: 304–310.

Avenarius HJ, Freund M, Dienhardt, et al: effect of recombinant human granulocyte colony-stimulating factor (rhG-CSF) on circulating platelets. Ann Hematol 1992; 65: 6–9.

Babikian VL, Kase CS, Pessin MS, et al: Intracerebral hemorrhage in stroke patients anticoagulated with heparin. Stroke 1989; 20: 1500–1503.

Baringarrementeria F, Cantu C, Balderrama J: Postpartum cerebral angiopathy with cerebral infarction due to ergonovine use. Stroke 1992; 23: 1364–1366.

Becker PS, Miller VT: Heparin-induced thrombocytopenia. Stroke 1989; 20: 1449–1459.

Boggild M: Intracerebral hemorrhage after dermal nitrate application. BMJ 1992; 305: 1000.

Bogousslavsky J, Regli F: Anticoagulant-induced intracerebral bleeding in brain ischemia. Acta Neurol Scand 1985; 71: 464–471.

Borgna-Pignatti C, Battisti L, Marradi P, et al: Transient neurologic disturbances in a child treated with moderate dose methotrexate. Br J Hematol 1992; 81: 448.

Bortolotto LA, Silva BH, Pilegi F: Cardiac and neurological complications in malignant hypertension due to oral contraceptive use. Blood Pressure 1994; 3: 319–321.

Bowton DL, Haddon WC, Prough DS, et al: Theophylline effect on the cerebral blood flow response to hypoxemia. Chest 1988; 94: 371–375.

Bruno A, Nolte KB, Chapin J: Stroke associated with ephedrine abuse. Neurology 1993; 43: 1313–1316.

Brust JCM, Richter RW: Stroke associated with addiction to heroin. JNNP 1976; 39: 194–199.

Buchanan DS, Brazinsky JH: Dural sinus and cerebral venous thrombosis. Arch Neurol 1970; 22: 440–444.

Caekebeke JFC, Saxena PR, Ferrari MD: Effect of sumatriptan on cranial blood flow velocity during and between migraine attacks. In Olesen J, Saxena PR (Eds.): 5-hydroxytryptamine mechanisms in primary headaches, New York, Raven Press, 1992, pp 273–277.

Caplan LR, Hier DB, Banks G: Current concepts of cerebrovascular disease—stroke: stroke and drug abuse. Stroke 1982; 13: 869–872.

Caramelli P, Mutarelli EG, Caramelli B, et al: Neurological complications after thromlbolytic treatment for acute myocardial infarction: emphasis on unprecedented manifestations. Acta Neurol Scand 1992; 85: 331–333.

Case records of the Massachusetts General Hospital: Case 27. NEJM 1993; 329: 117–124.

Cavazos JE, Caress JB, Chilukuri VR: Sumatriptan-induced stroke in sagittal sinus thrombosis. Lancet 1994; 343: 1105–1106.

Cerebral Embolism Study Group: Cardioembolic stroke, early anticoagulation, and brain hemorrhage. Arch Intern Med 1987; 147(4): 636–40.

Collaborative Group for the Study of Stroke in Young Women: Oral contraceptives and stroke in young women. JAMA 1975; 231: 718–722.

Collen D: Towards improved thrombolytic therapy. Lancet 1993; 342: 34–36.

Conci F, D'Angelico V, Tampieri D, et al: Intracerebral hemorrhage and angiographic beading following amphetamine abuse. Ital J Neurosci 1988; 9: 77–81.

Corby DG: Editorial comment. Obstet Gynecol 1981; 58: 737–740.

Dalakas MC: High dose intravenous immunoglobulin and serum viscosity: risk of precipitating thromboembolic events. Neurology 1994; 44: 223–226.

Daras M, Tuchman AJ, Marks S: Central nervous system infarction related to cocaine abuse. Stroke 1991; 22: 1320–1325.

Davies DM, Ferner RE, De Glanville H (Eds.): Davies' Textbook of Adverse Drug Reactions, 5th edition, Lippincott Williams & Wilkins, Baltimore, 1998.

de Bruijn SFTM, Stam J, Vandenbroucke JP, et al: Increased risk of cerebral venous sinus thrombosis with third-generation oral contraceptives. Lancet 1998; 351: 1404.

De Jaegere PP, Arnold AA, Balk AG, et al: Intracranial hemorrhage in association with thrombolytic therapy: incidence and clinical predictive factors. J Am Coll Cardiol 1992; 19: 189–294.

Delaney P, Estes M: Intracranial hemorrhage with amphetamine abuse. Neurology 1980; 30: 1125.

DeWys WD, Fowler EH: Report of vasculitis and blindness after intracarotid injection of 1,3-bis(2-chlorethyl)-1-nitrosourea (BCNU; NSC-409962) in dogs. Cancer Chemotherapy Reports 1973; 57: 33–40.

Diamond T, Gray WJ, Chee CP, et al: Subdural hematoma associated with long term oral anticoagulation. Br J Neurosurg 1988; 2: 351–355.

Dindar F, Platts ME: Intracranial venous thrombosis complicating oral contraception. CMAJ 1974; 111: 545–547.

Dohi S, Jones D, Hudak ML, et al: Effect of cocaine on pial arterioles in cats. Stroke 1990; 21: 1710–1714.

Doll DC, List AF, Greco FA, et al: Acute vascular ischemic events after cisplatin-based combination chemotherapy for germ-cell tumors of the testis. Ann Int Med 1986a; 105: 48–51.

Doll DC, Ringenberg QS, Yarbo JW: Vascular toxicity associated with antineoplastic agents. J Clin Oncol 1986b; 4: 1405–1407.

Donaldson JO, Ramsey JR: Carotid-dural arteriovenous fistula during use of oral contraceptives. Am J Obstet Gynecol 1983; 145: 106–107.

El Amrani M, Heinzlef O, Debrouker T, et al: Brain infarction following 5-fluorouracil and cisplatin therapy. Neurology 1998; 51: 899–901.

Ernst E, Hammerschmidt DE, Bagge U, et al: Leukocytes and the risk of ischemic disease. JAMA 1987; 257: 2318–2324.

Fagan Sc, Payne LW, Houtekier SC: Risk of cerebral hypoperfusion with antihypertensive therapy. DICP 1989; 23: 957–962.

Falkeborn M, Persson I, Terent A, et al: Hormone replacement therapy and the risk of stroke. Arch Int Med 1993; 153: 1201–1209.

Finney LA, Gholston D: Cerebral aneurysm rupture during anticoagulant therapy with survival. JAMA 1967; 200: 1127–1128.

Fogelholm R, Eskola K, Kiminkinen T, et al: Anticoagulant treatment as a risk factor for primary intracerebral hemorrhage. JNNP 1992; 55: 1121–1124.

Follezou JY, Chauveinc L, Guerin JM: Cerebral arterial disturbances in atransient encephalopathy induced by methotrexate. Medical Oncology & Tumor Pharmacotherapy 1993; 10: 181–183.

Forman HP, Levin S, Stewart B, et al: Cerebral vasculitis and hemorrhage in an adolescent taking diet pills containing phenylpropanolamine: case report and review of literature. Pediatrics 1989; 83: 737–741.

Frankle MA, Eichberg R, Zachariah SB: Anabolic androgenic steroids and a stroke in an athlete. Arch Phys Med Rehabil 1988; 69: 632–633.

Fraser I: Contraceptive choice for women with risk factors. Drug Safety 1993; 8: 271–279.

Fredericks RK, Lefkowitz DS, Challa VR, et al: Cerebral vasculitis associated with cocaine abuse. Stroke 1991; 22: 1437–1439.

Gandia D, Spielman M, Kac J, et al: Cerebrovascular accident associated with chemotherapy for oesophageal carcinoma. Eur J Cancer 1992; 28: 245.

Glick R, Hoying J, Cerullo L, et al: Phenylpropanolamine: an over-the-counter drug causing central nervous system vasculitis and intracerebral hemorrhage. Neurosurgery 1987; 20: 969–974.

Goldhirsch A, Joss R, Markwalder T-M, et al: Acute cerebrovascular accident after treatment with cis-platinum and methylprednisolone. Oncology 1983; 40: 344–345.

Graham DI: Ischemic brain damage following emergency blood pressure lowering in hypertensive patients. Acta Med Scand 1983; 678(suppl): 61–69.

Greenwald JG: Stroke, sickle cell trait, and oral contraceptives. Ann Int Med 1970; 72: 960.

Groome LJ, Goldenberg RL, Cliver SP, et al: Neonatal periventricular-intraventricular hemorrhage after maternal β-sympathomimetic tocolysis. Am J Obstet Gynecol 1992; 167: 873–879.

Gschwend J: Die Ovulationshemmer aus neurologischer Sicht. Schweiz Med Wochenschr 1976; 106: 644–647.

Hannaford PC, Croft PR, Kay CR: Oral contraceptives and stroke. Evidence from the Royal College of General Practitioner's Study. Stroke 1994; 25: 935–942.

Heinemann LA, Lewis MA, Spitzer WO, et al: Thromboembolic stroke in young women. A European case-control study on oral contraceptives. Transnational Research Group on Oral Contraceptives and the Health of Young Women. Contraception 1998; 57: 29–37.

Hemler RJB, Hoogeveen JH, Kraaier V, et al: A pharmacological model of cerebral ischemia. The effects of indomethacin on cerebral blood flow velocity, quantitative EEG and cognitive functions. Meth Find Exp Clin Pharmacol 1990; 12: 641–643.

Heye N, Hankey GJ: Amphetamine-associated stroke. Cerebrovasc Dis 1996; 6: 149–155.

Heyman A, Arons M, Quinn M, et al: The role of oral contraceptive agents in cerebral arterial occlusion. Neurology 1969; 19: 519–524.

Hirschl MM, Gwechenberger M, Zehetgruber M, et al: Severe complications following thrombolytic therapy of an acute thrombosis of a prosthetic mitral valve. Clinical Investigator 1994; 72: 466–469.

Horowitz BZ, Jadallah S, Derlet RW: Fatal intracranial bleeding associated with prehospital use of epinephrine. Ann Emergency Med 1996; 28: 725–727.

Hunt AC, Sutherland IC: Oral contraceptives and cerebral blood flow. Lancet 1968; 2: 1086.

Hutchinson EC, McCall AJ: Oral contraceptive use and cerebral blood flow. Lancet 1968; 2: 1299–1300.

Hylek EM, Singer DE: Risk factors for intracranial hemorrhage in outpatients taking warfarin. Ann Int Med 1994; 120: 897–902.

Iffy L: Postpartum intracerebral hemorrhage in a patient receiving bromocriptine. Pharmacoepidemiology and Drug Safety 1994; 3: 247–249.

Iijima S, Tsuji T, Sugita M, et al: Leukocyte activity and occurrence of tissue injury by G-CSF. Acta Obst Gynaec Jpn 1993; 45: 213–219.

Ikeda S, Sonoda K, Sumiyoshi M, et al: Acute cerebrovascular toxicity after chemotherapy with carboplatin and cyclophosphamide for advanced ovarian carcinoma. Int J Oncol 1999; 4: 52–53.

Inman WHW, Vessey MP, Westerholm B, et al: Thromboembolic disease and steroidal content of oral contraceptives. A report to the Committee on Safety of Drugs. BMJ 1970; 2: 203–209.

Inman WHW, Vessey MP: Investigation of deaths from pulmonary, coronary, and cerebral thrombosis and embolism in women of child-bearing age. BMJ 1968; 2: 193–199.

Inman WHW: Oral contraceptives and fatal subarachnoid hemorrhage. BMJ 1979; 2: 1468–1470.

Irey NS, McAllister HA, Henry JM: Oral contraceptives and stroke in young women: a clinicopathological correlation. Neurology 1978; 28: 1216–1219.

Jain KK: Stroke. D & MD Publications/IBC Communications Inc, Southborough, MA, 1998.

Jansen PA, Gribnau FW, Schulte BP, et al: Contribution of inappropriate treatment for hypertension to pathogenesis of stroke in the elderly. Br Med J (Clin Res Ed) 1986; 293: 914.

Janssens E, Hommel M, Mounier-Vehier F, et al: Postpartum cerebral angiopathy possibly due to bromocriptine therapy. Stroke 1995; 26: 128–130.

Jardine DS, Rogers K: Relationship of benzyl alcohol to kernicterus, intraventricular hemorrhage, and mortality in preterm infants. Pediatrics 1989 83: 153–160.

Jennett WB: Cerebral thrombosis and oral contraceptives. BMJ 1969; 3: 173.

Jick H, Porter J, Rothman KJ: Oral contraceptives and

nonfatal stroke in healthy young women. Ann Int Med 1978; 89: 58–60.

Johnson AG: NSAIDs and increased blood pressure. What is the clinical significance? Drug Safety 1997; 17: 277–89.

Kase CS, Pessin MS, Zivin JA, et al: Intracranial hemorrhage after coronary thrombolysis with tissue plasminogen activator. Am J Med 1992; 92: 384–390.

Katz M, Kroll D, Pak I, et al: Puerpural hypertension, stroke, and seizures after suppression of lactation with bromocriptine. Obstet Gynecol 1985; 62: 822–824.

Kaufman MJ, Levin JM, Ross MH: Cocaine-induced cerebral vasoconstriction detected in humans with magnetic resonance angiography. JAMA 1998; 279: 376–380.

Kjaer M, deFine Olivarius B, Waarst A: Cerebral ischemic lesions and oral contraception. Dan Med Bull 1971; 18: 129–137.

Klonoff DC, Andrews BT, Obana WG: Stroke associated with cocaine use. Arch Neurol 1989; 46: 989–993.

Krendel DA, Ditter SM, Frankel MR, et al: Biopsy-proven cerebral vasculitis associated with cocaine abuse. Neurology 1990; 40: 1090–1094.

Kukla LJ, McGuire WP, Lad T, et al: Acute vascular episodes associated with therapy for carcinomas of the upper aerodigestive tract with bleomycin, vincristine and cisplatin. Cancer Treat Rep 1982; 66: 369.

Kukla LJ, McGuire WP, Lad T, et al: Acute vascular episodes associated with therapy for the carcinoma of the upper aerodigestive tract with bleomycin, vincristine, and cisplatin. Cancer Treatment Reports 1982; 66: 369–370.

Landefeld CS, Goldman L: Major bleeding in outpatients treated with warfarin: incidence and prediction by factors known at the start of outpatient therapy. Am J Med 1989; 87: 144–152.

Laugharne JDE: Multiple cerebral infarction associated with neuroleptic-induced lupus anticoagulant. Behavioral Neurology 1994; 7: 185–187.

Le Coz P, Woimant F, Rougemont D, et al: Angiopathies cerebrales benignes et phenylpropanolamine. Rev Neurol (Paris) 1988; 144: 295–300.

Le Hello C, Cohen P, Bousser P, et al: Suspected hepatitis B vaccination related vasculitis. J Rheumatol 1999; 26: 191–194.

Lesko SM, Mitchell AA, Epstein MF, et al: Heparin as a risk factor for intraventricular hemorrhage in low-birth-weight infants. NEJM 1986; 314: 1156–1160.

Levine SR, Brust JCM, Futrell N, et al: Cerebrovascular complications of the use of "crack" form of alkaloidal cocaine. NEJM 1990; 323: 699–704.

Levine SR, Welch KMA: Cocaine and stroke. Stroke 1988; 19: 779–783.

Lewis IC, Philpott MG: Neurological complications in the Henoch-Schönlein syndrome. Arch Dis Child 1956; 31: 369–371.

Liard P, Lang R, Wildi E: Endocardites, lesions cerebrales et anticoagulants (etudes anatomo-clinique et statistique de 229 cases. Schweiz Arch Neurol Psychiatr 1993; 144: 39–61.

Lichtman MA, Rowe JM: Hyperleukocytic leukemias: rheological, clinical, and therapeutic considerations. Blood 1982; 60: 279–283.

Lidegaard O: Cerebrovascular deaths before and after the appearance of oral contraceptives. Acta Neurol Scand 1987; 75: 427–433.

Lidegaard O: Oral contraception and risk of cerebral thromboembolic attack: result of a case-control study. BMJ 1993; 306: 956–963.

Lieberman AN, Bloom W, Kishore PS, et al: Carotid artery occlusion following ingestion of LSD. Stroke 1974; 5: 213–215.

Lim HL, Teo CP, Wong YK, et al: L-asparaginase induced intracranial hemorrhage in acute lymphoblastic leukemia. Singapore Medical Journal 1998; 39: 76–78.

Longstreth WT, Swanson PD: Oral contraceptives and stroke. Stroke 1984; 15: 747–750.

Lorentz IT: Parietal lesion and "Enavid." BMJ 1962; 12: 1191.

Lucas C, Deplanque D, Sahli A, et al: Postpartum cerebral angiopathy associated with bromocriptine therapy. Three cases. Cerebrovascular Diseases 1996; 6(suppl 2): 88 (abstract).

Luman W, Gray RS: Adverse reactions associated with sumatriptan. Lancet 1993; 341: 1091–1092.

Maggioni AP, Franzosi MG, Santorio E, et al: The risk of stroke in patients with acute myocardial infarction after thrombolytic and antithrombotic treatments. NEJM 1992; 327: 1–6.

Mammen EF: Oral contraceptives and blood coagulation: a critical review. Am J Obstet Gynecol 1982; 142: 781–790.

Mandel MM, Strimmel WH: Bilateral carotid artery occlusion in a young adult. JAMA 1969; 208: 145–148.

Martinez del Prado P, Meana JA, Carrion JR: Acute cerebrovascular accident after treatment with cisplatin. Acta Oncol 1992; 31: 593–595.

Matsumo S, Murakami M, Kuroda Y, et al: A dural sinus thrombosis that developed during anticancer therapy.-report of two cases diagnosed by MRI. Gann No Rinsho 1992; 38: 1140–1146.

Mattle H, Kohler s, Huber P, et al: Anticoagulant-related intracranial extracerebral hemorrhage. J NNP 1989; 52: 829–837.

Maurer HJ: Kontrastmittelzwischenfälle bei neuroradiologischen Untersuchungen. Vasa 1991; 33(suppl): 293–294.

May A, Faiss J, Keidel M, et al: Zerebrale Angiitis oder zentrale Nebenwirkung nach lumbaler Myelographie (mit intrazerebral nachweisbaren Gefäss-Spasmen). Nervenarzt 1994; 65: 125–127.

McEnvoy AW, Kitchen ND, Thomas DGT: Intracerebral hemorrhage caused by drug abuse. Lancet 1998; 351: 1029.

McFarland HR: Regression of cerebral lesions after cessation of oral contraceptives. South Med J 1970; 63: 145–151.

McIntyre S, Gold R, Gean A, et al: A CNS vasculopathy as a manifestation of carbamazepine therapy? Neurology 1994; 44(suppl 3): A274 (abstract)

Mendizabal JE, Greiner F, Hamilton WJ, et al: Migranous stroke causing thalamic infarction and amnesia during treatment with propranolol. Headache 1997; 37: 594–596.

Michel M, Vincent F, Sigal R, et al: Cerebral vasculitis after interleukin-2 therapy for renal cell carcinoma. J Immunother Emphasis Tumor Immunol 1995; 18: 124–126.

Migita M, Fukunaga Y, Watanbe A, et al: Emperipolesis of neutrophils by megakaryocytes and thrombocytopenia observed in a case of Kostmann syndrome during intravenous administration of high-dose rh-G-CSF. Br J Hematol 1992,80: 413–415.

Moore PM, Cupps TR: Neurological complications of vasculitis. Ann Neurol 1983; 14: 155–167.

Morales A, Chaudhary S: Intravenous immunoglobulin, protein S deficiency and cerebral infarction. Pediatric Neurology 1994; 11: 141–142.

Moslet U, Hansen ES: A review of vitamin K, epilepsy and pregnancy. Acta Neurol Scand 1992; 85: 39–43.

Nagelberg SB, Laue L, Loriaux DL, et al: Cerebrovascular accident associated with testosterone therapy in a 21-year old hypogonadal man. NEJM 1986; 314: 649–650.

Nakao J, Chang WC, Murota SI, et al: Testosterone inhibits prostacyclin production by rat aortic smooth muscle cells in culture. Atherosclerosis 1981; 39: 203–209.

Nathan PE, Sonenblick D,Chakote V, et al: Headache, thrombolytic therapy, and chronic subdural hemorrhage. Angiology 1994; 45: 77–80.

Neuhaus KL, Essen RV, Tebbe U, et al: Safety observations from the pilot phase of the randomized r-hirudin for the improvement of thrombolysis (HIT-III) study. Circulation 1994; 90: 1638–1642.

Nighoghossian N, Derex L, Troullas P: Multiple intracerebral hemorrhage and vasospasm following antimigraine drug abuse. Headache 1998; 38: 478–480.

NINDS t-PA Study Group: Intracerebral hemorrhage after intravenous t-PA therapy for ischemic stroke. Stroke 1997; 28: 2109–2118.

Nolte KB, Brass LM, Fletterick CF: Intracranial hemorrhage associated with cocaine abuse. Neurology 1996; 46: 1291–1296.

O'Connor CM, Califf RM, Massey EW, et al: Stroke and acute myocardial infarction in the thrombolytic era: clinical correlates and long-term prognosis. J Am Coll Cardiol 1990; 16: 533–540.

Pectasides D, Barbounis V, Athanassiou A, et al: Cerebrovascular accidents following hormonochemotherapy in cancer patients. Am J Clin Oncol 1992; 15: 168–173.

Peterson PL, Roszler M, Jacobs I, et al: Neurovascular complications of cocaine abuse. J Neuropsychiatry 1991; 3: 143–149.

Pierce JR: Stroke following application of nicotine patch. Ann Pharmacother 1994; 28: 402.

Pihko H, Tyni T, Virkolaa K, et al: Transient ischemic lesions during induction chemotherapy for acute lymphoblastic leukemia. J Pediatr 1993; 123: 718–724.

Piper C, Mathias B: Orale Kontrazeptiva: unerwünschte Wirkungen in Bereich der inneren Medizin. Med Klin 1989; 84: 227–235.

Pizzolato GP, Sztajzel R, Burkhardt K, et al: Cerebral vasculitis during FK 506 treatment in a liver transplant patient. Neurology 1998; 50: 1154–1157.

Pohl M, Kornhuber B: Fruchtschädigung nach Antikoagulantienbehandlung in der Schwangerschaft. Med Klin 1966; 61: 964–965.

Popper H, Skvarc A, Ladurner G, et al: Zerebrale Komplikationen bei allergischer Vaskulitis. Nervenarzt 1978; 49: 720–723.

Prentice RL, Szatrowski TP, Kato H, et al: Leukocyte counts and cerebrovascular disease. J Chron Dis 1982; 35: 703–714.

Psaty BM, Heckbert SR, Atkins D, et al: A review of the association of estrogens and progestins with cardiovascular disease in postmenopausal women. Arch Int Med 1993; 153: 1421–1427.

Purvin VA, Dunn DW: Nitrate-induced transient ischemic attacks. Southern Med J 1981; 74: 1130–1131.

Ramachandaran S, Pellegrin FA, Ray RM, et al: The Walnut Creek Contraceptive Drug Study. J Reprod Med 1980; 25(suppl): 349–371.

Rasmussen KE: Retinal and cerebral fat emboli following lymphography with oily contrast media. Acta Radiol Diagn 1990; 10: 199.

Reichert EM, Fuller PW: Relationship of sodium bicarbonate to intraventricular hemorrhage in premature infants with respiratory distress syndrome. Nurs Res 1980; 29: 357–361.

Renzulli P, Tuchschmid P, Eich G, et al: Early vitamin K deficiency bleeding after maternal phenobarbital intake: management of massive intracranial hemorrhage by minimal surgical intervention. Eur J Ped 1998; 157: 663–665.

Roh JK, Park KS: Postpartum cerebral angiopathy with intracerebral hemorrhage in a patient receiving lisuride. Neurology 1998; 50: 1152–1154.

Rothwell PM, Grant R: Cerebral vasculitis following allopurinol treatment. Postgraduate Medical Journal 1996; 72: 119–120.

Royal College of General Practitioner's Oral Contraception Study: Mortality among oral-contraceptive users. Lancet 1977; 2: 727–731.

Rudolf J, Grond M, Stenzel C, et al: Incidence of space-occupying brain edema following systemic thrombolysis of acute supratentorial ischemia. Cerebrovasc Dis 1998; 8: 166–171.

Rumack CM, Guggenheim MA, Rumack BH, et al: Neonatal intracranial hemorrhage and maternal use of aspirin. Obstet Gynecol 1981; 58: 52S–56S.

Rumbaugh CL, Bergeron T, Scanlon RL, et al: Cerebral vascular changes secondary to amphetamine abuse in the experimental animal. Radiology 1971; 101: 345–351.

Russell RP, Sullivan MA: The pill and hypertension. Johns Hopkins Medical Journal 1970; 127: 287–293.

Sabin JA, Molins A, Turon A, et al: Migrana-infarto en pacientes tratados con blocqueadores β. Rev Clin Esp 1993; 192: 228–230.

Salanova V, Taubner R: Intracerebral hemorrhage and vasculitis secondary to amphetamine abuse. Postgrad Med J 1984; 60: 429–430.

Samniah N, Schlaeffer F: Cerebral infarction associated

with oral verapamil overdosage. J Toxicol 1988; 26: 365–369.

Samuels BL, Vogelsang NJ, Kennedy BJ: Severe vascular toxicity associated with vinblastine, bleomycin, and cisplatin chemotherapy. Cancer Chemotherapy Pharmacol 1987; 19: 253–256.

Schwartz SM, Siscovick DS, Longstreth WT Jr, et al: Use of low-dose oral contraceptives and stroke in young women. Ann Intern Med 1997; 127: 596–603.

Schwitter J, Agosti R, Ott P, et al: Small infarctions of cochlear, retinal, and encephalic tissue in young women. Stroke 1992; 23: 903–907.

Shah AR, Passalacqua BR: Sustained-release verapamil overdose causing stroke. Am J Med Sci 1992; 304: 357–359.

Shahar E, McGovern PG: Trials of streptokinase in severe acute ischemic stroke (letter). Lancet 1995; 345: 578.

Shimoda K, Okamura S, Harada N, et al: Identification of a functional receptor for granulocyte colony-stimulating factor on platelets. J Clin Invest 1993a; 91: 1310–1313.

Shimoda K, Okamura S, Inaba S, et al: Granulocyte colony-stimulating factor and platelet aggregation. Lancet 1993b; 341: 633.

Silbert PL, Knezevic PL, Bridge DT: Cerebral infarction complicating immunoglobulin therapy for polyneuritis cranialis. Neurology 1992; 42: 257–258.

Simmons MA, Adcock EW, Bard H, et al: Hypernatremia and intracranial hemorrhage in neonates. NEJM 1974; 291: 6–10.

Simoons ML, Maggioni AP, Knatterud G, et al: Individual risk assessment for intracranial hemorrhage during thrombolytic therapy. Lancet 1993; 342: 1523–1528.

Sissons C, Hall RD: Intracranial venous thrombosis complicating oral contraception. Lancet 1970; 2: 419.

Sloan MA, Kittner SJ, Rigamonti D, et al: Occurrence of stroke associated with use/abuse of drugs. Neurology 1991; 41: 1358–1364.

Sloan MA, Price TR, Petito CK, et al: Clinical features and pathogenesis of intracerebral hemorrhage after rt-PA and heparin therapy for acute myocardial infarction: the Thrombolysis in Myocardial Infarction (TIMI) II Pilot and Randomized Clinical Trial combined experience. Neurology 1995; 45: 649–58.

Sloan MA, Price TR, Terrin ML, et al: Ischemic cerebral infarction after rt-PA and heparin therapy for acute myocardial infarction. Stroke 1997; 28: 1107–1114.

Sloan MA: Thrombolysis and stroke: past and future. Arch Neurol 1987; 44: 748–768.

Soller RW, Stander H: Maternal drug exposure and perinatal intracranial hemorrhage. Obstet Gynecol 1981; 58: 735–737.

Sonntag VKH, Stein BM: Arteriopathic complications during treatment of subarachnoid hemorrhage with epsilon-aminocaproic acid. J Neurosurg 1974; 40: 480–485.

Stafford PJ, Strachan CJL, Vincent R, et al: Multiple microemboli after disintegration of clot during thrombolysis for acute myocardial infarction. BMJ 1989; 299: 1310–1312.

Steg RE, Lefkowitz DM: Cerebral infarction following intravenous immunoglobulin therapy for myasthenia gravis. Neurology 1994; 44: 1180–1.

Stampfer MJ, Willett WC, Colditz GA, et al: A prospective study of the past use of oral contraceptive agents and risk of cardiovascular diseases. NEJM 1988; 319: 1313–1317.

Strandgaard S: Cerebral ischemia caused by overzealous lowering of blood pressure. Danish Medical Bulletin 1987; 34(suppl 1): 5–7.

Stroke Prevention in Reversible Ischemia Trial (SPIRIT) Study Group: A randomized trial of anticoagulant versus aspirin after cerebral ischemia of presumed arterial origin. Ann Neurol 1997; 42: 857–865.

Sykes RS, Castle W, Palmer J: Sumatriptan-induced stroke in sagittal sinus thrombosis. Lancet 1994; 343: 1299–1300.

Thomas SHL: Drug-induced hypertension. Adverse Drug Reactions Bulletin 1993; 159: 559–562.

Thompson CM, Bayliff CD, Delamere K, et al: Intracerebral hemorrhage associated with phenylpropanolamine. Canad J Hosp Pharm 1998; 51: 88.

Thompson SG, Meade TW, Greenberg G: The use of hormonal replacement therapy and risk of stroke and myocardial infarction in women. J Epidemiol and Community Health 1989; 43: 173–178.

Thorogood M, Mann J, Murphy M, et al: Fatal stroke and use of oral contraceptives: findings from a case-control study. Am J Epidemiol 1992; 136: 35–45.

Urban P, Reynard C, Meier B: Thrombolysis and risk of stroke. Lancet 1992; 339: 817.

Vecchia CL, Franceschi S, Bruzzi P, et al: The relationship between oral contraceptive use, cancer and vascular diseases. Drug Safety 1990; 5: 436–446.

Vessey MP, Doll R: Investigation of relation between use of oral contraceptives and thromboembolic disease. A further report. BMJ 1969; 2: 651–657.

Vessey MP, Lawless M, Yeates D: Oral contraceptives and stroke: findings in a large prospective study. BMJ 1984; 289: 530–531.

Volpe J: Neonatal intracranial hemorrhage—iatrogenic etiology. NEJM 1974; 291: 43–45.

Voltz R, Rosen FV, Yousry T, et al: Reversible encephalopathy with cerebral vasospasm in a Guillain-Barré syndrome patient treated with intravenous immunoglobulin. Neurology 1996; 46: 250–251.

Wall JG, Weiss RB, Norton L, et al: Arterial thrombosis associated with adjuvant chemotherapy for breast carcinoma: a cancer and leukemia group B study. Am J Med 1989; 87: 501–504.

Walsh J, Wheeler HR, Geczy CL: Modulation of tissue factor on human monocytes by cisplatin and adriamcin. Br J Hematol 1992; 81: 480–488.

Weiss EB, Forman P, Rosenthal IM: Allopurinol-induced arteritis in partial HGPRTase deficiency. Arch Int Med 1978; 138: 1743–1744.

WHO Collaborative Study of Cardiovascular Disease and Steroid Hormone Contraception. Ischemic stroke and combined oral contraceptives: results of an international, multicenter, case-control study. Lancet 1996a; 348: 498–505.

WHO Collaborative Study of Cardiovascular Disease and Steroid Hormone Contraception. Hemorrhagic stroke, overall stroke risk, and combined oral contraceptives: results of an international, multicentre, case control study. Lancet 1996b; 348: 505–510.

Wijdicks EFM, Jack CR: Intracerebral hemorrhage after fibrinolytic therapy for acute myocardial infarction. Stroke 1993; 24: 554–557.

Wintzen AR, de Jonge H, Loeliger EA, et al: The risk of intracerebral hemorrhage during oral anticoagulation treatment: a population study. Ann Neurol 1984; 16: 553–558.

Wooten MR, Khangure MS, Murphy MJ: Intracerebral hemorrhage and vasculitis related to ephedrine abuse. Ann Neurol 1983; 13: 337–340.

Yu YJ, Cooper DR, Wellenstein DE, et al: Cerebral angiitis and intracerebral hemorrhage associated with methamphetamine abuse. J Neurosurg 1983; 58: 109.

Zachariah SB: Stroke after heavy marihuana smoking. Stroke 1991; 22: 406–409.

Chapter 10
Drug-Induced Disorders
of Cranial Nerves and Special Senses

Introduction

Cranial nerves and the special senses may be involved as a part of neurotoxicity of several drugs. This chapter is limited to the discussion of those adverse effects where the cranial nerve disturbances are the presenting or the predominant symptoms. It would be impossible to cover all the symptoms related to cranial nerves which are reported as adverse drug reactions. Among the special senses only disorders of vision, hearing, smell and taste are dealt with. For practical purposes the disorders will be described under the following headings:

- Drug-induced neuro-ophthalmological disorders
- Disorders of cranial nerves III–VII
- Drug-induced ototoxicity
- Recurrent laryngeal nerve palsy
- Drug-induced disorders of taste and smell

Drug-Induced Neuro-Ophthalmological Disorders

Drug-induced ocular side effects are numerous and are described in an encyclopedic work by Fraunfelder and Meyer (1989). In this section the following disorders will be described:

- Optic nerve disorders
  · optic neuropathy
  · optic (or retrobulbar) neuritis
  · optic atrophy
- Retinal degeneration or pigmentary changes
- Disorders of eye movements
- Cortical blindness

Some ocular manifestations are covered in other chapters: papilledema as a part of benign intracranial hypertension (Chapter 17), weakness of extraocular muscles (Chapter 12), and oculogyric crises (Chapter 8).

Optic Neuritis. The term "optic neuritis" means inflammation of the optic nerve but it does not explain the pathogenesis of the lesion. When it involves the part of the optic never within the eyeball, it is sometimes called "papillitis" and when it affects the portion behind the eyeball, it is called "retrobulbar neuritis." Optic neuropathy is a general term to indicate independent involvement of the optic nerve (excluding retinopathy) and is usually due to toxic or ischemic causes. Optic neuropathy is also a part of an epidemic reported from Cuba which also included sensorineural deafness, peripheral sensory neuropathy and dorsolateral myeloneuropathy (Romàn 1994). It was attributed to dietary deficiencies including those of micronutrients such as B-group vitamins but no toxic environmental chemicals or therapeutic drugs were implicated. This epidemic affected more than 50,000 persons. The risk was increased in those consuming tobacco and reducing with the use of vitamins (Cuba Neuropathy Field Investigation Team 1995).

Optic Atrophy. Damage to the complex structure of the optic nerve results in optic atrophy. This is seen as a thinning of the optic nerve (optic fascicle and tract), and is due to a reduction in parenchymal elements and a glial or fibrotic sclerosis. Primary optic atrophy is due to specific impairment of the neurons. Secondary optic atrophy, on the other hand, has many causes, the most common being retinal degeneration, inflammation, prolonged papilledema and glaucoma.

In adverse drug reaction reports, details of the optic nerve pathology are usually not available. Optic atrophy is a clear-cut finding but optic neuropathies are less well defined. The long-term follow-up may show either recovery or optic atrophy. Some drugs may affect the optic nerves only and spare the peripheral nerves or vice ver-

Table 10.1. Drugs that have been reported to cause toxic damage to the optic nerve.

Amiodarone*
Antimicrobials
  – Acyclovir
  – Chloramphenicol
  – Clioquinol
  – Dapsone
  – DDI (2'-3'-dideoxyinosine)
  – Ethambutol*
  – Isoniazid
  – Streptomycin
  – Sulfonamides
  – Tryparsamide
Antineoplastics
  – Cisplatin
  – 5-Fluorouracil
  – Paclitaxel
  – Vincristine
Clomiphene citrate (Purvin 1995b)
Corticosteroids
Cyproterone acetate (Markus et al 1992)
Ergotamine
GABA-mimetic antiepileptic agents
  – Progabide (Baulac et al 1998)
  – Vigabatrin*
Interferon-α*
Nicotinic acid (Callanan et al 1998)
Non-steroidal anti-inflammatory drugs
  – Ibuprofen*
  – Naproxen
OKT3 monoclonal antibody (Jin et al 1995)
Omeprazole
Oral contraceptives
Penicillamine
Quinine
Retinoids
Vaccines
  – DPT
  – Rabies
  – Hepatitis B
  – Influenza
  – Measles
  – Mumps
  – Rubella (live)

*Well documented.

sa; both may be involved or spinal cord may be involved in addition. Mechanism of toxicity and the reasons for these differential involvement are not known (Grant 1980). Visual evoked potentials should be used to monitor patients receiving drugs which are potentially toxic to the optic nerve. Drugs which have been reported to cause toxic damage to the optic nerve are shown in Table 10.1.

Retinal Degeneration or Pigmentary Changes. Drugs have been reported to cause retinal degeneration or pigmentary deposits are shown in Table 10.2.

Neuro-ophthalmic toxicity of some of the drugs listed in Tables 10.1 and 10.2 is described in the following pages.

Table 10.2. Drugs reported to be toxic to the retina.

Carbamazepine
Chloroquine
Desferoxamine*
Didanosine (Cobo et al 1996)
Granulocyte colony-stimulating factor (Matsumura et al 1997)
Growth hormone (Koller et al 1998)
Phenothiazines*: chlorpromazine and thioridazine
Quinine*
Sildenafil* (Viagra)
Tamoxifen
Trimethoprim

* Well documented.

Amiodarone. Amiodarone, a benzofuran derivative, is an α- and β-antagonist, with vasodilator and antiarrhythmic properties. Several adverse effects have been reported including peripheral neuritis (Chapter 11) and optic neuropathy. Feiner et al (1987) presented 13 cases of optic neuropathy following treatment with amiadarone. Other authors have added cases bringing the total to 20 (Gittinger and Asdourian 1987; Nazarian and Jacy 1988; DeWachter and Lievens 1988; Belec et al 1992; Krieg and Schipper 1992). No randomized study has been done to determine the true incidence of this complication but the incidence was higher than that found in age-matched general population.

Clinical features. This condition is less severe than ischemic optic neuropathy. The clinical picture is variable with onset from 1–72 months after start of therapy. The involvement can be unilateral or bilateral. All the cases with amiodarone-induced optic neuritis do not have visual loss. Some patients improve after discontinuation of the drug while others do not.

Pathomechanism. The pathomechanism of this condition is not clear. Mansour et al (1988) examined the optic nerve of a patient who was on amiadarone therapy but had no visual complaints after excision of the eyeball for melanoma. Sections of the retrobulbar optic nerve showed lamellar inclusions in large axons. The authors suggested that amiadarone may have chronic sub-clinical neurotoxic effect on the optic nerve and that this may be related to some forms of acute optic neuropathies.

Antimicrobials. A number of different antimicrobials have been associate with ocular toxicity.
- *Acyclovir.* A case of blindness following acyclovir treatment for herpes simplex has been reported (von Schultheiss and Sauter 1982). This patient died and autopsy showed necrotic vasculitis (considered to be drug-induced) involving both optic nerves.
- *Chloramphenicol.* Optic neuritis is the most common manifestation of chloramphenicol neurotoxicity. Twenty-seven patients reported in the English literature have been reviewed by Ramilo et al (1988). Most of these patients had peripheral neuropathy as well. Some had papilledema. Treatment was discontinuation of chloramphenicol and vitamin B-complex therapy, mainly B_{12}. Mechanism is not known but it may possibly be by interfering with vitamin B_{12} metabolism.
- *Clioquinol.* Optic atrophy associated with clioquinol is a part of subacute myelo-opticoneuropathy (see Chapter 24).
- *Dapsone.* This is used for the treatment of leprosy. Dapsone-induced motor peripheral neuropathy is well known (see Chapter 11). The first case of optic atrophy with loss of vision in addition to peripheral neuropathy in patient on high-dose dapsone therapy was reported by Homeida et al (1980). This complication is not reported in patients receiving normal doses of this drug.
- *Ethambutol.* This is a bacteriostatic antitubercular drug developed in 1962. Since then optic

neuritis has been reported as an adverse effect (Citron 1969; Barron et al 1974; Suzuki et al 1976; Jimnez-Lucho et al 1987; Kumar et al 1993). De Palma et al (1989) reported that 8 patients out of 84 treated for pulmonary tuberculosis with ethambutol presented with optic neuritis.

Early onset neuropathy is believed to be an idiosyncratic reaction (Karnik et al 1985) and is irreversible (Kahana 1987). Delayed onset neuropathy, on the other hand, is considered to be reversible (Nasemann et al 1989). The pathomechanism is presumed to be linked to the mode of action of this drug as a chelating agent and causing depletion of zinc in the optic nerve and impairing its metabolism. Hamard (1989) believes that optic disc swelling due to ethambutol is the clinical manifestation of a volumetric increase of the neural axons due to blockade of the axoplasmic transport without demyelinating lesions. This concept also explains the improvement after discontinuation of the drug.

The following are some of the recommended guidelines for prevention of ethambutol-induced optic neuropathy (Alvarez and Krop 1993):
- Recommended dose and duration should not be exceeded.
- Avoid use of this drug in patients with significantly reduced optic acuity prior to treatment.
- Patients should be informed that the drug may affect vision and if this happens, the drug should be stopped immediately. The patient should be referred to an ophthalmologist.

Dette et al (1991) recommend the use of visually evoked potentials for the early detection of preclinical changes of ethambutol-induced optic neuritis so that early discontinuation of the drug can be recommended. Baseline investigations and follow-up examination of patients on ethambutol therapy should include visual acuity testing with Snellen charts, automated threshold perimetry and optic fundus photography (Russo and Chaglasian 1994).
- *Isoniazid.* Optic atrophy has been reported as a complication of isoniazid during treatment of tuberculosis (Kiyosawa and Ishikawa 1981). The pathomechanism is related to pyridoxine deficiency and this complication can

be prevented by dietary supplementation with pyridoxine. One patient with combined ethambutol and isoniazid therapy for three months presented with mild sensory neuropathy and bilateral retrobulbar neuritis which progressed to optic atrophy (Leppert and Waespe 1988). The risk factors in this case were low serum zinc levels and slow acetylation of isoniazid. Most of the cases reported are associated with long-term isoniazid therapy but one case of optic neuritis with overdose of isoniazid has also been described (Lockman and Shum 1998). Bilateral fundal hyperemia was seen six hours following the overdose but cleared up after 16 hours following treatment with pyridoxine.

– *Streptomycin.* Streptomycin is known for toxic effect on the eight nerve but there are several reports of optic neuritis as well which have been reviewed by Walker (1961). This adverse effect was noted mostly when streptomycin was given intrathecally for tubercular meningitis although there are reports of optic neuritis developing during streptomycin therapy for other conditions.

– *Sulfonamides.* Optic neuritis has been reported as an adverse reaction to various sulfonamides but is usually reversible after discontinuation of the drug (Fraunfelder and Meyer 1989).

– *Tryparsamide.* This organic arsenical is used in the treatment of trypanosomiasis. The most serious and common adverse reactions to this drug involve the eye. About 10% of the patients taking this medications experience visual changes and if the medication is not discontinued the pathologic condition of the optic nerve may become irreversible and progress to blindness (Fraunfelder and Meyer 1989).

Antineoplastic Drugs. A number of antineoplastic drugs have been associated with ocular toxicity.

– *Chlorambucil.* Visual loss and optic atrophy has been reported after long-term use of chlorambucil in a patient with low-grade non-Hodgkin's lymphoma (Yiannakis and Larner 1993).

– *Fluorouracil.* Several cases of optic neuropa-

thy have been reported during long-term treatment with 5-fluorouracil (Adams et al 1984).

– *Cisplatin.* Bilateral optic neuritis has been reported in a patient after treatment of ovarian carcinoma with cisplatin/carboplatin combination (Caraceni et al 1997). This resolved one year after completion of the treatment and was considered to be more likely due to cisplatin rather than carboplatin. Cisplatin is administered intra-arterially in patients with brain tumors to increase the drug concentration at tumor site but this is associated with visual system toxic effects including retinal and optic nerve degeneration (Shimamura et al 1990). Retinal toxicity after high dose cisplatin therapy has been reported by Wilding et al (1985). Optic nerve toxicity and maculopathy after intra-arterial cisplatin does not appear to depend on the method of administration, whether it is supra-ophthalmic or infra-ophthalmic (Kupersmith et al 1988). Blindness due to optic neuritis was reported in a patient after treatment of glioblastoma with intra-arterial cisplatin therapy (Mansfield and Castillo 1994). Optic nerve toxicity can be monitored by visual evoked potentials (VEP) and alterations in VEP have been detected prior to visual loss (Maiese et al 1992).

– *Tamoxifen.* Tamoxifen is a non-steroidal antiestrogen used in the management of selected patients with breast cancer. It is well-tolerated without serious side effects. Retinopathy has been reported in patients treated mainly with high dose tamoxifen therapy for long periods (McKeown et al 1981). Even low-dose long-term treatment can induce retinopathy (Vinding and Nielsen 1983; Pavlidis et al 1992; Bentley et al 1992; Chern and Danis 1993). Costa et al (1990) reported a case of retinopathy seven years after completion of tamoxifen therapy. The pathomechanism of this toxic effect is not clear. It has been postulated that the cationic amphophilic nature of tamoxifen allows binding with polar lipids, interfering with their catabolism (Kaiser-Kupfer et al 1981).

– *Paclitaxel.* This is usually associated with peripheral neuropathy but a case of optic neuropathy has also been reported (Capri et al 1994). Loss of visual acuity was progressive during the treatment and was attributed to damage to the optic nerve. There was some recovery of function after completion of the treatment.

- *Vincristine.* The neurotoxicity of this antineoplastic agent consists mostly of peripheral neuropathy (see Chapter 11) and less often cranial neuropathies. Optic neuropathy has been reported in 9 patients by Munier et al (1992a). Postmortem histological examination of the optic nerve in one of these patients showed a primary toxic axonal injury followed by secondary retrograde degeneration, resulting in retinal nerve fiber atrophy and ganglia cell degeneration (Munier et al 1992b). Optic atrophy in this case was considered to be an idiosyncratic reaction to vincristine.

Carbamazepine. There are only two case reports in literature of retinotoxicity of carbamazepine (Nielsen and Syversen 1986). A few other cases have been reported to the manufacturer, Novartis, but no definite causal relationship has been established between the drug and this adverse effect. Impairment of color vision, however, is recognized as an early sign of neurotoxicity of antiepileptic drugs such as carbamazepine and phenytoin but valproic acid has not been reported to produce this effect (Bayer et al 1994).

Chloroquine. Significant ocular side effects including blindness have been reported with chloroquine and related drugs. Retinopathy has been reported with chloroquine (Sassani et al 1983; Marks 1982). The mechanism of this toxic effect is not understood. Since this drug is concentrated in the pigmented tissues, macular changes have been reported long after the drug therapy is stopped. Delayed-onset chloroquine retinopathy has been diagnosed in a rheumatoid arthritis patient 7 years after cessation of treatment (Ehrenfeld et al 1986). In one study reported recently (Lange et al 1994), retinopathy was not significantly associated with long-term once-weekly prophylactic use of chloroquine by 588 missionaries in West Africa. The median cumulative dose of chloroquine in these subjects was > 300 mg and 12 had taken the agent for 16–25 years. Hydroxychloroquine is considered to be safer than chloroquine but it has also been reported to produce retinopathy (Weiner et al 1991).

Corticosteroids. Various corticosteroids are reported to be associated with ocular complications including optic atrophy. A case of toxic optic neuropathy associated with use of prednisone has been reported (Teus et al 1991). There is no adequate documentation of the reported cases. Benign intracranial hypertension with papilledema, however, is a recognized complication of prolonged corticosteroid therapy.

Corticosteroids are also used in the treatment of optic neuritis of multiple sclerosis. A randomized controlled study found that oral prednisone is an ineffective treatment and increases the risk of new episodes of optic neuritis (Beck et al 1992) but I/V methylprednisone reduces the rate of development of multiple sclerosis over a 2-year period (Beck et al 1993).

Desferroxamine. This chelating agent is used in the treatment of iron-storage diseases and acute iron poisoning. Long-term intravenous or subcutaneous desferoxamine treatment is used in patients who develop massive tissue deposits of iron as a result of repeated blood transfusion used to treat chronic refractory anemias and may cause acute visual loss and toxic retrobulbar optic neuropathy has been reported (Olivieri et al 1986). Irreversible visual loss associated with optic neuropathy and retinal pigmentary degeneration has been reported after a single "challenge" dose of desferoxamine (Bene et al 1989). A case has been described where retinal pigmentary degeneration occurred after injection of subcutaneous desferoxamine (Mehta et al 1994).

Pathomechanism of desferoxamine neurotoxicity is not clear but it has been suggested that it may cause oxidative damage within the neural tissue by translocating copper (Pall et al 1989). Another possible mechanism is that zinc and iron depletion induced by desferoxamine may affect critical enzyme functions within the neural tissues which are dependent on these trace metals (De Virgilis et al 1988).

Interferon-α-2b. It is used for the treatment of chronic hepatitis as well as malignancies. Two cases of anterior ischemic optic neuropathy were reported following treatment in cancer patients were reported (Purvin 1995a). Both of these were treated with corticosteroids. One died due to progression of cancer and the in the other patient, the optic disc edema resolved considerably over a period of several months. One patient with chronic hepatitis C developed cotton wool patches on the retina after treatment with interferon-α resulting in considerable decrease of visual acuity of the other eye which showed ischemic changes of the fundus oculi on fluorescein angiography (Shahidullah et al 1995). There was slight improvement 18 months after cessation of the interferon therapy. In a study in Japan, retinal abnormalities were observed in 57% of the patients treated with interferon-α for chronic hepatitis C (Kawano et al 1996). The incidence was higher among patients with diabetes mellitus or hypertension.

Non-Steroidal Anti-Inflammatory Drugs. The role of these drugs in the causation of papilloedema, disc edema, and benign intracranial hypertension has been reviewed by Fraunfelder et al (1994) from the data reported to the National Registry of Ocular Side Effects. The overall pattern of retrobulbar optic neuritis and papillitis could not be differentiated from that seen in multiple sclerosis and drug cause-and-effect relationship could not be established. The largest number of cases were associated with propionic acid derivatives ibuprofen and naproxen. Fifty cases were reported in association with ibuprofen (43 optic neuritis and 7 papilledema) Decreased vision is reported by less than 5% of the patients using naproxen. Seventeen cases of optic neuritis and 5 cases of papilledema associated with naproxen were reported. Retinal pigmentary disorders and macular edema have also been reported. Naproxen is a photosensitizer and, theoretically, could enhance retinal disease.

Oral Contraceptives (OC). These are combination products of estrogens and progestogens. In addition to their use as oral contraceptives, they are used for treatment of amenorrhoea, dysmenorrhea, and premenstrual tension. Cerebrovascular disease as a complication of OC is described in Chapter 9. Benign intracranial hypertension with papilledema is a known complication (Chapter 17). Central retinal vascular occlusion

is associated with OC. Optic neuritis (ischemic pupillopathy) has also been described (Zhi-Hui and Shou-Jing 1988).

Omeprazole. This drug is used for the management of gastrointestinal ulcers. Several cases of visual impairment as an adverse reaction have been reported. In one case edematous papillitis was noted on fundoscopy and progressed to ischemic optic neuropathy with decreased vision (Schönhofer and Werner 1997). This was considered to be possibly due to drug-induced vasculitis but there is no supporting evidence and vasculitis confined to the eye is not known so far. A combined WHO and IMS International data analysis shows that the worldwide reporting rate for all visual complaints following use of omeprazole is 0.0008 per million treatment days (ADR Signals Analysis Project 1996). Although the background incidence of these complaints is not known, the reporting rates are not of serious concern in view of the widespread use of omeprazole.

Phenothiazines. The most significant ocular side effects are reported with long-term use of chlorpromazine and thioridazine probably because they are the most frequently prescribed drugs of this group. Retinal pigmentary changes and retinal degeneration has been reported (Ball and Caroff 1986; Hamilton 1985; Lam and Remick 1985; Mitchell and Brown 1995). Extensive chorioretinopathy has been reported to be associated with low dose thioridazine therapy as well (Neves et al 1990; Tekell et al 1996).

Pathomechanism. Phenothiazines combine with the retinal pigment and are slowly released and retinal changes may progress even after the drug is discontinued. A phototoxic process has been postulated to be involved in retinal degeneration.

Quinine. This alkaloid which is the oldest antimalarial drug is also used for the treatment of nocturnal leg cramps and myotonia congenital. Quinine-induced blindness is well known and is usually associated with overdosage (Guly and Driscoll 1992). Fundoscopy may be normal at first but constriction of retinal arteries, retinal edema, and a cherry red spot at macula may be seen later. Optic atrophy may develop weeks or months later (Canning and Hague 1988). Two cases of blindness have been described of which one was permanent (Waddell 1996).

Pathomechanism. Blindness is unlikely to be due to retinal arteriolar constriction but rather due to a direct toxic effect on the retina as shown by electroretinographic studies. It may be an idiosyncratic reaction in some cases.

Treatment. Suggested treatment includes stellate ganglia blocks, vasodilators, corticosteroids, and vitamin B. It is difficult to prove that any of these have significant clinical effects.

Sildenafil (Viagra). The drug is used for the treatment of impotence and has been associated with cerebrovascular ischemia (see Chapter 9). The drug was introduced in 1998 and is used extensively. Among the various adverse effects, visual complaints have been prominent. These are described as light sensitivity and seeing a bluish color tinge. No publications have yet appeared on this topic but the American Academy of Ophthalmology has warned about the adverse effects on the eye. The main concern is about permanent loss of vision in patients with existing retinal dysfunction. The effects are dose-related and are more likely to occur in patients who are taking larger than recommended doses of the drug.

Vaccines. Optic neuritis associated with vaccines is usually transient and associated with other neurological complications such as encephalomyelitis and Guillain-Barré syndrome. Bilateral optic neuritis with has been reported following small pox and diphtheria-tetanus toxoid vaccinations (McReynolds et al 1953). Optic neuritis with reversible blindness has been reported following influenza vaccination (Perry et al 1979; Hara et al 1983; Ray and Dreizin 1996; Hull and Bates 1997). Optic atrophy has been reported after swine influenza vaccination (Cangemi and Bergen 1980; Macoul 1982). A case of optic neuritis and myelitis was reported following a booster dose of tetanus toxoid (Topaloglu et al 1992). Recombinant hepatitis B vaccine has been reported to be associated with optic neuritis and visual loss (Albitar et al 1997). Multiple lesions of the retinal pigment epithelium with visual impairment has been reported after hepatitis B vaccination (Brézin et al 1993).

Vigabatrin. It is a GABA-mimetic antiepileptic drug. Several cases of ocular adverse effects such as visual field constriction have been reported following the use of vigabatrin. (Eke et al 1997; Blackwell et al 1997; Wong et al 1997; Wilson and Brodie 1997). Four cases of vigabatrin-associated retinal cone system dysfunction manifested by blurred vision and investigated by electroretinography have also been published (Krauss et al 1998). One case of unilateral optic atrophy was confirmed by impairment of visual evoked potential and improved after discontinuation of vigabatrin and treatment with dexamethasone (Crofts et al 1997). In a case of unilateral ischemic optic neuropathy with impairment of vision following use of vigabatrin, the pathomechanism was considered to be allergic vasculitis and this was confirmed by a positive lymphocyte transformation test for vigabatrin (Dieterle et al 1994). The patient recovered after discontinuation of vigabatrin and treatment with cortisone.

Epidemiology. Since the start of the clinical trials of vigabatrin in 1995, health authorities in UK have received 41 reports of visual field defects associated with the use of vigabatrin. These have been reported form one month to several years after start of the therapy. The manufacturer (Hoechst Marion Roussel) has started several trials to investigate whether vigabatrin is associated with visual field defects. More than 140,000 patients have been treated with vigabatrin since its introduction in 1989. According to the manufacturer, visual field defects have been reported with a frequency of < 0.1% and a causal association cannot be proven from the case reports (Backstrom et al 1997).

Pathomechanism. One of the explanations offered is that vigabatrin and other agents increase the persistence of GABA and cause visual field constriction by unknown mechanisms (Harding 1997). Another hypothesis is that chronic exposure to GABA and other antiepileptic agents such as phenobarbital which interact with $GABA_A$ receptors leads to removal of the receptor subunits from the surface of neurons and downregulation of GABA binding sites (Sieghart 1995). With this background, introduction of GABA mimetics leads to high concentrations of GABA which can be toxic to neural cells including the retinal cells.

Prevention. The patients at risk of developing visual impairment should be identified at an early stage. Visual field testing should be done routinely to monitor patients on vigabatrin therapy. Visual evoked potential detect optic nerve involvement but are normal in retinopathy which is detected by electroretinographic abnormalities. patients on multiple antiepileptic drugs which include other GABA-modulating drugs should have baseline studies to assess visual function prior to start of vigabatrin.

Drug-Induced Disorders of Eye Movements

Several disturbances of eye movements are associated with drugs but only nystagmus and ophthalmoplegia will be considered here:

Nystagmus

Various types of ocular oscillations described as nystagmus in relation to drugs are positional, downbeat, upbeat, gaze evoked, and periodic alternating nystagmus. Most of these disturbances are probably due to a pharmacologically induced transient dysfunction of the vestibulo-cerebellar flocculus loop (Esser and Brandt 1983). Some of the drugs for which nystagmus has been reported as an adverse reaction are listed in Table 10.3.

Paralysis of Cranial Nerves III to VII

Ophthalmoplegia. Ophthalmoplegia or paralysis of eye muscles may be external or internal. Drug-induced external ophthalmoplegia may be due to involvement of muscles or the neuromuscular junction (see Chapter 13).

External ophthalmoplegia with absent vestibulo-ocular reflexes in an unconscious patient may suggest structural brainstem pathology and this has been reported with the following medications:

- Amitriptyline (Smith 1979)
- Barbiturates (Edis and Mastaglia 1977)

Table 10.3. Drugs reported to induce nystagmus.

Amiodarone
Amitriptyline
Aspirin
Baclofen
Barbiturates
Benzodiazepines
Bromide
Bupivacaine
Carbamazepine
Cephalosporins
Chloral hydrate
Chloroquine
Chlorpromazine
Cytosine arabinoside
Disulfiram
Fenfluramine
Fluorouracil
Glutethimide
Ibuprofen
Isoniazid
Ketamine
Lithium carbonate
Melatonin overdose (Balentine and Hagman 1997)
Meperidine
Meprobamate
Metrizamide
Nalidixic acid
Nitrofurantoin
Perhexiline
Phenelzine
Phenytoin
Piperazine
Quinine
Streptomycin
Valproic acid

- Carbamazepine overdosage (Ng et al 1991; Mullaly 1982; Noda and Umezaki 1982)
- Cisplatin intracarotid infusion (Alderson et al 1996)
- Dilantin (Spector et al 1976)

Internal ophthalmoplegia is due to lesions of the nuclei of the cranial nerves III, IV, and VI which supply the ocular muscles. Internuclear ophthalmoplegia is due to lesions of structures between the nuclei in the brainstem, e. g., involvement of medial longitudinal fasciculus with failure of conjugate movements. The following drugs have been reported to produce internuclear ophthalmoplegia:

- Benzodiazepines
- Fenfluramine (Carreres et al 1992)

– Fluorouracil
– Lithium (Deleu and Ebinger 1989)

Paralysis of the VI (Abducent) Cranial Nerve

Abducent nerve has the longest free-hanging course of all the intracranial nerves and mechanical factors also predispose to abducent palsy such as occurs in rise of intracranial pressure. The following are example of drug-induced abducent palsy:
– Complication of myelography with iopamidol (Bell et al 1992, Bell and McIlwaine 1990).
– A case of reversible bilateral lateral rectus palsy has been described in association with high dose cytosine arabinoside therapy (Ventura et al 1986).
– Four patients developed unilateral or bilateral abducent nerve palsy while receiving cyclosporin and ganciclovir following allogeneic bone marrow transplantation (Openshaw et al 1997).
– One patient developed unilateral abducent palsy as a manifestation of post-lumbar puncture syndrome following intrathecal administration of prednisolone (Dumont et al 1998).

Paralysis of the VII (Facial Nerve)

The following are examples of drug-induced facial palsy (Bell's palsy):
– One patient developed facial palsy after sulfasalazine therapy but recovered after withdrawal of the drug (Magnus et al 1993).
– A few case shave been reported following hepatitis B vaccination (Ganry et al 1992).
– A case of peripheral facial nerve paralysis has been reported following local upper dental anesthesia using articaine (Bernsen 1993). The patient made a complete recovery within 10 weeks.
– One patient developed facial palsy after carotid endarterectomy performed with local infiltration of 1% lidocaine and 0.5% bupivacaine around the carotid artery in the neck (Szocik

et al 1995). The patient recovered 12 hours after surgery.
– Two patients with HIV infection developed facial neuropathy following treatment with didanosine (Gottfried et al 1994). One of the these patients had a trochlear nerve palsy as well. The symptoms of cranial neuropathy improved in both patients after didanosine was discontinued.
– Insulin-like growth factor-1 therapy in a child with growth hormone deficiency (Wollmann and Ranke 1994). The child recovered after discontinuation of the therapy.

Various mechanisms have been postulated but the most likely is an immunologic reaction. Facial nerve swelling is likely to result in compression in the bony facial canal and paralysis which frequently recovers spontaneously after the swelling subsides.

Cortical Blindness

The term cortical blindness indicates loss of site due to bilateral lesions in the occipital lobes. It is rare but severe adverse reaction to drugs. Drugs which have been reported to be induce cortical blindness are shown in Table 10.4.
– *Cisplatin.* Cortical blindness and seizures possibly related to cisplatin have been reported (Young et al 1993). The possible pathomechanism is similar to that for cisplatin-encephalopathy (see Chapter 3).
– *Cyclosporin.* Reversible cortical blindness has been reported in bone marrow transplant patients receiving cyclosporin therapy (Edwards et al 1995; Ghalie et al 1990; Rubin 1989). Visual impairment and bilateral occipital lobe white matter abnormalities correlated

Table 10.4. Drugs reported to induce cortical blindness.

Cisplatin
Cyclosporine
Diatrizoate-meglu mine
Interferon-α
Nifedipine
Sulfonamides
Ta crolismus (FK506)
Vinblasti ne

with the degree, duration, and rate of elevation in blood pressure from baseline. This leads to the hypothesis that these reversible abnormalities are due to cerebral edema incited by hypertension (Singh et al 1999). Hypertension may be drug induced and visual abnormalities may be prevented by aggressive management of hypertension which occurs prior to the onset of visual symptoms. There may be no need to discontinue cyclosporin or further imaging studies if there is a rapid clinical improvement. A case report of permanent blindness after cyclosporin neurotoxicity and review of the 10 cases in the literature is presented by Esterl et al (1996).

- *Diatrizoate-meglumine.* This is an iodinated contrast material for angiography. Lantos (1989) reported four cases of cortical blindness following cerebral angiography. CT scan showed abnormal contrast enhancement in occipital regions in all the cases indicating that there was disruption of the BBB likely due to the contrast material.

- *Interferon-α.* A case of cortical blindness during therapy with interferon-α has been reported (Merimsky et al 1992). CT scan excluded structural damage to the brain indicating that toxic or metabolic reactions may have caused this adverse effect.

- *Nifedipine.* Cortical blindness was reported following treatment of hypertension with nifedipine (Morton and Hickey 1992). Bilateral occipital lobe infarction was demonstrated on CT. The infarction was likely due to hypotension induced by nifedipine.

- *Tacrolismus (FK506).* This is an immunosuppressive medication used after organ transplantation and is similar to cyclosporin in action. It is reported to induce an encephalopathy and a case of cortical blindness was reported (Eidelman et al 1991). A second case was reported of a patient on FK506 therapy who developed cortical blindness 8 days after liver transplantation (Shutter et al 1993). MRI showed white matter lesions similar to those seen in cyclosporin leukoencephalopathy (see Chapter 3). The patient recovered vision after discontinuation of FK506 and treatment with methylprednisone although the white matter lesions persisted.

Drug-Induced Ototoxicity

This section includes drug-induced disorders of the end organs of the vestibulocochlear nerve (VIII) in the inner ear. Drugs may induce hearing loss (cochlear) and/or vestibular dysfunction. Drug-induced hearing loss is usually sensorineural. Only aspects of ototoxicity relevant to neurology are reviewed in this section.

Tinnitus. Most ototoxic drugs cause hearing loss by damaging the cochlea, particularly the auditory hair cells and stria vascularis, a specialized epithelial organ within the inner ear responsible for homeostasis of fluids and electrolytes. Tinnitus can be an early symptom before onset of hearing loss and has been reviewed by Seligman et al (1996). Tinnitus has been reported with several drugs (see Table 10.5) and is difficult to evaluate because of the subjective nature of the complaints. It is not necessarily accompanied by hearing loss and usually resolves when the drug is discontinued. Many of the ototoxic drugs listed in Table 10.7 produce tinnitus also and there is an overlap in the drugs listed in Tables 10.5 and 10.7.

Vertigo. The vestibular system is of fundamental importance in the maintenance of equilibrium. It has connections with the medulla oblongata, the cerebellum, the oculomotor system, and the cerebral cortex. Vertigo is an illusionary sense of motion in which the subject feels that the motion is internal or that the objects in the surroundings are rotating or tilting. Vertigo is often caused by an imbalance of neuronal activity between the two labyrinths or between the vestibular nuclei on each side of the brainstem. Vertigo as an adverse effect of drugs as well as management of vertigo has been reviewed by Rascol et al (1995). Symptoms of drug-induced vestibular toxicity can be vertigo, loss of balance, nausea and vomiting. Drugs which induce vertigo are shown in Table 10.6.

Ototoxic Drugs

Ototoxicity of the drugs was documented as early as the nineteenth century with the use of quinine and salicylates as therapeutic agents. The

Table 10.5. Drugs that induce tinnitus.

Anesthetics
  Lidocaine
Antiepileptic drugs
  Carbamazepine
  Phenytoin
  Valproic acid
Antihistaminics
Antimicrobials
  Aminoglycosides
  Macrolide antibiotics
  Sulfonamides
  Tetracyclines
  Vancomycin
Antimalarial drugs
  Chloroquine
  Primaquine
  Quinine
Antineoplastic drugs
  Cisplatin
  Tamoxifen
  Vincristine
Antiulcer drugs
  Cimetidine
  Famotidine
  Omeprazole
Benzodiazepine withdrawal
Cardiovascular drugs
  Antiarrhythmics
  Antihypertensives
    Diazoxide
    Enalapril
CNS stimulants
  Amphetamine
  Caffeine
Diuretics
  Bumetanide
  Ethacrynic acid
  Furosemide
  Torasemide
Non-steroidal anti-inflammatory drugs
  Salicylates
Opioids

Table 10.6. Drugs that induce vertigo.

Ototoxic drugs (see Table 10.7)
Drugs inducing a central vestibular syndrome
  Antiepileptic drugs
  Anxiolytics
  Neuroleptics
  Opioids
  Tricyclic antidepressants
Drugs producing pseudovertigo of nonvestibular origin
  Drugs that induce orthostatic hypotension
  Drugs that disturb vigilance
    Sedatives
    Hypoglycemic agents

medical profession became fully aware of ototoxicity in 1940s when streptomycin was introduced for the treatment of tuberculosis. In the modern setting ototoxicity is most frequently encountered with aminoglycoside antibiotics. Drugs which have been reported to be associated with ototoxicity are listed in Table 10.7.

Table 10.7. Drugs reportedly associated with ototoxicity.

Aminoglycoside antibiotics*
  Amikacin
  Gentamicin
  Kanamycin
  Neomycin
  Netilmicin
  Streptomycin
  Tobramycin
Antibiotics (nonaminoglycoside)
  Ampicillin
  Azithromycin
  Cephalosporins
  Chloramphenicol
  Erythromycin*
  Minocycline
  Polymixins
  Sulfonamides
  Vancomycin
  Viomycin
Antiepileptic drugs
  Valproic acid (Armon et al 1990)
Antiinflammatory drugs: salicylates*
Antimalarials
  Quinine*
  Chloroquine
Antineoplastic agents
  Carboplatin*
  Cisplatin*
  Cytosine arabinoside
  Nitrogen mustard
  Paclitaxel
Diuretics
  Ethacrynic acid
  Furosemide
Other drugs
  Beta-adrenergic receptor blockers
  Calcium channel blockers
  Carbimazole
  Desferoxamine*
  Interferon
  Local Anesthetics: Lidocaine
  Muromonanmab CD3 (Hartnick et al 1997)
  Metrizamide
  Oral contraceptives

*Well documented.

Aminoglycoside Antibiotics

Amikacin. It is derived from kanamycin and has similar pharmacokinetics. Both drugs are more cochleotoxic than vestibulotoxic and both are nephrotoxic.

Gentamicin. The chemical structure of gentamicin is related to that of kanamycin and neomycin. The is the most widely used aminoglycoside antibiotic currently. When administered to patients with renal insufficiency at high doses, it causes vestibular disorders in 2.5 to 5% of them, some of them only unilateral (Jao and Jackson 1964). Reports of cochlear changes are less frequent (El Bakri et al 1998; Lu et al 1996). Intratympanic instillation of gentamicin has been used for vestibular ablation in treatment of Meniere's disease (Magnusson and Padoan 1991).

Pathomechanism. Ototoxicity likely results from rapid uptake of the drug and exposure of the inner ear tissues to the drug. The toxic effects are due to the metabolized or activated form of the drug through formation of an iron-gentamycin complex that, in turn, produces free radicals. This provides the rationale for the proposed treatment of gentamycin ototoxicity with free radical scavengers (Minor 1998). Basile et al (1996) have shown that aminoglycoside-induced hearing loss is mediated through an excitotoxic process and opens up the prospects of reduction of ototoxicity by NMDA (N-methyl-D-aspartate) antagonists.

Kanamycin. Changes produced by kanamycin are mainly cochlear as shown by clinical and experimental studies. Hearing loss usually occurs at the highest frequencies and is preceded by tinnitus. Renal function impairment potentiates the ototoxic effects of kanamycin, which may continue after the medication is discontinued. The drug accumulates in the inner ear and the elimination is slow. One of the proposed mechanisms of action of kanamycin is through combination of the drug with polypeptides, which may inhibit the course of protein synthesis. In this manner, the drug may have a direct effect on the nutritional status of the hair cells and of the cochlear nerve, eventually causing degeneration of the organ of Corti (Lundquist and Wersall 1966).

Neomycin. Neomycin is considered to be one of the most ototoxic drugs used currently and the damage is limited mostly to the cochlear portion with sensorineural loss affecting high tones and sometimes it is total and irreversible (Leach 1962). Deafness has been reported following intravesical instillation of neomycin in patients with end-stage renal disease (Gerharz et al 1995). Deafness has been reported in a child following bladder irrigation with 1% neomycin solution (De Jong et al 1993).

Netilmicin. It is a new semisynthetic aminoglycoside derived from gentamicin and has low ototoxicity (Vesterhauge et al 1980). Netilmicin does not cause the phenomenon of aminoglycosideinduced ototoxicity because it does not seem to affect the hair cells of the basal turn of the cochlea.

Streptomycin. Soon after streptomycin was started to be used around 1945 at dose of 2 to 3 g/day, it was found to destroy the function of the vestibular system within a few weeks. The vestibulotoxicity of streptomycin was subsequently confirmed by animal experimental studies. On rare occasions streptomycin was used for vestibular ablation in Meniere's disease. Cochlear changes with hearing impairment were less common. The mechanism of action of streptomycin on the receptor cells of the vestibular system is explained on the structural and biochemical actions of the drug, i. e., action on the cell membrane, inhibition of protein synthesis and ribosomal function, mitochondrial alteration of the vestibular receptor cells (Duvall and Wersäll 1964).

Tobramycin. It has a low incidence of ototoxicity. In a series of 3506 patients who utilized tobramycin, only 21 showed signs of ototoxicity with auditory and vestibular disturbances distributed equally (Bendush et al 1977).

Antibiotics (Nonaminoglycoside)

Ampicillin. Intravenous high-dose ampicillin therapy has been reported to be associated with a high percentage of bilateral sensorineural hearing loss in patients with Hemophilus influenzae meningitis (Gamstrop and Klockhoff 1974). The role of ampicillin in ototoxicity cannot be ascertained because meningitis can also cause deafness.

Azithromycin. This is new antibiotic which is used against Mycobacterium avium infections in AIDS patients. Bilateral sensorineural hearing loss has been reported in 3/21 (14%) patients 30–90 days after beginning azithromycin therapy as a part of three drug regimen, where the other two drugs were clofazimine and ethambutol (Wallace et al 1994). In two of these patients hearing loss recovered after discontinuation of azithromycin therapy and one patient who was rechallenged with this drug developed hearing loss again. No further cases of hearing loss were reported after azithromycin was substituted by clarithromycin in the same three-dose regimen. Intravenous azithromycin is more likely to induce ototoxicity due to higher peak serum concentrations (Bizjak et al 1999).

Cephalosporins. Ototoxicity has been reported in two patients with renal failure while on cephalexin therapy (Sennasael et al 1982). Studies in experimental animals with cephazolin show that the drug accumulates in perilymph but does not produce any lesions.

Chloramphenicol. A case of nerve deafness following an unusually high dose of chloramphenicolin a child was reported (Gargye and Dutta 1959). Sporadic cases have been reported of hearing impairment after use of chloramphenicol ear drops. The ototoxic effect may be due to propylene glycol which is used as vehicle in ear drops.

Erythromycin. Ototoxicity with erythromycin is rare. Ototoxicity of erythromycin is dose-related and occurs in patients with renal or liver disease. However, it has been reported in patients who are free from predisposing factors and may be idiosyncratic (Sacristan et al 1993a). At high serum concentrations of this drug, the amount reaching the cochlea may be sufficient to affect the hair cells. Hearing loss develops between 8 hours and 8 days of treatment and disappears from 24 hours to 14 days after discontinuation of the drug (Cramer 1986), although some irreversible cases have been reported (Dylewski 1986). Intravenous administration of erythromycin in renal transplantation patients has been reported to result in clinically significant hearing loss in one-third of patients (Vasquez et al 1993). Improvement in hearing occurred in all patients within 5 days of discontinuation of therapy. The mechanism of erythromycin-induced ototoxicity is not known but instillation of this drug into the middle ears of animals has been shown to alter the hair cells of the cochlea (Stupp et al 1973). Auditory evoked potential studies have shown erythromycin-induced hearing loss to be attributable to a functional disorder of the peripheral parts of the auditory system (Sacristan et al 1993b). Mogfod and Pallett (1994) have reported a case of erythromycin-induced deafness in a patient with renal impairment. Cimetidine, a comedication was considered to have aggravated the deafness by increasing the serum and otic concentrations of erythromycin.

Minocycline. It is a semisynthetic derivative of tetracycline. Several investigators have reported the occurrence of vestibular symptoms during treatment with minocycline, though no cochlear symptoms appear. The frequency of this adverse effect is reported to be as high as 86% (Jacobson and Daniel 1975). Experimental studies in guinea pigs exposed to minocycline have failed to show any lesions of the organ of Corti (Kepenis et al 1975) but the validity of these studies is questionable because the serum concentrations of the drug were low and this species may not be a suitable subject for these studies.

Polymyxin B. Ototoxicity may occur in patients with renal insufficiency when blood concentration of Polymyxin B is greater than 5 µg/ml (Horton and Pankey 1981). Vestibular changes have been observed in experimental animals but the organ of Corti and vestibular neuroepithelium remained histologically normal (Riskaer et al 1956).

Sulfonamides. Vertigo, ataxia, and tinnitus are known as adverse reactions of sulfonamides. Vertigo has been observed in patients treated with sulfamethoxazole/trimethoprim. No animal experimental studies are available regarding oto-toxicity of sulfonamides.

Vancomycin. The most serious toxic effect attributed to vancomycin are tinnitus, decreased auditory acuity and deafness, which have been reported to occur when serum concentrations exceed 90 to 100 mg/ml (Brown and Wise 1982). Vancomycin ototoxicity occurs in patients treated with massive doses, in those with renal failure, or in patients who have received other oto-toxic drugs concomitantly. The hearing loss is often reversible with discontinuation of the drug.

Viomycin. In a study of patients treated for tuberculosis with streptomycin or viomycin, the latter was found to be more ototoxic with greater involvement of the vestibular system than the cochlea (Daly and Cohen 1965). Ototoxicity has been confirmed by experimental studies on animals.

Antiinflammatory Drugs

Salicylates. Aspirin is one of the most widely used drugs. Among the documented adverse effects of aspirin are tinnitus and hearing loss. Dose-related deafness occurred in 32 of the 2974 hospital patients given aspirin reported by the Boston Collaborative Drug Surveillance Program (Porter and Jick 1977).

Significant hearing loss at relatively low serum salicylate concentrations (below 40 mg/dl) has been reported in patients receiving 300 mg of aspirin daily. This hearing loss was reversible within one week of stopping the salicylate (Jardini et al 1978). Experimental studies on several animal species have shown depression of cochlear electrical activity, which may explain the hearing loss detected in patients treated with salicylate. These changes are reversible as indicated by the absence of histological changes in the organ of Corti.

Pathomechanism. The mechanism of ototoxicity of salicylates is not fully understood. Clinically and electrophysiologically the cochlea appears to be the site of toxic effects (Evans and Borerwe 1982). Aspirin-induced hearing loss in experimental animals has been used as a model of sensorineural hearing loss. A single dose of salicylate has been shown to interfere with the ability of cochlea to generate a neural action potential (AP) whereas the cochlear microphonic is unaffected. This decrease in AP affects the synaptic transmission in the auditory nerve but is reversible. Salicylate intoxication produces biochemical changes in the endolymph and perilymph which disturbs the inner ear homeostasis. Prostaglandins, through their stimulatory effect on the adenyl cyclase system, may affect the cell membrane Na^+, K^+ ATPase pump which affects AP generation (Miller 1985). Vasoconstriction within the cochlear microvasculature may be mediated through the prostaglandin biosynthetic pathway. Decreased sensitivity may be the result of inhibited prostaglandin synthesis in the cochlea (Jung et al 1988). If antiprostaglandin effects are important in the etiology of ototoxicity, other NSAIDs may be expected to induce such clinical effects. There are reports associating hearing loss, tinnitus, and vertigo with naproxen, indomethacin, ibuprofen etc. (Brien 1993).

Antimalarials

Quinine. The most common cochlearvestibular symptoms observed during quinine administration are hyperacusis and tinnitus, which occur with doses of about 2 g/day. The hearing loss is of a sensorineural type and usually recovers after discontinuation of the drug but may be irreversible in some cases.

The ototoxicity of quinine in guinea pig is similar to that of sodium salicylate. Labyrinthine changes may be explained by the occurrence of ischemia or hemorrhages. These vascular changes support the hypothesis of Hawkins (1973) that ototoxic action first occurs at the level of vascular structures such as the stria vascularis and planum semilunatum which contain melanin. The lesions occur in the secretary and reabsorption tissue and not in the receptor cells. Another hypothesis is that quinine has an effect on the contractile structure of the outer hair cells of the organ of Corti (Karlsson and Flock 1990). In studies on healthy human volunteers reversible quinine-induced hearing impairment, concentration-effect relationship was consistent and was formulation and time-dependent but independent of the route of administration (Paintaud et al 1994).

Chloroquine. This is another cinchona derivative which may cause transitory deafness predominantly at acute frequencies and accompanied by tinnitus, as well as irreversible deafness (Hart and Naunton 1964).

Antineoplastic Drugs

Carboplatin. Hearing loss with high-dose carboplatin is common in patients. It occurs in nearly all of the patients who have received prior treatment with other ototoxic agents. In one study of children with neuroblastoma who received carboplatin therapy prior to receiving bone marrow transplantation, bilateral hearing loss developed in all cases and hearing aids were recommended for 81.8% of these (Parsons et al 1998).

Cisplatin. Cisplatin-induced ototoxicity appears to be mainly confined to auditory function with a few reports of vestibular toxicity. Symptoms of ototoxicity include deafness, tinnitus and otalgia. The overall incidence of hearing loss, in a review of eight studies in adults, was 69%, and that of tinnitus 7% (Moroso and Blair 1983). A recent study of long-term follow-up after cisplatin indicates that ototoxicity persists in 20% of the patients (Bokemeyer et al 1998). The hearing loss is usually irreversible. Some important features of ototoxicity of cisplatin are:
- The elevated thresholds for hearing are not reversible.
- Cumulative effect is not observed in all cases.
- The use of diuretics does not reduce the incidence of ototoxicity.
- There is a considerable interpatient variability in the hearing loss.
  Risk factors for cisplatin ototoxicity are:
- Hearing loss tends to be more severe in patients who have received previous radiotherapy encompassing the ear (Skinner et al 1990).
- Exposure to loud noises and previous hearing losses may be risk factors for the ototoxic effects.

- Children < 5 years and the elderly who have renal impairment are at risk for hearing loss.
- Ototoxicity is accentuated in children with brain tumors who receive radiotherapy prior to chemotherapy (Granowetter et al 1983) but not in patients where chemotherapy precedes radiotherapy (Kretschmar et al 1990).

Pathomechanism. This is not well understood. Some authors have suggested that endocochlear potential is reduced during cisplatin administration in experimental animals, implicating that stria vascularis is the site of ototoxicity (Laurell and Engstrom 1989). Others have observed significant reductions in the value of cochlear microphonic potential without significant reduction in the value of endocochlear potential (Konishi et al 1979). McAlpine and Johnstone (1990) concluded that cisplatin causes hearing loss by blocking the outer hair cell transduction channels.

Cytosine Arabinoside (ARA-C). Neurotoxicity of high dose ARA-C therapy including vertigo and nystagmus is well known. Hearing loss has been reported as a complication of low dose ARA-C therapy by Cersosimo et al (1987).

Nitrogen Mustard. Hearing changes have been reported in patients receiving nitrogen mustard but no vertigo has been reported. Experimental studies have shown that there is no significant hearing loss with systemic administration of nitrogen mustard at usual doses of 14 mg/kg body weight. However, at high sublethal doses, as is the case with regional perfusions including the ear the drug may induce sensorineural hearing loss due to toxic effect on the hair cells of the organ of Corti.

Paclitaxel/Vinorelbine. One case of ototoxicity with this regimen has been reported (Tibaldi et al 1998). The hearing loss did not resolve after discontinuation of the therapy.

Loop Diuretics

Loop diuretics act by blocking active sodium reabsorption in the ascending part of the loop of

Henle. Two drugs of this class are usually used: ethacrinic acid and furosemide.

Ethacrynic Acid. The first patient to develop ototoxicity from the use of this drug had bilateral sensorimotor loss (Maher and Schreiner 1965). This patient died and examination of cochlea revealed loss of outer cells in the basal turn. Most of the cases of hearing loss have been reported in patients with impaired renal function where the concentration of the drug in the labyrinthine fluid is higher because of poor excretion. The hearing loss is usually reversible but cases of irreversible hearing loss have also been reported (Rybak 1988). Pillay et al (1969) reported 5 cases of deafness in uremic patients following treatment with ethacrynic acid and in 3 the deafness was permanent.

The pathomechanism of hearing loss with ethacrynic acid is not known but there are several hypotheses. One of these is based on the similarities between the renal glomerulus and the stria vascularis of the cochlea. The loop diuretics may have a similar action on the stria vascularis and cause sodium and water accumulation inducing electrolyte changes in the endolymph as well as damage to the stria vascularis. Ethacrynic acid also inhibits the enzyme adenylate cyclase in the stria vascularis and reduces the cochlear potentials. This enzyme is responsible for the production of cyclic AMP and its inhibition is an important mechanism of action of loop diuretics.

Furosemide. Several investigators have reported reversible sensorineural hearing loss with the use of furosemide, with some patients also developing vertigo and tinnitus (Schwartz et al 1970; Cooperman and Rubin 1973). Furosemide has essentially no vestibulotoxic effect. Furosemide does not accumulate in the perilymph and this may explain the absence of histological lesions after chronic administration of the drug and the reversibility of the hearing loss.

Pathomechanism of hearing loss induced by furosemide is not directly mediated by a change in electrolyte balance. Furosemide has a reversible effect on oxidative phosphorylation in the outer hair cells of the basal cochlear turn (Akiyoshi 1981). This may explain the possible functional alterations of the cells.

Other Drugs

α-**adrenoreceptor Blockers.** Practolol, propranolol, and metoprolol are drugs of this group which have been used for treatment of cardiac arrhythmias. Cases of sensorineural hearing loss have been reported after treatment with proctolol (Jones et al 1977). Tinnitus has been reported with propranolol (Lloyd-Mostyn 1969). In a study of 18 patients with propranolol, one case of hearing loss was reported by McLean et al (1967) where recovery occurred after 6 months. Animal experimental studies have shown that propranolol produces a dose-dependent reduction of auditory response (Wiederhold 1985). Faldt et al (1984) reported loss of hearing in a patient during treatment with metoprolol and it cleared up after the drug was discontinued.

Calcium Channel Blockers. The Spanish system of pharmacovigilance has reported 8 patients who developed tinnitus during calcium antagonist therapy (Narvaez et al 1994). These patients received nifedipine (n = 2), verapamil (n = 2), nicardipine (1), nitrendipine (1), diltiazem (1), and cinnarizine (1). Five of these patients were on calcium channel blocker monotherapy and tinnitus resolved 126 days after discontinuation of the drug involved in each case.

Carbimazole. A case of hearing loss and tinnitus is described in a patient with Graves disease treated with carbimazole (Hill et al 1994). Carbimazole hypersensitivity was diagnosed in this case. The patient developed serological evidence of lupus. The drug was withdrawn and replaced with another thiourea derivative. The hearing loss gradually resolved but some tinnitus persisted.

Desferoxamine. Of the 89 patients with transfusion dependent anemia who were receiving desferoxamine

Interferon (IFN). In a prospective follow-up cohort study of auditory function in 49 patients receiving IFN, auditory disability (tinnitus, hearing loss or both) occurs in 22 (45%) patients (Kanda et al 1994). These adverse effects developed in the late stage of treatment and resolved in all patients within 7 to 14 days after discontinuation of IFN. The authors stated that auditory disability was attributable to IFN for the following reasons:

- The frequency of auditory disability was unexpectedly high.
- Rapid improvement after discontinuation of drug.
- Ototoxicity appeared to be dose-related.
- There were no other potential causes of ototoxicity in these patients. However, interaction of IFN with antipyretics received by these patients in the early phase might have contributed to this adverse reaction.

Pathomechanism. The pathomechanism of this adverse reaction is not clear. Two mechanisms have been proposed:

- Thrombocytopenia induced by IFN may have cause a vascular accident in the inner ear.
- IFN

Local Anesthetics. Lidocaine is commonly used as a local anesthetic. It has been used for alleviation of tinnitus and vertigo in Meniere's disease. However, vestibular dysfunction has also been reported as an adverse reaction to intravenous lidocaine. Lidocaine applied locally to the middle ear diffuses through the round window and into the inner ear and alters the activity of the hair cells of the organ of Corti. It may temporarily alter the efficiency of the transduction mechanism of the cochlea, possibly causing a simultaneous cellular injury. There is controversy regarding the reversibility of these effects.

Oral Contraceptives (OC). Oral contraceptives are frequently related to changes in the auditory system only or in the vestibular system only or in both systems simultaneously. Hearing loss occurs during prolonged treatment with OCs and it s evolution is unpredictable, with possibility of improving, stabilizing, or deteriorating (Dvorak 1980). The ototoxic mechanism of oral contraceptives has been related to vascular changes.

The pathomechanism is not known. The symptoms may be due to a reduction in blood supply to the central part of the vestibular system located in the brainstem. Cerebrovascular disease aggravated by OC may involve the internal auditory artery.

Prevention of Drug Ototoxicity

General Measures. These vary according to the drugs used and the reversibility. Antibiotic-induced ototoxicity is mostly reversible whereas antineoplastic drug-induced ototoxicity is mostly not reversible. Attempts at reducing the ototoxicity of drugs consist of modifying the dosage schedules, using less toxic derivatives of original drugs, and giving compounds concomitantly to counteract the neurotoxicity. Vitamin A and vitamin B complex have been used but there is no proof of their efficacy. For practical purposes the most important measures are avoidance of risk factors and early detection of neurotoxicity so that the drug may either be discontinued or the dosage reduced. Monitoring of auditory and vestibular functions is recommended during treatment with ototoxic drugs. A shortened monitoring protocol has been suggested for use with patients unable to tolerate lengthy audiometric testing protocols (Fausti et al 1992).

Potential New Treatments. Several other measures have been proposed but not fully investigated. These include the following:

- Free radical scavengers
- NMDA antagonists
- Neurotrophic factors. Several studies show that specific neurotrophic factors (NTFs) protect spiral ganglion neurons (SGNs) from ototoxic drugs in vitro and in vivo (Jain 2000). SGNs are required to relay the signal to the central nervous system even when a cochlear implant is used to replace hair-cell function or in the case that cochlear sensory epithelium can be stimulated to regenerate new hair cells successfully (Gao 1998). NTFs have potential therapeutic value in prevention and treatment of hearing impairment.

Recurrent Laryngeal Nerve Palsy

This is a branch of the vagus or the X cranial nerve. All of the reports of laryngeal nerve palsy are following vincristine (Erdmann 1990; Alfredsunder et al 1992; Annino et al 1992). Peripheral neuropathy is a well known complication of vincristine and may be present in these cases or recurrent laryngeal palsy may be an isolated finding. The manifestation is vocal cord paralysis with hoarseness of voice, dysphagia, and neck pain. Orofacial pain reported in patients on vincristine therapy may also possibly be due to involvement of trigeminal and glossopharyngeal nerves (McCarthy and Skillings 1992). Diagnosis is by indirect laryngoscopy. Stridor may occur and children may require tracheal intubation as a supportive measure. Early withdrawal of the drug usually leads to recovery.

Drug-Induced Disorders of Taste and Smell

A large number of drugs affect the taste and smell sensations. There is either a report of total loss of taste or, more often, alteration of taste sensation with or without disturbances of smell. Various expressions are used by the patients for describing taste and smell alterations and a system for classifying these, based on the findings, is shown in Table 10.8.

Epidemiology. The true incidence of drug-induced taste and smell disturbances is difficult to determine because of the infrequency of reporting. Even for agents that are considered to rarely cause taste and smell disturbances, the true incidence may be greater than 3% (Ackerman and Kasbekar 1997). There are no further reports appearing in the literature during the past decade on some of the older drugs which are known to cause taste disturbances and are still prescribed.

Disturbances of Taste

Disturbances of taste may involve loss or distortion of function. Dysgeusia is a general term used to describe taste disturbances and dysosmia implies distortion of smell. Loss of taste (ageusia) means the ability to detect as salt, sweet, sour, and bitter substances whereas hypogeusia means diminished ability to do so. Distortion of taste (phantageusia) may be in response to intake of food or medicines or not associated with any of these when it may be due to gustatory hallucinations. Other terms that are used are cacosmia means interpretation of normal odors as foul and parosmia which is perception of an odor that is not present. The commonest disorder of taste, other than actual taste loss, associated with drugs is "metallic taste" and this is more clearly specified and described with regard to onset by most of the patients. Anosmia may be associated with weight loss due to decrease of appetite resulting from loss of perception of flavor of food. Smell acuity reflects the ability to detect and recognize vapors which can be evaluated clinically. Drug-induced disturbances of taste can usually be linked to the drug used and affect the taste receptors over the entire tongue and palate.

Disturbances of Smell

Dysosmia is a general term used to describe smell disturbances. Loss of smell (anosmia) is inability to detect or recognize vapors at the primary or accessory areas of olfaction. Complete loss of smell is rare and most drug-induced smell disorders involve reduced ability (hyposmia) to smell familiar vapors such as those of perfumes. Drug-induced olfactory disorders are usually bi-

Table 10.8. A simple classification of loss and distortion of taste and smell function.

Disturbance	Taste	Definition	Smell
Loss	Ageusia	Inability to detect any stimuli	Anosmia
Diminished function	Hypogeusia	Decreased ability to detect stimuli	Hyposmia
Disturbance (unspecified)	Dysgeusia	Either decreased or increased or distorted perception of stimuli	Dysosmia
Distortion	Phantageusia	Distorted perception of stimuli	Phantosmia

lateral whereas unilateral anosmia is usually due to head injury or other syndromes unrelated to drug use. Smell and taste disorders frequently coexist. Patients with loss of smell have impairment of taste sensation as well.

Pathology of Smell and Taste Disturbances

Injury and impairment of the smell and taste sensory systems may occur at various levels and both sensations may be affected by the same drug. Three levels described by Henkin (1944) are as follows:
– *Central nervous system*. This is involved in less than 5% of cases.
– *Neural transmission*. Disorders of sensory neural transmission contributes to less than 5% of the total drug-related taste and smell pathology.
– *Receptors*. Taste and smell receptor dysfunction comprise the bulk of drug-related smell and taste dysfunction. Receptor injury impairs the initial step of these sensory process. These are further subdivided as:
  · Receptor pathology in 45% of cases
  · Impairment of receptor-mediated mechanisms in 45% of cases

Drugs may affect the receptors directly or indirectly by producing vitamin and essential element (zinc and copper) deficiencies. Zinc metalloproteins (gustin and lumicarmine for taste, a gustin-like protein for smell) are critical for maintaining receptor integrity. Molecular events underlying these disturbances can involve alteration of primary, secondary, or tertiary receptor protein structure. Subsequent events may be as follows (Henkin 1994b).
– Decreased receptor sensitivity
– Inhibition of receptor turnover
– Inactivation of events of receptor-coupled on system which normally involve G protein synthesis, cyclic adenosine monophosphate (cAMP) activity, and activation of sodium and/or calcium ion channels. Drug-induced impairment of these events can lead to lack of generation of action potential which is trans-mitted along taste/smell nerve pathways to the CNS
– Drug-induced events in the receptor-coupled off mode usually involve taste and smell distortions. These may involve a direct receptor pathology or a binding abnormality due to activation of an inhibitory G protein or receptor kinases or cytochrome p450 proteins. The receptor is not erased or turned off and the smell or taste may persist in a distorted manner.

Drugs Reported to Induce Disorders of Smell and Taste

Disorders of smell and taste have been reported with a large number of pharmaceuticals. It would be impossible to list all of these. Only drugs where the frequency of these disorders is reported at 1% or higher are listed in Table 10.9.

Pathomechanism of Drug-Induced Taste Disorders

Our knowledge of how drugs can modify the taste is very limited because taste is a very subjective sensation and cannot be verified objectively. The knowledge of neurotransmitters responsible for relaying the taste and olfactory information from the periphery to the brain is still incomplete. Evaluation of drug-induced taste disturbances is difficult because some of the complaints are due to the taste of the drug itself rather than a pathologic change in the taste system. Even if the galenic preparation masks the unpleasant taste of the drug, it may reach the taste receptors by being excreted in the saliva or by vascular route. Furthermore, the patients have diseases that contribute to or can cause smell and taste disturbances. Possible mechanisms to explain the effect of drugs on taste and smell have been are listed in Table 10.10. The role of genetic factors in the pathogenesis of drug-induced smell and taste disturbances has not been defined but it is likely that genetic factors interacting with environmental factors may increase the susceptibility to drug-induced smell and taste disturbances.

Table 10.9. Drugs reported to induce disorders of taste and smell with a frequency of occurrence of 1% or more. This is based on publications from 1980–1998 plus drug safety data released by pharmaceutical manufacturers. Collective reviews of this topic during this period were also consulted (Mott and Leopold 1991; Schiffman 1991; Griffin 1992; Henkin 1994a; Ackerman and Kasbekar 1997).

Anesthetics, local: dysgeusia due to nerve injury during dental anesthesia
  benzocaine
  lidocaine
  procaine
Anorectic drugs
  amphetamines: dysgeusia, hyposmia
  fenfluramine: dysgeusia
  mazindol: dysgeusia
  phendimetrazine: dysgeusia
Antiasthmatics
  flunisolide: dysgeusia, hypogeusia, hyposmia
Antihistaminics
  terfandine:dysgeusia
  loratadine: dysgeusia
  promethazine: hypogeusia, hyposmia
Antimicrobial agents
Antifungals
  griseofulvin: dysgeusia
  terbinafine: hypogeusia, metallic taste
Anthelminthics
  levamisole: taste alteration
Antiprotozoals
  metronidazole: metallic taste, hypogeusia
  pentamidine: hyposmia, metallic taste, hypogeusia
Antivirals
  didanosine: dysgeusia
  foscarnet: dysgeusia
  idoxyuridine: dysgeusia
  interferon-alpha: phantogeusia, anosmia
  zalcitabine: taste distortion
  zidovudine: dysgeusia
Cephalosporins
  cefacetrile: hypogeusia
  cefadroxil: dysgeusia
  cefamandole: dysgeusia
  cefpodoxime: dysgeusia
  cefalexin: dysgeusia
Chlorhexidine mouth wash: hyposmia, dysgeusia
Penicillins
  ampicillin: hypogeusia
  procaine penicillin: hypogeusia
  piperacillin: hypogeusia
Quinolones
  enoxacin: phantogeusia
  ofloxacin: taste and smell distortions
Tetracyclines
  minocycline: dysgeusia
Antineoplastics
  bleomycin: hypogeusia
  doxorubicin: hypogeusia
  5-fluorouracil: bitter phantogeusia
  gallium: dysgeusia
  interleukin-2: hyogeusia, hyposmia

  methotrexate: hypogeusia
  vincristine: hypogeusia
Antirheumatic drugs
  gold: hypogeusia, phantogeusia
  penicillamine: hypogeusia, dysgeusia
Antismoking agents
  nicotine polacrilex: dysgeusia
Cardiovascular drugs
  ACE inhibitors
    captopril: sweet and salt phantogeusia, hypogeusia
    enalapril: hypogeusia, dysgeusia
    fosinopril: hypogeusia, dysgeusia
    lisiopril: hypogeusia, dysgeusia
  AT_1 (angiotensin receptor subtype 1) antagonists
    losartan: dysgeusia
  calcium channel inhibitors
    amlodipine: dysgeusia, dysosmia
    nifedipine: dysosmia, hypogeusmia
    diltiazem: hypogeusia
  diuretics
    acetazolamide: dysgeusia
    amiloride: hypogeusia
    ethacrynic acid: hypogeusia
    metolazone: bitter phantogeusia
    riamterene: hypogeusia
  antiarrhythmics
    amiodarone: abnormal taste and smell
    flecainide: dysgeusia, altered taste
    moracizine: bitter phantogeusia
    procainamide: bitter phantogeusia
  antihyperlipidemica
    cholestyramine: hyposmia
    gemfibrozil: hyposmia
    lovastatin: hyposmia
    pravastatin: hyposmia
Other agents
  diazoxide: hypogeusia
  isosorbide nitrates: bitter phantogeusia
  labetalol: dysgeusia
  nitroglycerin: hypogeusia
  phenindione: dysgeusia
  topical silver nitrate (chronic): hypogeusia, anosmia
Drugs for endocrine disorders
  antithyroid drugs
    carbamizole: hypogeusia, hyposmia
    methimazole: hypogeusia
  antihyperglycemic agents
    tolbutamide: taste alterations
    glipzicid: severe taste changes
  antihypoglycemic
    diazoxide: taste loss
  glucocorticoids: hypogeusia, hyposmia
Drugs for gastrointestinal disorders
  famotidine: dysgeusia

Table 10.9 continued

granisetron (antiemetic): dysgeusia
scopolamine (antispasmodic): hyposmia, hypogeusia
Drugs for neurological disorders
  antiparkinsonian drugs
    bromocriptine: phantosmia
    levodopa: dysosmia, hypogeusia, dysgeusia
    pergolide: dysgeusia
  antiepileptic drugs
    carbamazepine: ageusia, bitter phantogeusia
    felbamate: dysgeusia
  antimigraine drugs
    sumatriptan: taste and smell disturbances
  muscle relaxants
    baclofen: hypogeusia
    cyclobenzaprine: ageusia
Nasal decongestants
  oxmetazoline: hyposmia
  phenylephrine: hyposmia
  pseudoephedrine: dysgeusia
Non-steroidal anti-iflammatory drugs
  aspirin: hypogeusia, dysgeusia
  diclofenac: taste disorder
  etodolac: dysgeusia
  flurbiprofen: taste change, dysosmia
  ibuprofen: hypogeusia
  indomethacin: hypogeusia

nabometone: taste alteration
phenylbutazone: hypogeusia
piroxicam: taste alteration
sulindac: metallic bitter taste
Psychotropic drugs
  anxiolytics/hypnotics
    alprazolam: hypogeusia
    estazolam: dysgeusia
    flurazepam: dysgeusia
    oxazepam: hypogeusia
    zolpidem: dysgeusia
  antidepressants
    amitriptyline: hypogeusia
    bupropion: dysgeusia
    clomipramine: dysgeusia
    desipramine: dysgeusia
    imipramine: hypogeusia
    paroxetine: dysgeusia
    sertraline: dysgeusia
    trazodone: phantogeusia
  antipsychotics
    fluphenazine: phantogeusia
    risperidone: bitter phantogeusia
    lithium: dysgeusia, metallic taste
Retinoids
  etidronate: hypogeusia
  etiretinate: dysgeusia

Diagnosis. The diagnosis of problematic because of the subjective nature of the complaints. History of use of medications that are associated with smell and taste disturbances is important and these drugs should be considered in the differential diagnosis.

Differential diagnosis. Drug-induced taste and smell disturbances should be differentiated from those associated with several diseases shown in Table 10.11 and 10.12 respectively. Drug-induced olfactory disorders are usually bilateral whereas unilateral anosmia is usually due to head injury or other syndromes unrelated to drug use. Smell and taste disorders frequently coexist. Patients with loss of smell have impairment of taste sensation as well.

Diagnostic procedures. Diagnostic work-up of a patient with smell or taste impairment is quite extensive because the complaints are subjective and objective assessment is difficult. There are four important components of clinical evaluation of a patient with smell and taste disturbance:

– History is the most important step because it gives the etiological clue, e. g., the offending drug.

– Physical examination. Examination of the ear, nose and throat as well as neurological examination.

– Special examination of taste and smell. Smell acuity reflects the ability to detect and recog-

Table 10.11. Diseases that affect taste.

Bell's palsy
Cancer
Depression
Diabetes mellitus
Guillain-Barré syndrome
HIV infection
Hyperaldosteronism
Hypothyroidism
Meningitis
Migraine headaches
Multiple sclerosis
Parkinson's disease
Periodontal disease (gingivitis and periodontitis)
Pernicious anemia
Xerostomia (dry mouth)
Zinc deficiency

Table 10.10. Pathomechanisms of drug-induced disturbances of smell and taste.

Depletion of mineral and vitamins
Zinc depletion: captopril, enalapril, diuretics
Copper depletion: penicillamine
Vitamin A inhibition: cholesterol-lowering drugs
Disturbances of sensory receptors
  – Ion channel disturbances
    • sodium channels: amiloride, spironolactone, lithium
    • calcium channels: calcium channel blockers, e.g., nifedipine
  – IInhibition of sensory receptor turnover: calithromycin, chlorhexidine
  – Reduction of permeability of taste cell membrane: amphotericin B
  – Disruption of the integrity of lipids in the receptor cell
  – membranes: clofibrates
  – Inhibition of protein synthesis: aminoglycoside antibiotics
  – Inhibition of cDNA synthesis: penicillins
  – Inhibition of ATP-dependent reactions: aspirin
  – Inhibition of cAMP: metalazone, dipyridamole
  – Catecholamine alterations: anorexiants, β-blockers
  – Inhibition of cytochrome P450: quinolone antibiotics, terbinafine, antihistaminics
  – Olfactory receptor injury: nasal decongestants
  – Glossitis-inhibiting receptor cell turnover: antineoplastic drugs
Interference with axonal transport: colchicine
Inhibition of receptor-coupled off events: antivirals, retinoids, antiepileptics, antipsychotics
Inhibition of receptor-coupled on events (action potentials): antiarrhythmics, antihypoglycemics
Prostaglandin inhibition: non-steroidal anti-inflammatory drugs
Hypothyroidism-induced cytotoxic effects: antithyroid drugs
Mucosal death with decreased regeneration

nize vapors which can be evaluated clinically. Psychophysiologic approach to testing involves measurement of physical parameters such as blood pressure after exposure to odors. Electrogustometry (application of weak electrical currents to taste bud areas in the oral cavity) provides a more objective assessment of taste than simple testing with salt, bitter and sweet substances (Frank and Smith 1991).

– Laboratory tests. The tests that are used for this purpose are:
  · Computed tomography of the head is particularly useful for a patient with smell disorder. Particular attention is paid to the nasal cavities, anterior cranial fossa and nasal sinuses. Apart from anatomical abnormalities, neoplasms in these locations should also be ruled out. Further imaging studies such as MRI is indicated according to the lesion suspected.
  · Electroencephalography and olfactory evoked potentials. These have been used mainly in establishing the sensory function in patients with neurodegenerative disease and for localization of epileptic foci. They have a role in evaluation of a patient where the cause of olfactory impairment is not certain. Because of some technical problems, gustatory evoked potentials have not become a routine investigation for taste disorders in humans.
  · Biopsy of the olfactory neuroepithelium can be obtained by a needle and is generally a safe procedure. It is useful for demonstrating changes that occur in steroid-dependent anosmia, posttraumatic anosmia, postviral olfactory dysfunction and congenital anosmia.

Prevention. Drug-induced smell and taste disturbances can be minimized by avoiding the use of drugs known to induce such disturbances in patients with diseases that make them susceptible to smell and taste disorders. Good nutritional support with zinc supplementation may reduce the possibility of onset of drug-induced smell and taste disorders. Good oral hygiene with prevention of dry mouth may reduce the incidence of taste disturbances. Once a patient shows signs

Table 10.12. Disorders that can cause smell disturbances.

Local disorders
Allergic rhinitis
Atrophic rhinitis
Chronic sinusitis
Cleft palate
Deviated nasal septum and septoplasty
Nasal polyposis
Neoplasms of the nose and nasal sinuses
Paget's disease involving facial and maxillomanibular
    region
Viral rhinitis

Systemic disorders
Adrenal disorders
Aging
Cancer
Diabetes mellitus
Hepatic disease
HIV infection
Hypothyroidism
Kallmann's syndrome (anosmia, hypogonadism)
Malnutrition, zinc deficiency
Organic solvent exposure
Renal disease
Sjögren's syndrome

Neurological and psychiatric disorders
Alzheimer's disease
Congenital anosmia
Depression
Down's syndrome
Epilepsy: olfactory hallucinations
Head injury
Huntington's chorea
Korsakoff psychosis
Parkinson's disease
Pick's disease
Schizophrenia
Shy-Drager syndrome
Tumors of the anterior cranial fossa

of such disturbance, an early discontinuation of the offending drug may prevent complete loss or irreversible distortion of smell or taste.

Prognosis and Complications. Most of the disorders of taste and smell are dose-related and resolve after discontinuation of the drug. In some cases the loss of smell or taste or their distortion may be irreversible. Complications of loss of taste is weight loss due to poor eating and inappropriate intake of salt in patients who should have salt restriction because of a cardiovascular disorder.

Management. Treatment of smell and taste disturbances is mostly limited to zinc supplementation with variable results, reduction of dose of the offending drug or substitution of the offending drug by another one in the same therapeutic category. If the drug-induced disturbances are severe enough to impair the quality of life and the drug is not required for a serious or life-threatening condition, it may be discontinued. Treatment with zinc may correct hyposmia and hypogeusia associated with drug effect. Treatment with drugs that stimulate cAMP synthesis (theophylline, fluoride, and magnesium) has been used in some cases with good results.

References

Ackerman BH, Kasbekar N: Disturbances of taste and smell induced by drugs. Pharmacotherapy 1997; 17: 482–496.

Adams JW, et al: Recurrent acute toxic optic neuropathy secondary to 5-FU. Cancer Treat Rep 1984; 68: 565.

ADR Signals Analysis Project (ASAP) Team: Omeprazole and visual disorders: seeing alternatives. Pharmacoepidemiol Drug Safety 1996; 5: 27–32.

Akiyoshi M: Effect of loop diuretics on hair cells of the cochlea in guinea pig: histological and histochemical study. Scand Audiol 1981; (suppl 14): 185–199.

Albitar S, Bourgeon B, Genin R, et al: Bilateral retrobulbar optic neuritis with hepatitis B vaccination. Nephrology Dialysis Transplantation 1997; 12: 2169–2170.

Alderson LM, Noonan PT, Choi IS, et al: Regional subacute cranial neuropathies following internal carotid cisplatin infusion. Neurology 1996; 47: 1088–1090.

Alfredsunder P, Hochman MC, Kaplan BH: Low-dose vincristine-associated bilateral vocal cord paralysis. New York State J Med 1992; 92: 268–269.

Alvarez KL, Krop LC: Ethambutol-induced ocular toxicity revisited. Ann Pharmacother 1993; 27: 102–103.

Annino DJ, Macarthur CJ, Friedman EM: Vincristine-induced recurrent laryngeal nerve paralysis. Laryngoscope 1992; 102: 1260–1262.

Armon C, Brown E, Carwile S, et al: Sensorineural hearing loss: a reversible effect of valproic acid. Neurology 1990; 40: 1896–1898.

Backstrom JT, Hinkle RL, Flicker MR: Severe persistent visual field constriction associated with vigabatrin; manufacturers have started several studies. BMJ 1997; 314: 1694–1695.

Balentine J, Hagman J: More on melatonin. J Am Acad Child Adolesc Psychiat 1997; 36: 1013.

Ball WA, Caroff SN: Retinopathy, tardive dyskinesia and low-dose thioridine. Am J Psychiatry 1986; 143: 256.

Barron GJ, Tepper L, Irvine G: Ocular toxicity from ethambutol. Am J Ophthalmol 1974; 77: 256.

Basile A, Huaang JM, Xie C, et al: N-methyl-D-aspartate

antagonists limit aminoglycoside antibiotic-induced hearing loss. Nature Medicine 1996; 2: 1338–1343.

Baulac M, Normann JP, Lanoè Y: Severe visual-field constriction and side effects of GABA-mimetic antiepileptic drugs. Lancet 1998; 352: 546.

Bayer AU, Kuehn M, Thiel HJ, et al: Color vision test for early detection of antiepileptic drug-induced neurotoxicity (abstract). Neurology 1994; 44(suppl 2): A294.

Beck RW, Cleary PA, Anderson MM, et al: A randomized controlled trial of corticosteroids in the treatment of acute optic neuritis. NEJM 1992; 326: 581–588.

Beck RW, Cleary PA, Trobe JD, et al: The effect of corticosteroids for acute optic neuritis on the subsequent development of multiple sclerosis. NEJM 1993; 329: 1764–1769.

Belec L, Devila G, Bleibel JM, et al: Bilateral optic neuropathy during prolonged treatment with amiodarone. Annales Med Int (Paris) 1992; 143: 349–351.

Bell JA, Dowd TC, McIlwaine GC, et al: Postmyelographic abducent nerve palsy in association with contrast agent iopamidol. J Clin Neuro-Ophthalmology 1990; 10: 115–117.

Bell JA, McIlwaine GC: Postmyelographic lateral rectus palsy associated with iopamidol. BMJ 1990; 300: 1343–1344.

Bendush CL, Senior SL, Woller HO: Evaluation of nephrotoxic and ototoxic effects of tobramycin in worldwide study. Med J Austral 1977; (suppl 2): 22–26.

Bene C, Manzler A, Bene D, et al: Irreversible ocular toxicity from single "challenge" dose of desferoxamine. Clinical Nephrology 1989; 31: 45–48.

Bentley CR, Davies G, Aclimandos WA: Tamoxifen retinopathy: a rare but serious complication. BMJ 1992; 304: 495–496.

Bernsen PLJA: Peripheral facial nerve paralysis after local upper dental anesthesia. Eur Neurol 1993; 33: 90–91.

Bizjak ED, Haugh MT, Schilz RJ, et al: Intravenous azithromycin-induced ototoxicity. Pharmacotherapy 1999; 19: 245–248.

Blackwell N, Hayllar J, Kelly G: Severe persistent visual field constriction associated with vigabatrin: patients taking vigabatrin should have regular visual field testing. BMJ 1997; 314: 1694.

Bokemeyer C, Berger CC, Hartman JT, et al: Analysis of risk factors for cisplatin-induced ototoxicity in patients with testicular cancer. Brit J Cancer 1998; 77: 1355–1362.

Brézin AP, Lautier-Frau M, Hamedani M, et al: Visual loss and eosinophilia after recombinant hepatitis B vaccine. Lancet 1993; 342: 563–564.

Brien J: Ototoxicity associated with salicylates. Drug Safety 1993; 9: 143–148.

Brown R, Wise R: Vancomycin: a reappraisal. BMJ 1982; 284: 1508–1509.

Callanan D, Blodi BA, Martin D: Macular edema associated with nicotinic acid (Niacin) JAMA; 279: 1702.

Cangemi FE, Bergen RL: Optic atrophy following swine flu vaccination. Ann Ophthalmol 1980; 12: 857.

Canning CR, Hague S: Ocular quinine toxicity. Br J Ophthalmol 1988; 72: 23–26.

Capri G, Munzone E, Terenzi E, et al: Optic nerve disturbances: a new form of paclitaxel neurotoxicity (letter). J Natl Cancer Inst 1994; 86: 1099–1101.

CARA-Ceni A, Martini C, Spatti G, et al: Recovering optic neuritis during systemic cisplatin and carboplatin chemotherapy. Acta Neurolog Scand 1997; 96: 260–261.

Carreres ML, Garrido JL, Rico MG, et al: Toxic inter-nuclear ophthalmoplegia related to obesity treatment. Ann Pharmacother 1992; 26: 1457–1458.

Cersosimo RJ, Carter RT, Mathews SJ, et al: Acute cerebellar syndrome, conjunctivitis, and hearing loss associated with low-dose cytarabine administration. Drug Intell Clin Pharm 1987; 21: 798–803.

Chern S, Danis RP: Retinopathy associated with low-dose tamoxifen. Am J Ophthalmol 1993; 116: 372–373.

Christiansson JK, Hannesson OB, Sveinsson O, et al: Bilateral anterior uveitis and retinal hemorrhages after administration of trimethoprim. Acta Ophthalmologica Scandinavica 1997; 75: 314–315.

Citron KM: Ethambutol: a review with special reference to ocular toxicity. Tubercle 1969; 50: 32.

Cobo J, Ruiz MF, Figueoa MS, et al: Retinal toxicity associated with didanosine in HIV-infected adults. AIDS 1996; 10: 1297–1300.

Cooperman LB, Rubin IL: Toxicity of ethacrynic acid and furosemide. Am Heart J 1973; 85: 831–834.

Costa RH, Dhooge MR, Van Wing F, et al: Tamoxifen retinopathy—a case report. Bull Soc Belge Ophtalmol 1990; 238: 161–168.

Cramer R: Erythromycin ototoxicity. Drug Intell Clin Pharm 1986; 20: 764–765.

Crofts K, Brennan R, Kearney P, et al: Vigabatrin-induced optic neuropathy. J Neurol 1997; 244: 666–667.

Cuba Neuropathy Field Investigation Team. Epidemic Neuropathy in Cuba—Clinical characterization and risk factors. NEJM 1995; 333: 1176–1182.

Daly JF, Cohen NL: Viomycin ototoxicity in man: a cupulometric study. Ann Otol 1965; 53: 150–163.

De Jong TPVM, Donckerwolcke RAMG, Boemers TM: Neomycin toxicity in bladder irrigation. J Urol 1993; 150: 1199.

de Oliveira JAA: Audiovestibular Toxicity of Drugs. Boca Raton, Florida, CRC Press, 1989.

De Palma P, Franco F, Bragliani G, et al: The incidence of optic neuropathy in 84 patients treated with ethambutol. Metabol Pediatr Syst Ophthalmol 1989; 12: 80–82.

De Virgilis S, Congia M, Turco MP, et al: Depletion of trace elements and acute ocular toxicity induced by desferrioxamine in patients with thalassemia. Arch Dis Child 1988; 63: 250–255.

Deleu D, Ebinger G: Lithium-induced internuclear ophthalmoplegia. Clin Neuropharmacol 1989; 12: 224–226.

Dette TM, Spitznas M, Gobbels M, et al: Visually evoked cortical potentials for early detection of optic neuritis in ethambutol therapy. Fortschr Ophthalmol 1991; 88: 546–548.

DeWachter A, Lievens H: Amiodarone and optic neuropathy. Bull Soc Belg Ophtalmol 1988; 227: 47–50.

Dieterle L, Becker EW, Berg PA, et al: Allergic vasculitis

due to gamma-vinyl GABA treatment. Nervenarzt 1994; 65: 122–124.

Dumont D, Hariz H, Maynieu P, et al: Abducens palsy after an intrathecal glucocorticoid injection: evidence for a role of intracranial hypotension. Revue du Rheumatisme 1998; 65: 352–354.

Duvall AJ, Wersäll J: Site of action of streptomycin upon inner ear sensory cells. Acta Otolarygol 1964; 57: 581.

Dvorak K: Hormonal contraception and hearing disorders. Cesk Gynekol 1980; 45: 653–655.

Dylewski J: Irreversible sensorineural hearing loss due to erythromycin. Canad Med Assoc J 1988; 139: 230–231.

Edis RH, Mastaglia FL: Vertical gaze palsy in barbiturate intoxication. BMJ 1977; 1: 144–145.

Edwards LL, Wsolek ZK, Normand MM: Neurophysiologic evaluation of cyclosporine toxicity associated with bone marrow transplantation. Acta Neurol Scand 1995; 92: 423–429.

Ehrenfeld M, Nesher R, Merin S: Delayed onset chloroquine retinopathy. Brit J Ophthalmol 1986; 70: 281.

Eidelman BM, Abu-Elmagd K, Wilson J, et al: Neurologic complications of FK506. Transplant Proc 1991; 23: 3175–3178.

Eke T, Talbot JF, Lawden MC: Severe persistent visual field constriction associated with vigabatrin. BMJ 1997; 314: 180–181.

El Bakri F, Pallett A, Smith AG, et al: Ototoxicity induced by once-daily gentamicin. Lancet 1998; 351: 1407.

Erdmann H: Einseitige Parese des Nervus recurrens durch Vincristin. Med Klin 1990; 85: 154–155.

Esser J, Brandt T: Pharmakologisch verursachte Augenbewegungsstörungen—Differentialdiagnose und Wirkungsmechanismen. Fortschr Neurol Psychiatr 1983; 51: 41–56.

Esterl RM, Gupta N, Garvin PJ: Permanent blindness after cyclosporine neurotoxicity in a kidney-pancreas transplant recipient. Clin Neuropharmacol 1996; 19: 259–266.

Evans EF, Borerwe TA: Ototoxic effects of salicylates on the responses of single cochlear nerve fibers and on the cochlear potentials. Br J Audiol 1982; 16: 101–108.

Fäldt R, Liedholm H, Aursnes J: β-blockers and loss of hearing. BMJ 1984; 289: 1490–1492.

Faldt R, Liedholm H, Aursnes J. Beta blockers and loss of hearing. Br Med J (Clin Res Ed) 1984; 289: 1490–2.

Fausti SA, Henry JA, Schaffer HI, et al: High frequency audiometric monitoring for early detection of aminoglycoside ototoxicity. J Infect dis 1992; 165: 1026–1032.

Feiner LA, Younge BR, Kazmier FJ, et al: Optic neuropathy and amiodarone therapy. Mayo Clin Proc 1987; 62: 701–717.

Frank ME, Smith DV: Electrogustometry. In Getchell TV, et al (Eds.): Smell and taste in health and disease, New York, Raven Press, 1991, pp 503–514.

Fraunfelder FT, Meyer SM: Drug-induced ocular side effects and drug interactions (3rd ed), Philadelphia, Lea & Febiger, 1989.

Fraunfelder FT, Samples JR, Fraunfelder FW: Possible optic nerve side effects associated with nonsteroidal anti-inflammatory drugs. J Toxicol Cut & Ocular Toxicol 1994; 13: 311–316.

Freedman MH, Boyden M, Taylor M, et al: Neurotoxicity associated with desferoxamine therapy. Toxicology 1988; 49: 283–290.

Gamstrop I, Klockhoff I: Bilateral, severe, sensorimotor hearing loss after hemophilus influenzae meningitis in childhood. Neuropaediatrie 1974; 5: 121.

Gao WQ: Therapeutic potential of neurotrophins for treatment of hearing loss. Mol Neurobiol 1998; 17 (1–3): 17–31

Ganry O, Rerailler F, Vercelletto M, et al: Paralysie faciale périphérique faisant suite à une vaccination contre l'hépatite B. Therapie 1992; 47: 433–447.

Gargye AK, Dutta DV: Nerve deafness following chloromycetin therapy. Ind J Pediatr 1959; 26: 265.

Gerharz EW, Weingärtner K, Melekos MD, et al: Neomycin-induced perception deafness following bladder irrigation in patients with end-stage renal disease. Brit J Urology 1995; 76: 479–481.

Ghalie R, Fitzsimmons WE, Bennett D, et al: Cortical blindness: a rare complication of cyclosporine therapy. Bone Marrow Transplantation 1990; 6: 147–149.

Gittinger JW, Asdourian GK: Papillopathy caused by amiadarone. Arch Ophthalmology 1987; 105: 349–351.

Gottfried M, Hunter K, deSilva S, et al: Cranial neuropathy associated with 2',3'-dideoxyinosine therapy for HIV infection. Neurology 1994; 44(suppl 2): 249.

Granowetter L, Rosenstock JG, Packer RG: Enhanced cis-platinum neurotoxicity in pediatric patient with brain tumors. J Neuro-Oncology 1983; 1: 293–297.

Grant WM: The peripheral visual system as a target. In Spencer PS, Schaumburg HH (Eds.): Experimental and clinical neurotoxicology, Baltimore, Williams and Wilkins, 1980, pp 77–91.

Griffin JP: Drug-induced disorders of taste. Adv Drug React Toxicol Rev 1992; 11: 229–239.

Guerin A, London G, Marchais S, et al: Acute deafness and desferrioxamine. Lancet 1985; ii: 39.

Guly U, Driscoll P: The management of quinine-induced blindness. Arch Emerg Med 1992; 9: 317–322.

Hamard H: Ethambutol and the optic nerve. Bull Soc Ophtalmol Fr 1989; 89: 1001–1003.

Hamilton JD: Thioridazine retinopathy within the upper dosage limit. Psychosomatics 1985; 26: 823.

Hara Y, Wakano R, Sakaguchi K: A case of optic neuritis after influenza vaccination. Folia Ophthalmol Jpn 1983; 34: 1980.

Harding GFA: Severe persistent visual field constriction associated with vigabatrin. BMJ 1997; 314: 1694.

Hart CW, Naunton RF: The ototoxicity of chloroquine phosphate. Arch Otolaryngol 1964; 80: 407–412.

Hartnick CJ, Cohen AF, Smith RV: Reversible sensorineural hearing loss after renal transplant immunosuppression with OKT3 (muromonab-cd3). Ann Otol Rhinol Laryngol 1997; 106: 640–642.

Hawkins JE: Ototoxic mechanisms, a working hypothesis. Audiology 1973; 12: 383.

Henkin RI: Concepts of therapy in taste and smell dysfunction: repair of primary sensory receptor function as primary treatment. In Kurihara K, WT L (Eds.): Olfaction and taste 11, Tokyo, Springer-Verlag, 1994b, pp. 568–573.

Henkin RI: Drug-induced taste and smell disorders. Drug Safety 1994: 11: 318–377.

Hill D, Whittet H, Simpson H: Hearing loss and tinnitus with carbimazole. BMJ 1994; 309: 929.

Homeida M, Babikr A, Daneshmend DK: Dapsone-induced optic atrophy and motor neuropathy. BMJ 1980; 281: 1180.

Horton JA, Pankey GA: Polymyxin B: Med Clin North Am 1981; 66: 135.

Hull TP, Bates JH: Optic neuritis after influenza vaccination. Am J Ophthalmology 1997; 124: 703–704.

Jacobson JA, Daniel B: Vestibular reactions associated with minocycline. Antimicrobial Agents Chemotherapy 1975; 8: 453.

Jain KK: Neurotrophic Factors. Jain Pharmabiotech Publications, Basel, Switzerland, 2000 (in press).

Jao RL, Jackson GC: Gentamicin sulfate, a new antibiotic against gram-negative bacilli. JAMA 1964; 189: 817–822.

Jardini L, Findlay R, Burgi E, et al: Auditory changes associated with moderate blood salicylate levels. Rheumatol Rehabilitation 1978; 1: 233–236.

Jimnez-Lucho VE, Del Busto R, Odel J: Isoniazid and ethambutol as causes of optic neuropathy. Eur J Resp Dis 1987; 71: 42–45.

Jin DC, Kim SY, Lee JM, et al: Visual loss complicating OKT3 monoconal antibody transplant recipient. nephrology Dialysis Transplantation 1995; 10: 2144–2146.

Jones RFM, Hammond VT, Wright D, et al: Practolol and deafness. J Laryngol Otol 1977; 91: 963–972.

Jung TTK, Woo HY, Baer W, et al: Effect of non-steroidal anti-inflammatory drugs on the hearing and prostaglandin levels in the perilymph. Otol Head Neck Surg 1988; 99: 154–155.

Kahana LM: Toxic ocular effects of ethambutol. Canad Med Assoc J 1987; 137: 212–216.

Kaiser-Kupfer MI, Kupfer TC, Rodreques MM: A clinicopathological report. Ophthalmology 1981; 88: 89–93.

Kanda Y, Shigeno K, Kinoshita N, et al: Sudden hearing loss associated with interferon. Lancet 1994; 343: 1134–1135.

Karlsson KK, Flock A: Quinine causes isolated outer hair cells to change length. Neurosci Lett 1990; 116: 101–105.

Karnik AM, Al-Shamali MA, Fewech FF: A case of ocular toxicity to ethambutol: an idiosyncratic reaction. Postgrad Med J 1985; 61: 811–813.

Kawano T, Shigehira M, Uto H, et al: Retinal complications during interferon therapy for chronic hepatitis C. Am J Gastroenterol 1996; 91: 309–313.

Kepenis V, Yuda N, Gordon G, et al: Assessment of ototoxic potential of minocycline in guinea pigs. Toxicol Appl Pharmacol 1975; 34: 327–339.

Kiyosawa M, Ishikawa S: A case of isoniazid optic neuropathy. Neuro-Ophthalmology 1981; 2: 67.

Koller EA, Green L, Gertner JM, et al: Retinal changes mimicking diabetic retinopathy in two non-diabetic, growth hormone-treated patients. J Clin Endocrinol Met 1998; 83: 2380–2383.

Konishi T: Some observations on negative endocochlear potentials during anoxia. Acta Otolarygol 1979; 87: 506–516.

Krauss GL, Johnson MA, Miller NR, et al: Vigabatrin-associated retinal cone system dysfunction: electroretinogram and ophthalmic findings. Neurology 1998; 50: 614–618.

Kretschmar CS, Warren MP, Lavally BL, et al: Ototoxicity of radiation and cisplatin for children with central nervous system tumors. J Clin Oncol 1990; 8: 1191–1198.

Krieg P, Schipper I: Bilaterale Optikusneuropathie nach Amiodarone-Therapie. Klin Mbl Augenheilk 1992; 200: 128–132.

Kumar A, Sandramouli S, Verma L, et al: Ocular ethambutol toxicity: is it reversible? J Clin Neuro-ophthalmology 1993; 13: 15–17.

Kupersmith MJ, Frohman LP, Choi IS, et al: Visual system toxicity following intra-arterial chemotherapy. Neurology 1988; 38: 284–289.

Kupersmith MJ, Seiple WH, Holopigian K, et al: Maculopathy caused by intra-arterially administered cisplatin and intravenously administered carmustine. Am J Ophthalmol 1992; 113: 435–438.

Lam RW, Remick RA: Pigmentary retinopathy associated with low-dose thioridazine retinopathy. Canad Med Assoc J 1985; 132: 737.

Lange WR, Frankenfield DL, Moriarty-Sheehan M, et al: No evidence of chloroquine-associated retinopathy among missionaries on long-term malaria prophylaxis. Am J Trop Med & Hyg 1994; 51: 389–392.

Lantos G: Cortical blindness due to osmotic disruption of the blood-brain barrier by angiographic contrast material: CT and MRI studies. Neurology 1989; 39: 567–571.

Laurell G, Engstrom B: The ototoxic effect of cisplatin on guinea pigs in relation to dosage. Hearing Res 1989; 38: 27–34.

Leach WB: Ototoxicity of neomycin and other antibiotics. J Laryngol Otol 1962; 76: 774.

Leppert D, Waespe W: Neurotoxicity of antituberculous drugs in a patient with active tuberclulosis. Ital J Neurosci 1988; 9: 31–34.

Lloyd-Mostyn RH: Tinnitus and propranolol. BMJ 1969; 2: 766.

Lockman P, Shum S: Optic neuritis in acute isoniazid overdose (abstract). J Toxicol-Clin Toxicol 1998; 36: 475.

Lu CMC, James SH, Lien YHH: Acute massive gentamicin intoxication in a patient with end-stage renal disease. Am J Kid Dis 1996; 28: 767–771.

Lundqvist PG, Wersäll J: Kanamycin-induced changes in cochlear hair cells of the guinea pig. Z Zellforsch Mikrosk Anat 1966; 72: 543.

Macoul KL: Bilateral optic atrophy and blindness following swine influenza vaccination. Ann Ophthalmol 1982; 14: 398.

Magnus JH, Elverland HH, Olsen EG, et al: Facial palsy and partial accomodative insufficiency associated with sulfasalazine treatment in a patient with ankylosing spondylitis. Scand J Rheumatol 1993; 22: 199–201.

Magnusson M, Padoan S: Delayed onset of ototoxic effects of gentmicin in treatment of Meniere's disease. Acta Otolarygol 1991; 111: 671–676.

Maher JF, Schreiner GE. Studies on ethacrynic acid in patients with refractory edema. Ann Int Med 1965; 62: 15–29.

Maiese K, Walker RW, Gargan R, et al: Intra-arterial cis-platin-associated optic and otic toxicity. Arch Neurol 1992; 49: 83–86.

Mansfield SH, Castillo M: MR of cis-platinum-induced optic neuritis. AAJNR 1994; 15: 1178–1180.

Mansour AM, Puklin JE, O'Grady R: Optic nerve ultra-structure following amiodarone therapy. J Clin Neuro-Ophthalmology 1988; 8: 231–237.

Marks JS: Chloroquine retinopathy: Is there a safe daily dose? Ann Rheum Dis 1982; 41: 52.

Markus H, Polkey M: Visual loss and optic atrophy asso-ciated with cyproterone acetate. BMJ 1992; 305: 159.

Matsumura T, Maruyama-Tabata H, Kuwahara Y, et al: Subretinal hemorrhage after granulocyte colony-stim-ulating factor. Lancet 1997; 350: 336.

McAlpine D, Johnstone BM: The ototoxic mechanisms of cisplatin. Hearing Research 1990; 47: 191–204.

McCarthy CM, Skillings JR: Jaw and other orofacial pain in patients receiving vincristine for the treatment of cancer. Oral Surg Oral Med Oral Pathol 1992; 74: 299–304.

McKeown CA, Swart M, Blom J, et al: Tamoxifen reti-nopathy. Br J Ophthalmol 1981; 65: 177–179.

McLean CE, Stoughton PV, Kavey KS: Experiences with b-adrenergic blockade. Vasc Surg 1967; 1: 108.

McReynolds WU, Havener WH, Petrohelos MA: Bilat-eral optic neuritis following small pox vaccination and diphtheria tetanus toxoid. Am J Dis Child 1953; 86: 601.

Mehta AM, Engstrom RE, Krieger AE: Desferoxamine-associated retinopathy after subcutaneous injection. Am J Ophthalmol 1994; 118: 260–262.

Merimsky O, Nisipeanu P, Loewenstein A, et al: Interfer-on-related cortical blindness. Cancer Chemother Phar-macol 1992; 29: 329–330.

Miller JJ: Non-steroidal anti-inflammatory drugs. In Miller JJ (Ed.): CRC handbook on ototoxicity, Boca Raton, CRC Press, 1985, pp 73–85.

Minor LB: Gentamicin-induced bilateral vestibular func-tion. JAMA 1998; 279: 541–544.

Mitchell AC, Brown KW: Clorpromazine-induced retino-pathy. Brit J Psychiatry 1995; 166: 822–823.

Mogford N, Pallett A: Erythromycin deafness and cime-tidine treatment. BMJ 1994; 309: 1620.

Moroso MJ, Blair RL: A review of cisplatinum ototoxi-city. J Otolarygology 1983; 12: 365.

Morton C, Hickey-Dwyer M: Cortical blindness after ni-fedipine treatment. BMJ 1992; 305: 693.

Mott AE, Leopold DA: Disorders of taste and smell. Med Clin North Am 1991; 75: 1321–1353.

Mullaly WJ: Carbamazepine-induced ophthalmoplegia. Arch Neurol 1982; 39: 64.

Munier F, Perentes E, Herbort CP, et al: Selective loss of optic nerve β-tubulin in vincristine-induced blindness. Am J Med 1992b; 93: 232–233.

Munier F, Uffer S, Herbort CP, et al: Bilateral loss of ret-inal ganglion cells secondary to vincristine therapy. Klin Monatsbl Augenheilkd 1992a; 200: 550–554.

Narvaez M, Figuera A, Caplla D, et al: Tinnitus with cal-cium channel blockers. Lancet 1994; 343: 1229–1230.

Nasemann J, Zrenner E, Riedel KG: Recovery after se-vere ethambutol intoxication: psychophysical and electrophysiological correlations. Doc Ophthalmol 1989; 71: 179–192.

Nazarian SM, Jay WM: Bilateral optic neuropathy asso-ciated with amiodarone therapy. J Clin Neuro-Oph-thalmology 1988; 8: 25–28.

Neves MS, Jordon K, Dragt H: Extensive retinopathy as-sociated with very low dose thioridazine. Eye 1990; 4: 767–770.

Ng K, Silbert PL, Edis RH: Complete external ophthal-moplegia and asterixis with carbamazepine toxicity. Aust NZ J Med 1991; 21: 886–887.

Nielsen NV, Syversen K: Possible retinotoxic effect of carbamazepine. Acta Ophthalmol (Copenh) 1986; 64(3): 287–90.

Noda S, Umezaki H: Carbmazepine-induced ophthalmo-plegia. Neurology 1982; 32: 1320.

Olivieri NF, Buncic JR, Chew e, et al: Visual and auditory neurotoxicity in patients receiving subcutaneous de-feroxamine infusions. NEJM 1986; 314: 869–873.

Openshaw H, Slatikin NE, Smith E: Eye movement dis-orders in bone marrow transplant patients on cyclospo-rin and ganciclovir. Bone Marrow Transplantation 1997; 19: 503–505.

Paintaud G, Alvan G, Berninger E, et al: The concentra-tion-effect relationship of quinine-induced hearing im-pairment. Clin Pharmacol Ther 1994; 55: 317–323.

Pall H, Bloke Dr, Winyard P, et al: Ocular toxicity of des-ferrioxamine—an example of copper promoted auto-oxidative damage? Br J Ophthalmol 1989; 73: 42–47.

Parsons SK, Neault MW, Lehmann LE, et al: Severe oto-toxicity following carboplatin-containing condition-ing regimen for autologous marrow transplantation for neuroblastoma. Bone Marrow Transplantation 1998; 22: 669–674.

Pavlidis NA, Petris C, Briassoulis E, et al: Clear evidence that long-term, low-dose tamoxifen treatment can in-duce ocular toxicity. Cancer 1992; 69: 2961–2964.

Perry HD, Mallen FJ, Grodin RW, et al: Reversible blind-ness in optic neuritis associated with influenza vacci-nation. Ann Ophthalmol 1979; 11: 545–550.

Pillay VKG, Schwartz FD, Aimi K, et al: Transient and permanent deafness following treatment with ethacrynic acid in renal failure. Lancet 1969; i: 77–79.

Porter J, Jick H: Drug induced anaphylaxis, convulsions, deafness and extrapyramidal symptoms. Lancet 1977; 1: 578–587.

Porter JB, Jaswon MS, Huens ER, et al: Desferrioxamine toxicity: evaluation of risk factors in thalassemic pa-tients and guidelines for safe dosage. Br J Hematol 1989; 73: 403–409.

Purvin VA: Anterior ischemic optic neuropathy second-ary to interferon α. Arch Ophthalmology 1995a; 113: 1041–1044.

Purvin VA: Visual disturbances secondary to clomiphene citrate. Arch Ophthalmology 1995b; 113: 482–484.

Ramilo O, Kinane BT, McCracken GH: Chloramphenicol neurotoxicity. Pediatr Infect Dis J 1988; 7: 358–359.

Rascol O, Hain TC, Brefel C, et al: Antivertigo medications and drug-induced vertigo. Drugs 1995; 50: 777–791.

Ray CL, Dreizin IJ: Bilateral optic neuropathy associated with influenza vaccination. J Neuro-Ophthalmol 1996; 16: 182–184.

Riskaer N, Christensen E, Petersen PV, et al: The ototoxicity of neomycin. Acta Otolaryngol 1956; 46: 137.

Romàn GC: An epidemic in Cuba of optic neuropathy, sensorineural deafness, peripheral sensory neuropathy and dorsolateral myeloneuropathy. J Neurol Sci 1994; 127: 11–28.

Rubin AM: Transient cortical blindness and occipital seizures with cyclosporine toxicity. Transplantation 1989; 47: 572–573.

Russo PA, Chaglasian MA: Toxic optic neuropathy associated with ethambutol: implications for current therapy. J Am Optometric Assoc 1994; 65: 332–338.

Rybak LP: Ototoxicity of ethacrynic acid. J Laryngol Otol 1988; 102: 518–520.

Sacristan JA, De Cos MA, Soto J, et al: Ototoxicity of erythromycin in man: electrophysiologic approach. Am J Otology 1993b; 14: 186–187.

Sacristan JA, Soto JA, de Cos MA: Erythromycin-induced hypacusis: 11 new cases and literature review. Ann Pharmacother 1993a; 27: 950–955.

Sassani JW, et al: Progressive chloroquine retinopathy. Ann Ophthalmol 1983; 15: 19.

Schiffman SS: Drugs affecting taste and smell. In Getchell TV, et al (Eds.): Smell and taste in health and disease, New York, Raven Press, 1991, pp 845–850.

Schönhofer PS, Werner B: Ocular damage associated with proton pump inhibitors. BMJ 1997; 314: 1805.

Schwartz GH, David DS, Rigio RR, et al: Ototoxicity induced by furosemide. NEJM 1970; 282: 1413–1414.

Seligman H, Podoshin L, Ben-David J, et al: Drug-induced tinnitus and other hearing disorders. Drug Safety 1996; 14: 198–212.

Sennasael J, Verbeeln D, Lauwers S: Ototoxicity associated with cephalexin in two patients with renal failure. Lancet 1982; ii: 1154.

Shahidullah AB, Cerruli MA, Berman DH: Interferon may cause retinopathy during hepatitis therapy. Am J Gastroenterol 1995; 90: 1543.

Shimamura Y, Chikama M, Tanimoto T, et al: Optic nerve degeneration caused by supraophthalmic carotid artery infusion with cisplatin and ACNU. J Neurosurg 1990; 72: 285–288.

Shutter LA, Green JP, Newman NJ, et al: Cortical blindness and white matter lesions in a patient receiving FK506 after liver transplantation. Neurology 1993; 43: 2417–2418.

Sieghart W: Structure and pharmacology of g-aminobutyric acid receptor sub-types. Pharmacol Rev 1995; 47: 181–234.

Singh MK, Jichici D, Sachdeo K, et al: Reversible Visual Impairment from Cyclosporine / FK506 Induced Hypertension. Presented at American Academy of Neurology Meeting, 20 April 1999, Toronto, Canada.

Skinner R, Pearson HA, Amineddine HA, et al: Ototoxi-

city of cisplatinum in children and adolescents. Br J Cancer 1990; 61: 927–931.

Smith MS: Amitriptyline ophthalmoplegia. Ann Int Med 1979; 91: 793.

Spector RH, Davidof RA, Schwartman RJ: Phenytoin-induced ophthalmoplegia. Neurology 1976; 26: 1031–1034.

Stupp H, Kupper K, Laglerr F, et al: Inner ear concentrations and ototoxicity of different antibiotics in local and systemic application. Audiology 1973; 12: 350–363.

Suzuki M, Majima Y, Hiramitsu T, et al: Optic neuropathy induced by the use of ethambutol. Folia Ophthal Jpn 1976; 27: 111–115.

Szocik JF, Kellog W, Wakefield TW: Temporary facial nerve palsy during carotid endarterectomy under local anesthesia. Anesthesia and Analgesia 1995; 81: 1106–1107.

Tekell JL, Arturo Silva J, Maas JA, et al: Thioridazine-induced retinopathy. Am J Psychiatry 1996; 153: 1234–1235.

Teus MA, Teruel JL, Pascuel J, et al: Corticosteroid-induced toxic optic neuropathy. Am J Ophthalmol 1991; 112: 605–606.

Tibaldi C, Pazzagli I, Berrettini S, et al: A case of ototoxicity in a patient with metastatic carcinoma of the breast treated with paclitaxel and vinorelbine. Eur J Cancer 1998; 34(Part A): 1133.

Tobias JD, bozeman PM: Vincristine-induced recurrent laryngeal nerve paralysis in children. Intensive Care Med 1991; 17: 304–305.

Topaloglu H, Berker M, Kansu T, et al: Optic neuritis and myelitis after booster tetanus toxoid vaccination. Lancet 1992; 339: 178–179.

Urba S, Forastiere AA: Retrobulbar neuritis in a patient treated with intraarterial cisplatin for head and neck cancer. Cancer 1988; 62: 2094–2097.

Vasquez EM, Maddux MS, Sanchez J, et al: Clinically significant hearing loss in renal allograft recipients treated with intravenous erythromycin. Arch Int Med 1993; 153: 879–882.

Ventura GJ, Keating MJ, Castellanos AM, et al: Reversible bilateral lateral rectus muscle palsy associated with high-dose cytosine arabinoside and mitoxandrone therapy. Cancer 1986; 58: 1633–1635.

Vesterhauge S, Johsen NJ, Thomsen J, et al: Netilmicin treatment followed by monitoring of vestibular and auditory functions using highly sensitive methods. Scand J Infect Dis 1980; (suppl 23): 117–121.

Vinding T, Nielsen NV: Retinopathy caused by treatment with tamoxifen in low dose. Acta Ophthalmol 1983; 61: 45–50.

von Schulthess GK, Sauter C: Acyclovir and herpes zoster. Lancet 1982; 305: 1349.

Waddell K: Blindness from quinine as an antimalarial. Trans Roy Soc Trop Med Hyg 1996; 90: 331–332.

Walker GF: Blindness during streptomycin and chloramphenicol therapy. Brit J Ophthalmol 1961; 45: 555–559.

Wallace MR, Miller LK, Nguyen MT, et al: Ototoxicity with azithromycin (letter). Lancet 1994; 343: 241.

Weiner A, Sandberg MA, Gaudio AR, et al: Hydroxychloroquine retinopathy. Am J Ophthalmol 1991; 112: 528–34.

Wiederhold ML: Effects of propranolol and other adrenergic drugs on responses of the cochlea, auditory nerve, and brain stem to acoustic stimuli. In Miller JJ: Handbook of ototoxicity, Boca Raton, CRC Press, 1985, pp 277.

Wilding G, Caruso R, Lawrence TS, et al: Retinal toxicity after high-dose cisplatin therapy. J Clin Oncol 1985; 3: 1683–1689.

Wilson EA, Brodie M: Severe persistent visual field constriction associated with vigabatrin: chronic refractory epilepsy may have a role in causing these unusual lesions. BMJ 1997; 314: 1693.

Wollmann HA, Ranke MB: Bell's Palsy after onset of insulin-like growth factor therapy in a patient with growth hormone receptor deficiency. Act Paediatr Suppl 1994; 399: 148–149.

Wong IGK, Mawar CE, Sander JWAS: Severe persistent visual field constriction associated with vigabatrin: reaction might be dose-dependent. BMJ 1997; 314: 1693–1694.

Yiannakis PH, Larner A: Visual failure and optic atrophy associated with chlorambucil therapy. BMJ 1993; 306: 109.

Young DC, Mitchell A, Kessler J, et al: Cortical blindness and seizures possibly related to cisplatin, vinblastine, and bleomycin treatment of ovarian dysgerminoma. J Am Osteopathic Assoc 1993; 93: 502–504.

Zhi-Hui L, Shou-Jing F: Ischemic pupillopathy and contraceptives. Chinese Medical Journal 1988; 101: 446–447.

Chapter 11
Drug-Induced Peripheral Neuropathies

Introduction

"Peripheral neuropathy" is a general term referring to any disorder that affects the peripheral nervous system (PNS) including infections, toxins, metabolic disturbances, and trauma. The peripheral nervous system is defined as those portions of the motor neurons, autonomic neurons and primary sensory neurons that extend outside the central nervous system (CNS) and are associated with Schwann cells or ganglionic satellite cells. CNS and PNS are interconnected because the bodies of many PNS neurons lie within the CNS and some peripheral sensory neurons have central projections. The term "polyneuropathy" means involvement of more than several peripheral nerves including cranial nerves. However, both these terms are used commonly to mean peripheral neuropathy and the same practice is followed in this chapter.

Several drugs induce peripheral neuropathy commonly referred to as toxic neuropathy. It is important to consider drug exposure in the differential diagnosis of patients who present with symptoms of peripheral neuropathies. Identification of drug as a cause is important as many of these neuropathies are reversible when the offending drugs are discontinued. An understanding of pathomechanism of drug-induced neuropathies helps in the prevention and management. Several drugs mentioned in this chapter have adverse effects involving other systems besides the peripheral nervous system. It is beyond the scope of this book to list all such effects and only those are mentioned which have a bearing on the pathomechanism of peripheral neuropathies.

Although a broad definition the peripheral nervous system includes cranial and spinal nerves, drug-induced disorders of these nerves are described separately in Chapter 10 (cranial nerves and special senses) and Chapter 14 (disorders of the spine and the spinal cord). Autonomic dysfunction may occur in peripheral nerve disease and several drugs produce autonomic neuropathies (McLeod 1993) which are described in Chapter 18. Neuromuscular disorders and myopathies are described in Chapter 12. Drugs associated with neuropathy are shown in Table 11.1.

Pathophysiological Classification

A popular classification that enables clinicopathological and electrodiagnostic correlations is an anatomical one with two overall types, focal and generalized. This is applicable to drug-induced peripheral neuropathy and is shown in Table 11.2. Neuropathies with initially axonal degeneration present with predominantly sensory symptoms affecting distal portions of long nerves and then progress proximally. These are referred to as distal axonopathies. If myelin sheath, which is derived from Schwann cells is involved, symptoms of both motor and sensory neuron involvement are present. These disorders are referred to as myelinopathies (demyelinating neuropathies). If neural cell bodies are the primary targets, symptoms may begin anywhere but are restricted to either motor or sensory neurons. These disorders are called neuronopathies. Various lesion sites that can produce a neuropathic disorder are shown in Figure 11.1. There are variations in clinical presentations and biopsy abnormalities among patients treated with the

Table 11.1. Drugs reported to be associated with peripheral neuropathy.

Antineoplastic (chemotherapy)
5-Azacytidine
5-Fluouracil
Cisplatin
Cytarabine (Ara-C) high dose
Etoposide (VP-16)
Gemcitabine
Hexamethylmelamine
Ifosphamide
Misonidazole
Suramin
Teniposide (VM-26)
Taxoids
Vinca alkaloids

Antimicrobials
Antiviral nucleoside analogs
Chloroquine
Chloramphenicol
Clioquinol
Dapsone
Ethambutol
Fluoroquinolones
Isoniazid
Mefloquine
Metronidazole
Nitrofurantoin
Podophyllum Resin
Sulfonamides

Cardiovascular drugs
Amiodarone
Enalapril
Hydralazine
HMG-CoA reductase inhibitors: statins

Perhexiline

CNS Drugs
Amitriptyline
Antiepileptic drugs
Chlorprothixene
Gangliosides
Lithium
Nitrous oxide
Phenelzine
Thalidomide

Miscellaneous drugs
Allopurinol
Almitrine
Anticoagulants
Arsenic
Botulinum toxin
Cimetidine
Colchicine
Disulfiram
Etretinate
FK506
Gold
Interferon-α-2B
Interferon-α-2A
Interleukin-2
Lipid lowering agents
Oral contraceptives
Pencillamine
Pyridoxine abuse
Sulphasalazine
Tacrolismus
Tryptophan
Vaccines

Table 11.2. Anatomical classification of peripheral neuropathy.

Overall type	Anatomical subtype
Symmetrical generalized (Polyneuropathy)	Distal axonopathies
	Myelinopathies
	Neuronopathies (motor)
	Neuronopathies (sensory)
	Autonomic
Focal	Focal mononeuropathy or multiple mononeuropathy

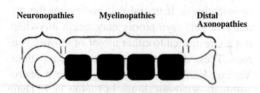

Figure 11.1. Sites of various lesions that produce a neuropathic disorder.

same drug and reflect more than one mechanism of drug-induced nerve injury.

Epidemiology

The exact incidence of drug-induced neuropathy is difficult to determine. Milder forms are overlooked and subclinical forms are more common than generally appreciated. About 2% to 4% of peripheral neuropathies seen in neurological clinics are caused by drugs.

Pathomechanisms of Drug-Induced Neuropathies

Predisposing Factors in the Peripheral Nerves. The following anatomical and physiological features of the peripheral nerves make them more susceptible than the brain to the effects of toxins and drugs:

- Peripheral nerves depend on blood flow which is not autoregulated. Instead the flow is critically dependent on extraneural factors such as blood pressure and blood viscosity. Drug-induced hypotension may interfere with microcirculation, oxygenation, and metabolism of peripheral nerves.
- Dorsal root ganglia of the peripheral somatic nervous system lack an efficient vascular barrier to many large molecular substances. This is an important pathomechanism in toxic lesions with preferential localization to ganglia, i.e., doxorubicin intoxication.
- Endothelial cells of the epineural vessels contain fenestrations and there are open junctions between adjoining cells which allow the escape of proteins from the blood into the extracellular space. Protein-bound drugs can, thus, gain access to the epineurium.
- Endoneural vascular permeability has certain similarities to the vascular permeability in the CNS but compared with the blood-brain barrier, the blood-nerve barrier is less efficient. This implies that toxic agents and pharmaceutical products may have easier access to the parenchyma in the nerves than to brain parenchyma.
- Lack of lymphatics in the endoneural nerve fascicles impedes the removal of toxic substances which have gained access to the endoneural fluid. The toxins can spread both centrifugally and centripetally along the nerve fascicles and cause widespread damage.
- The sink action of CSF which helps to dilute the toxins in the CNS is lacking in the peripheral nerves which are exposed to higher concentrations of ingested toxic substances.

Drugs can produce peripheral neuropathies in several ways of which the following are known:
- *Direct neurotoxicity.* This is an expected dose-related effect of some drugs such as chemotherapeutic agents (see the following section). Injury to myelin may occur such as in hexachlorophene neuropathy with intramyelinic edema and splitting of myelin lamellae.
- *Drug-induced vitamin deficiencies.* Deficien-

cy of some vitamins is a known cause of peripheral neuropathy. Some examples of this are:
- Pyridoxine (vitamin B6) deficiency produced by isoniazid
- Folate deficiency produced by anticonvulsants
- Vitamin B12 deficiency due to prolonged use of chloramphenicol
- Riboflavin deficiency
- *Interference with metabolic processes in nerves.* Examples of this are:
- Nitrofurans can interfere with pyruvate oxidation by competing with thiamine pyrophosphate
- Perhexiline can interfere with lipid metabolism
- Drugs which inhibit cholesterol synthesis interfere with axonal transport and can induce neuropathies
- *Immune mechanisms.* An example of this is neuropathy induced by zimeldine.
- *Drug-induced peripheral vascular disease.* Drug-induced vasculitis is offered as an explanation of cimetidine neuropathy. Vasospasm due to ergot compounds may produce an ischemic neuropathy.
- *Increase of permeability of diffusion barrier.* Drugs which increase the permeability of diffusion barrier can lead to vasogenic edema in the peripheral nerves. There is outpouring of macromolecules into the endoneurium. The increase of endoneural pressure can disturb the microcirculation and impair nerve function.
- *Anticoagulant-induced hemorrhage.* When such a hemorrhage occurs in confined anatomical spaces, it can lead to a compression neuropathy. Anticoagulant femoral neuropathy is an example.
- *Local damage to nerves by drug application.* The following are examples of this:
- Faulty injection of drugs around and into peripheral nerves.
- Local anesthetics can cause endoneural edema, elicit mast cell reaction, and result in endoneural and perineural fibrosis.
- Mononeuropathy associated with intrale-

sional vinblastine treatment of AIDS Kaposi sarcoma.
- Regional neurotoxicity. Infusion of cisplatin into the internal or external iliac artery may produce an acute lumbosacral plexopathy or mononeuropathy within 24 hours.

The principal pathological process in drug-induced neuropathies is axonal degeneration in the form of the "dying back" phenomenon. The induced disturbance interferes with axonal flow and supply of nutrients to the distal axons, so that the malfunction first appears most distally in the axon and gradually spreads proximally towards the cell body. Less commonly there is segmental demyelination exemplified by postvaccinial polyneuropathy and perhexiline neuropathy in which Schwann cells and myelin sheaths are primarily affected, whereas the axons are largely spared.

Predisposing Factors. The following factors predispose to the development of drug-induced peripheral neuropathy:
- *Genetic predisposition* and preexisting sensory motor hereditary neuropathies.
- *Variations in drug pharmacokinetics:*
  - Slow acetylators of isoniazid are more likely to develop peripheral neuropathy.
  - Patients with renal and hepatic dysfunction can accumulate toxic concentrations of drugs.
- *Underlying diseases.* Patients with diabetes mellitus, rheumatoid arthritis, alcoholism, and subclinical vitamin deficiencies are more prone to develop drug-induced peripheral neuropathies as the peripheral nerves may already be affected in these patients.
- *Patients with subclinical nerve entrapments.* Nerves passing through tight compartments are more susceptible to entrapment neuropathies during treatment with some drugs. Carpal tunnel syndrome has been reported after β-blocker therapy in hypertensive patients.

Chemotherapy-Induced Neuropathy. This should be considered in the context of overall causes of neuropathy in patients with malignant disease which are as follows (Amato and Collins 1998):
- Direct effect of malignancy

- Invasion by tumor
  - Compression of nerves by tumor
- Paraneoplastic mechanisms: remote effects of cancer
  - Immunologic pathogenesis
  - Monoclonal gammopathy
  - Neuropathy associated with lymphoma
- Complications of therapy
  - Toxic effects of chemotherapy
  - Effect of immunosuppressive agents
  - Radiation-induced effects
  - Infections

Mechanisms related to chemotherapeutic drug actions. These drugs can produce peripheral neuropathies in several ways of which the following are known:
- Direct neurotoxicity as a dose-related effect of chemotherapeutic agents. Examples of this are:
  - Doxorubicin has a direct effect on chromosomal DNA due to intercalation of the compound into DNA double-helix and breakdown of nucleic acid, thus impairing protein synthesis of neurons.
  - Vinca alkaloids produce depolymerization of microtubules and accumulation of neurofilaments blocks the axonal flow.
  - Injury to myelin may occur such as in hexachlorophene neuropathy with intramyelinic edema and splitting of myelin lamellae.
- Vitamin deficiencies induced by antineoplastic drugs may cause of peripheral neuropathy.
- Interference with metabolic processes in nerves
- Local damage to nerves by drug application. The following are examples of this:
  - Mononeuropathy associated with intralesional vinblastine treatment of AIDS Kaposi sarcoma.
  - Regional neurotoxicity. Infusion of cisplatin into the internal or external iliac artery may produce an acute lumbosacral plexopathy or mononeuropathy within 24 hours.

Clinicopathological correlations of chemotherapy-induced neuropathy are shown in Table 11.3.

Table 11.3. Mechanism of neurotoxicity and clinical features of chemotherapy-induced peripheral neuropathy.

Drug	Mechanism of neurotoxicity	Clinical features
Vinca alkaloids: vincristine	vinblastine	vinorelbine
Cisplatin	Preferential damage to DRG ganglia: binds to and cross-links neuronal DNA, inhibits protein synthesis and impairs axonal transport	Axonal neuropathy affecting predominantly large myelinated sensory fibers (Postma and Heimans 1998)
Taxanes: paclitaxel	docetaxel	Promote axonal microtubule assembly; interfere with axonal transport
Suramin	Axonal neuropathy: inhibition of NTF binding?	Symmetric, predominantly sensory neuropathy
	Demyelinating neuropathy: immunological mechanisms?	Subacute, sensorimotor neuropathy with diffuse weakness (proximal > distal)
Ara-C high dose	Selective Schwann cell toxicity	Pure sensory neuropathy; brachial plexopathy
Etoposide (VP-16)	Selective DRG toxicity?	Sensory predominant neuropathy; autonomic neuropathy

DRG = dorsal root ganglia, NTF = neurotrophic factor.

Antineoplastic Agents

Peripheral neuropathy is well known with several chemotherapeutic agents. Only those agents documented to produce neuropathy frequently are discussed in this section. Other chemotherapeutic agents which normally do not produce peripheral neuropathy may do so at high doses. For example, 4% of patients with hematological malignancies who receive etoposide prior to autologous bone marrow transplantation subsequently develop a sensory polyneuropathy (Imrie et al 1994). Patients should be evaluated prior to chemotherapy for chronic diseases such as nutritional disorders which lead to silent peripheral neuropathies and for paraneoplastic syndromes involving peripheral nerves. electrodiagnostic studies are helpful in assessing these patients. Sural nerve biopsies are used occasionally. Current management of peripheral neuropathy due to chemotherapy involves various approaches which vary according to the drug used. The chemotherapeutic drug is usually discontinued when a patient develops peripheral neuropathy and some of these patients recover. General measures include use of analgesics. The following section will include management of cisplatin-induced neuropathy as an example of special management strategies.

Cisplatin (Cis-diamine-dichloroplatinum)

This is widely used either alone or in combination with other antineoplastic agents for its effectiveness in the treatment of malignant tumors of the testis, ovaries, neck, and bladder. Sensory peripheral neuropathy following cisplatin therapy is well known during the past decade and is the most frequent reason for stopping this treatment. Peripheral neuropathy was found in 14/115 (12%) patients treated for testicular cancer with cisplatin-based therapy for a median follow-up of 6 years (Bokemeyer et al 1993). Cisplatin affects mainly the large sensory nerve fibers but involvement of small diameter nerve fibers and motor fibers has also been reported (Ongerboer et al 1985; Pages et al 1986). Krarup-Hansen et al (1993) carried out an electrophysiological and histological study of cisplatin-induced neuropathy in humans. Their findings do not suggest that cisplatin causes a primary distal lesion with sparing of more proximal parts of the peripheral nerves. Their findings were consistent with a neuropathy affecting mainly the large sensory neurons. Brainstem and somatosensory evoked potentials and H-reflexes suggested that the brainstem and the spinal cord were affected as well.

The presenting symptoms are paresthesias and dysaesthesias in hands and feet which can spread proximally, become painful and even unbearable. Sensory ataxia may occur. The neuropathy is dose-related and is reported to occur in 70% to 100% of patients at a cumulative dose of 540–600 mg/m^2 (Sghirlanzoni et al 1992; Thompson et al 1984). Sebille et al (1990), however, reported a lower incidence of peripheral neuropathy (14%) in patients with head and neck cancer who were given continuous cisplatin infusion for 4 days and no other neurotoxic chemotherapeutic agents were combined with this treatment. Clinical progression of the symptoms may occur for two to three months after which the symptoms may remain stationary or even improve, possibly due to some kind of adaptation. Clinical and neurophysiological signs of progression of polyneuropathy up to three months (Hilkens et al 1994) and up to six months (Lo-Monaco et al 1992) after discontinuation of cisplatin has also been reported. In a retrospective study of 45 patients with cisplatin-induced neuropathy, there was a high incidence of deterioration after withdrawal and frequently symptoms related to nerve-root demyelination such as electric shock-like sensation and muscle cramps were reported (Siegel and Haim 1990).

Degeneration of myelinated as well as unmyelinated axons has been human sural nerve biopsies. Tomiwa et al (1986) have suggested that the primary toxic effect of platinum is disruption of RNA mechanisms which could be a precursor of axon degeneration. Dorsal root ganglia seem to have a major involvement. There is accumulation of platinum in peripheral nerves but not in the brain or the spinal cord. Pathological findings in the peripheral nerves have been correlated with platinum toxicity and the highest concentrations are found in dorsal root ganglia (Gregg et al 1992).

Prevention and Management. Cisplatin-induced neuropathy is dependent on the intensity of the total dose as well as that of the single dose. The use of less neurotoxic schedules (Same total dose but lesser single doses) may prevent or reduce sensory nerve damage (Cavaletti et al 1992). However, even low-dose cisplatin therapy is associated with a 10% incidence of peripheral neuropathy (Greenspan and Treat 1988). Sensory nerve action potential amplitude and sensory latency of ulnar nerve are the two best objective parameters that can be utilized to monitor patients for adverse nerve conduction side effects of cisplatin (Ashraf et al 1990). Various approaches to management are:

– *Corticosteroids.* These have been used for prevention of sensory neuropathy but there is not evidence of their efficacy.

– *Glutamate.* Boyle et al (1999) report the use of a rat model of cytotoxic neuropathy to evaluate the role of glutamate as a possible neuroprotectant for these two drugs. In cytotoxic treated animals, supplementation with oral sodium glutamate before chemotherapy protected against both sensory and motor neuropathy. Similar doses of glutamate did not impair the cytotoxic efficacy of paclitaxel or cisplatin against a transplantable rat mammary adenocarcinoma grown subcutaneously in rats. These findings suggest that glutamate warrants clinical trial as a neuroprotectant in patients receiving paclitaxel or cisplatin.

– *Org 2766.* This is an ACTH(4–9) analog which enhances repair mechanisms after damage to peripheral nerves and has been shown to prevent peripheral neuropathy when given concomitantly with cisplatin without interfering with cytotoxic effect. It appears to protect against cisplatin induced neurotoxicity directly at cellular level (Windebank et al 1994: Hol et al 1994). Russell et al (1995) have shown that cisplatin and ACTH(4–9) affect fast axonal transport by specific mechanisms which appear related to their observed neurotoxic and neuroprotective roles, respectively. Hovestadt et al (1992) have recommended that Org 2766 treatment should be continued up to four months after the last cycle of cisplatin to prevent late-onset neuropathy. A double-blind, placebo-controlled, multicenter study has shown that Org 2766 cannot completely prevent cisplatin neurotoxicity in young men with testicular cancer but nerve damage can be ameliorated (van Gerven et al 1994).

- *Reduced glutathione*. This is a sulfur-containing compound which has been shown to protect against cisplatin-induced nephrotoxicity (Di Re et al 1990). It has also been shown to reduce peripheral neurotoxicity, possibly by improving the renal function and preventing accumulation of cisplatin (Pirovano et al 1992). Glutathione may have a direct neuroprotective effect but no data is available to show its uptake by the peripheral nerves.

- *Vitamin E*. Cisplatin neuropathy is similar to that caused by vitamin E deficiency and vitamin E has been used to reduce its severity (Nudelman 1991).

- *Amifostine* (Ethyol®, Alza/US Bioscience). Amifostine is a prodrug that is dephosphorylated by alkaline phosphatase in tissues to a pharmacologically active free thiol metabolite that can reduce the toxic effects of cisplatin. The ability to differentially protect normal tissues is attributed to the higher capillary alkaline phosphatase activity, higher pH and better vascularity of normal tissues relative to tumor tissue, which results in a more rapid generation of the active thiol metabolite as well as a higher rate constant for uptake. The higher concentration of free thiol in normal tissues is available to bind to, and thereby detoxify, reactive metabolites of cisplatin; and also can act as a scavenger of free radicals that may be generated in tissues exposed to cisplatin. Results from a multicenter phase III trial of women with advance ovarian cancer receiving combination chemotherapy with cisplatin plus cyclophosphamide showed that amifostine pretreatment was associated with moderate but significant reductions in cisplatin-associated peripheral neuropathy, tinnitus and nephrotoxicity, while achieving equivalent pathological response rates and median survival. Amifostine also protects against radiation therapy (Werner-Wasik 1999). This was the first neuroprotective agent approved to enhance the clinical effectiveness of cisplatin.

- *Neurotrophic factors (NTFs)*. Various NTFs investigated for the treatment of chemothera-

py-induced peripheral neuropathy include nerve growth factor (NGF), insulin-like growth factor (IGF)-1 and neurotrophin-3 (NT-3). None of these NTFs are yet approved but the rationale of their use and clinical trials have been reviewed by Jain (1999). Apfel et al (1992) have reported an animal study suggesting that nerve growth factor prevents neurotoxicity from cisplatin. Hol and Bär (1995) have found it to be effective in protecting a dorsal root ganglion model from cisplatin toxicity. NGF is the only agent reported to prevent, rather than partially protect, cisplatin-induced neuropathy in an experimental model (Alberts and Noel 1995). NT-3 treatment has been shown to correct an abnormal cytoplasmic distribution of neurofilament protein in large sensory neurons in dorsal root ganglia and the reduction in the number of myelinated fibers in sural nerves caused by cisplatin (Gao et al 1995). The NT-3-dependent reversal of cisplatin neurotoxicity thus suggests the possible use of NT-3 in the treatment of peripheral sensory neuropathy. Indirect evidence is provided by the study showing that NT-3 administration attenuates deficits of pyridoxine-induced large fiber sensory neuropathy in adult rats (Helgren et al 1997). This type of neuropathy resembles that seen with cisplatin and pyridoxine was selected as a neurotoxic agent because it produces specific, marked impairment of proprioceptive function without producing profound systemic toxicity.

Cytarabine

Cytosine arabinoside (Ara-C) is a chemotherapeutic agent used to treat leukemias and non-Hodgkin's lymphomas. Peripheral neuropathy, though uncommon, is reported with high dose therapy (more than 200 mg/m² body surface area per day). Lower extremities are more involved than the upper ones. The symptoms may begin a few days to 2 weeks after start of treatment. The nerve lesions documented are mostly axonal (Montalbetti et al 1992) and less often demyelinating (Nevill et al 1989). Ara-C may act directly as an axonal toxin inhibiting myelin basic proteins. Demylinating polyneuropathy has been reported in 1% of patients treated with high-dose Ara-C (Openshaw et al 1996).

Suramin

Suramin is an experimental antineoplastic agent that is currently being tested in clinical trials for a number of human cancers. In previous clinical trials, it has been noted that a significant percentage of patients treated with suramin develop a peripheral neuropathy. Both the cytotoxic (chemotherapeutic) and neurotoxic mechanisms of action of this compound are unknown. Gill and Windebank (1998) have presented experimental evidence that both effects may be due to extensive disruption in glycolipid transport and/or metabolism. Suramin treated dorsal root ganglion cultures revealed an accumulation of the GM_1 ganglioside and ceramide. Exposure of cultures to suramin, a cell permeable ceramide analog, or sphingomyelinase lead to apoptotic cell death demonstrated by electron microscopy, bisbenzimide staining and DNA laddering on gel electrophoresis. Furthermore, a significant increase in intracellular ceramide preceded cell death in suramin treated neurons. These finding suggest that suramin induced ceramide accumulation within neurons leads to apoptotic cell death.

A prospective study has shown that suramin-induced peripheral neuropathy usually has two patterns: distal axonal neuropathy and an inflammatory demyelinating neuropathy that is partially reversible (Chaudhry et al 1996). Neurological monitoring for development of neuropathy will improve the safety of suramin use.

Taxoids

Two taxoids are commonly used in chemotherapy: paclitaxel (Taxol) and docetaxel (Taxotere).

Paclitaxel. This is a unique mitotic inhibitor that enhances microtubular assembly and prevents depolymerization. It is approved for the treatment of ovarian cancer that is refractory to other chemotherapeutic agents. Mixed sensory and motor neuropathy is dose-dependent toxicity now that neutropenia can be controlled with granulocyte colony-stimulating factor, allowing higher doses of the drug (Chaudhry et al 1994). The neuropathy is predominantly sensory. Nerve conduction studies showed a marked reduction of sensory amplitude potential in major nerve trunks with normal motor amplitude in median and ulnar nerves. Motor neuropathy has been reported in 17% of patients who received docetaxel or paclitaxel for ovarian, breast or non-small cell lung cancer (Freilich et al 1996). The weakness mostly resolved after discontinuation of the treatment. Sural nerve biopsy in a case of taxol neuropathy showed severe nerve fiber loss with axonal atrophy and secondary demyelination (Sahenk et al 1994).

Peripheral neuropathy is the main side effect with cycles of paclitaxel at standard doses (175 mg/m^2 for 21 days). Administration of a single high-dose paclitaxel (HDP) is a novel approach for the treatment of cancer. Iniguez et al (1998) have prospectively measured neurotoxicity induced by HDP during a phase I trial in patients treated with escalating doses of paclitaxel by 24-hour infusion. Peripheral neuropathy induced by HDP was moderate and reversible but severe peripheral neuropathy was seen in patients who had received previous neurotoxic chemotherapy. Peripheral neuropathy. The neuropathy is dose-related as indicated in a study where 100% of the patients receiving 250–300 mg/m^2 via a 3 hour infusion every three weeks developed neuropathic symptoms compared to only 50% in the group receiving a dose of 135 mg/m^2 (Postma et al 1995). Combination of paclitaxel infused over 3 hours in patients with gynecologic cancers, followed immediately by cisplatin, is associated with 71% incidence of neurotoxicity which is considered to be unacceptable (Connelley et al 1996).

Docetaxel. This has similar mechanism of action as paclitaxel with some differences. It is twice as potent as paclitaxel in preventing microtubule depolymerization and has a greater promise as an antineoplastic agent. Docetaxel induced sensorimotor peripheral neuropathy is similar to that induced by paclitaxel and has been reported in 11% of the patients with a wide rage of doses

(New et al 1996). It is also dose-dependent and disabling at higher doses (Hilkens et al 1996). Combination of docetaxel and cisplatin induces a dose-dependent neuropathy that is more severe than that seen with the use of either agent alone (Hilkens et al 1997).

Vinca Alkaloids

Vincristine

This is a vinca alkaloid and is used mainly as a chemotherapeutic agent for Hodgkin's disease. Vincristine neuropathy has been reported by several authors (Haggard et al 1968; Bradley et al 1970; Casey et al 1973). This neuropathy is painful, is usually of mixed sensory and motor type, with marked depression of tendon reflexes but with little objective sensory loss. However, motor weakness is the most serious manifestation of this neuropathy. The manifestations are mostly reversible after discontinuation of vincristine and do not recur if the dose is reduced. Neurotoxicity has been found to be not troublesome in patients maintained on long term vincristine neuropathy with dose not exceeding 12 mg in 18–24 week periods (Postma et al 1993). Vincristine toxicity may be precipitated by interaction with itraconazole used concomitantly as an antifungal prophylaxis (Böhme et al 1994).

Clinical, electrophysiological, and pathologic studies all indicate that the dominant neuromuscular lesion caused by vincristine in humans is peripheral neuropathy. Predominant lesion seen on sural nerve biopsy of human patients is axonal degeneration but in guinea pigs myopathic changes are more prominent than neuropathy (Bradley 1970). Pathomechanism is similar to that of vinblastine-induced block of axon flow by binding to tubulin as shown in experimental animals by Paulson and McLure (1975).

The neuropathy involves both sensory and motor fibers, although small sensory fibers are especially affected. Virtually all patients have some degree of neuropathy, which is the dose-limiting toxicity. The clinical features resemble those of other axonal neuropathies and the earliest symptoms are usually paresthesias in the fingertips and feet and muscle cramps. These symptoms may occur after several weeks of treatment or even after the drug has been discontinued, and progress for several months before improving. Children tend to recover more quickly than adults. Severe neuropathies are particularly likely to develop in older patients who are cachectic, patients who have received prior radiation to the peripheral nerves or concomitant hemopoietic colony-stimulating factors (Weintrub et al 1996). Patients with hereditary neuropathies may be at increased risk of developing peripheral neuropathy on exposure to vincristine and this has been demonstrated in case of Charcot-Marie-Tooth disease type 1A (Graf et al 1996). Vincristine may also cause focal neuropathies. Autonomic neuropathy is also common in patients receiving vincristine.

Management. Patients with mild neuropathies can receive full doses of vincristine, but when the neuropathies increase in severity and interfere with neurologic function, reduction in dose or discontinuation of the drug may be necessary. The neurotoxicity is dose-related and cumulative with repeated dosage such that the drug therapy has to be stopped after a cumulative dose of 30 to 50 mg (Legha 1986). The neurotoxicity is usually reversible on interruption of the therapy, but the recovery is slow and takes several months. There are no specific antidotes which have established usefulness against neurotoxicity. The following therapies are either used or in development.

- *Glutamine*: There are anecdotal reports that glutamine may help some patients with vincristine neuropathy.

- *Org 2766*: In a randomized, double-blind, placebo-controlled pilot study on patients with lymphoma who were treated with combination chemotherapy containing vincristine and vinblastine, sensory disturbances occurred more often in the placebo group than in the org 2766-treated group (van Kooten et al 1992).

- IGF-1: This has been shown to prevent vincristine-neuropathy in mice (Contreras et al 1997) and is currently in clinical trials for chemotherapy-induced peripheral neuropathy.

Vinorelbine

The related vinca alkaloids vindesine, vinblastine, and vinorelbine tend to have less neurotoxicity. This may be related to differences in lipid solubility, plasma clearance, terminal half life, and sensitivities of axoplasmic transport (Forsyth and Cascino 1995). Vinorelbine is a semisynthetic vinca alkaloid. There is a high incidence of dose-dependent vinorelbine neurotoxicity in patients who receive an intensified regimen of the agent for treatment of advanced breast cancer. In one study all patients who received intravenous vinorelbine 25 mg/week for 24 weeks developed a sensorimotor distal symmetrical axonal neuropathy which was moderate in most patients but severe in 33.3% (Pace et al 1996). The drug was not discontinued in any patient because of neuropathy and follow-up data after 6 months showed that neuropathy was partially reversible. Combination of vinorelbine with paclitaxel is not recommended as it produces severe neurotoxicity (Parimoo et al 1996).

Antimicrobial Agents

Antiviral Nucleoside Analogs

A number of these compounds inhibit viral reverse transcriptase activity and are used as anti-HIV-1 drugs. Dideocytidine (ddC, Zalcitibine), dideoxynosine (ddI), stavudine, and lamivudine are accompanied by varying degrees of neurotoxicity. Peripheral neuropathies caused by these drugs are similar to those of HIV-associated distal sensory neuropathy. This condition, which presents as a pain, numbness. burning and/or dysaesthesia initially in the feet, is often multifactorial in its origin. In contrast to HIV-associated neuropathy which evolves over months, drug-induced neuropathy progresses over weeks. Approximately 10% of patients receiving stavudine or zalcitabine and 1 to 2% of didanosine recipients may have to discontinue therapy with these agents due to neuropathy (Moyle and Sadler 1998). Drug withdrawal eventually leads to recovery although it may be incomplete and peripheral neuropathy may continue to improve

for several weeks after cessation of the offending drug.

Zidovudine (formerly AZT) causes myopathy but not neuropathy and neither ddC nor ddI cause myopathy. Long term treatment will all antiviral nucleoside analogs produces mitochondrial toxicity (Lewis and Dalakas 1995). DdC and ddI decrease mitochondrial DNA (mtDNA), cause destruction of mitochondria and increase lactate production in neuronal cell lines. Rabbits treated with ddC develop an axonopathy with abnormal Schwann cell mitochondria and decreased myelin mRNA in vivo.

Risk factors for the development of peripheral neuropathy with antiviral nucleoside analogs are:

- AIDS patients with pre-existing neuropathy are at risk of exacerbation of neuropathic symptoms when treated with these agents which inhibit mitochondrial DNA polymerase in vitro and cause mitochondrial changes in the peripheral nerves in animals (Anderson et al 1994).
- Patients in the advanced stages of AIDS low CD4+ cell count (< 100 cells/mm^3) are more susceptible to drug-induced neuropathy.
- Use of other neurotoxic agents including high alcohol (ethanol) consumption and nutritional deficiencies such as low serum hydroxocobalamin levels predispose to development of these adverse effects.
- High-dose regimens are more likely to produce these adverse effects.
- Combination antiretroviral therapy may have overlapping peripheral neuropathy toxicity and may increase the likelihood of developing this complication. In a clinical trial, ZDV-ddC combination was associated with the highest rate of distal sensory neuropathy (Simpson et al 1998).

Dideoxycytidine (ddC). Painful sensory neuropathy has been reported to result from treatment with ddC (Dubinsky et al 1989; Berger et al 1993). It is temporally related to treatment with ddC and begins to resolve after its discontinuation. It is a dose-limiting toxic effect but the pathomechanism is not known. Peripheral neuropathy develops in 34% of patients treated with ddC but in only 4% of comparable patients treated with zidovudine alone (Blum et al 1996). The decision to continue treatment in patients developing new sensory symptoms is difficult because of the similarity of ddC neuropathy to HIV-related distal, predominantly sensory neuropathy which develops in 30–60% of AIDS patients.

Dideoxynosine (ddI). Painful sensory neuropathy has been reported as an adverse effect of ddI (Connolly et al 1991; Kieburtz et al 1992). LeLacheur and Simon (1991) reported a patient who developed severe neuropathy following the administration of ddI which was given shortly after the patient was removed from a clinical trial of ddC. The rapid development of toxicity in this case indicates that this adverse effect is additive or synergistic for these agents.

Lamivudine. This is the least potent inhibitor of gamma DNA polymerase and the least toxic to mitochondria in vitro. Cupler and Dalakas (1995) have reported a patient with HIV infection who experienced exacerbation of his underlying peripheral neuropathy when treated with lamivudine.

Management. Patients at increased risk of peripheral neuropathy should avoid the use of the neurotoxic nucleoside analogues or be more carefully monitored during therapy. Management of this problem includes patient education. Prompt withdrawal of the likely causative agent (giving consideration not to leave the patient on a sub-optimal therapy regimen). Analgesic agents, augmented with tricyclic antidepressants or anticonvulsant agents, may be used when pain is severe. New agents that may assist in managing this condition include levacecarnine (acetyl-L-carnitine) and nerve growth factors such as recombinant human nerve growth factor.

Chloramphenicol

Prolonged high-dose therapy with this antibiotic can produce a distal symmetric sensory neuropathy involving the lower extremities and optic neuropathy (Ramilo et al 1988). Motor fibers are usually spared. Chloramphenicol is usually given in short courses to avoid other hematological complications and neuropathy is rare. It occurs in less than 30% of the patients treated. The pathomechanism is not known but interference with vitamin

B$_{12}$ activity has been proposed. Recovery usually follows discontinuation of therapy. preventive measures are periodic visual acuity screening and questioning the patients regarding paresthesias during the course of chloramphenicol treatment. The value of prophylactic vitamin B complex therapy is not proven.

Chloroquine

It is an antimalarial agent which is also used in the treatment of some connective tissue and dermatological conditions such as lupus erythematosus. Main adverse effect is myopathy but peripheral neuropathy has also been described (Loftus 1963). Sural nerve biopsies of these patients have shown segmental demyelination and involvement of Schwann cells (Tegnér et al 1988). Estes et al (1987) reported both axonal neuropathy and segmental demyelination in a patient with chloroquine neuromyotoxicity. Curvilinear bodies noted in pericytes on electron microscopy were considered to be diagnostic of chloroquine neuropathy. Neuropathy improves after discontinuation of treatment in most of the cases.

Clioquinol

This has been associated with myelooptic neuropathy and is described in Chapter 24.

Dapsone

This is used mainly in the treatment of leprosy and also various other dermatological conditions. Motor neuropathy has been reported in patients taking high doses for conditions other than leprosy (Waldinger et al 1984; Arhens et al 1986) and in patients with leprosy (Allday and Barnes 1951; Jacob et al 1992) where involvement of the peripheral nerves by the disease had been ruled out. The clinical picture of neuropathy caused by dapsone is usually that of progressive muscle weakness and wasting involving the distal muscles of the extremities. Fernandez-Obregon and Forconi (1988) described two patients with peripheral neuropathy following use of dapsone for dermatitis herpetiformis. Both patients had normal motor nerve conduction velocities and absence of muscle wasting which ruled out dapsone-induced neuropathy. Dapsone was also ruled out as a cause in a patients who developed sensory polyneuropathy during treatment of dermatitis herpetiformis associated with enteropathy on the basis of clinical and electrophysiological findings and the patient improved in spite of continuous dapsone therapy (Dillmann et al 1991).

Dapsone has a primary, if not exclusive effect on soma and axons of motor neurons rather than on the Schwann cells and myelin (Gutmann et al 1976). The drug has been detected autoradiographically in nerves of patients with leprosy. The pathomechanism of this phenomenon may be dose-related toxicity or an idiosyncratic reaction. Dapsone metabolism, like that of isoniazid, involves acetylation. Slow acetylators are more liable to develop this complication (Koller et al 1977). Pretreatment screening of patients for slow acetylation may be helpful in determining those patients who are at increased risk for the development of neurotoxicity. Recovery from neuropathy is good but may take months to years.

Ethambutol

This is used for the treatment of tuberculosis. Peripheral neuropathy has been reported in 3.8% of patients on this therapy (Ando et al 1982). Sensory disturbances were more frequent in lower than upper limbs, muscular weakness was noted in about one-third and visual changes (optic neuritis) were recognized in nearly one-half of the patients. The major pathological change is axonal degeneration although occasionally segmental demyelination and some evidence of remyelination may be present (Takeuchi et al 1980). The neurotoxic effects are reversible in most patients.

Fluoroquinolones

Various antibiotics belong to this category include norfloxacin, ciprofloxacin and temafloxacin. Occasional cases of peripheral neuropathy

have been reported in association with fluoroquinolones (Aoun et al 1992). Two cases of painful dysthesias associated with ciprofloxacin treatment have been reported (Zehnder et al 1995). Paresthesia was the most common peripheral nerve disorder associated with fluoroquinolone treatment for bacterial infection in a survey conducted in Sweden (Hedenmalm and Spigset 1996). Predisposing factors for peripheral nerve disorders in patients on fluoroquinolone therapy are:
– Impaired renal function
– Diabetes mellitus
– Lymphatic malignancy
– Treatment with another drug known to cause neuropathy.

Isoniazid (INH)

It is one of the most effective antituberculous drugs. INH polyneuropathy occurs in approximately 2% of patients receiving conventional doses (3 to 5 mg/kg), and its incidence increases with higher doses. Symptoms appear in about 6 months and are characterized by paresthesias, impaired sensation in distal part of the lower extremities, and weakness. The main pathological process is axonal degeneration affecting both myelinated and unmyelinated fibers, accompanied by prominent axonal regeneration (Ochoa 1970). Mild sensory neuropathy may be accompanied by retrobulbar neuritis as in a case reported by Leppert and Waespe (1988).

The following factors should be taken into consideration to explain the pathomechanism of INH neuropathy:
– INH interferes with the metabolism of pyridoxine which is an essential cofactor in protein, carbohydrate and fatty acid metabolism. Pyridoxine is also involved in the synthesis of sphingomyelin. Pyridoxine deficiency interferes with vitamin B_6-dependent enzymes and vitamin B_6 deficiency may be the culprit (Blakemore 1980).
– Neurotoxicity might be a direct effect of INH since this compound can easily penetrate into a nerve due to the fact that only 40% of it is protein bound.
– Patients who are rapid acetylators seldom de-

velop neuropathy whereas slow acetylators do as they maintain higher blood levels of free INH for a longer time (Hughes et al 1954).
- Patients with low zinc level are at special risk for developing neurotoxicity from INH.
- Immune mechanisms initiated by the tubercle bacillus rather than INH may be the culprit.

After absorption INH is acetylated in the liver by an enzyme acetyl transferase. INH neuropathy can be prevented by use of vitamin B_{6m} (10 mg daily). Usually recommended doses of 100–200 mg of pyridoxine can exacerbate INH neuropathy and should be avoided (Nisar et al 1990).

Mefloquine

This is used for chemoprophylaxis of malaria. Only one case of paresthesias and painful dysesthesias associated with mefloquine has been reported in literature (Olson et al 1992). The patient recovered after discontinuation of mefloquine. Nerve conduction studies were unremarkable. There are several spontaneous reports of paresthesias associated with this drug in the safety data base of the manufacturer (Hoffmann La Roche, Basel) and in some of these cases there was mixed sensory and motor peripheral neuropathy. EMG and/or nerve biopsy showed axonal degeneration in cases where the causal relation to the drug was considered possible. There was partial improvement of the symptoms in these cases after discontinuation of the drug. On this basis mefloquine should be added to the list of drugs which can induce peripheral neuropathy.

Metronidazole

It is an antiprotozoal and antiaerobic bacterial agent used widely for the treatment of amebiasis, trichomoniasis vaginitis, and Crohn's disease. A predominantly sensory type of neuropathy has been reported in patients treated with metronidazole for several months (Bradley et al 1977; Coxon and Pallis 1976). Takeuchi et al (1988) have reviewed the reports of metronidazole neuropathy in literature and presented a case where electron microscopy confirmed the axonal de-

generation of both the myelinated and unmyelinated fibers. Peripheral neuropathy was reported in an old man treated for *Heliobacter pylori* infection with metronidazole (Learned-Coughlin 1994). The symptoms improved 4 weeks after finishing the medication. Most of the cases reported received more than 1.5 g/day of metronidazole for more than a month. One case was reported of peripheral neuropathy in a patient who received repeated short courses of 2 g/metronidazole for 5 days every other month (Dreger et al 1998). The patient recovered completely four months after discontinuation of metronidazole.

The incident of metronidazole-induced neuropathy is not known but up to 50% of the patients may have evidence of peripheral nerve dysfunction. A proposed mechanism of metronidazole-induced peripheral neuropathy is metronidazole binding to RNA in nerve cells which has been documented in rats (Bradley et al 1977). Binding of neuronal RNA may inhibit neuronal protein synthesis, resulting in peripheral axonal degeneration. Metronidazole-induced neuropathy is generally reversible although the recovery may take up to two years.

Nitrofurantoin

This is broad spectrum antimicrobial agent used for urinary tract infections. Renal failure is a major risk factor for the development of this toxic neuropathy and toxic levels of nitrofurantoin have been reported in patients with renal insufficiency who develop symptoms of a sensory-motor neuropathy the course of treatment (Loughridge 1962). Nitrofurantoin can unmask peripheral neuropathy in a type 2 diabetic patients.

Initial symptoms are distal paresthesias and sensory loss. Weakness which invariably follows sensory loss may be pronounced and resemble that of Guillain-Barré syndrome. A slight decrease in nerve conduction velocity and electrophysiologic evidence of denervation has been found in a proportion of treated subjects without symptoms (Toole et al 1968).

Histological studies show axonal degeneration with alterations in dorsal root ganglia and chromolytic changes in anterior horn cells. The presumed pathomechanism is dose-dependent depletion of glutathione due to conjugation of drug metabolites with glutathione (Spielberg et al 1981). Patients with glutathione synthetase deficiency are more susceptible to nitrofurantoin toxicity.

Prevention of nitrofurantoi--induced neuropathy is likely best accomplished by awareness of this complication and avoidance of nitrofurantoin in patients with renal insufficiency. The drug should be discontinued at the onset of symptoms such as numbness and tingling.

Podophyllum Resin

Podophyllum resins are used as topical solutions for the treatment of genital condyloma acuminata and several derivatives are used as antineoplastic agents and carry similar risks of neurotoxicity as vincristine and etoposide. Neurotoxicity may occur after absorption from local application and an axonal sensorimotor neuropathy occurs in combination with encephalopathy. Multiorganfailure may occur. The neuropathy may progress for several months after cessation of application of the drug and improvement may take months.

Prevention is by avoiding application over ulcerated or bleeding areas. Immediate treatment includes local irrigation to remove the residual drug and supportive medical treatment.

Sulfonamides

The older sulfonamides were neurotox but the newer compounds have a low rate of adverse reactions which seldom involve the nervous system. Occasional cases of peripheral neuropathy have been reported in association with trimethoprim-sulfamethoxazole (Craven and Donofrio 1992).

E7010 is a novel sulfonamide which exhibits a broad spectrum of antitumor activity against human tumor xenografts. In a phase I study, the dose-limiting toxicity was peripheral neuropathy (Yamamoto et al 1998).

Cardiovascular Drugs

Antiarrhythmic drugs in particular are associated with peripheral neuropathy. In one study, electrophysiological investigations revealed polyneuropathy in 25% of the patients who had been taking antiarrhythmic agents for 6 months to 10 years (Beghi 1994). However, clinical manifestations of polyneuropathy were present in only 3% of the patients. The incidence was similar with various agents which included amiodarone, propafenone, atenolol, verapamil, mexiletine and flecainide, singly or in combination. In comparison, only 18% of the patients with cardiovascular disorders not treated with antiarrhythmic drugs had electrophysiological polyneuropathy.

Amiodarone

This drug is used in the treatment of cardiac arrhythmias. Sensory-motor neuropathy is a common finding in patients on this therapy. This complication has been reported in approximately 6% of patients treated for several months with amiadarone (Charness et al 1984). There is symmetric sensory impairment, absent tendon reflexes, and sensory ataxia. Muscle wasting and weakness may occur progressing to quadriplegia. Severe forms of this neuropathy may not improve after discontinuation of the drug.

There is segmental demyelination and sural nerve biopsies show characteristic amidiarone-induced lamellated inclusion in many cell types. Pathomechanism is based on lipophilic properties of this drug and its capacity to penetrate lysozymes and bind irreversibly to polar lipids. There is accumulation of lipids within lysozymes in neural tissues including peripheral nerves. Besser et al (1994) found that storage of amiodarone in muscle cells results in a proximal myopathy, storage in Schwann cells results in a secondary neuropathy, and storage in Purkinje cells may be responsible for cerebellar gait disorders. Therefore, these authors term the clinical picture neurotoxic amiodarone syndrome rather than amiodarone neuropathy.

Hydralazine

This is an antihypertensive drug which may produce sensory neuropathy in 15% of the patients. The usual manifestations are paresthesias without clinical signs. Axonal degeneration has been described in some patients. Slow acetylators are more likely to develop this complications. Pathomechanism may be based on pyridoxine deficiency as hydralazine is structurally related to isoniazid. Symptoms usually improve after withdrawal of the drug or vitamin B$_6$ replacement (Sterman and Schaumburg 1980).

Perhexiline

This is an antianginal agent. Painful neuropathy is commonly seen in patients treated with 300–400 mg/d for 4 months to one year (Bousser et al 1976). In 15% of the patients on perhexiline, the initial complaints are painful paresthesias; muscle weakness, loss of tendon reflexes and ataxia may develop later (Wijesekera et al 1980). Autonomic abnormalities (postural hypotension) has also been described (Fraser et al 1977). Sensory symptoms occur in nearly all of the cases. Most of the adverse effects are reversible but the recovery may be prolonged and incomplete.

There is marked reduction of conduction velocity of peripheral nerves in these patients suggesting segmental demyelination. This has been confirmed by a clinicopathological study by Said (1978) who found that segmental demyelination involves 16–90% of myelinated fibers with axonal degeneration in only 3–20%. Electron microscopy showed lipid inclusions in many structures including Schwann cells. The explanation for this is that perhexiline, like amidiorone, is a lipophilic drug capable of penetrating lysozymes.

Perhexiline neuropathy is induced by excessive drug levels either due to slow metabolism or an overdose or renal or hepatic insufficiency (Laplane and Bousser 1981). Susceptibility to the adverse effects of this drug is probably genetically determined depending on its oxidation rate. Shah et al (1982) have shown that patients who develop perhexiline neuropathy have also impaired oxidation of debrisoquine. They suggested that patients at risk of developing neuropathy can be identified by a test dose (10 mg) of debrisoquine and estimating the ratio of the drug to its metabolite in urine.

Miscellaneous Cardiovascular Drugs

Peripheral neuropathy has been reported in patients using enalapril (Hormigo and Alves 1982; Ahmad 1995a), captopril (Samanta and Burden 1984), and flecainide (Palace et al 1992). The underlying cardiovascular disease plays some role in the development of peripheral neuropathy. Up to 25% of the cardiac patients, regardless of the antiarrhythmic used, develop peripheral neuropathies (Beghi et al 1994). Most of these patients are asymptomatic and are discovered to have electrophysiologic abnormalities. For comparison, 18% of cardiac patients who are not on treatment with antiarrhythmic drugs also have evidence of peripheral nerve dysfunction.

Central Nervous System (CNS) Drugs

Amitriptyline

This is a tricyclic antidepressant which is commonly used for the treatment of painful neuropathies. It has been associated with a number of cases of sensorimotor neuropathy with axonal degeneration, mainly in the elderly patients and those on high doses for long terms (Isaacs and Carlish 1963). Acute polyneuropathy has also been reported after amitriptyline overdose (LeWitt and Formo 1985; Leys et al 1987). Meadows et al (1982) reported a case where paresthesias were relieved by use of pyridoxine. They speculated that their patient belonged to a subgroup of individuals who rapidly metabolized amitriptyline to the primary amine desmethylnortriptyline, which would then bind with the aldehyde moiety pyridoxal phosphate leading to pyridoxine deficiency.

Protriptyline which is similar in structure and

metabolism has also been reported to be associated with a similar type of peripheral neuropathy (Stept and Subramony 1988).

Antiepileptic Drugs

Phenytoin is a widely used anticonvulsant drug and can cause an asymptomatic neuropathy which rarely becomes symptomatic. The manifestations are distal sensory loss, lower limb areflexia, and mildly reduced conduction velocities of peripheral nerves (So and Penry 1981). One mechanism of phenytoin-induced neurotoxicity is glutathione depletion which has been demonstrated in the rat peripheral nerve (Raya et al 1995).

Lovelace and Horwitz (1968) reported an incidence of lower limb areflexia of 18% after at least 5 years of phenytoin therapy rising to 50% after more than 15 years. Axonal shrinkage with secondary demyelination but without loss of nerve fibers has been reported on sural nerve biopsy of a patient with moderately severe neuropathy after 30 years of phenytoin use and high blood levels of the drug (Ramirez et al 1986). There was clinical improvement after discontinuation of the drug.

Use of carbamazepine, primidone and phenobarbital in epileptic patients has also been shown to be associated with sensory neuropathy. More than 50% of patients treated with one or more antiepileptic drugs show either symptoms of neuropathy or electrophysiological abnormalities (Bono et al 1993). One case of a newer antiepileptic gabapentin has been reported in a patient where this drug was being used for relief of head pain (Gould 1998).

Chlorprothixene

This is a neuroleptic used in psychiatry. Luisto et al (1992) reviewed 7 reports of polyneuropathy as an adverse reaction to high doses of this drug (500 mg/day) and added 7 of their own patients with similar manifestations. The initial symptoms were sensory: numbness or pain in limbs and motor weakness developed later.

Symptoms cleared up gradually in 6–14 months after discontinuation of the drug. Electromyographic studies were consistent with axonal neuropathy. Chlorprothixene has been shown to block axonal transport in animal studies (Lavoie 1987). It inhibits the action of calmodulin, a calcium-binding protein, which is widely distributed in the nervous tissue.

Gangliosides

These substances have a role in promoting nerve repair in mammalian cells by increasing collateral sprouting. Gangliosides have been used for the treatment of peripheral neuropathies. One case of motor neuropathy with multifocal conduction blocks has been reported following ganglioside therapy (Garcia-Monco et al 1992). Several cases of acute motor polyneuropathy have been reported from Spain (Figueras et al 1992). Other cases of demyelinating polyradiculoneuritis (Guillain-Barré syndrome) have been reported following ganglioside treatment (see Chapter 22).

Antibodies against asiato-GM$_1$ ganglioside were present in CSF suggesting that this may be an immune-mediated neuropathy. Antibodies to GM$_1$ ganglioside are found in some patients with the Guillain-Barré syndrome and multifocal motor neuropathy, and may alter neuronal excitability. Benatar et al (1999) measured voltage-gated sodium channel (VGSC) function by Na$^+$ influx in a motor neuronal cell line (NSC19) in which they demonstrated GM$_1$ ganglioside and tetrodotoxin-sensitive VGSC function.

Lithium

Lithium carbonate is used for acute mania and to reduce the severity of manic depressive episodes. CNS intoxication by lithium is well known but peripheral neuropathy is rare (Chang et al 1988; Vanhooren et al 1990). This is a sensory-motor neuropathy with predominance of motor symptoms and signs. Paresthesias but not pain is a frequent complaint. The signs and symptoms of lithium-induced neuropathy are not usually recognized until the acute CNS disorder has resolved. Recovery begins after drug withdrawal but may not be complete. Axonal degeneration was documented in a case reported by Pamphlet and MacKenzie (1982).

Sural nerve biopsies show axonal degeneration and loss of mxelinated fibers. Licht et al (1997) have shown diminution of the caliber of axons and nerve fibers in sural nerves of rats with raised serum levels of lithium. Pathomechanism of lithium neuropathy is not known. Electromyographic abnormalities are noted in asymptomatic patients on therapeutic doses of lithium and overdose is not the only factor for development of neuropathy. Lithium can cause hypothyroidism and two cases have been reported of patients on lithium therapy who developed carpal tunnel syndrome via this adverse effect (Deahl 1988). In a recent study, comparing lithium-treated with non-lithium treated patients, Podnar et al (1993) suggested that lithium, if used within therapeutic levels is just one among many factors which lead contribute to proximal neuropathy in psychiatric patients.

Lithium-induced neuropathy may be prevented by frequent monitoring of lithium levels particularly in patients with renal dysfunction or pre-existing neuropathy. Hemodialyis may lower serum lithium levels in case of intoxication but does not immediately lower tissue lithium levels. There is no evidence that hemodialysis improves the peripheral nerve function.

Nitrous Oxide

Nitrous oxide intoxication occurs in individuals either through contamination of the operating room or by recreational use of this gas. Anesthetists and dentists are at risk of exposure to this. Chronic repeated exposure produces a predominantly sensory polyneuropathy with radicular, rather than distal distribution of numbness (Layzer et al 1978; Nevins 1980). This is an axonal rather than a demyelinating neuropathy. Potential of nitrous oxide to inactivate vitamin B_{12} (Deacon et al 1978) and resemblance to subacute combined degeneration of spinal cord suggests B_{12} deficiency as a pathogenetic factor.

Phenelzine

This is an antidepressant of monoamine oxidase inhibitor type. Two patients with generalized sensory-motor neuropathy and a clear relationship to phenelzine have been reported (Goodheart et al 1991). The electrophysiological abnormalities in these cases were consistent with axonal neuropathy and both patients recovered after discontinuation of the drug. Heller and Friedman (1983) described pyridoxine deficiency associated with long-term phenelzine therapy. Since phenelzine, like hydralazine and isoniazid, is a hydrazine capable of reducing pyridoxine levels in the rat, it is possible that phenelzine, like hydralazine and isoniazid, may cause a pyridoxine-responsive peripheral neuropathy in humans.

Thalidomide

This was introduced as a sedative-hypnotic drug in 1955 but its use ended in disastrous embropathic effect, leading to its withdrawal in 1961. Less known is the fact that this drug caused an "epidemic" of peripheral neuropathy in Europe in 1960 and 1961. This drug is presumed to have an anti-inflammatory effect and continues to be used for a number of inflammatory and dermatologic conditions. It has been found to be useful in controlling erythema nodosum leprosum. Thalidomide neuropathy has not been reported in patients with leprosy who invariably have neuritis due to the basic disease (Jakeman and Smith 1994).

In earlier cases the neuropathy was reported in 0.5% of the cases and the initial symptoms were sensory with motor weakness occurring later affecting proximal more than the distal muscles (Fullerton and Kremer 1961). Follow-up of these cases for 4 to 6 years showed a poor recovery from sensory symptoms; 25% recovered fully, 25% partially, and 50% remained unchanged (Fullerton and O'Sullivan 1968). After reintroduction of this drug the frequency of polyneuropathy has been found to be 25% or higher (Knop et al 1983; Wulff et al 1985; Heney et al 1991). Harland et al (1993) consider peripheral neuropathy to be a frequent but unpredictable adverse reaction not related to dose of thalidomide. In a prospective clinical and electromyographic survey in 29 patients treated with thalidomide, neuropathy appeared in 11 patients and a decrease of 50% of the amplitude of sensory action potential seemed to be predictive (Colamarino et al 1992). Ochonisky et al (1994) reported that nine (21%) of 42 patients who received thalidomide for various dermatologic conditions developed neuropathy; 3 of these patients recovered incompletely after thalidomide withdrawal. The mean duration of symptoms before the initial appearance of symptoms ranged from 1–24 months. Crawford (1992) suggested electrophysiological monitoring of patients on thalidomide therapy and recommended that the drug should be stopped at an early stage of peripheral nerve involvement to offer the best chances for recovery.

The pathology is axonal degeneration and degenerative changes in the posterior columns of the spinal cord (Klinghardt 1965). The predominant effect is on large fibers (Chapon et al 1985). Pathomechanism of thalidomide toxicity is not well understood. One hypothesis is that the product of thalidomide hydrolysis inhibits glutamic acid metabolizing enzymes involved in protein synthesis in the peripheral nervous system (Fabro et al 1965). A comparison has also been made with the toxic action of methyl mercury upon the RNA of the neural perikaryon, binding amines and acylating aliphatic amines associated with ribosomal function (Cavanagh 1973). Serum samples of patients with thalidomide neuropathy produced morphologic changes in cultured dorsal root ganglion cells (Aronson et al 1984). These observed changes support the postulate that thalidomide induces primary neuronal degeneration.

Hess et al (1986) performed a prospective clinical and electrophysiological follow-up on patients under thalidomide treatment in order to detect the earliest possible drug-induced peripheral neuropathy. No single reliable neurophysiological parameter for detection of thalidomide-induced neuropathy could be found. Pharmacogenetic classification with regard to hydroxylation and acetylation phenotypes was then performed in some patients and interpreted with relation to thalidomide neurotoxicity. A possible relationship between slow acetylators and development of thalidomide-induced neuropathy was found.

Miscellaneous Drugs

Allopurinol

This drug is widely used for the treatment of hyperuricemia. Cases of allopurinol-induced peripheral neuropathies have been reported following long-term use of the drug (Azulay et al 1993). The symptoms and signs regress after withdrawal of the drug. This neuropathy is usually of sensory-motor type and sural biopsy shows a demyelinating neuropathy and to a lesser extent axonal degeneration. Pathomechanism is unknown.

Almitrine

This is a chemoreceptor agonist used in the treatment of chronic obstructive pulmonary disease (COPD) to improve the arterial blood oxygenation. Painful neuropathy may appear two months after start of therapy. The onset is insidious, beginning with symmetrical glove and stocking sensory loss in legs, and loss of tendon reflexes (Gherardi et al 1985). In another series of 46 patients with COPD who received almitrine (Bouche et al 1989), polyneuropathy appeared between 9–25 months after start of treatment. Patients began to improve 3–6 months after withdrawal of the drug. Recovery was usually complete in 12 months.

The precise prevalence of this adverse effect is not known but more than 150 cases of peripheral neuropathy have been reported in association with this drug since 1985. Symptoms of peripheral neuropathy due to hypoxia are common in patients with COPD and complicates the assessment of cases treated with almitrine. Allen and Prowse (1989) carried out a double-blind prospective study of the effect of almitrine versus placebo on 12 patients with COPD who were free from peripheral neuropathy before the start of the study. None of the seven patients on placebo developed any signs or symptoms of peripheral neuropathy. Three of the five patients who received almitrine developed peripheral neuropathy during the 12 months of study and a fourth who continued to receive almitrine developed neuropathy at 18 months.

Sural nerve biopsy specimens show that the pathology is mainly axonal degeneration affecting mostly large myelinated fibers. Regeneration is prominent during recovery. The pathomechanism is poorly understood. The drug is lipophilic, diffuses widely through the tissues, undergoes extensive hepatic metabolism, and is excreted in bile. The drug has been detected in plasma up to 20 weeks after discontinuation of therapy indicating that the drug is slowly released from peripheral sites (McLeod et al 1983). It is conceivable that delayed detoxification in certain individuals can produce neurotoxicity. Belec et al (1989) performed oxidative phenotyping in 15 patients with almitrine neuropathy using dextromethorphan, a test compound subject to oxidative metabolism similar to debrisoquine. They concluded that susceptibility to develop almitrine neuropathy, in contrast to perhexiline neuropathy, is not related to a poor metabolizer phenotype.

Anticoagulants

Femoral neuropathy due to hemorrhagic complication of anticoagulant therapy is well known and over 40 cases have been reported in literature and reviewed by Olesen (1989). Further three cases have been reported (Piazza et al 1990; Niakan et al 1991; Puechal et al 1992). These patients suffered a typical femoral neuropathy with severe pain in the hip region aggravated by extension, sensory disturbances in cutaneous innervation zone of the femoral nerve, quadriceps paresis, and loss of patellar reflex.

Pathomechanism is compression-hypoxia of the femoral nerve behind the inguinal ligament by a hematoma beneath the tight non-distensible iliac fascia. This hematoma can be detected by computer tomography of the inguinal region. Recommended treatment of this complication is as follows:

- Discontinue anticoagulant therapy and take measures to stop the bleeding, e. g., protamine.
- Immobilize the patient for a few days with hip

flexed and externally rotated to reduce nerve compression.
- Surgical decompression may be considered if there is no response to conservative treatment.
- Physical therapy should be starting after several days when the patient is ambulatory to facilitate the absorption of the hematoma and for the rehabilitation of the muscles.

Arsenic

The most frequent neurologic complication of inorganic arsenic poisoning is distal symmetrical polyneuropathy which may appear acutely after ingestion of a massive dose or may develop insidiously after chronic environmental or industrial exposure (Heyman et al 1956; Chuttani et al 1967; Murphy 1981). Arsenic is a constituent of some unconventional drugs history of ingestion of such drugs should be elicited during investigation of a patient with peripheral neuropathy. It is usually a chronic poisoning but acute and subacute forms of presentation are also documented. A case of chronic arsenic intoxication associated with macrocytosis and neuropathy, without anemia has been reported (Heaven et al 1994). Removal of the source of exposure resulted in resolution of macrocytosis and slight improvement of neuropathy. This case emphasizes that arsenic intoxication should be considered in patients with macrocytosis with peripheral neuropathy, even in the absence of anemia.

Diagnosis. Arsenic neuropathy is usually symmetrical with involvement of both sensory and motor fibers. Clinical presentation may resemble Guillain-Barré syndrome or muscular dystrophy. Electrophysiological studies show a delay in sensory conduction velocity along with reduction of the amplitude of evoked potentials. The pathology is axonal degeneration with involvement of large myelinated fibers (Le Quesne and McLeod 1977), although segmental demyelination has also been described. There are no specific clinical features and laboratory analysis is required for confirmation of arsenic poisoning. The human biological samples of choice are urine and hair. Various methods of arsenic anal-

ysis done in specialized laboratories have been reviewed by Stoeppler and Vahter and are:
- Neutron activation analysis. This is the most sensitive method but is not easily available.
- Determination of total arsenic in biological matrices using atomic absorption spectrometry.
- Regular flame absorption spectrophotometry is not useful as the air-acetylene flame interferes with the sensitive resonance lines for arsenic.
- Analysis of arsenic metabolites.
- The presence of arsenic within myelinated fibers has been documented by laser microprobe mass analysis (Goebel et al 1990).

Treatment. Chelation therapy with dimercaprol (British Anti-Lewisite, BAL) should no longer be used because it is considerably toxic and increases the arsenic content of the brain, possibly by forming a lipophilic complex which readily passes the blood brain barrier (Kreppel et al 1990). Dimercaptosuccinic acid (DMSA) is the antidote of choice in the treatment of arsenic poisoning (Inns and Rice 1993).

Dimercaptosuccinic acid

Botulinum Toxin

Brachial plexus neuropathy has been reported following botulinum toxin injection for the treatment of cervical or upper extremity dystonia (Tarsy 1997; Sheean et al 1995; Vieregge and Kompf 1993; Sampaio et al 1993; Glanzman et al 1990). In addition to these, several other reports are filed with the manufacturer—Allergan Pharmaceuticals Inc. Considering the extensive worldwide use of therapeutic botulinum toxin A injection, the incidence is considered to be rare. The mechanism of brachial plexopathy is not clear. An immune mediated mechanism is suspected.

The manifestation can be radiating pain or painless weakness of the upper extremity and may occur on the side of the injection or on the opposite side. Weakness and EMG abnormalities are usually confined to C5 and C6 nerve root distribution. The onset is usually within a few weeks and recovery takes place with a few months. Readministration of botulinum toxin

has not been associated with recurrence of brachial plexopathy but unexplained pain in the shoulder region after an injection of botulinum toxin contraindicates a second injection.

Cholesterol-Lowering Agents

The most commonly used cholesterol-lowering agents act by inhibiting hydroxymethylglutaryl coenzyme A (HMG-CoA) reductase, the rate limiting enzyme in cholesterol synthesis. The drugs in this category include simvastatin, lovastatin and pravastatin. There are isolated case reports of sensory neuropathy with lovastatin (Jacobs 1994; Ahmad 1995b). Simvastatin has also been associated with peripheral neuropathy in several cases (Phan et al 1995). The electrophysiological and pathological features of the neuropathy were those of axonal degeneration. Most of these recovered after cessation of therapy and in a few cases there was recurrence of symptoms after re-exposure to the drug.

Possible mechanisms by which cholesterol-lowering agents could damage peripheral nerves is interference with cholesterol which is an essential component of human cell membranes. Inhibition of cholesterol synthesis can reduce axon transport which is an early indicator of neurite degeneration. Simvastatin not only blocks the synthesis of cholesterol but also that of dolichol and ubiquinone which is a key enzyme in the mitochondrial respiratory chain. Intracellular deficiency of ubiquinone disturbs energy utilization of the neuron. Mitochondrial abnormalities have been reported in the muscle biopsies of patients treated with simvastatin who develop myopathy (see Chapter 13) which improve following administration of ubiquinone. Ziajka and Wehmeier (1998) have reported a case of a peripheral neuropathy induced and exacerbated by several commonly used HMG-CoA reductase inhibitors including lovastatin, simvastatin, pravastatin, and atorvastatin, and the vitamin niacin. This case shows the cross-reactivity of the neuropathic process to different HMG-CoA reductase inhibitors, and it is the first reported case of a peripheral neuropathy exacerbated by the use of niacin. Jeppesen et al (1999) have reviewed seven cases of reversible peripheral neuropathy apparently caused by statins reported during 1995–1998 and added report seven additional cases associated with long-term statin therapy, in which other causes of neuropathy were thoroughly excluded. The neuropathy in all cases was axonal with involvement of both thick and thin nerve fibers. The symptoms of neuropathy persisted during an observation period lasting from 10 weeks to 1 year in four cases after statin treatment had been withdrawn.

There are isolated case reports of sensory neuropathy with benzafibrates which are also used for lowering cholesterol. Motor neuropathy has been reported with clofibrate (Gabriel and Pierce 1976) and cases of paresthesias have been reported to various health authorities around the world including the World Health Organization. The documentation of these cases is insufficient for adequate assessment. Ellis et al (1994) reported a case of peripheral neuropathy with benzafibrate which was substantiated by nerve conduction studies suggesting a sensory neuropathy of axonal type. The symptoms resolved on discontinuation of benzafibrate.

Cimetidine

Peripheral neuropathy has been reported following cimetidine—a H_2-receptor antagonist used for the prophylaxis and treatment of gastroduodenal ulcers (Vincent et al 1988). A rapidly developing pure motor neuropathy characterized by severe weakness, areflexia, and muscle atrophy has been reported within days after initiation of therapy (Walls et al 1980). Pouget et al (1986) reported a case of peripheral neuropathy with pain and symmetric motor neuropathy, predominant distally and in the lower limbs, four days after beginning cimetidine therapy. Motor function began to recover with a week after discontinuation of the drug and recovery was complete within five months. Electrophysiological studies showed an axonal neuropathy and morphometric studies revealed loss of large myelinated fibers in some fascicles while other fascicles were normal. Microvasculitis was present in the epineurium.

Small-vessel immune-complex vasculitis plays a role in the pathogenesis of cimetidine-induced peripheral neuropathy. Neuropathy improves within several weeks after discontinuation of the drug.

Colchicine

Colchicine has been used for the treatment of gout for over 200 years but neuromuscular toxicity has been recognized only recently. The main adverse effect is a myopathy but peripheral neuropathy is occasionally associated (Kuncl et al 1987). This is a sensory-motor neuropathy with axonal degeneration, particularly of the large fibers as seen in sural nerve biopsy specimens. Colchicine toxicity occurs in patients who have elevated drug levels because of mild renal insufficiency. The pathomechanism is based on colchicine binding to tubulin in the same way as vinblastine and has been used experimentally to block axon transport (Paulson and McLure 1975).

Disulfiram

Disulfiram (antabuse) has been in use for the treatment of alcoholism since 1947 and occasionally produces peripheral neuropathy (Moddel 1978) which should be distinguished from alcoholic neuropathy. A systematic review of adverse reactions to disulfiram in Denmark indicates that neuropathy is a frequent complication (Enghusen Poulsen et al 1992). The incidence is dose-related and most patients receiving more than 500 mg/day develop nerve damage after 6 months (Mokri et al 1981). Disulfamine-induced peripheral neuropathy does not occur below a dose of 250 mg/d (Dano et al 1996). The initial symptoms are sensory but muscle weakness, more marked proximally, may occur if the drug is continued. Optic neuritis and encephalopathy are other manifestations of neurotoxicity of disulfiram but not necessarily in patients who develop neuropathy. Improvement takes place over a period of months after the drug is discontinued. However, there are instances of severe motor deficits of disulfiram neuropathy where the patients did not recover (Klugkist and Preuss 1992).

Frisoni and Di Monda (1989) have reviewed 37 cases of disulfiram neuropathy reported from 1971–1988 and reached the following conclusions:
- Disulfiram neuropathy is a dose-dependent phenomenon
- Recovery depends primarily on the initial degree of impairment
- Chloral hydrate as a comedication can potentiate disufiram-induced neuropathy and concomitant use with disulfiram should be avoided.

Nerve conduction velocity may be slightly reduced suggesting primary axonal pathology. Axonal degeneration is the usual finding in sural nerve biopsies (Bouldin et al 1980). In some cases electron microscopy examination reveals axons distended by neurofilaments (Bergouignan et al 1988). The pathomechanism involves carbon disulfide, a neurotoxin produced during metabolism of disulfiram. Axonal swelling and accumulation of neurofilaments similar to that in disulfiram neuropathy has been induced in experimental animals treated with carbon disulfide (Seppalainen and Haltia 1980). Carbon disulfide causes neuropathy by reacting with amino groups to form dithiocarbonates which also chelate with the trace metals of enzyme systems, particularly affecting glycolytic processes (Ansbacher et al 1982).

Etretinate

This is a retinoid used for the treatment of psoriasis. Peripheral neuropathy has been reported after long term use of the drug (Hammer et al 1993; Danon et al 1986). This is a sensory neuropathy and proximal axons or dorsal root ganglia are probable target sites. Reversal of signs and symptoms after discontinuation of the drug favors a toxic rather than an idiopathic or disease related sensory neuropathy.

Gold

Gold, usually in the form of sodium aurothiomalate, has been in use for the treatment of rheuma-

toid arthritis since 1927. There are systemic toxic effects but peripheral neuropathy is rare; 4 patients (0.5%) among 900 patients (Hartfall et al 1937).

Encephalopathy and cranial as well as peripheral neuropathies have been described (Fam et al 1984). Koh and Boey (1992) reported a patient with rheumatoid arthritis who developed rapid onset of a sensorimotor neuropathy whilst on treatment with intra-muscular gold (sodium aurothiomalate). The patient's condition improved after cessation of gold therapy. Polyneuropathy resembling Guillain-Barré syndrome develops in some patients (see Chapter 22). Rarely a dose-related distal sensorimotor neuropathy may develop. Sural nerve biopsies have shown a mixture of axonal degeneration and segmental demyelination in these patients (Katrak et al 1980). Myokymia and autonomic dysfunction may occur in these patients. Improvement generally occurs after the drug is discontinued.

Drug-induced neuropathies need to be distinguished from varied manifestations of rheumatoid neuropathies. Pathomechanism of gold neuropathy is presumed to be a dose-dependent direct toxic effect as both axonal degeneration and segmental demyelination have been produced in nerves of hens with aurothiomalate. In case of Guillain-Barré syndrome, neuropathy is considered to be immune-mediated.

Interferons

Interferons are glycoproteins secreted in the body in response to viral infections and are presumed to confer protection on other cells against viral infection. Two types of interferons have been identified: Type 1 (interferon-α and interferon-β) and type 2 (interferon-γ). Interferon-α has been developed mostly for applications in virology and oncology. Interferon-β 1b is approved for the treatment of multiple sclerosis.

Peripheral neuropathy is a rare neurologic side effect of interferon. Cases of axonal neuropathy have been reported during treatment with interferon α-2a in patients with chronic leukemia (Cudillo et al 1990) and chronic hepatitic C (Negoro et al 1994; Sakajiri and Takamori 1992;

Tambini et al 1997). In a case of peripheral neuropathy which developed during treatment with interferon-α for chronic hepatitis C, the onset was insidious, beginning symmetrically in the hands with paresthesia (Quattrini et al 1997). Neurophysiological investigation revealed a predominantly sensory axonal neuropathy. A sural nerve biopsy confirmed primary axonal damage. Immunofluorescence studies showed increased expression of HLA-DR molecules prevalently on Schwann cells of non-myelin-forming type.

Interferon α-2b treatment may exacerbate a pre-existing neuropathy. La Civita et al (1996) have described a hepatitis B virus (HBV) positive patient with mixed cryoglobulinemia with recurrent purpura, mild sensory peripheral neuropathy, and active hepatitis who was treated with interferon α-2b. Rapid improvement of the purpura, liver enzymes, and cryocrit, and disappearance of serum HBV DNA were observed after four weeks of treatment. However, concomitant aggravation of the neuropathy required discontinuation of interferon therapy.

Interleukin-2

Interleukin-2 (IL-2) is an immunomodulating cytokine used in the treatment of renal cell carcinoma, melanoma and other malignant conditions. Neurological adverse effect mainly involve the CNS and include encephalopathy and cerebral edema. Two cases of brachial plexopathy have been reported by Loh et al (1992) which presented during treatment of cancer patients by IL-2 and where other causes such as invasion by tumor metastases was ruled out. These patients recovered completely after discontinuation of therapy. Electrophysiological examination showed active degeneration, indicating some axon loss. Rapid and complete recovery, however, suggests a demyelinating element. The pathomechanism is postulated to be focal immune-mediated demyelination.

Carpal tunnel syndrome has also been associated with IL-2 and is considered to result from increased vascular permeability and soft tissue edema which leads to compression of the median nerve at the wrist (Puduvalli et al 1996; Heys et al 1992). This usually resolves after conclusion of IL-2 treatment and resolution of limb edema.

Lidocaine

Subarachnoid lidocaine has been used for anesthesia and peripheral nerve root involvement resulting in persistent peripheral neuropathy has been linked to it (Phillips et al 1969). Transient peripheral nerve disturbances have been recorded following subarachnoid anesthesia with 5% lidocaine hyperbaric solution (Schneider et al 1993). Exposure of rat sciatic nerve to 2.5% lidocaine results in selective damage to the unmyelinated fiber Schwann cells (Powell et al 1988). Neurotoxic effects of lidocaine are dose-dependent and increase with duration of drug exposure. Possible pathomechanisms are altered peripheral nerve permeability, nerve fascicular edema, and increased endoneural fluid pressure.

Oral Contraceptives

Oral contraceptives may result in folate and vitamin B_{12} deficiency. The development of megaloblastic anemia is rare and neurological complication of this have not been described. Kornberg et al (1989) have described a case of a young women who developed megaloblastic anemia and peripheral sensory-motor polyneuropathy after 4 years of oral contraceptive use. She had low levels of folate and B_{12} and she recovered after vitamin therapy.

Subdermal contraceptive implants (Norplant) are now used as an alternative to the pill. Seventy to 80% of women using Norplant have reported side effects, such as uterine bleeding, headache, mastalgia, and local pain at the site of insertion. Hueston and Locke (1995) reported two patients who presented with peripheral neuropathy associated with the implants. One patient responded to removal of the device. The second patient, whose symptoms were thought to be related to trauma, was successfully treated with non-steroidal anti-inflammatory agents. There are case reports of peripheral nerve injury during removal of implants and a case of sensorimotor ulnar neuropathy associated with subdermal contraceptive implant has been reported (Marin and McMillian 1998).

Pyridoxine

Pyridoxine is a water-soluble vitamin that functions as a coenzyme in several essential metabolic reactions and plays an important role in maintaining lipid membrane integrity. Pyridoxine has been prescribed for the treatment of INH-induced neuropathy, pyridoxine-dependent epilepsy, carpal tunnel syndrome and many other disorders. Normal daily requirement of pyridoxine (vitamin B_6) are 2 to 4 mg/day. Megavitamin therapy with pyridoxine (2 to 6 g/day) has been used for the treatment of several disorders none of which has been shown to be due to pyridoxine deficiency.

Schaumburg et al (1983) were the first to describe severe sensory neuropathy due to pyridoxine megadosage, the salient features of which were ataxia and absence of motor weakness. On electrophysiological examination, absence of nerve action potentials and preservation of motor conduction velocity are characteristic. Sural nerve biopsies showed axonal degeneration of both large and small diameter fibers. In a further study, Parry and Bredesen (1985) reported 16 patients who developed sensory neuropathy with lower doses of pyridoxine, as low as 200 mg/day. The clinical patterns were similar to that of neuropathy resulting from higher doses. Improvement usually occurs after discontinuation of pyridoxine therapy but there are reports of cases where sensory abnormalities were profound and persisted at the time of follow-up an year later (Albin and Albers 1990). Further cases of peripheral neuropathy associated long-term megadose pyridoxine therapy have been reported and this topic has been reviewed by Bendlich and Cohen (1990) as well as Bernstein (1990).

The pathomechanism is based on direct neurotoxicity of pyridoxine. Windebank et al (1984) found that, in cell cultures of dorsal root ganglia, pyridoxine inhibited outgrowth of neurites at low concentrations (10^{-3}–10^{-4} mol/L) and resulted in cell death at higher concentrations. Mont-

petit et al (1988) found accumulation of neurofilaments in proximal axons and microtubule-neurofilament dissociation in the cyton and axons of dorsal root ganglia. They suggested that this is due to increased neurofilament protein synthesis and results in mechanical obstruction of axon transport. Various experimental studies suggest that high doses of pyridoxine produces a ganglion neuropathy. The findings of a study on healthy human volunteers by Berger et al (1992) suggest that (1) pyridoxine-induced neuropathy is dose-related, (2) quantitative sensory threshold abnormalities precede changes in nerve conduction studies, (3) symptoms continue to progress for 2 to 3 weeks despite stopping pyridoxine, and (4) a dose-dependent vulnerability may exist among nerve fibers of different caliber when exposed to pyridoxine.

Public and physician education is important for prevention of pyridoxine-induced neuropathy. Megadoses as a dietary supplement without any medical rationale should be discouraged.

Pencillamine

Pencillamine has been used successfully for the treatment of rheumatoid arthritis for several years. Immune-mediated adverse reactions such as thrombocytopenia, glomerulonephritis, myasthenia gravis, and systemic lupus erythematosus are known with this drug. Guillain-Barré syndrome has been described as a complication (see Chapter 22). Pedersen and Hogenhaven (1990) described a case of motor neuropathy within 2 months of start of pencillamine therapy. The patient recovered after discontinuation of the drug. Mayr et al (1983) reported polyneuropathy six weeks after commencing therapy with D-Penicillamine[Penicillamine] in a patient with chronic rheumatoid arthritis. The patient developed bilateral oculomotor palsy and axonal peripheral neuropathy with high levels of antinuclear antibodies and antibodies against native DNA. The appearance of polyneuropathy after repeated administration of penicillamine, the regression of symptoms with rapid decrease in antinuclear antibodies after discontinuation of the drug indicate the causal relationship.

Pyridoxine deficiency has been suggested as a possible pathomechanism as pencillamine is a pyridoxine antagonist and recovery followed use of pyridoxine in one case.

Sulphasalazine

This is an enteric drug used for the treatment of ulcerative colitis. It is poorly absorbed but several systemic side effects have been reported. Peripheral neuropathy is a well known complication (Hebal and Greenberg 1988; Price et al 1985; Smith et al 1982; Wallace 1970). Sulphasalazine is split by colonic bacteria into 5-aminosalicylic acid and sulfapyridine moieties. The latter is absorbed and causes a reversible sensory-motor neuropathy with delayed recovery. A case of peripheral neuropathy due to mesalzine (enteric coated 5-aminosalicylic acid) has been reported (Woodward 1989). The patient recovered after discontinuation of the drug.

Tacrolismus

FK506 is an important immunosuppressant that has shown great promise in the treatment of autoimmune diseases. Approximately 5% of patients receiving FK506 develop major central nervous system toxicity, but the peripheral nerves are usually spared. During 1990–1991, some 1000 patients received liver transplants under FK506 immunosuppression. Of these, three patients developed severe multifocal demyelinating sensorimotor polyneuropathy 2–10 weeks after initiation of FK506 therapy and improvement followed plasmapheresis or intravenous immunoglobulin (IVIG), suggesting an immune-mediated cause (Wilson et al 1994). Another liver transplant patient developed demyelinating sensorimotor polyneuropathy 8 weeks after start of FK506 therapy (Bronster et al 1995). FK506 was discontinued and therapy was replaced by cyclosporin and azathioprine. The patient recovered and had no sequelae at follow-up one year later.

Tryptophan

This substance is known for the epidemic of eosinophilia-myalgia syndrome (see Chapter 20). Heiman-Patterson et al (1990) have presented 3 patients who presented with peripheral neuropathy associated with tryptophan use. These neuropathies were predominantly motor and maximal in the lower extremities. Electrophysiological studies showed marked multifocal conduction blocks indicating segmental demyelination. Sural nerve biopsies showed axonal degeneration. The cause of this neuropathy is unknown but may include immune mechanisms, or toxicity of eosinophils, L-tryptophan, its metabolic products, or contaminants within L-tryptophan products.

Vaccines

Neurological complications of vaccination are well known. Postvaccinal leukoencephalomyelitis is described in Chapter 3. Tetanus toxoid is reported to produce brachial plexus neuropathy (Beghi et al 1985) and relapsing demyelinating neuropathy (Pollard and Selby 1978). There is a case report of systemic vasculitis following influenza virus vaccine and manifesting as sensory-motor polyneuropathy (Gavaghan and Webber 1993). A plexus neuropathy was reported subsequent to a vaccination against tick-borne encephalitis (TBE) followed by an inoculation of tetanus toxoid six days later (Sander et al 1995). Decrease of T-helper cells and a significant lowered CD4/CD8 ratio could be detected indicating a possible link between an altered immune state and post-vaccinal neuropathy.

Prevention of Drug-Induced Peripheral Neuropathy

The following measures are aimed at reducing the frequency of occurrence of drug-induced neuropathies:
- The most important step in prevention is the awareness of drugs being a cause of peripheral neuropathy. If a patient is on a drug known to

cause peripheral neuropathy, monitoring should be instituted for any early symptoms and signs. If there is occult neuropathy, decision regarding possible discontinuation of the drug should be made.
- Most of the drug-induced neuropathies are dose-dependent. Care should be taken not to use any more than the minimum necessary dose of these drugs.
- If the pathomechanism of a particular drug-induced neuropathy is known and if it can be corrected, steps should be taken at the earliest stage to do so before considering discontinuation of the drug. An example is vitamin deficiency which should be verified by laboratory examination and appropriate vitamin supplement should be given.
- Care should be taken in administering drugs known to cause dose-dependent peripheral neuropathy to patients with known risk factors or systemic disease which slows the excretion of drugs and raise serum levels.

Management of Drug-Induced Peripheral Neuropathy

The general measures have been reviewed by Olesen and Jensen (1991) and are as follows:
- Discontinue the offending drug while the improvement is still possible.
- Promote the excretion of the drug. For example 2,3-dimercaptopropanol (BAL) can promote excretion of metals such as gold.
- In cases with presumed immunological etiology, plasmapheresis and immunosuppressive treatment with corticosteroids should be considered.
- If vitamin deficiency is identified, appropriate vitamin should be given.
- Autonomic dysfunction accompanying peripheral neuropathy should be treated symptomatically.
- The following measures can be considered for the treatment of painful peripheral neuropathy:
  · Peripherally acting analgesics, e. g., acetaminophen
  · Centrally acting analgesics

· Transcutaneous electrical stimulation
- Physical therapy should be instituted early in the management of these patients.

References

Ahmad S: Enalapril and peripheral neuropathy. JAGS 1995a; 43: 1182.

Ahmad S: Lovastatin and peripheral neuropathy. American Heart Journal 1995b; 130: 1321.

Alberts DS, Noel JK: Cisplatin-associated neurotoxicity: can it be prevented? Anticancer Drugs 1995; 6: 369–383.

Albin RL, Albers W: Long-term follow-up of pyridoxine-induced acute sensory neuropathy-neuronopathy. Neurology 1990; 40: 1319.

Allday EJ, Barnes J: Toxic effects of diamino diphenyl sulphone in the treatment of leprosy. Lancet 1951; 2: 205–206.

Allen MB, Prowse K: Peripheral nerve function in patients with chronic bronchitis receiving almitrine or placebo. Thorax 1989; 236: 29–33.

Amato AA, Collins MP: Neuropathies associated with malignancy. Semin Neurol 1998; 18: 125–144.

Anderson TD, Davidovich A, Feldman D, et al: Mitochondrial schwannopathy and peripheral myelinopathy in a rabbit model of dideooxycytidine neurotoxicity. Lab Invest 1994; 70: 724–739.

Ando K, Ohashi T, Matsuoka Y, et al: Neuropathies due to antituberculous drugs. Saishin Igaku 1982; 25: 901–915.

Ansbacher LE, Bosch EP, Cancilla PA: Disulfiram neuropathy: a neurofilamentous distal axonopathy. Neurology 1982; 32: 424–428.

Aoun M, Jacquy C, Debusscher L, et al: Peripheral neuropathy associated with fluoroquinolones. Lancet 1992; 340: 127.

Apfel SC, Arezzo JC, Lipson L, et al: Nerve growth factor prevents experimental cisplatin neuropathy. Ann Neurol 1992; 31: 76–80.

Arhens EM, Meckler RJ, Callen JP: Dapsone-induced peripheral neuropathy. Int J Dermatol 1986; 25: 314–316.

Aronson IK, Yu R, West DP, et al: Thalidomide-induced peripheral neuropathy. Effect of serum factor on nerve cultures. Arch Dermatol 1984; 120: 1466–1470.

Ashraf M, Riggs JE, Weardon S, et al: Prospective study of nerve conduction parameters and serum magnesium following cisplatin therapy. Gynecol Oncol 1990; 37: 29–33.

Azulay JP, Blin O, Valentin P, et al: Regression of allopurinol-induced neuropathy after drug withdrawal. Eur Neurol 1993; 33: 193–194.

Beghi E: Antiarrhythmic drugs and polyneuropathy. JNNP 1994; 57: 340–343.

Beghi E, Kurland LT, Mulder DW, et al: Brachial plexus neuropathy in the population of Rochester, Minnesota, 1970–1981. Ann Neurol 1985; 18: 320–3.

Belec L, Larrey D, De Cremoux H, et al: Extensive oxidative metabolism of dextromethorphan in patients with almitrine neuropathy. Br J Clin Pharmacol 1989; 27: 387–390.

Benatar M, Willison HJ, Vincent A: Immune-mediated peripheral neuropathies and voltage-gated sodiums channels. Muscle Nerve 1999; 22: 108–110.

Bendlich A, Cohen M: Vitamin B$_6$ safety issues. Ann NY Acad Sci 1990; 585: 321–330.

Berger AR, Arezzo JC, Schaumberg HH, et al: 2',3'-Dideocytidine (ddC) toxic neuropathy. Neurology 1993; 43: 358–362.

Berger AR, Schaumburg HH, Schroeder C, et al: Dose response, coasting, and differential fiber vulnerability in human toxic neuropathy. Neurology 1992; 42: 1367–1370.

Bergouignan FX, Vital C, Henry P, et al: Disulfiram neuropathy. J Neurol 1988; 235: 382–383.

Bernstein AL: Vitamin B$_6$ in clinical neurology. Ann NY Acad Sci 1990; 585: 250–260.

Besser R, Treese N, Bohl J, et al: Klinische neurophysiologische and bioptische Befunde beim neurotoxischen Amiodaronsyndrom. Med Klin 1994; 89: 367–372.

Blakemore WF: Isoniazid. In Spencer PS, Schaumberg HH (Eds.): Neurotoxicology, Baltimore, Williams and Wilkins, 1980, pp 476–489.

Blum AS, Dal Pan GJ, Feinberg J, et al: Low-dose zalcitabine-related toxic neuropathy: frequency, natural history, and risk factors. Neurology 1996; 46: 999–1003.

Böhme A, Ganser A, Bergmann L, et al: Unusual severe vincristin-induced neurotoxicity in four patients with all simultaneously receiving antifungal prophylaxis with itraconazole. Onkologie 1994: 17 (suppl 2): 13.

Bokemeyer C, Frank B, van Rhee J, et al: Peripheral neuropathy following cancer chemotherapy. Tumor Diagnostic Therapie 1993; 14: 232–237.

Bono A, Beghi E, Bogliun G, et al: Antiepileptic drugs and peripheral nerve function: a multicenter screening investigation of 141 patients with chronic treatment. Epilepsia 1993; 34: 323–331.

Bouche P, Lacombez L, Leger JM, et al: Peripheral neuropathies during treatment with almitrine: report of 46 cases. J Neurol 1989; 236: 29–33.

Bouldin TW, Hall CD, Krigman MR: Pathology of disulfiram neuropathy. J Neuropath Exp Neurol 1980; 6: 155.

Bousser MG, Bouche P, Brochard C, et al: Neuropathies périphériques au malate de perhexiline. A propos de 7 observations. Coeur Med Interne 1976; 15: 181.

Boyle FM, Wheeler HR, Shenfield GM: Amelioration of experimental cisplatin and paclitaxel neuropathy with glutamate. J Neurooncol 1999; 41: 107–116.

Bradley WG, Karlsson IJ, Rassol CG: Metronidazole neuropathy. BMJ 1977; 2: 610–611.

Bradley WG, Lassman LP, Pearce GW, et al: The neuromyopathy of vincristine in man: clinical, electrophysiological and pathological studies. J Neurol Sci 1970; 10: 107–131.

Bradley WG: The neuromyopathy of vincristine in the guinea pig: an electrophysiological and pathological study. J Neurol Sci 1970; 10: 133–162.

Bronster DJ, Yonover P, Stein J, et al: Demyelinating sensorimotor polyneuropathy after administration of FK506. Transplantation 1995; 59: 1066–1068.

Brunner KW, Young CW: a methylhydrazine derivative in Hodgkin's disease and other malignant neoplasms: therapeutic and toxic effects studied in 51 patients. Ann Int Med 1965; 63: 69–86.

Casey EB, Jellife AM, Le Quesne PM, et al: Vincristine neuropathy. Brain 1973; 96: 69–86.

Cavaletti G, Marzorati L, Bogliun G, et al: Cisplatin-induced peripheral neurotoxicity is dependent on total-dose intensity and single-dose intensity. Cancer 1992; 69: 203–207.

Cavanagh JB: Peripheral neuropathy caused by chemical agents. CRC Crit Rev Toxicol 1973; 2: 365–380.

Chang YC, Yip PK, Chiu YYN, et al: Severe generalized polyneuropathy in lithium intoxication. Eur Neurol 1988; 39–41: 1988.

Chapon F, Lechevalier B, da Silva DC, et al: Neuropathies à la thalidomide. Rev Neurol (Paris) 1985; 141: 719.

Charness M, Morady F, Scheinman M: Frequent neurologic toxicity associated with amiodarone therapy. Neurology 1984; 34: 669.

Chaudhry V, Eisenberger MA, Sinibaldi VJ, et al: A prospective study of suramin-induced peripheral neuropathy. Brain 1996; 119: 2039–2052.

Chaudhry V, Rowinsky EK, Sartorius SE, et al: Peripheral neuropathy from taxol and cisplatin combination chemotherapy: clinical and electrophysiological studies. Ann Neurol 1994; 35: 304–311.

Chuttani PN, Chawla LS, Sharma TD: Arsenical neuropathy. Neurology 1967; 17: 269–274.

Colamarino R, Clavelou P, Roger H, et al: Neuropathies liées au thalidomide: bilan d'une étude prospective clinique et électromyographique. Revue de Médecine Interne 1992; 13(suppl 6): S47.

Connelly E, Markman M, Kennedy A, et al: Paclitaxel delivered as a 3-hr infusion with cisplatin in patients with gynaecologic cancers: unexpected incidence of neurotoxicity. Gynecologic Oncology 1996; 62: 166–168.

Connolly KJ, Allan JD, Fitch H, et al: Phase I study of 2',3'-dideoxycytidine administered orally twice daily to patients with AIDS or AIDS-related complex and hematologic intolerance to zidovudine. Am J Med 1991; 91: 471–478.

Contreras PC, Vaught JL, Gruner JA, et al: Insulin-like growth factor-I prevents development of a vincristine neuropathy in mice. Brain Res 1997; 774: 20–26.

Coxon A, Pallis CA: Metronidazole neuropathy. JNNP 1976; 39: 403.

Craven W, Donofrio PD: Sensory and autonomic polyneuropathy associated with trimethoprim-sulfamethoxazole (abstract). Ann Neurol 1992; 32: 281–282.

Crawford CL: Thalidomide neuropathy. NEJM 1992; 327: 735.

Creaven PJ, Mihich E: The clinical toxicity of anticancer drugs and its prediction. Seminars in Oncology 1977; 4: 147–163.

Cudillo L, Cantonetti M, Venditti A, et al: Peripheral neuropathy during treatment with α-2 interferon. Hematologia 1990; 75: 485–486.

Cupler EJ, Dalakas MC: Exacerbation of peripheral neuropathy by lamivudine. Lancet 1995; 345: 460–461.

Dano P, Tammam D, Brosset C, et al: Peripheral neuropathies caused by disulfiram. Rev Neurol (Paris) 1996; 152: 294–295.

Danon MJ, Carpenter S, Weiss V, et al: Sensory neuropathy associated with long term etretinate therapy. Neurology 1986; 36(suppl 1): 321.

Deacon R, Perry J, Lumb M, et al: Selective inactivation of vitamin B₁₂ in rats by nitrous oxide. Lancet 1978; 2: 1023–1024.

Deahl MP: Lithium-induced carpal tunnel syndrome. Br J Psychiatry 1988; 153: 250–251.

Di Re F, Bohm S, Oriana S, et al: Efficacy and safety of high-dose cisplatin and cyclophosphamide with glutathione protection in the treatment of bulky advanced epithelial ovarian cancer. Cancer Chemother Pharmlacol 1990; 25: 355–360.

Dillmann U, Krämer G, Goebel HH: Polyneuropathie bei Dermatitis hepetiformis Duhring. Nervenarzt 1991; 62: 516–518.

Dreger LM, Gleason PP, Chaudry TK, et al: Intermittent-dose metronidazole-induced peripheral neuropathy. Ann Pharmacotherapy 1998; 32: 267–268.

Dubinsky RM, Yarchoan R, Dalakas M, et al: Reversible axonal neuropathy from the treatment of AIDS and related disorders with 2',3'-dideoxycytidine (ddC). Muscle & Nerve 1989; 12: 856–860.

Ellis CJ, Wallis WE, Caruana M: Peripheral neuropathy with benzafibrate. BMJ 1994; 309: 929.

So EL, Penry JK: Adverse effects of phenytoin on peripheral nerves and neuromuscular junction: a review. Epilepsia 1981; 22: 467–473.

Enghusen Poulsen H, Loft S, Andersen JR, et al: Disulfiram therapy—adverse drug reactions and interactions. Acta Psychiatr Scand Suppl 1992; 369: 59–66.

Estes ML, Ewing-Wilson D, Chou SM, et al: Chloroquine neuromyotoxicity. Am J Med 1987; 82: 447–455.

Fabro S, Schumacker H, Smith RL, et al: The metabolism of thalidomide: some biological effects of thalidomide and its metabolites. Br J Pharmacol 1965; 25: 352–362.

Fam AG, Gordon DA, Sarkozi J, et al: Neurologic complications associated with gold therapy for rheumatoid arthritis. J Rheumatol 1984; 11: 700.

Fernandez-Obregon AC, Forconi RJ: Neurologic symptoms posing as dapsone-induced polyneuropathy in two patients with dermatitis herpetiformis. Cutis 1988; 41: 347–350.

Figueras A, Morales-Olivas FJ, Capella D, et al: Bovine gangliosides and acute motor polyneuropathy. BMJ 1992; 305: 1330–1331.

Forsyth PA, Cascino TL: Neurologic complications of chemotherapy. In Wiley RG (Ed.): Neurologic complications of cancer, New York, Marcel Dekker, 1995, pp. 241–266.

Fraser DM, Campbell IW, Miller HC: Peripheral and autonomic neuropathy after treatment with perhexiline maleate. BMJ 1977; 3: 675–676.

Freilich RJ, Balmaceda C, Seidman AD, et al: Motor neuropathy due to docetaxel and paclitaxel Neurology 1996; 47: 115–117.

Frisoni GB, Di Monda V: Disulfiram neuropathy: a review (1971–1988) and report of a case. Alcohol Alcohol 1989; 24: 429–437.

Fullerton PM, Kremer M: Neuropathy after intake of thalidomide. BMJ 1961; 2: 855.

Fullerton PM, O'Sullivan DJ: Thalidomide neuropathy: a clinical, electrophysiological and histological follow-up. JNNP 1968; 31: 543.

Gabriel R, Pierce JMS: Clofibrate-induced myopathy and neuropathy. Lancet 1976; ii: 906.

Gao WQ, Dybdal N, Shinsky N: Neurotrophin-3 reverses experimental cisplatin-induced peripheral sensory neuropathy. Ann Neurol 1995; 38: 30–37.

Garcia-Monco JC, Baldarrain MG, Ayani I, et al: Neuropatia motora multifocal tras la administracion de gangliosidos. Med Clin 1992; 99: 345–346.

Gavaghan T, Webber CK: Severe systemic vasculitic syndrome post influenza vaccination. New Zealand Journal of Medicine 1993; 23: 220.

Gherardi R, Louarn F, Benvenuti C, et al: Peripheral neuropathy in patients treated with almitrine dimesylate. The Lancet 1985; 1: 1247–1250.

Gill JS, Windebank AJ: Suramin induced ceramide accumulation leads to apoptotic cell death in dorsal root ganglion neurons. Cell Death Differ 1998; 5: 876–83.

Glanzman RL, Gelb DJ, Drury I, Bromberg MB, et al: Brachial plexopathy after botulinum toxin injections. Neurology 1990; 40: 1143.

Goebel HH, Schmidt PF, Bohl J, et al: Polyneuropathy due to acute arsenic intoxication: biopsy studies. J Neuropathol Exp Neurol 1990; 49: 137–149.

Goodheart RS, Dunne JW, Edis RH: Phenelzine-associated neuropathy. Austr NZ J Med 1991; 21: 339–340.

Gould HJ: Gabapentin-induced polyneuropathy. Pain 1998; 74: 341–343.

Graf WD, Chance PF, Lensch MW, et al: Severe vincristine neuropathy in Charcot-Marie-Tooth disease type 1A. Cancer 1996; 77: 1356–1362.

Greenspan A, Treat J: Peripheral neuropathy and low dose cisplatin. Am J Clin Oncol 1988; 11.660–662.

Gregg RW, Molepo JM, Montpetit VJA, et al: Cisplatin neurotoxicity: the relationship between dosage, time, and platinum concentration in neurologic tissues, and morphologic evidence of toxicity. J Clin Oncol 1992; 10: 795–803.

Gutmann L, Martin J, Welton W: Dapsone motor neuropathy—an axonal disease. Neurology 1976; 26: 514.

Haggard ME, Fernbach DJ, Holcomb TM, et al: Vincristine in acute leukemia of childhood. Cancer 1968; 22: 438–444.

Hamers R, van der Hoop RG, Traber J, et al: Beneficial effects of calcium entry blocker nimodepine on cisplatin-induced neuropathy in the rat (abstract). Proc ASCO 1990; 9: 140.

Hammer CJ, Carter CC, Hanifin JM: Peripheral neuropathy during etretinate therapy for psoriasis. J Am Acad Dermatol 1993; 28: 272–273.

Harland CC, Steventon GB, Marsden JR: Thalidomide induced neuropathy and drug metabolic polymorphism. Clin Res 1993; 41: 496A.

Hartfall SJ, Garland HG, Goldie W: Gold treatment of arthritis. A review of 900 cases. Lancet 1937; 2: 838.

Heaven R, Duncan M, Vukelja SJ: Arsenic intoxication presenting with macrocytosis and peripheral neuropathy, without anemia. Acta Haematol 1994; 92: 142–143.

Hebal FM, Greenberg GR: Treatment of ulcerative colitis with oral 5-aminosalicylic acid including patients with adverse reactions to sulphasalazine. Am J Gastroenterol 1988; 83: 15–19.

Hedenmalm K, Spigset O: Peripheral sensory disturbances related to treatment with fluoroquinolones. J Animicrob Chemotherapy 1996; 37: 831–837.

Heiman-Patterson TD, Bird SJ, Parry GJ, et al: Peripheral neuropathy associated with eosinophilia-myalgia syndrome. Ann Neurol 1990; 28: 522–528.

Helgren ME, Cliffer KD, Torrento K, et al: Neurotrophin-3 administration attenuates deficits of pyridoxine-induced large-fiber sensory neuropathy. J Neuroscience 1997; 17: 372–382.

Heller CA, Friedman PA: Pyridoxine deficiency and peripheral neuropathy associated with long-term phenelzine therapy. Am J Med 1983; 75: 887–888.

Heney D, Norfolk DR, Wheeldon J, et al: Thalidomide treatment for chronic graft-versus-host disease. Br J Hematol 1991; 78: 23–27.

Hess CW, Hunziker T, Kupfer A, et al: Thalidomide-induced peripheral neuropathy. A prospective clinical, neurophysiological and pharmacogenetic evaluation. J Neurol 1986; 233: 83–89.

Heys SD, Mills K, Eremin O: Bilateral carpal tunnelsyndrome associated with interleukin-2 therapy. Postgrad Med J 1992; 68: 587.

Hilkens PHE, Planting AST, van der Burg MEL, et al: Clinical course and risk factors of neurotoxicity following cisplatin in an intensive dosing schedule. Eur J Neurol 1994; 1: 45–50.

Hilkens PHE, Pronk LC, Verweij J, et al: Peripheral neuropathy induced by combination chemotherapy of docetaxel and cisplatin. Brit J Cancer 1997; 75: 417–422.

Hilkens PHE, Verweij J, Stoter G, et al: Peripheral neurotoxicity induced by docetaxel. Neurology 1996; 46: 104–108.

Hol EM, Bär PR: Cisplatin neuropathy. Neurology 1995; 45: 596.

Hol EM, Mandys V, Sodaar P, et al: Protection by an ACTH$_{4-9}$ analogue against the toxic effects of cisplatin and taxol on sensory neurons and glial cells in vitro. J Neurosci Res 1994; 39: 178–185.

Hormigo A, Elvis M: Peripheral neuropathy in a patient receiving enalapril.BMJ 1992; 305: 1332.

Hovestadt A, van der Burg MEL, Verbiest HBC, et al: The course of neuropathy after cesation of cisplatin treatment, combined with Org 2766 or placebo. J Neurol 1992; 239: 143–146.

Hueston WJ, Locke KT, et al: Norplant neuropathy: peripheral neurologic symptoms associated with subdermal contraceptive implants. J Fam Pract 1995; 40: 184–186.

Hughes HB, Biehl JP, Jones AP, et al: Metabolism of isoniazid in man as related to the occurrence of periph-

eral neuropathy. Am Rev Tuberc Pulm Dis 1954; 70: 266.

Imrie KR, Couture F, Turner CC, et al: Peripheral neuropathy following high-dose etoposide and autologous bone marrow transplantation. Bone Marrow Transplantation 1994; 13: 77–79.

Iniguez C, Larrode P, Mayordomo JI, et al: Reversible peripheral neuropathy induced by a single administration of high-dose paclitaxel. Neurology 1998; 51: 868–870.

Inns RH, Rice P: Efficacy of dimercapto chelating agents for the treatment of poisoning by percutaneously applied dichloro(2-chlorovinyl)arsine in rabbits. Hum Exp Toxicol 1993; 12: 241–246.

Isaacs AD, Carlish S: Peripheral neuropathy after amitriptyline. BMJ 1963; 1: 1739.

Jackson DV, Wells HB, Atkins JN, et al: Amelioration lof vincristine neurotoxicity by glutamic acid. Am J Med 1988; 84: 1016–1022.

Jacob AJ, Rajendran A, Menezes J, et al: Dapsone induced motor polyneuropathy. Southeast Asian J Trop Med Public Health 1992; 23: 341–3.

Jacobs MB: HMG-CoA reductase inhibitor therapy and peripheral neuropathy. Ann Int Med 1994; 120: 970.

Jain KK: Neurotrophic factors. Jain PharmaBiotech Publications, Basel, 1999.

Jakeman P, Smith WCS: Thalidomide in leprosy reaction. Lancet 1994; 343: 432–433.

Jeppesen U, Gaist D, Smith T, et al: Statins and peripheral neuropathy. Eur J Clin Pharmacol 1999; 54: 835–838.

Katrak SM, Pollock M, O'Brien CP, et al: Clinical and morphological features of gold neuropathy. Brain 1980; 103: 671–693.

Kieburtz KD, Seidlin M, Lambert JS, et al: extended follow-up of peripheral neuropathy in patients with AIDS and AIDS-related complex treated with dideoxycytidine. J Acq Immune Def Synd 1992; 5: 60–64.

Klinghardt GW: Ein Beitrag der experimentellen Neuropathologie zur Toxitätsprufung neuer Chemotherapeutica. Mitt Max Planck Ges 1965; 3: 142.

Klugkist H, Preuss S: Disulfiram-Neuropathie. Dtsch Med Wschr 1992; 117: 1278–1282.

Knop J, Bonsmann G, Hepple R: Thalidomide in the treatment of 60 cases of chronic discoid lupus erythematosus. Br J Dermatol 1983; 108: 461–466.

Koh WH, Boey ML: Polyneuropathy following intramuscular sodium aurothiomalate for rheumatoid arthritis—a case report. Ann Acad Med Singapore 1992; 21: 821–822.

Koller WC, Gehlmann K, Malkinson FD, et al: Dapsone-induced neuropathy. Arch Neurol 1977; 34: 644

Kornberg A, Segal R, Theitler J, et al: Folic acid deficiency, megaloblastilc anemia and peripheral neuropathy due to oral contraceptives. Isr J Med Sci 1989; 25: 142–145.

Krarup-Hansen A, Fugleholm K, Helweg-Larsen S, et al: Examination of distal involvement in cisplatin-induced neuropathy in man. Brain 1993; 116: 1017–1041.

Kreppel H, Reichl FX, Szinicz L, et al: Efficacy of various dithiol compounds in acute As$_2$O$_3$ poisoning in mice. Arch Toxicol 1990; 64: 387–392.

Kuncl RW, Duncan G, Watson D, et al: Colchicine myopathy and neuropathy. NEJM 1987; 316: 1562–1568.

La Civita L, Zignego AL, Lombardini F, et al: Exacerbation of peripheral neuropathy during α-interferon therapy in a patient with mixed cryoglobulinemia and hepatitis B virus infection. J Rheumatol 1996; 23: 1641–1643.

Laplane D, Bousser M: Polyneuropathy during perhexiline maleate therapy. Int J Neurol 1981; 15: 293–300.

Lavoie PA: Penfluridol, chlorprothixene and haloperidol block fast axonal transport in order of potency consistent with a mechanism related to inhibition of calmodulin. Neuropharmacology 1987; 26: 1359–1365.

Layzer RB, Fishman RA, Schafer JA: Neuropathy following abuse of nitrous oxide. Neurology 1978; 28: 504–508.

Learned-Coughlin S: Peripheral neuropathy induced by metronidazole. Ann Pharmacother 1994; 28: 536.

Legha SS: Vincristine neurotoxicity. Pathophysiology and management. Med Toxicol 1986; 1: 421–427.

LeLacheur SF, Simon GL: Exacerbation of dideoxycytidine-induced neuropathy with Dideoxynosine. J Acq Immune Def Synd 1991; 4: 538–539.

Leppert D, Waespe W: Neurotoxicity of antituberculous drugs in a patient with active tuberculosis. Ital J Neurosci 1988; 9: 31–34.

Le Quesne PM, McLeod J: Peripheral neuropathy following a single exposure to arsenic. J Neurol Sci 1977; 32: 437–451.

Lewis W, Dalakas MC: Mitochondrial toxicity of antiviral drugs. Nature Medicine 1995; 1: 417–422.

Leys D, Pasquier F, Lamblin MD, et al: Acute polyradiculopathy after amitriptyline overdose. BMJ 1987; 294: 608.

Licht RW, Smith D, Braendgaard H: The effect of chronic lithium treatment on the calibre of axons and nerve fibres in the rat sural nerve. Eur Neuropsychopharmacol 1997; 7: 95–98.

Loftus LR: Peripheral neuropathy following chloroquine therapy. Canad Med Assoc J 1963; 89: 917–920.

Loh FL, Herkovitz S, Berger AR, et al: Brachial plexopathy associated with interleukin-2 therapy. Neurology 1992; 42: 462–462.

LoMonaco M, Milone M, Batocchi AP, et al: Cisplatin neuropathy: clinical course and neurophysiological findings. J Neurol 1992; 239: 199–204.

Loughridge LW: Peripheral neuropathy due to nitrofurantoin. Lancet 1962; 2: 1133.

Lovelace RE, Horwitz SJ: Peripheral neuropathy in long-term diphenylhydantoin therapy. Arch Neurol 1968; 18: 69–77.

Luisto M: Polyneuropathy caused by chlorprothixene. Acta Psychiatr Scand 1992; 85: 246–248.

Marin R, McMillian D: Ulnar neuropathy associated with subdermal contraceptive implant. South Med J 1998; 91: 875–878.

Mayr N, Graninger W, Wessely P: A chemically induced polyneuropathy in chronic polyarthritis treated with D-Penicillamine? Wien Klin Wochenschr 1983; 95(3): 86–88.

McLeod CM, Thomas RW, Bartley EA, et al: Effects and handling of almitrine bimesylate in healthy subjects. Eur J Resp Dis 1983; 64(suppl 126): 275–289.

McLeod JG: Autonomic dysfunction in peripheral nerve disease. J Clin Neurophysiol 1993; 10: 51–60.

Meadows GG, Huff MR, Fredericks S: Amitriptyline-related peripheral neuropathy relieved during pyridoxine hydrochloride administration. Drug Intell Clin Pharm 1982; 16: 876–7.

Moddel G, Bilbao JM, Payne D, et al: Disulfiram neuropathy. Arch Neurol 1978; 35: 658.

Mokri B, Ohnishi A, Dyck PJ: Disulfiram neuropathy. Neurology 1981: 31: 730–735.

Montpetit VJ, Clapin DF, Tryphonas L, et al: Alteration of neuronal cytoskeletal organization in dorsal root ganglia associated with pyridoxine neurotoxicity. Acta Neuropathol (Berl) 1988; 76(1): 71–81.

Montalbetti L, Brambilla PG, Trotti G, et al: Polyneuritis after HD Ara-C therapy for malignant lymphoma. Ital J Neurol Sci 1992; 13: 85.

Montepetit VJA, Clapin DF, Tryphonas L, et al: Alterations in neuronal cytoskeletal organization in dorsal root ganglia associated with pyridoxine neurotoxicity. Acta Neuropathol 1988; 76: 71.

Moyle GJ, Sadler M: Peripheral neuropathy with nucleoside antiretrovirals: risk factors, incidence and management. Drug Safety 1998; 19: 481–494.

Murphy MJ, Lyon LW, Taylor JW: Subacute arsenic neuropathy: clinical and electrophysiological observations. JNNP 1981; 44: 896–900.

Negoro K, Fukusako T, Morimatsu M, et al: Acute axonal polyneuropathy during interferon a-2a therapy for chronic hepatitis type C. Muscle & Nerve 1994; 17: 1351–1352.

Nevill TJ, Benstead TJ, McCormick CW, et al: Horner's syndrome and demyelinating peripheral neuropathy caused by hilgh dose cytosine arabinoside. Am J Hematol 1989; 32: 314–315.

Nevins MA: Neuropathy after nitrous oxide abuse. JAMA 1980; 244: 2264.

New PZ, Jackson CE, Rinaldi D, et al: Peripheral neuropathy secondary to docetaxel (Taxotere). Neurology 1996; 46: 108–111.

Niakan E, Carbone J, Adams M, et al: Anticoagulants, iliopsoas hematoma, and femoral nerve compression. Am Fam Phys 1991; 44: 2100–2102.

Nisar M, Watkin SW, Bucknall RC, et al: Exacerbation of isoniazid-induced peripheral neuropathy by pyridoxine. Thorax 1990; 45: 419–420.

Nudelman KL: Preventing chemotherapy-induced neuropathy. West J Med 1991; 155: 70.

Ochoa J: Isoniazid neuropathy in man: quantitative electron microscopic study. Brain 1970; 93: 831–850.

Ochonisky S, Verroust J, Bastuji-Garin S, et al: Thalidomide neuropathy. Incidence and clinico-electrophysiologic findings in 42 patients. Arch Dermatol 1994; 130: 66–69.

Olesen LL: Femoral neuropathy due to anticoagulation. J Int Med 1989; 226: 279–280.

Olesen LL, Jensen TS: Prevention and management of drug-induced peripheral neuropathy. Drug Safety 1991; 6: 302–314.

Olson PE, Kennedy CH, Morte PD: Paresthesias and mefloquine prophylaxis. Ann Int Med 1992; 117: 1058–1059.

Openshaw H, Slatkin NE, Stein AS, et al: Acute polyneuropathy after high dose cytosine arabinoside in patients with leukemia. Cancer 1996; 78: 1899–1905.

Pace A, Bove L, Nistico C, et al: Vinorelbine neurotoxicity: clinical and neurophysiological findings in 23 patients. J Neurol Neurosurg Psychiatry 1996; 61: 409–411.

Pages M, Pages AM, Bories-Azeau L: Severe sensorimotor neuropathy after cisplatin therapy. JNNP 1986; 49: 333–334.

Palace J, Shah R, Clough C: Flecainide-induced peripheral neuropathy. BMJ 1992; 305: 810.

Pamphlet R, MacKenzie RA: Severe peripheral neuropathy due to lithium intoxication. JNNP 1982; 45: 656–661.

Parimoo D, Jeffers S, Muggia FM, et al: Severe neurotoxicity from vinorelbine-paclitaxel combination. JNCI 1996; 88: 1079–1080.

Parry GJ, Bredesen DE: Sensory neuropathy with low dose pyridoxine. Neurology 1985; 35: 1466–1468.

Paulson JC, McLure WO: Inhibition of axoplasmic transport by colchicine, podophyllotoxin and vinblastine: an effect on microtubules. Ann NY Acad Sc 1975; 253: 517.

Pedersen PB, Hogenhaven H: Pencillamin-induced neuropathy in rheumatoid arthritis. Acta Neurol Scand 1990; 81: 188–190.

Phan T, McLeod JG, Pollard JD, et al: Peripheral neuropathy associated with simvastatin. JNNP 1995; 58: 625–628.

Phillips OC, Ebner H, Nelson AT, et al: Neurologic complications following spinal anesthesia with lidocaine: a prospective review of 10,440 cases. Anesthesiology 1969; 30: 284–289.

Piazza I, Girardi A, Giunta G, et al: Femoral nerve palsy secondary to anticoagulant induced iliacus hematoma. A case report. Int Angiol 1990; 9: 125–126.

Pirovano C, Balzarini A, Böhm S, et al: Peripheral neurotoxicity following high-dose cisplatin with glutathione: clinical and neuropsychological assessment. Tumori 1992; 78: 253–257.

Podnar S, Vodusek DB, Zvan V: Lithium and peripheral nervous system. Acta Neurol Scand 1993; 88: 417–421.

Pollard JD, Selby G: Relapsing neuropathy due to tetanus toxoid. J Neurol Sci 1978; 37: 113–125.

Postma TJ, Benard BA, Huijens PC, et al: Long term effects of vincristine on peripheral nervous system. J Neuro-oncology 1993; 15: 23–27.

Postma TJ, Heimans JJ, Muller MJ, et al: Pitfalls in grading severity of chemotherapy-induced peripheral neuropathy. Ann Oncol 1998; 9: 739–744.

Postma TJ, Vermorken JB, Liefting AJ, et al: Paclitaxel-induced neuropathy. Ann Oncol 1995; 6: 489–494.

Pouget J, Pellissier JF, Jean P, et al: Peripheral neuropathy during treatment with cimetidine. Rev Neurol (Paris) 1986; 142: 34–41.

Powell HC, Kalichman MW, Garrett RS, et al: Selective vulnerability of unmyelinated fiber Schwann cells in nerves exposed to local anesthetics. Lab Invest 1988; 59: 271–280.

Price TR: Sensorimotor neuropathy with sulphasalazine. Postgrad Med J 1985; 61: 147–148.

Puduvalli V, Sella A, Austin S, et al: Carpal tunnel syndrome associated with interleukin-2 therapy. Cancer 1996; 77: 1189.

Puechal X, Liote F, Kuntz D: Bilateral femoral neuropahy caused by iliacus hematoma during anticoagulation after cardiac catheterization. Am Heart J 1992; 123: 262–263.

Quattrini A, Comi G, Nemni R, et al: Axonal neuropathy associated with interferon-α treatment for hepatitis C: HLA-DR immunoreactivity in Schwann cells. Acta Neuropathol (Berl) 1997; 94: 504–508.

Ramilo O, Kinane BT, McKracken GH: Chloramphenicol neurotoxicity. Ped Infect Dis 1988; 7: 358–359.

Ramirez JA, Mendell JR, Warmolts JR, et al: Phenytoin neuropathy: structural changes in the sural nerve. Ann Neurol 1986; 19: 162.

Raya A, Gallego J, Bosch-Morell F, et al: Phenytoin-induced glutathione depletion in rat peripheral nerve. Free Radicl Biology & Medicine 1995; 19: 665–667.

Russell JW, Windebank AJ, McNiven MA, et al: Effect of cisplatin and ACTH$_{4-9}$ on neural transport in cisplatin induced neurotoxicity. Brain Res 1995; 676: 258–267.

Sahenk Z, Barohn R, New P, et al: Taxol neuropathy. Arch Neurol 1994; 51: 726–729.

Said G: Perhexiline neuropathy: a clinicopathological study. Ann Neurol 1978; 3: 259–266.

Sakajiri K, Takamori M: Multiple mononeuropathy during recombinant interferon-α-2a therapy for chronic hepatitis. Clin neurol (Tokyo) 1992; 32: 1041–1043.

Samanta A, Burden AC: Fever, myalgia, and arthralgia in a patient on captopril and allopurinol. Lancet 1984; 1: 679.

Sampaio C, Castro-Caldas A, Sales-Luis MI, et al: Brachial plexopathy after Botulinum toxin administration for cervical dystonia. J Neurol Neurosurg Psychiatry 1993; 56: 220.

Sander D, Scholz C, Eiben P, et al: Plexus neuropathy following vaccination against tick-borne encephalitis and tetanus due to a sports related altered immune state. Neurol Res 1995; 17: 316–319.

Schaumburg H, Kaplan J, Windeback A, et al: Sensory neuropathy from pyridoxine abuse. NEJM 1983; 309: 445–448.

Schneider M, Ettlin T, Kaufmann M, et al: Transient neurologic toxicity after hyperbaric subarachnoid anesthesia with 5% lidocaine. Anesth Analg 1993; 76: 1154–1157.

Sebille A, St-Guily JL, Angelard B, et al: Low prevalence of cisplatin-induced neuropathy after 4-day continuous infusion in head and neck cancer. Cancer 1990; 65: 2644–2647.

Seppalainen AM, Haltia M: Carbon dilsulfide. In Spencer PS, Schaumburg H (Eds.): Experimental and clinical neurotoxicology, Baltimore, Williams and Wilkins, 1980, pp 356–373.

Shah RR, Oates NN, Idle JR, et al: Impaired oxidation of

debrisoquine in patients with perhexiline neuropathy. BMJ 1982; 184: 295–299.

Sheean GL, Murray NMF, Marsden CD: Pain and remote weakness in limbs injected with botulinum toxin A for writer's cramp. Lancet 1995; 346: 154–156.

Shirlanzoni A, Silvani A, Scaioli V, et al: Cisplatin neuropathy in brain tumor chemotherapy. Ital J Neurol Sci 1992; 13: 311–315,

Siegel T, Haim N: Cisplatin-induced peripheral neuropathy. Cancer 1990; 66: 1117–1123.

Simpson DM, Katzenstein DA, Hughes MD, et al: Neuromuscular function in HIV infection: analysis of a placebo-controlled combination antiretroviral trial. AIDS Clinical Group 175/801 Study Team. AIDS 1998; 12: 2425–2432.

Smith AG, Windeback AJ: Effect of ACTH analogs on cilsplatin neurotoxicity using embryonic rat dorsalroot ganglia explant as an in vitro model (abstract). Neurology 1992; 42: 29P.

Smith MD, Gibson GE, Rowland R: Combined hepatotoxicity and neurotoxicity following sulphasalazine administration. Austr NZ J Med 1982; 12: 76–80.

Spielberg SP, Gordon GB, Lombardi L: Nitrofurantoin cytotoxicity. J Clin Invest 1981; 67: 37–41.

Stept M, Subramony SH: Peripheral neuropathy associated with protriptyline. J Am Acad Child Adolesc Psychiatry 1988; 27: 377–380.

Sterman AB, Schaumburg H: Neurotoxicity of selected drugs. In Spencer PS, Schaumburg H (Eds.): Experimental and clinical neurotoxicology, Baltimore, Williams and Wilkins, 1980.

Stoeppler M, Vahter M: In Stoeppler M, Herber RFM (Eds.) Trace element analysis in biological specimens, Amsterdam, Elsevier Science, 1994.

Takeuchi H, Takahashi M, Kang J, et al: Ethambutol neuropathy: clinical and electroneuromyographic studies. Folia Psychiatr Neuolog Jpn 1980; 34: 45–55.

Takeuchi H, Yamada A, Touge T, et al: Metronidazole neuropathy: a case report. Jpn J Psychiatr Neurol 1988; 42: 291–295.

Tambini R, Quattrini A, Fracassetti O, et al: Axonal neuropathy in a patient receiving interferon-α therapy for chronic hepatitis C. J Rheumatol 1997; 24: 1656–1657.

Tarsy D: Brachial plexus neuropathy after botulinum toxin injection. Neurology 1997; 49: 1176–1177.

Tegnér R, Tomé FMS, Godeau P, et al: Morphological study of peripheral nerve changes induced by chloroquine treatment. Acta Neuropathol 1988; 75: 253–260.

Tomiwa K, Nolan C, Cavanagh JB: The effects of cisplatin on rat spinal ganglia: a study by light and electron microscopy and by morphometry. Acta Neuropathol 1986; 69: 295.

Toole JF, Gergen JA, Hayes DM, et al: Neural effects of nitrofurantoin. Arch Neurol 1968; 18: 680–687.

Tugwell P, James SL: Peripheral neuropathy and ethambutol. Postgrad Med J 1972,48: 667–670.

van Gerven JMA, Hovenstadt A, Moll JWB, et al: The effects of an ACTH (4–9) analogue on the development of cisplatin neuropathy in testicular cancer: a randomized trial. J Neurol 1994; 241: 432–435.

van Kooten B, van Diemen HAM, Groenhout KM, et al: A pilot study on the influence of a corticotropin (4–9) analogue on vinca alkaloid-induced neuropathy. Arch Neurol 1992; 49: 1027–1031.

Vanhooren G, Dehaene I, Zandycke MV, et al: Polyneuropathy in lithium intoxication. Muscle & Nerve 1990; 204–208.

Vieregge P, Kompf D: Brachial plexopathy after botulinum toxin administration for cervical dystonia (letter). JNNP 1993; 56: 1383–1339.

Vincent D, Penicaud-Vedrine A, Rancurel G, et al: Peripheral neuropathy in treatment with cimetidine. Presse Med 1988; 17: 589–590.

Waldinger TP, Siegle RJ, Weber W, et al: Dapsone-induced peripheral neuropathy—case report and review. Arch Dermatol 1984; 120: 356.

Wallace IW: Neurotoxicity associated with a reaction to sulphasalazine. Practitioner 1970; 204: 850–851.

Walls TJ, Pearce SJ, Venables GS: Motor neuropathy associated with cimetidine. BMJ 1980; 281: 974–975.

Weintrub M, Adde MA, Venzon DJ, et al: Severe atypical neuropathy associated with administration of hematopoietic colony-stimulating factors and vincristine. J Clin Oncol 1996; 14: 935–40.

Werner-Wasik M: Future development of amifostine as a radioprotectant. Semin Oncol 1999; 26(2, suppl 7): 129–34.

Whisnant JP, Espinosa RE, Kierland RR, et al: Chloroquine neuromyopathy. Proc Mayo Clin 1963; 39: 719.

Wijesekera JC, Critchley EMR, Fahim Y, et al: Peripheral neuropathy due to perhexiline maleate. J Neurol Sc 1980; 46: 303–309.

Williams MH, Bradley WG: An assessment of dapsone toxicity in the guinea pig. Br J Dermatol 1972; 86: 650.

Wilson JR, Conwit RA, Eidelman BH, et al: Sensorimotor neuropathy resembling CIDP in patients receiving FK506. Muscle Nerve 1994; 17: 528–532.

Windebank AJ, Blexrud M, Low PA, et al: Reversible, selective neurotoxicity in pyridoxine in vivo and in vitro (abstract). Neurology 1984; 34: 137.

Windebank AJ, Smith AG, Russel JW: The effect of NGF, CNTF, and ACTH analogs on cis-platinum neurotoxicity in vitro. Neurology 1994; 44: 488–494.

Woodward DK: Peripheral neuropathy and mesalazine. BMJ 1989; 299: 1224.

Wulff CH, Hoyer H, Asboe-Hansen G, et al: Development of polyneuropathy during thalidomide therapy. Br J Dermatol 1985; 112: 475–480.

Yamamoto K, Noda K, Yoshimura A, et al: Phase I study of E7010. Cancer Chemother Pharmacol 1998; 42: 127–134.

Zehnder D, Hoigne R, Neftel KA, et al: Painful dysaesthesias with ciprofloxacin. BMJ 1995; 310: 1204.

Ziajka PE, Wehmeier T: Peripheral neuropathy and lipid-lowering therapy. South Med J 1998; 91: 667–668.

Chapter 12
Drug-Induced Neuromuscular Disorders

Introduction

Drug-induced neuromuscular disorders should be differentiated from drug-induced myopathies (Chapter 13) and drug-induced polyneuropathies (Chapters 10, 11, and 22). Drug-induced neuromuscular blockade may present in any of the following ways (Howard 1990):

- Prolonged duration of neuromuscular blockade
- Post-operative respiratory depression
- Unmasking or aggravation of myasthenia gravis
- Drug-induced reversible myasthenic syndromes with no evidence of pre-existing defect of neuromuscular transmission.

Prolonged Duration of Neuromuscular Blockade

The duration of neuromuscular blockade may be longer and more pronounced than that intended and would be considered as a complication. Various causes for this are:

- Genetic factors with impairment of the metabolic pathways for the drug
- Systemic diseases such as hepatic and renal impairment leading to impaired metabolism and excretion of the neuromuscular blocking agent
- Patients with neuromuscular diseases such as myasthenia gravis and Lambert-Eaton syndrome

Postoperative Respiratory Depression

This is the commonest clinical manifestation of drug-induced neuromuscular blockade. Drugs such as aminoglycoside antibiotics given prior to surgery may delay the recovery of strength of muscles, particularly those of respiration. Assisted respiration is used in the management of such patients. Calcium gluconate infusion is used to overcome the presynaptic component of block and parenteral neostigmine is used to counteract the postsynaptic curare-like effect (Argov and Mastaglia 1979).

Unmasking or Aggravation of Myasthenia Gravis

Several drugs which affect neuromuscular transmission have been reported to precipitate myasthenia gravis in predisposed patients: aminoglycoside antibiotics, chloroquine, procainamide, phenytoin, lithium, etc. D-Penicillamine produces deterioration in myasthenia gravis and it use is contra-indicated in these patients.

Lambert-Eaton myasthenic syndrome is due to reduced release of ACh from motor nerve terminals. These patients have an exaggerated response to neuromuscular blocking agents and the disease may be first recognized when there is prolonged apnea after use of neuromuscular blocking agents during surgery.

Drug-Induced Reversible Myasthenic Syndromes

Drugs may produce a reversible myasthenic syndrome in a patient with no evidence of pre-existing disorder of neuromuscular transmission. Such a syndrome can be distinguished from naturally occurring myasthenia gravis which is associated with the presence of acetylcholine receptor antibodies. Myasthenic symptoms manifest soon after start of drug therapy and resolve after the drug is withdrawn.

Acute external ophthalmoplegia is seen in the following conditions and should be differentiated:

– Myasthenia gravis
– Ophthalmoplegic migraine
– Third cranial nerve palsy
– Guillain-Barré syndrome (Miller-Fisher variant)
– Wernicke's encephalopathy
– Drug induced, e. g.,
  · phenytoin intoxication
  · blocking agent-corticosteroid myopathy

Pathomechanism of Drug-Induced Neuromuscular Disorders

Some drugs produce neuromuscular effects through an immunological action. Others affect neuromuscular transmission directly. There are four possible mechanisms as proposed by Argov and Mastaglia (1979):

1. Presynaptic local anesthetic-like action, e. g., propranolol.
2. Postsynaptic receptor blockade, e. g., D-penicillamine.
3. Combination of 1 and 2. Postsynaptic curare-like action, e. g., aminoglycoside antibiotics.
4. Interference with muscle-membrane conductance, e. g., quinine.

Drugs that Impair Neuromuscular Transmission

Various drugs which have been alleged to impair neuromuscular transmission are listed in Table 12.1. Most of these reports are anecdotal and there are few in vitro evaluations of drugs on human or animal neuromuscular preparation.

Anesthetics

Various causes for prolonged duration of neuromuscular weakness following anesthesia are:
– Inheritable disorders such as pseudocholinesterase deficiency. Pseudocholinesterase hydrolyses acetylcholine as well as succinylcholine and mivacurium. A deficiency of this enzyme, therefore, results in an abnormally prolonged muscle relaxation if succinylcholine and mivacurium are administered.
– Systemic diseases with hepatic and renal impairment lead to impaired metabolism and excretion of neuromuscular blocking agents and prolong their action.
– Patients with neuromuscular diseases such as myasthenia gravis and Lambert-Eaton syndrome are at risk.
– Certain drugs such as anticholinesterases, monoamine oxidase inhibitors can decrease the activity of pseudocholinesterase and prolong neuromuscular weakness.

General anesthetics may potentiate neuromuscular blocking in patients with myasthenia gravis (Baraka et al 1971). Short-acting anesthetics such as ketamine and diazepam can enhance the effect of neuromuscular blocking agents. Intravenous injection of local anesthetic such as lidocaine is likely to potentiate the effect of neuromuscular blocking agents by both presynaptic as well as post synaptic effects with a reduction in ACh release (Mathews and Quillam 1964).

Antibiotics

There are several hundred reports of muscular weakness resulting from effect of antibiotics on

Table 12.1. Drugs reported to impair neuromuscular transmission.

Anesthetics*
- diazepam
- halothane
- ketamine
- lidocaine
- methoxyflurane

Antibiotics*
- amikacin
- ampicillin
- ciprofloxacin
- clindamycin
- colistimethate
- colistin
- kanamycin
- lincomycin
- neomycin
- netilmicin
- penicillin
- polymyxin B
- streptomycin
- sulfonamide
- tetracycline
- tobramycin
- vancomycin

Anticonvulsants
- barbiturates
- carbamazepine
- ethosuximide
- mephenytoin
- phenytoin
- trimethadione

Botulinum toxin*

Cardiovascular drugs*
- antiarrhythmic drugs
  • bretylium
  • cebenzoline
- calcium channel blockers
  • verapamil
  • diltiazem
- procainamide
- quinine and quinidine
- β-blockers
  • atenolol
  • betaxolol
  • labetalol
  • metoprolol
  • nadolol
  • oxyprenolol
  • pindolol
  • practolol
  • propranolol
  • timolol
  • ganglia blocking agents
    (e. g., trimetaphan)

Chloroquine*

D-Penicillamine*

Endocrine preparations

- corticosteroids*
- levonorgestrel implant*
- thyroid hormone

Interferon-α*

Neuromuscular blocking agents*
  (non depolarizing)
- Steroidal
  • vercuronium
  • pancuronium
- Non-steroidal
  • benzylisoquinolinium
  • non-benzylisoquinolinium

Psychotropic drugs
- chlorpromazine
- lithium

Miscellaneous drugs
- diuretics
- DL-carnitine
- iodinated contrast media
- ketoprofen
- sodium lactate
- tetanus antitoxin
- trihexphenidyl (Artane)

*Well documented.

the neuromuscular junction in otherwise normal patients, those receiving neuromuscular blocking agents, those with myasthenia gravis, and those receiving drugs toxic to the neuromuscular junction (McQuillan et al 1968; Pittinger et al 1970; Albiero et al 1978; Burkett et al 1979). Since the description of first cases by Hokkanen and Toivakka (1969), aminoglycoside antibiotics have been well recognized for producing neuromuscular weakness. This is related to the dose and the serum levels and is partially reversible by cholinesterase inhibitors, calcium infusion and aminopyridines (Maeno and Enomoto 1978). These drugs act presynaptically or post-synaptically or at both sites. Clinically only gentamicin, kanamycin, neomycin, tobramycin, and streptomycin have been implicated in producing muscle weakness in non-myasthenic patients. Erythromycin therapy in normal volunteers has demonstrated a facilitatory response with repetitive nerve stimulation suggesting a presynaptic neuromuscular block (Herishanu and Taustein 1971). Lincomycin and clindamycin differ in structure only slightly from aminoglycosides but both can cause neuromuscular blockage that is not readily reversed with cholinesterase inhibitors (Samuelson et al 1975). Vancomycin has been reported to potentiate suxamethonium chloride-induced neuromuscular blockade (Albrecht and Lanier 1993). Penicillins and sulfonamides have been reported to cause transient worsening of myasthenic weakness and to potentiate the effect of neuromuscular blocking agents. Ampicillin has been reported to aggravate the weakness of myasthenia gravis (Argov et al 1986). Tetracycline analogs may exacerbate myasthenia gravis but the mechanism is not clear (Gibbels 1967).

Two fluoroquinolones, ciprofloxacin (Moore et al 1988) and norfloxacin (Rauser and Ariano 1990), have been reported to exacerbate myasthenia gravis. Neuromuscular weakness has been reported with polymyxin B (Pohlman 1966). This drug reduces ACh release and to a lesser degree produce postjunctional block of ACh receptors (Durant and Lambert 1981). Large doses of clindamycin can result in prolonged neuromuscular blockade (Al Ahdal and Bevan 1995).

Anticonvulsants

Symptomatic myasthenia gravis has been reported in previously asymptomatic patients receiving a variety of anticonvulsant medications including phenytoin (Brumlik and Jacobs 1974), trimethadione (Peterson 1966; Booker et al 1970) and barbiturates (Osserman and Genkins 1971).

Experimentally phenytoin has been shown to reduce the release of ACh from nerve terminals. Trimethadione may induce an autoimmune disorder directed towards the neuromuscular junction. Barbiturates and ethosuximide produce postsynaptic neuromuscular block while carbamazepine exerts its effects presynaptically (Alderdice and Trommer 1980). There have been no clinical reports of such adverse reactions to carbamazepine or ethosuximide.

Botulinum Toxin

Local injection of botulinum A toxin is widely used in the treatment of focal dystonias such as blepharospasm and spastic torticollis. Botulinum toxin has a potent effect in blocking acetylcholine release at presynaptic level. It has a dose dependent effect on neurotransmission in muscles distant from the site of injection. Girlanda et al (1992), who have confirmed these effects, recommend that patients undergoing treatment with botulinum toxin should be monitored carefully particularly when high accumulative dose is used and comedications impairing neuromuscular transmission are used. A case is reported of unmasking of Lambert-Eaton syndrome following periorbital injection of botulinum toxin for blepharospasm and weakness of pelvic muscles (Erbguth et al 1993). This resolved within 8 weeks. Blepharospasm recurred 20 weeks later following repeat injection of botulinum toxin. Further investigations revealed an underlying adenocarcinoma of the lung which was removed with recovery of muscle weakness. The authors recommended caution in the use of botulinum toxin for focal dystonia in patients with neuromuscular disorders. Myasthenia gravis is a theoretical contraindication for the use of botulinum toxin. A life-threatening reaction due to antiacetyl choline-receptor antibody has been reported in a myasthenic patient after injection of botulinum toxin (Borodic 1998). this patient had a previous botulinum toxin injection which masked the results of the tensilon test.

Cardiovascular Drugs

Several cardiovascular drugs have been reported to affect the muscle strength of patients with myasthenia gravis. These include the following:

Antiarrhythmic Drugs. The following antiarrhythmic drugs have been reported to induce neuromuscular weakness:
- *Bretylium,* used for refractory ventricular arrhythmias, has been reported to cause weakness and potentiate the neuromuscular blockade of competitive neuromuscular blocking agents (Campbell and Montuschi 1960).
- *Cibenzoline* therapy for ventricular arrhythmia has been associated with a myasthenia-like syndrome in a patient with renal failure who was receiving continuous peritoneal dialysis (Wakutani et al 1998). For some un-

known reasons, patients on peritoneal dialysis are unable to eliminate cibenzoline from the blood. If this adverse effects occurs, it is recommended to either discontinue the drug or use hemodialysis in stead of peritoneal dialysis.

– *Procainamide* is reported to produce worsening of strength in patients with myasthenia gravis (Drachman and Skom 1965). It is postulated to act at the presynaptic membrane with impaired formation of ACh.

– *Quinidine* is a stereoisomer of quinine and at one time formed the basis of a provocative test for the diagnosis of myasthenia gravis. It can aggravate or unmask myasthenia gravis (Shy et al 1985). The effect is presynaptic with impairment of formation and release of ACh.

Calcium Channel Blockers. There is conflicting information on the adverse effects of calcium channel blockers on neuromuscular conduction. Low concentrations of verapamil and diltiazem increase potency of the neuromuscular blocking agents (Bikhazi et al 1983).

Verapamil is an antiarrhythmic drug which acts mainly at the atrioventricular node and blocks calcium channels that are specific to cardiac and smooth muscles but its effect on the striated muscle and the neuromuscular junction is less well studied. There is experimental evidence that verapamil may have actions at presynaptic and postsynaptic sites at the motor end-plate. Swash and Ingram (1992) reported a patient in whom verapamil severely exacerbated pre-existing myasthenia gravis.

Diltiazem is an antagonist of voltage operated calcium channels and has been shown to reduce ACh release in experiments performed *in vitro* (Chang et al 1988). Diltiazem has been reported to aggravate and precipitate Lambert-Eaton syndrome (Ueno and Hara 1992).

β-Blockers. Some β-adrenergic blocking agents have been implicated in causing worsening of strength in myasthenic patients. Atenolol, labetalol, metoprolol, nadolol, propranolol, and timolol cause a dose-dependent reduction in efficacy of neuromuscular transmission in normal rat skeletal muscle (Howard et al 1987). Propranolol has the most effect and atenolol the least

effect on neuromuscular transmission. The mechanism of β-blocker-induced neuromuscular blockade is not clear but one possibility is that these drugs specifically block β-adrenergic receptors whose activity is important for neuromuscular transmission.

Propranolol, oxyprenolol, and practolol, and timolol have been reported to induce a myasthenic syndrome or to unmask myasthenia gravis (Herishanu and Rosenberg 1975; Hughes and Zacharias 1976; Verkijk 1985). Transient diplopia has been reported in several patients receiving a variety of β-blockers (Weber 1982). Confavreux et al (1990) have reported a case of myasthenia gravis precipitated by acetbutalol therapy which had a fulminant course despite drug withdrawal. Even those drugs instilled topically on the cornea are capable of producing such weakness.

Ganglia Blocking Agents. Trimetaphan is used in hypertensive emergencies and there are isolated reports that it can produce neuromuscular weakness. It has been reported to cause acute respiratory paralysis, probably due to curare-like action at the neuromuscular junction (Dale and Schroeder 1976).

Chloroquine

Chloroquine is used primarily as an antimalarial but in higher doses it is also used in the treatment of collagen vascular disorders including rheumatoid arthritis. Neurological disorders caused by this drug include optic neuritis (see Chapter 10), peripheral neuropathy (see Chapter 11), myopathy (see Chapter 13), and myasthenia-like syndromes (De Bleecker et al 1991; Sghirlanzoni et al 1988). These authors propose an autoimmune mediated mechanism through induction of ACh receptor antibodies. In a previously reported case, direct toxic effect of chloroquine on the neuromuscular junction was considered (Robberecht et al 1989). Sieb et al (1992) reported a case of Lambert-Eaton syndrome which manifested during a four month prophylactic use of chloroquine but the pathogenesis remains uncertain.

Speak (1993) has reviewed 12 published case reports where chloroquine has unmasked or aggravated myasthenia gravis or induced a myasthenia-like syndrome. Approximately half of these relate to high-dose, long-term therapy. The other half relate to low-dose short-term malaria prophylaxis.

D-*Penicillamine*

D-Penicillamine (DP) is used in the treatment of rheumatoid arthritis, Wilson's disease, and cystinuria. A number of autoimmune disorders have been reported in patients receiving DP and these include myasthenia gravis (Bucknall et al 1975). A literature survey revealed 150 cases of DP-induced myasthenia gravis (Dubost et al 1992). DP-induced myasthenia gravis is clinically similar to the idiopathic form and it is distinguishable from the idiopathic form only by the high remission rate after DP is discontinued (Albers et al 1980). A genetic susceptibility to the development of DP-induced myasthenia gravis in patients with rheumatoid arthritis is suggested by the abnormal distribution of HLA-DR antigens (Delamere et al 1983).

DP-induced myasthenia gravis is usually mild and may be restricted to ocular muscles manifested by diplopia and/or ptosis (Ferbert 1989; Liu and Bienfang 1990; Ferro et al 1993). Experimental studies on animals provide no evidence that DP has any direct and clinically significant effect on neuromuscular transmission. It is more likely that DP acts by a reversible effect on the immune system rather than by unmasking latent disease (Vincent et al 1978).

The diagnosis of DP-induced myasthenia gravis can be confirmed by response to cholinesterase inhibitors, electromyographic abnormalities, and elevated serum AChR antibodies. DP should be discontinued in patients who develop myasthenia gravis. Long-term cholinesterase inhibitor treatment is indicated only in those patients with additional extraocular manifestations.

Endocrine Preparations

Corticosteroids. Exacerbation of myasthenia gravis can occur after start of high-dose steroid therapy for this disease (Scoppetta et al 1979). Direct effect of corticosteroids has been shown in experimental muscle-nerve preparations (Wilson et al 1974) but none of these are seen in clinical situations. Enhanced lymphocyte transformation has been noted in vitro in patients with prednisone-induced aggravation of myasthenia gravis and it has been postulated that immunologically non-reactive lymphocytes are destroyed by corticosteroids, with enhanced proliferation of sensitized lymphocytes (Abramsky et al 1975). It is advisable to hospitalize patients with myasthenia gravis at the start of corticosteroid therapy. Most of the adverse effects can be managed by adjusting the dosage of cholinesterase inhibitors but plasma exchange may be used to prevent or reduce the severity of steroid-induced exacerbations.

Levonorgestrel Implant (Norplant). There are several cases reported to FDA of myasthenia-like syndrome following levonorgestrel implants. In one case, symptoms started four months after the implant and myasthenia gravis was diagnosed 8 months later (Brittain and Lange 1995). This patient had strongly positive anti-acetylcholine receptor antibodies, a positive tensilon test and electromyographic findings characteristic of myasthenia gravis. There was improvement with pyridostigmine therapy and the dose could be lowered after removal of the levonorgestrel implant.

Thyroid Hormone. The relation of thyroid gland to myasthenia gravis is well known. Thyroid hormone and antithyroid medications have been reported to aggravate the weakness of patients with myasthenia gravis (McEachern and Parnell 1948) but this is not considered to a be problem with newer therapies.

Interferon-α

Myasthenia gravis was first reported as a complication of treatment with interferon-α-2b for cancer of bladder (Batocchi et al 1995). The diagnosis of myasthenia was confirmed by edrophonium testing and a positive anti-acetylcholine receptor antibody test. Interferon was discontinued and the patient was treated with pyridostigmine and prednisone. One year later, the patient was asymptomatic with pyridostigmine alone and anti-acetylcholine antibodies were still detectable. Several other cases have been reported during treatment of chronic hepatitis C with interferon-α-2b (Mase et al 1996; Uyama et al 1996). In two cases myasthenia was confined to the ocular muscles (Piccolo et al 1996; Rohde et al 1996).

Neuromuscular Blocking Agents

Neuromuscular blocking agents may be polarizing or depolarizing. The latter are used more commonly in clinical practice. Neuromuscular blocking drugs are designed to resemble acetylcholine structurally which allows the to interact with the cholinergic site on the nicotinic receptors at the neuromuscular junction. The ratio of the dose which produces an adverse effect to that required for neuromuscular blocking effect is termed safety ratio and has been measured for most of the non-depolarizing muscle relaxants (NDMR). Factors which affect the recovery from neuromuscular blockade are (Watling and Dasta 1994):

- Concomitant drug use
- Duration of therapy
- End organ function
- Severity of underlying disease
- Availability of neuromuscular monitoring devices

Predisposing Factors for Prolongation of Neuromuscular Blockade. Because of the wide margin of safety for neuromuscular transmission under physiological circumstances, clinically manifest neuromuscular paralysis is uncommon. It is likely to occur when the safety margin is reduced such as in myasthenia gravis or when the following predisposing factors exist:

- Electrolyte disturbances: hypokalemia, hypocalcemia
- Concomitant use of muscle relaxants
- Abnormally high drug concentrations in patients with renal impairment
- Elderly persons
- Patients with disorders of immune function

- Overdose of neuromuscular blocking agents
- Generalized muscular weakness has been observed following prolonged use of muscle relaxants to eliminate competitive muscular effort in mechanically ventilated patients.
- Concomitant use of corticosteroids. Pancuronium bromide and vercuronium bromide are structurally similar to corticosteroids. Corticosteroids have often been administered to patients with post-ventilation paralysis. This has led to the speculation that they may potentiate the effects of muscle relaxants in the development of prolonged myasthenic syndrome (Benzing and Bove 1992).
- Drug interactions
  - with other drugs themselves can induce neuromuscular blockade by themselves
  - cimetidine
  - magnesium

Examples of Prolonged Neuromuscular Blockade. The following are some of the reports of prolonged neuromuscular blockade:

Atracurium besilate. Cases of prolonged paralysis has been reported after infusion of atracurium besilate for neuromuscular blockade was stopped (Branney et al 1994; Hoey et al 1995; Rubio and Seelig 1996). *Vercuronium bromide.* Benzing et al (1990) reported the case of a child who developed a myasthenic syndrome after receiving muscle relaxants for one week and took six weeks to recover. Other cases of long-term paralysis following vercuronium infusion have been reported (Lagasse et al 1990; Vanderheyden et al 1992). Neuromuscular paralysis after the long-term administration of vercuronium as muscle relaxant is associated with metabolic acidosis, elevated plasma magnesium concentrations and presence of renal failure with high plasma concentrations of 3-desacetylvercuronium (Segredo et al 1992). Other causes for the prolonged action of vercuronium are renal and hepatic dysfunction following cardiac arrest (Sanders and Aucker 1996), mitochondrial myopathy (Naguib et al 1996), and interaction with magnesium sulfate used for the treatment of preeclampsia (Kwan et al 1996).

Drug Interactions with Neuromuscular Blockers. These have been reviewed by Feldman and Karalliedde (1996). Various sites of interactions include actions on motor nerve conduction and spinal reflexes, acetylcholine (ACh) synthesis, mobilization and release, sensitivity of motor end plate to ACh and ease of propagation of the motor action potential. Additive effects occur when two non-depolarizing muscle relaxants are administered together. In spite of the numerous possibilities, clinically significant interactions are uncommon in practice. Some examples of interactions of neuromuscular blockers with other drugs are as follows:

- Drugs that interact by affecting ACh formation or release: aminoglycosides, calcium antagonists, magnesium sulfate and procaine.
- Drugs that interact by inhibiting plasma cholinesterase: metaclopramide, oral contraceptives and tacrine.
- Drugs that interfere with muscle contractility: volatile anesthetics, clindamycin and dantrolene.

Differential Diagnosis. Prolonged paralysis after the use of neuromuscular junction blocking agents as an adjunct to anesthesia may lead to neurogenic atrophy (Gooch et al 1991). NDMR-induced paralysis should be differentiated from polyneuropathy and myopathy. The following important points of distinction have been pointed out by Zochodne and Ramsay (1994):

- Polyneuropathy in patients in intensive care is not associated with neuromuscular blocking agents
- Polyneuropathy is usually associated with systemic sepsis and multiple organ failure
- Polyneuropathy is not associated with elevated CK levels as is the case with necrotizing myopathy
- Polyneuropathy is usually not associated with neuromuscular transmission deficit.

Prevention. From the information currently available restrain should be exercised in the routine use of neuromuscular blocking agents as they may compromise rather than facilitate the establishment of spontaneous respiratory function (Gazmuri et al 1992). Abel et al (1994) consider that an ideal muscle relaxant should have the following properties but none of the current-

ly available drugs has reached this ideal standard:

- It should affect specifically at the nicotinic receptor of the motor end plate and lack effect on all the other organ systems
- It should have a rapid and reliable onset of action as well as a predictable duration of action
- It duration of action should not be affected by the medical condition of the patient
- Reversal of neuromuscular blockade should not be required.

Psychotropic Drugs

Chlorpromazine. Chlorpromazine was first reported to produce acute exacerbation of muscle weakness in a myasthenic schizophrenic patient (McQuillan et al 1963). Chlorpromazine has been shown to produce postsynaptic block in a nerve-muscle preparation (Argov and Yaari 1979). Phenothiazines (chlorpromazine and promazine) can antagonize ACh and prolong the effect of succinylcholine.

Lithium. There are several reports of unmasking of myasthenia gravis (Neil et al 1976) and prolongation of effect of neuromuscular blocking agents (Borden et al 1974; Hill et al 1976). It is considered to act mainly at presynaptic level by substituting lithium ions for sodium ions at the nerve terminal. Some investigators have postulated a progressive accumulation of lithium inside the presynaptic nerve terminal, where it serves as a competitive cation for calcium, resulting in an inhibition of ACh synthesis and release (Vizi et al 1972).

Miscellaneous Drugs

A number of drugs are described briefly here where the evidence for association of neuromuscular disorders with the drug is based on occasional case reports.

Diuretics. Diuretics aggravate the weakness in patients with myasthenia gravis probably by wasting potassium as these patients are sensitive to hypokalemia (Jenkins et al 1970).

DL-Carnitine. DL-carnitine, but not L-carnitine, has been reported to worsen the muscle strength in patients undergoing renal dialysis (Bazzato et al 1981). The exact mechanism of this is not known but it is postulated to be due to a presynaptic block or postsynaptic block by accumulation of acylcarnitine esters (De Grandis et al 1980).

Iodinated Contrast Media. Intravenous infusion of iodinated contrast media has been reported to aggravate the muscle strength in patients with myasthenia gravis or to precipitate a myasthenic crisis (Canal and Franceschi 1983; Chagnac et al 1985). The mechanism of these adverse reactions is not known. There is one report of a patient with Lambert-Eaton syndrome who developed respiratory insufficiency after intravenous injection of iodinated contrast material and the postulated mechanism was hypocalcemia due to direct binding by the contrast agent resulting in further presynaptic blockade (Van den Bergh et al 1986).

Ketoprofen. McDowell and McConnel (1985) reported cholinergic crisis in a patient with myasthenia precipitated by ketoprofen, a non-steroidal anti-inflammatory agent. Such a reaction has not been reported by other drugs in this category.

Sodium Lactate. The intravenous infusion of sodium lactate is reported to worsen muscular strength in patients with myasthenia gravis (Engel et al 1974). The mechanism is unknown but may be related to transient hypocalcemia due to sodium lactate.

Trihexyphenidyl (Artane). Trihexyphenidyl has been reported to have unmasked myasthenia gravis in a patient where the concentration of ACh antibody paralleled the degree of weakness (Ueno et al 1987).

Management

The possibility of drug-induced disorder of neuromuscular transmission should be considered in any patient presenting with a myasthenic syndrome. Tensilon test, single-fiber electromyographic studies, and ACh receptor antibody studies should be performed in all cases. Recovery after withdrawal of the drug indicates drug-induced disorder rather than unmasking of myasthenia gravis. Calcium gluconate has been recommended to reverse the presynaptic component of the neuromuscular block but there is no agreement on the dose or rate of administration. Neostigmine may be used to counteract the postsynaptic component of the neuromuscular block.

In spite of the information that several drugs interfere with neuromuscular transmission, there is no absolute contraindication for any drug with the exception of D-penicillamine.

References

Abel M, Book J, Eisenkraft JB: Adverse effects of non-depolarizing neuromuscular blocking agents. Drug Safety 1994; 10: 420–438.

Abramsky O, Aharanov A, Titelbaum D: Myasthenia gravis and acetylcholine receptors. Arch Neurol 1975; 32: 684–687.

Al Ahdal O, Bevan DR: Clindamycin-induced neuromuscular blockade. Canad J Anes 1995; 42: 614–615.

Albers JW, Hodach RJ, Kimmel DW, et al: Penicillamine-associated myasthenia gravis. Neurology 1980; 30: 1246–1250.

Albiero L, Bamonte F, Ongini E, et al: Comparison of neuromuscular effects and acute toxicity of some aminoglycoside antibiotics. Arch Int Pharmacodyn Ther 1978; 233: 343–350.

Albrecht RF, Lanier WL: Potentiation of succinylcholine-induced phase II block by vancomycin. Anesthesia Analgesia 1993; 77: 1300–1302.

Alderdice MT, Trommer BA: Differential effects of anticonvulsants phenobarbital, ethosuximide and carbamazepine on neuromuscular transmission. J Pharmacol Exp Ther 1980; 215: 92–96.

Argov Z, Brenner T, Abramsky O: Ampicillin may aggravate clinical and experimental myasthenia gravis. Arch Neurol 1986; 43: 255–256.

Argov Z, Mastaglia FL: Disorders of neuromuscular transmission caused by drugs. NEJM 1979; 301: 409–413.

Argov Z, Yaari Y: The action of chlorpromazine at an isolated cholinergic synapse. Brain Res 1979; 164: 227–236.

Baraka A, Afifi A, Muallem M, et al: Neuromuscular effects of halothane, suxamethonium, and tubocurarine in a myasthenic undergoing thymectomy. Br J Anesth 1971; 43: 91–95.

Batocchi AP, Evoli A, Servidei S, et al: Myasthenia gravis

during interferon α therapy. Neurology 1995; 45: 382–383.

Bazzato G, Coli U, Landini S, et al: Myasthenia like syndrome after D,L-carnitine but not L-carnitine. Lancet 1981; 1: 209.

Benzing G, Bove KE: Sedating drugs and neuromuscular blockade during mechanical ventilation. JAMA 1992; 267: 1775.

Benzing G, Iannaccone ST, Bove KE, et al: Prolonged myasthemic syndrome after one week of muscle relaxants. Pediatr Neurol 1990; 6: 190–196.

Bikhazi GB, Leung I, Foldes EF: Ca-channel blockers increase potency of neuromuscular blocking agents in vivo. Anesthesiology 1983; 59: A269.

Booker HE, Chun RWM, Sanguino M: Myasthenia gravis syndrome associated with trimethadione. JAMA 1970; 21: 2262–2263.

Borden H, Clark MT, Katz H: The use of pancuronium bromide in patients receiving lithium carbonate. Can Anesth Soc J 1974; 21: 79–82.

Borodic G: Myasthenia crisis after botulinum toxin. Lancet 1998; 352: 1832.

Branney SW, Haenel JB, Moore FA, et al: Prolonged paralysis with atracurium infusion: a case report. Crit Care Med 1994; 22: 1699–1701.

Brittain J, Lange LS: Myasthenia gravis and levonorgestrel implant. Lancet 1995; 346: 1556.

Brumlik J, Jacobs RS: Myasthenia gravis associated with diphenylhydantoin therapy for epilepsy. Canad J Neurosci 1974; 1: 127–129.

Bucknall RC, Dixon AStJ, Glick EN, et al: Myasthenia gravis associated with penicillamine treatment for rheumatoid arthritis. BMJ 1975; 1: 600–602.

Burkett L, Bikhase GB, Thomas KC, et al: Mutual potentiation of the neuromuscular effects of antibiotics and relaxants. Aneth Analg 1979; 58: 107–115.

Campbell EDR, Montuschi E: Muscle weakness caused by bretylium tosylate. Lancet 1960; 2: 789.

Canal N, Franceschi M: Myasthenic crisis precipitated by iothalamic acid. Lancet 1983; 1: 1288.

Chagnac Y, Hadanin M, Goldhammeer Y: Myasthenic crisis after intravenous administration of iodinated contrast agent. Neurology 1985; 35: 1219–1220.

Chang CC, Lin SO, Hong SJ, et al: Neuromuscular block by verapamil and diltiazem and inhibition of acetylcholine release. Brain Res 1988; 454: 332–339.

Confavreux C, Charles N, Aimard G: Fulminant myasthenia gravis soon after initiation of acebutalol therapy. Eur Neurol 1990; 30: 279–281.

Dale RC, Schroeder ET: Respiratory paralysis during treatment of hypertension with trimethaphan camsylate. Arch Int Med 1976; 136: 816–818.

De Bleecker J, De Reuck J, Quatacker J, et al: Persisting chloroquine-induced myasthenia? Acta Clin Belg 1991; 46: 401–406.

De Grandis D, Mezzina C, Fiaschi A, et al: Myasthenia due to carnitine treatment. J Neurol Sci 1980; 46: 365–371.

Delamere JP, Jobson S, Mackintosh LP, et al: Penicillamine-induced myasthenia in rheumatoid arthritis: its clinical and genetic features. Ann Rheum Dis 1983; 42: 500–504.

Drachman DA, Skom JA: Procainamide—a hazard in myasthenia gravis. Arch Neurol 1965; 13: 316–320.

Drosos AA, Christou L, Galanopoulou V, et al: D-penicillamine induced myasthenia gravis: clinical, serological and genetic findings. Clin Exp Rheumatol 1993; 11: 387–391.

Dubost JJ, Soubrier M, Bouchet F, et al: Complications neuromusculaires de la D.Penicillamine dans la polyarthrite rhumatoide. Rev Neurol 1992; 148: 207–211.

Durant NN, Lambert JJ: The action of polymyxin B at neuromuscular junction. Br J Pharmacol 1981; 72: 41–47.

Engel WK, Festoff BW, Patten BM, et al: Myasthenia gravis. Ann Int Med 1974; 81: 225–246.

Erbguth F, Claus D, Engelhardt A, et al: Systemic effects of local botulinum toxin injections unmasks the subclinical Lambert-Eaton myasthenic syndrome. JNNP 1993; 56: 1235–1236.

Feldman S, Karalliedde L: Drug interactions with neuromuscualr blockers. Drug Safety 1996; 15: 261–273.

Ferbert A: D-Penicillamine-induzierte okuläre Myasthenie bei Psoriasisarthritis. Nervenarzt 1989; 60: 576–579.

Ferro J, Susano R, Gomez C, et al: Miastenia inducida por penicilamina: existe interaccion con los antidepresivos triciclos? Rev Clin Esp 1993; 192: 70–71.

Fogdall RP, Miller RD: Prolongation of pancuronium-induced neuromuscular blockade by clindamycin. Anesthesiology 1974; 41: 407–408.

Gazmuri RJ, Hanif S, Wagner D: Persistent paralysis after vecuronium administration. NEJM 1992; 327: 1881.

Gibbels E: Weitere Beobachtungen zur Nebenwirkung intravenoser Reverin-Gabe bei Myasthenia gravis pseudoparalytica. Deutsch Med Wochenschr 1967; 92: 1153–1154.

Girlanda P, Vita G, Nicolosi C, et al: Botulinum toxin therapy: distant effects on neuromuscular transmission and autonomic nervous system. JNNP 1992; 55: 844–845.

Gooch JL, Suchyta MR, Baslbierz JM, et al: Prolonged paralysis after treatment with neuromuscular junction blocking agents. Crit Care Med 1991; 19: 1125–1131.

Herishanu Y, Rosenberg P: Beta blockers and myasthenia gravis. Ann Int Med 1975; 83: 834–835.

Herishanu Y, Taustein I: The elctromyographic changes induced by antibiotics: a preliminary study. Conf Neurol 1971; 33: 41–45.

Hill GE, Wong KC, Hodges MR: Potentiation of succinylcholine neuromuscular blockade by lithium carbonate. Anesthesiology 1976; 44: 439–442.

Hoey LL, Joslin SM, Nahum A, et al: Prolonged neuromuscular blockade in two critically ill patients treated with atracurium. Pharmacotherapy 1995; 15: 254–259.

Hokkanen E, Toivakka E: Streptomycin-induced neuromuscular fatigue in myasthenia gravis. Ann Clin Res 1969; 1: 220–226.

Howard JF, Johnson BR, Quint SR: The effects of β-adrenergic agonists on neuromuscular transmission in rat skeletal muscle. Soc Neurosci Abstr 1987; 13: 147.

Howard JF: Adverse drug effects on neuromuscular transmission. Sem Neurol 1990; 10: 89–102.

Hughes RO, Zacharias FJ: Myasthenic syndrome during treatment with practolol. Br Med J 1976; 1: 460–461.

Jenkins RB, Witorsch P, Smythe NPD: Aspects of treatment of crisis in myasthenia gravis. South Med J 1970; 63; 1127–1130.

Kwan WF, Lee C, Chen BJ: A non-invasive method for the differential diagnosis of vercuronium-induced and magnesium-induced protracted neuromuscular block in a severely preeclamptic patient. J Clin Anes 1996; 8: 392–397.

Lagasse RS, Katz RI, Peterson M, et al: Prolonged neuromuscular blockade following vercuronium infusion. J Clin Anesth 1990; 2: 269–271.

Liu GT, Bienfang DC: Penicillamine-induced ocular myasthenia gravis in rheumatoid arthritis. J Clin Neuro-Ophthalmol 1990; 10: 201–205.

Maeno T, Enomoto K: Reversal of streptomycin-induced muscle paralysis by 3,4-diaminopyridine. J Pharm Pharmacol 1978; 30: 249–250.

Mase G, Zorzon M, Vitrani B, et al: Development of myasthenia gravis during interferon-α treatment for anti-HCV positive chronic hepatitis. JNNP 1996; 60: 348–349.

Mathews EK, Quillam JP: Effect of central depressant drugs on acetylcholine release. Br J Pharmacol 1964; 22: 415–440.

McDowell IFW, McConnell JB: Cholinergic crisis in myasthenia gravis precipitated by ketoprofen. BMJ 1985; 291: 1094.

McEachern D, Parnell JL: Relationship of hyperthyroidism to myasthenia gravis. J Clin Endocrinol 1948; 8: 842–850.

McQuillan MP, Canter HE, O'Rourke JR: Myasthenic syndrome associated with antibiotics. Arch Neurol 1968; 18; 402–415.

McQuillan MP, Gross M, Johns RJ: Chlorpromazine-induced weakness in myasthenia gravis. Arch Neurol 1963; 8: 286–290.

Moore B, Safani M, Keesey J: Possible exacerbation of myasthenia by ciprofloxacin. Lancet 1988; 1: 882.

Naguib M, El Dawlatly AA, Ashour M, et al: Sensitivity to mivacurium in a patient with mitochondrial myopathy. Anesthesiology 1996; 84: 1506–1509.

Neil JF, Himmelhoch JM, Licata SM: Emergence of myasthenia gravis during treatment with lithium carbonate. Arch Gen Psychiatry 1976; 33: 1090–1092.

Osserman KE, Genkins G: Studies in myasthenia gravis: review of twenty-year experience in over 1200 patients. Mt Sinai J Med 1971; 38: 497–572.

Peterson HDC: Association of trimethadione therapy and myasthenia gravis. NEJM 1966; 274: 506–507.

Piccolo G, Franciotta D, Versino M, et al: Myasthenia gravis in a patient with chronic active hepatitis C during interferon-α treatment. JNNP 1996; 60: 348.

Pittinger CB, Eryasa Y, Adamson R: Antibiotic-induced paralysis. Anesth Analg 1970; 49: 487–501.

Pohlman G: Respiratory arrest associated with intravenous administration of polymyxin B sulfate. JAMA 1966; 196: 181–183.

Rauser EH, Ariano RE, Anderson BA: Exacerbation of myasthenia gravis by norfloxacin. Ann Pharmacother 1990; 24: 207–208.

Robberecht W, Bednarik J, Bourgeois P, et al: Myasthenic syndrome caused by direct effect of chloroquine on neuromuscular junction. Arch Neurol 1989; 46: 464–468.

Rohde D, Sliwka U, Schweizer K, et al: Oculo-bulbar myasthenia gravis induced by cytokine treatment of a patient with metastasizing renal cell carcinoma. Eur J Clin Pharmacol 1996; 50: 471–473.

Rubio ER, Seelig CB: Persistent paralysis after prolonged atracurium in the absence of corticosteroids. South Med J 1996; 89: 624–626.

Samuelson RJ, Giesecke AH Jr, Kallus FT, et al: Lincomycin-curare interaction. Anesth Analg 1975; 54: 103–105.

Sanders KA, Aucker R: Early recognition of risk factors for persistent effects of vecuronium. South Med J 1996; 89: 411–414.

Scoppetta C, Tonali P, Evoli A, et al: Treatment of myasthenia gravis: Report on 139 patients. J Neurol 1979; 222: 11–21.

Segredo V, Caldwell JE, Matthay MA, et al: Persistent paralysis in critically ill patients after long-term administration of vecuronium. NEJM 1992; 327: 524–528.

Sghirlanzoni A, Mantsgazza R, Mora M, et al: Chloroquine myopathy and myasthenia-like syndrome. Muscle & Nerve 1988; 11: 114–119.

Shy ME, Lange DJ, Howard JF, et al: Quinidine exacerbating myasthenia gravis: a case report and intracellular recordings. Ann Neurol 1985; 18: 120.

Sieb JP, Dengler R, Jerusalem F: Das nichtparaneoplastische Lambert-Eaton-Syndrom. Nervenarzt 1992; 63: 234–239.

Speak G: Malaria and myasthenics. Pharmaceutical Journal 1993; 251: 302.

Swash M, Ingram DA: Adverse effects of verapamil in myasthenia gravis. Muscle & Nerve 1992; 15: 396–398.

Ueno S, Hara Y: Lambert-Eaton myasthenic syndrome without anti-calcium channel antibody: adverse effect of calcium antagonist diltiazem. JNNP 1992; 55: 409–410.

Ueno S, Takahashi M, Kajiyama K, et al: Parkinson's disease and myasthenia gravis: adverse effect of trihexiphenidyl on neuromuscular transmission. Neurology 1987; 37: 832–838.

Uyama E, Fujki N, Uchino M: Exacerbation of myasthenia gravis during interferon-α treatment. J Neurol Sci 1996; 144: 221–222.

Van den Bergh P, Kelly JJ Jr, Carter B, et al: Intravascular contrast media and neuromuscular junction disorders. Ann Neurol 1986; 19: 206–207.

Vanderheyden BA, Reynolds HN, Gerold KB, et al: Prolonged paralysis after long-term vecuronium infusion. Crit Care Med 1992; 20: 304–307.

Verkijk A: Worsening of myasthenia gravis with timolol maleate eye drops. Ann Neurol 1985; 17: 211–212.

Vincent A, Newsom-Davis J, Martin V: Anti-acetylcholine receptor antibodies in D-penicillamine-associated myasthenia gravis. Lancet 1978; 1: 1254.

Vizi ES, Illes P, Ronai A, et al: The effect of lithium on acetylcholine release and synthesis. Neuropharmacology 1972; 11: 521–530.

Wakutani Y, Matushima E, Son A, et al: Myasthenia-like syndrome due to adverse effects of cibenzoline in a patient with chronic renal failure. Muscle and Nerve 1998; 21: 416–417.

Watling SM, Dasta JF: Prolonged paralysis in intensive care unit patients after the use of neuromuscular blocking agents: a review of the literature. Crit Care Med 1994; 22: 884–893.

Weber JCP: Beta-adrenoceptor antagonists and diplopia. Lancet 1982; 2: 826–827.

Wilson RW, Ward MD, Johns TR: Corticosteroids—a direct effect at neuromuscular junction. Neurology 1974; 24: 1091–1095.

Zochodne DW, Ramsay DA: Acute quadriplegic myopathy (letter). Neurology 1994; 44: 988.

Chapter 13
Drug-Induced Myopathies

Introduction

Several therapeutic drugs are known to produce adverse effects on the skeletal muscle or the neuromuscular apparatus or the peripheral nerves. Effect of alcohol (one of the oldest drugs known) in causing muscle weakness has been recognized since the middle of nineteenth century. Adverse effects of pharmaceuticals on muscles has been recognized mostly within the last 50 years.

Clinical manifestations of drug-induced myopathies range from muscle pain to serious sequelae such as rhabdomyolysis. Although some categories of drugs are associated with specific

Table 13.1. Clinical manifestations of drug-induced myopathies.

Myalgia: muscle pain, stiffness or cramps without neurological signs
Myotonia: Delayed relaxation of skeletal muscle after a voluntary contraction
Painless proximal myopathy characterized by muscle weakness
Painful myopathies
 – with drug-induced polymyositis
 – without polymyositis
Focal myopathy with focal area of damage due to injections
Myokymia or rhythmic rippling of muscles corresponding to widespread myokymic discharges seen on EMG
Hypokalemic myopathy associated with weakness of muscles due to drug-induced hypokalemia
Mitochondrial myopathy is associated with inhibition of mitochondrial DNA and is characterized by ragged red fibers
Rhabdomyolysis: acute muscle necrosis with myoglobinuria and systemic complications
Malignant hyperthermia
Secondary effects of myopathies
 – Renal shutdown in rhabdomyolysis
 – Compartment syndromes due to myositis (Chow and Chow 1993)

forms of myopathies, a drug can cause more than one type of myopathy and this term is used in a broad sense to report adverse effect of drugs on muscles. The term myopathy usually refers to skeletal muscle although rarely it is attached to cardiac muscle as "cardiac myopathy". Adverse effects on the neuromuscular apparatus are described in Chapter 12 and on the peripheral nerves in Chapter 11. Clinical manifestations of drug-induced myopathies are shown in Table 13.1.

Myalgia (Muscle Pain)

Muscle pain, stiffness, and cramps are the most common medical complaints. These are subjective symptoms and is difficult to evaluate them in the absence of associated myositis, muscle spasm, or peripheral neuropathy. These may be the first symptom of these disorders and may precede the evolution of objective signs. Drug-induced muscle pain may be due to the following mechanisms:

– *Mechanical pain.* This may be due to mechanical displacement of the muscle by a hematoma, spasm or rigidity, or secondary to a drug-induced movement disorder.
– *Inflammatory pain.* This may be due to myositis or rhabdomyolysis.
– *Ischemic pain.* This may be due to drug-induced spasm or vasculitis involving the peripheral arteries.
– *Enhanced prostaglandin synthesis.* Drugs which enhance prostaglandin synthesis may cause muscle pain. This pain is usually relieved by prostaglandin inhibitors such as piroxicam. A case of myalgia due to ACE inhibitors has been described and postulated to be due to increased bradykinin concentrations,

Table 13.2. Drugs reported to induce myalgia or muscle cramps.

Angiotensin-converting enzyme (ACE) inhibitors
Anticholinesterases
Antimony compounds: sodium stibogluconate,
    meglumine antimonate
Beta-adrenergic agonists
Calcium antagonists
Captopril
Carbimazole, treatment of hyperthyroidism
Cimetidine
Clofibrate
Colchicine
Corticosteroids, withdrawal
Cytotoxic drugs
Danazol
Dexamethasone
Diuretics
D-Penicillamine
Enalapril
Filgrastim (granulocyte colony-stimulating factor)
Gold compounds
Labetalol
Levamisole (Buecher et al 1996)
Lithium
Losartan potassium
L-tryptophan
Metolazone
Nifedipine
Pindolol
Procainamide
Rifampicin
Salbutamol
Suxamethonium chloride (van der Berg and Iqbal
    1996)
Zidovudine
Zimeldine

stimulating arachidonic acid release, or inhibiting the destruction of cyclooxygenase (Peppers 1995).

– *Decrease in serum calcium with influx into muscle cells.* This mechanis has been proposed for suxamethonium-induced myalgia (Book et al 1994). High intracellular calcium ion concentration may cause damage to muscle spindles by asynchronous muscle bundle contractions.

– *Referred pain.* This may occur with drug-induced peripheral neuropathies.

Drugs which have been reported to cause myalgia or muscle cramps in the absence of a demonstrable neurological or muscular disorders are shown in Table 13.2.

Drug-Induced Myotonic Disorders

Some drugs can induce or exacerbate myotonia in humans or experimental animals (Kwiecinski et al 1981). These drugs are listed in Table 13.3. Myotonia develops in fast-twitch fibers and requires intact muscle innervation. The pathogenesis is not well understood.

Depolarizing muscle relaxants such as suxamethonium can markedly exacerbate myotonia during general anesthesia. Therefore, non-depolarizing relaxants should be used in patients with known myotonia (Mastaglia 1992). Other drugs which exacerbate myotonia are the β_2-adrenergic blockers and β_2-adrenergic agonists (Sholl et al 1985).

Table 13.3. Drugs which induce or unmask myotonic disorders.

Anesthetic propofol (Kinney and Harrison 1996)*
β-agonists
    – fenoterol
    – ritodrine
β-blockers
Clofibrate
Depolarizing muscle relaxants*
Diazacholesterol
Diuretics*
    – frusemide
    – ethacrynic acid
    – mersalyl
    – acetazolamide
Iodine compounds
Propanolol
Vincristine

* Well documented.

Myositis. Drugs which induce myositis are shown in Table 13.4. Myositis is generally considered to be an idiopathic inflammatory disorder of muscles. Recent findings indicate that environmental agents acting on genetically susceptible persons lead to physiologic responses involving immune activation and subsequent tissue damage that is recognized as myositic syndromes. Persons receiving the antirheumatic drug D-Penicillamine can develop a syndrome that is clinically, pathologically, and serologically indistinguishable from polymyositis. The syndrome resolves when drug therapy is discontin-

Table 13.4. Drugs reported to cause myositis.

Alcohol
Amiodarone (Bonnet et al 1995)
Chloroquine*
Cimetidine
Cocaine
Colchicine
Corticosteroids*
D-Penicillamine* (Chappel and Willems 1996)
Interferon-α (Solis et al 1996)
Interleukin-2 (Finger et al 1995)
Ipecac
Lipid-lowering agents*
  – lovastatin
  – pravastatin (Schalke et al 1992)
L-Tryptophan*
Pentazocine (Kim and Song 1996)
Phenobarbital
Procainamide
Tranilast (Arase et al 1990)
Zidovudine

*Well documented. The rest of the list is based on isolated case reports.

ued. Because HLA types of persons who develop myositis associated with D-Penicillamine differs from those persons whose myositis is not associated with D-Penicillamine exposure, individual factors such as immunologic or metabolizer genes, or other cofactors may account for the finding that myositis develops in only a few persons exposed to these agents.

Pathological Types of Myopathies

Correlation of structural lesions in muscles and clinical manifestations is usually not possible but an attempt has been made by Stoltenburg-Didinger and Neuhaus (1987) as shown in Table 13.5.

The following pathological types of myopathies are generally recognized:

– Necrotizing myopathies
– Mitochondrial myopathies
– Inflammatory myopathies
– Autophagic myopathies
– Focal myopathies

Table 13.5. Correlation of structural lesions and clinical manifestations in drug-induced myopathies (modified from Stoltenberg-Didinger and Neuhaus 1987).

Structural/Functional Effects	Principal Clinical Manifestations	Examples/Drugs
A. *Toxic effects on muscle structure*		
1. Muscle fiber necrosis. Damage to intracytoplasmic membrane	Painless proximal muscle weakness	Chloroquine
2. Muscle fiber necrosis and sarcolemmal damage	Muscle pain and swelling. Proximal muscle weakness, elevated CK, myoglobinuria	Clofibrate
3. Myofibrillary damage	Proximal muscle weakness with decrease of muscle contractility	Emetine
4. Type 2 fiber atrophy	Chronic proximal muscle weakness	Cortisone
B. *Toxic effect on muscle function*		
1. Contractility	Genetic predisposition. Increased CK. Hyperthermia. Muscle weakness and pain. Neuroleptic malignant syndrome	Inhalation anesthetics
2. Energy metabolism (mitochondrial myopathy)	Muscle weakness, muscle pain on exertion	Zidovudine
3. Neuromuscular conduction	Myasthenic reaction	(see Chapter 12)

Necrotizing Myopathies. These myopathies evolve slowly with involvement of proximal muscles at first which may proceed on to generalized muscle weakness. Pain is experienced usually in cases with rapid evolution. Examples of drugs associated with this type of myopathy are epoxy-aminocaproic acid and cholesterol-lowering drugs.

Mitochondrial Myopathy. This is characterized by ragged red fibers. An example is the myopathy seen in AIDS patients on long-term therapy with zidovudine which inhibits mitochondrial DNA replication.

Inflammatory Myopathy. This myopathy is indistinguishable from other types of polymyositis clinically and pathologically except that improvement follows discontinuation of drug therapy. An example of this type of myopathy is that caused by penicillamine. Eosinophilia-myalgia syndrome associated with use of tryptophan is described in Chapter 20.

Autophagic Myopathy. Drugs with amphophilic cationic properties interfere with lysozymal digestion and lead to autophagous degeneration and accumulation of phospholipids in muscles and other tissues. Examples of this type of myopathy is that caused by chloroquine which produces peripheral neuropathy as well.

Focal Myopathy. Localized areas of muscle damage follow intramuscular injection as a result of needle insertion (needle myopathy). Fibrous myopathy has been reported following the injection of drugs listed in Table 13.6. Myopathy may be due to traumatic necrosis, hematoma formation, low-grade infection or local toxic effect of injected drugs. Repeated intramuscular injec-

Table 13.6. Fibrous myopathy following drug injection.

Antibiotics
Botulinum toxin
Butorphanol (Wagner and Cohen 1991)
Chloroquine (Aguayo and Hudgson 1970)
Chlorpromazine (Cohen 1972)
D-Propoxyphene (Restrepo et al 1993)
Drug abuse
Meperidine (Aberfeld et al 1968)
Paraldehyde (Lane and Mastaglia 1978)
Pentazocine (Adams et al 1983)

tion may lead to fibrosis and contractures. A progressive fibrous myopathy may result from chronic intramuscular drug abuse. Johnson et al (1976) described patients who presented with contractures of hips and knees after abusing meperidine and other agents for years. Soft tissues of thighs and buttocks were "wood hard," EMG showed absence of action potentials in affected muscles, and biopsy revealed extensive replacement of muscle with dense, acellular fibrous tissue. This complication may mimic other rheumatic disorders and early recognition may prevent disability. Good functional results can be obtained by excision of areas of fibrosis.

Critical Illness Myopathy

This has reported in critically ill patients treated with high-dose intravenous corticosteroids and non-depolarizing neuromuscular junction-blocking agents in the intensive care (Gutmann and Gutmann 1999). Minimizing the use of these agents may prove helpful in preventing the occurrence of these disorders. However, comatose and critically ill patients have been reported to develop muscle weakness or paralysis (quadriplegia) during the course of sepsis and multiple-organ failure where drugs such as steroids, neuromuscular-blocking agents and aminoglycosides were not responsible for paralysis (Latronico et al 1996). These patients may become completely paralyzed because of non-drug-induced neuromuscular disorders. The diagnosis is important to avoid unnecessary investigations and unreasonably pessimistic prognosis. Electromyography is essential for the diagnosis and for planning further clinical management. Biopsy needs to be done only when it is necessary.

Pathomechanism of Drug-Induced Myopathies

These myopathies are mostly due to toxic effect of the drugs on the muscles as a primary event as evidenced by elevation of serum CK. Excessive neural driving or accumulation of ACh at neuromuscular junction by cholinesterase inhibitors such as phencyclidine. Finally, other drug-induced disturbances may produce myopathies as a secondary event.

Direct Effect of Drugs on Muscle. These are as follows:

- Effect on the muscle plasma membrane which is the most exposed part of the muscle and is vulnerable to toxins. Disturbances of ionic permeability of the membrane increases entry of calcium into the cell leading to myofibrillary contracture and initiating a chain of events which leads to cell death. Drug-induced changes in electrical properties of muscle plasma membrane can produce myalgia, cramps, and myotonia. Uncoupling of oxidative phosphorylation can produce mitochondrial myopathy.
- Interference with protein synthesis and degradation in muscles. Emetine can inhibit protein synthesis and mitochondrial respiration leading to disruption of cell membrane if high concentrations of drug are present.
- Autophagic degeneration and phospholipid accumulation in muscles, e. g., chloroquine-induced myopathy. There may be disruption of microtubule-dependent cytoskeletal network that interacts with lysozymes as in the case of colchicine-induced myopathy.
- Infiltration of muscles with neutrophils, e. g., as an effect of drugs such as granulocyte colony-stimulating factor.

Indirect Effects of Drugs on Muscle. These are due to other drug-induced disorders as follows:

- Electrolyte disturbances such as in hypokalemia and hyponatremia.
- Drug-induced immune disturbances leading to myositis.
- Drug-induced metabolic disorders, e. g., carnitine deficiency associated with pivampicillin (Rose et al 1992).

Effect on Muscle Plasma Membrane. This is the most exposed part of the muscle and is vulnerable to toxins (Pritchard 1979). Disturbances of ionic permeability of the membrane increases entry of calcium into the cell leading to myofibrillary contracture and initiating a chain of

events which leads to cell death (Steer and Mastaglia 1986).

Hypokalemic Myopathy

This is caused by the following drugs:
- Amphotericin B
- Carbenoxolone
- Diuretics
- Licorice (Shintani et al 1992)
- Purgatives

Diuretics are the most common cause of hypokalemic myopathy. Hypokalemic myopathy differs from hypokalemic periodic paralysis (HPP) as follows:

- There is an underlying cause such as a drug or disease. In HPP the cause of hypokalemia is unexplained.
- Muscle glycogen is absent whereas in HPP muscle is overloaded with glycogen.
- Enzymes derived from muscles are elevated and rhabdomyolysis may occur whereas such an event is not a presenting feature in HPP.
- It requires a large quantity of therapeutic potassium supplementation for an extended term till recovery.

Drugs that Induce Myopathy

There is a considerable amount of literature on this topic including some excellent reviews such as that by Mastaglia (1992). Drugs which have been reported to cause myopathy are listed in Table 13.7.

Amiodarone

The neurologic adverse effects of this antiarrhythmic agent are tremor, ataxia, and neuropathy associated with myopathy (Roth et al 1990; Clouston and Donnelly 1984). The pathologic feature is a vacuolar myopathy. Vacuoles are present in both type 1 and type 2 fibers and on electron microscopy correspond to autophagic vacuoles of varied size. These changes disappear on discontinuation of the drug.

Table 13.7. Drugs reported to cause myopathy.

Alcohol
Amiodarone*
Carbimazole
Chloroquine*
Cholesterol-lowering agents*
Cimetidine
Clozapine (Scelsa et al 1996)
Colchicine* (Sinsawaiwong et al 1997; Lee et al 1997)
Corticosteroids*
Cyclosporine
D-Penicillamine
Emetine
Epsilon-aminocaproic acid*
Germanium
Glycyrrhizin (licorice)*
Gold salts
Growth hormone
Interferon-α-2b (Arai et al 1995; Dippel et al 1998)
Ipecac
Labetalol (Willis et al 1990)
Leuprolide acetate
Omeprazole (Sarrot-Reynauld et al 1996)
Perhexiline
Phenybutazone
Phenytoin
Propylthiouracil
Pyrazinamide (Fernandez-Sola et al 1996)
Retinoids: Etiretinate, tretinoin and isotretinoin
    (Fiallo et al 1996).
Tranilast
Vincristine
Zidovudine*

*Well documented.

Carbimazole

Three cases of myopathy has been reported in association with carbimazole and manifested by muscular pain and increase of serum CK. Improvement occurred after reduction of dose of carbimazole.

Chloroquine

This antimalarial and antirheumatic drug may cause myopathy or peripheral neuropathy (see Chapter 11). Estes et al (1987), after reviewing the literature and adding six of their own cases, concluded that:

– Chloroquine or hydrochloroquine (a less toxic substitute) may cause reversible vacuolar myopathy with acid phosphatase positive vacuoles mainly in type 1 fibers.

– There is insidious development of painless muscle weakness, particularly of proximal muscles associated with muscle wasting.

– There is associated cardiac muscle involvement and the diagnosis can be made by endomyocardial biopsy in addition to skeletal muscle biopsy.

– Characteristic ultrastructural changes consist of curvilinear body formation are present in all affected tissues and help to distinguish it from polymyositis, steroid myopathy, and SLE, conditions in which these bodies are absent.

– Possible pathomechanism is lysozymal accumulation of the drug with subsequent enzyme inhibition and rise of intralysozymal pH. When pH rises above 7.4, activities of most acidic lysozymal hydrolases are inhibited leading to accumulation of phospholipids, glycogen, and curvilinear body formation.

– The myopathy is reversible if the drug is withdrawn but recovery may take several months.

A retrospective review of 214 patients who received chloroquine or hydroxychloroquine for rheumatic disorders identified three patients who developed myopathy out of a total of 303 patient years of treatment (Avina-Zubieta et al 1995). All of the three patients had received chloroquine for 12–18 months and the incidence of myopathy was 1 in 100 patient years. All patients improved within 8 weeks of discontinuation of therapy.

Cholesterol-Lowering Agents

Several drugs are used to lower LDL serum cholesterol, raise HDL cholesterol, retard the progression of atherosclerosis and reduce the mortality and morbidity of cardiovascular diseases. Myopathy has been described with a number of cholesterol-lowering agents: fibric acid derivatives (clofibrate, benzafibrate, gemfibrozil), 3-hydroxy-3-methylglutaryl coenzyme A (HMG-CoA) reductase inhibitors (Lovastatin, simvastatin, pravastatin), and nicotinic acid. Another HMG-CoA reductase inhibitor, fluvastatin has been studied, both as a monotherapy and in combination with niacin, but no case of myopathy was observed (Jacobson et al 1994).

Clinical Features. Most patients with cholesterol-lowering agent myopathy (CLAM) myopathy complain of muscle cramps and weakness; myotonia and elevated creatine kinase (CK) are common findings. It may proceed on to rhabdomyolysis.

Although a transient increase in serum creatine kinase is common after treatment with lovastatin, clinically manifest myopathy has been reported in less than 1% of patients on this drug. Pravastatin, another slightly different drug of this category, is associated with dermatomyositis (Schalke et al 1992).

Polymyositis has been reported in a patient on fenofibrate therapy (Sauvaget et al 1991). Gemfibrozil alone has been reported to be associated with myopathy (Magarian et al 1991). Other fibric acid deratives such as clofibrate (Hattori et al 1990), and benzafibrate (Inoue et al 1992) have also been reported to induce myopathy. Necrotising myopathy has been described in a patient on fenofibrate therapy (Berger et al 1993). Similar complication has been reported with use of nicotinic acid as well (Litin and Anderson 1989).

Combined drug use increases the risk of myopathy. Combination of lovastatin with gemfibrozil has also been reported to induce myopathy (Chucrallah et al 1992). The incidence of myopathy with this combination is severe enough to discontinue treatment in 3% of patients (Glueck et al 1992). Drug-interaction also increases the risk of lovastatin-induced myopathy when it is coadministered with cyclosporine in patients with a kidney or heart transplant and hyperlipidemia (Arellano and Krupp 1991).

Pathomechanism. The pathomechanism of these myopathic changes is poorly understood. One explanation is that cholesterol is a major constituent of the muscle membrane, which is affected with an increase in "membrane fluidity" in patients receiving a variety of cholesterol-lowering drugs. This may result in unstable sarcolemma, myotonic discharges, and increased levels of sarcoplasmic enzymes or myoglobinu-

ria (London et al 1991). Simvastatin-induced myopathy in rabbits shows myotonic discharges on EMG, myonecrosis, and raised serum CK levels suggesting that the pathomechanism of myopathy is lesions of muscle surface membrane (Nakahara et al 1992a). HMG-CoA reductase inhibitors have been shown to produce dose-related myocytotoxicity in rats and this effect was potentiated by the concomitant use of cyclosporine (Smith et al 1991).

Cimetidine

This is a histamine H_2-receptor antagonist which has a possible role as an immunomodulator in addition to an inhibitory action on gastric acid secretion. Polymyositis has been reported in addition to acute interstitial nephritis in a patient on cimetidine therapy (Watson et al 1983). Muscle biopsy showed fragmentation of muscle fibers, areas of regeneration and lymphocytic infiltrates. Immunologic studies of B and T cells suggested activation of cell-mediated immune system in the pathogenesis of both myopathy and nephritis. Steroid therapy resulted in improvement of the condition.

Colchicine

Colchicine is used mainly in the treatment of gout but also for familial mediterranean fever, primary biliary cirrhosis, and proliferative vitreoretinopathy. Myopathy and neuropathy has been described as a complication of its use (Younger et al 1991; Kuncl et al 1987; Riggs et al 1986). It is more likely to occur in patients with renal dysfunction leading to elevated plasma drug levels (Older et al 1992). Colchicine-induced myopathy has been reported in renal transplant patients receiving cyclosporin (Jonsson et al 1992; Rieger et al 1990). Cyclosporine may interfere with hepatic metabolism or renal clearance of colchicine and myopathy may present acutely (van der Naalt et al 1992). Colchicine-induced myopathy may be rapid in onset and this may be due to concomitant use of drugs such as cimetidine and calcium channel blockers which inhibit cytochrome P450 system (Schiff and Drislane 1992).

Serum CK levels are usually elevated 10- to 20-fold and pathologically the myopathy is of vacuolar type marked accumulation of lysozymes and autophagic vacuoles unrelated to necrosis. Striking accumulation of large amounts of granular substance immunoreactive for tubulins has been observed in skeletal muscle fibers in a case of colchicine myopathy (Himmelman and Schröder 1992). The pathomechanism involves disruption of a microtubule-dependent cytoskeletal network that interacts with lysozymes. Recovery usually occurs after withdrawal of the drug.

Corticosteroids

Chronic myopathy caused by corticosteroids excess whether endogenous or exogenous is well known and has been described in the course of Cushing's syndrome (Muller and Kugelberg 1959). This disease has been reported in the course of various diseases treated with corticosteroids for long periods; SLE (Dubois 1958), rheumatoid arthritis (Fryberg et al 1958), bronchial asthma (Dunenci et al 1959) and polymyositis (Askari et al 1976). Corticosteroids induce a painless myopathy with slow onset of proximal muscle weakness of the lower extremities and seldom of the upper extremities. Steroid myopathy, as manifested by clinically detectable proximal muscle weakness, is seen in as many as 60% of those receiving steroids (Batchelor et al 1997).

Pathomechanism. The basic cellular action of corticosteroids seems to be an inhibition of messenger RNA synthesis, which, in turn influences the translation and synthesis of muscle specific proteins (Karpati 1984). Myopathy is more likely to develop in patients treated with 9-α-fluorinated corticosteroids such as triamcinolone, betamethasone, and dexamethasone (Dropcho and Soong 1991). Serum levels of CK and other enzymes are normal in steroid myopathy and if CK is elevated another type of myopathy should be considered. EMG shows myopathic changes in proximal muscles with reduction in motor unit duration and amplitude without spontaneous muscle fiber potentials. Muscle biopsy shows a characteristic atrophy of type 2 muscle fibers. Fast-twitching glycolytic (type 2b) fibers are more susceptible but the cause is uncertain. Denervation and disuse due to physical inactivity increase the susceptibility to corticosteroid myopathy.

Clinical Features. Acute myopathy may occur less often within a week after onset of treatment with high dose corticosteroids. Such myopathy involving respiratory muscles has been described in patients with asthma and chronic obstructive pulmonary disease (Decramer and Stas 1992; Dekhuijzen and Decramer 1992). Patients with status asthmaticus treated with high dose corticosteroids in combination with neuromuscular blockade induced by steroidal muscle relaxants are more prone to develop myopathy which is also referred to as "blocking agent-corticosteroid" myopathy (Griffin et al 1992; Waclawik et al 1992; Hirano et al 1992; Danon and Carpenter 1991; Shee 1990). One case of ophthalmoplegia in this setting has been described by Sitwell et al (1991). Even without combination with neuromuscular blocking agents, high parenteral doses of corticosteroids may produce acute myopathy in patients with myasthenia gravis (Panegyres et al 1993).

Management. Corticosteroid myopathy is usually reversible if the drug is withdrawn or the dose is reduce or if prednisone is substituted. Corticosteroid-induced muscle atrophy and weakness can be partially prevented or reversed by a program of physical exercises.

Cyclosporin

Myopathy has been reported in patients treated with cyclosporin (Noppen et al 1987; Goy et al 1989). Symptoms were generalized severe muscle pain and weakness. Serum CK was elevated. EMG showed myopathic changes and muscle biopsy showed atrophic muscle fibers, segmentary necrosis with accumulation of glycogen (Fernandez-Sola et al 1990). Electron microscopy showed lipid vacuoles and abnormal mitochondria. Arellano and Krupp (1991) reviewed 29 cases reported up to end of 29 cases (published as well as unpublished) and occurring mostly in transplant patients. Two patterns were identified: myopathy and rhabdomyolysis (see under the appropriate section). Myopathy occurred in a dose dependent manner and subsided on reduction of dose or discontinuation of the drug. In the postmarketing surveillance of these authors, the incidence rate in 3017 patients was found to 0.17% in one year. Causal relation in these cases could not be assessed. In a double-blind randomized study (Arnadottir et al 1994), low dose simvastatin (10 mg per day) was found to be well tolerated and efficacious for the treatment of hypercholesterolemia in renal transplant patients.

D-*Penicillamine (DP)*

DP can cause autoimmune adverse reactions such as pemphigus, nephritis, neuromuscular disorders, SLE, and Sjögren's syndrome. Polymyositis has been reported in 1.2% of patients with rheumatoid arthritis treated with DP (Takahashi et al 1986). The most common clinical manifestations were muscle weakness and dysphagia. Discontinuation of DP and treatment with steroids resulted in improvement. Biopsy of striated muscle frequently showed perivascular mononuclear cell infiltration suggesting cell-mediated immunity in the pathogenesis of this adverse effect. Whether DP treatment is the sole cause of polymyositis or whether it acts as a trigger for the development of a secondary or overlap type of autoimmune disorder in patients who already have a primary autoimmune disorder remains unknown. Polymyositis appears to be an idiosyncratic reaction to DP that does not have a relation to dose or the duration of treatment (Aydintug et al 1991). When polymyositis develops in patients with rheumatoid arthritis, it is generally advisable to temporarily interrupt or discontinue treatment with DP if corticosteroids are administered (Carroll et al 1987).

Emetine *(see also below "Ipecac")*

This is the principal alkaloid of ipecac which is used for treating amoebiasis and also as an emetic and is abused by patients with anorexia nervosa. Reversible generalized muscle weakness is known as an adverse effect of this drug (Bennett et al 1982; Mateer et al 1985; Palmer et al 1985). Serum CK was elevated up to 14-fold in some cases but was normal in other cases. Muscle biopsy shows muscle necrosis with type 2 fiber atrophy. Gradual recovery occurred in the reported cases after withdrawal of the drug.

The pathomechanism is inhibition of protein synthesis and mitochondrial respiration by emetine and disruption of cell membrane by high concentrations of the drug (Duane and Engel 1970).

Epsilon-Aminocaproic Acid

Epsilon-aminocaproic acid (EACA) is an antifibrinolytic agent used in the treatment of patients with subarachnoid hemorrhage. Myopathy is recognized as a complication of long-term (4–6 weeks) treatment with doses of over 18 g/day (Britt et al 1980). Muscle biopsy shows fiber necrosis with selective involvement of type 1 fibers. Pathomechanism of EACA-induced myopathy is not known. EACA is an analog of lysine and may substitute for it in the cellular membranes, thus impairing their function.

Germanium

In recent years anti-tumor activity of a few germanium preparations has been reported in Japan and such preparations are used widely in over-the-counter remedies. Germanium-induced myopathy has been reported by Higuchi et al (1989). Prominent histochemical findings were a vacuolar myopathy with lipid excess, increased acid phosphatase activity, and decreased cytochrome oxidase activity. Ultrastructural examination showed it to be a mitochondrial myopathy. The findings were replicated in animal studies by the authors.

Glycyrrhizin (Licorice)

Licorice is used widely as a Chinese medicine and contains glycyrrhizin (GL) as the main ingredient. Licorice is also used as a sweetener and in several foods and drugs in Europe and USA. GL-induced hypokalemic myopathy (GIHP) was first reported by Cayley (1950). Shintani et al (1992) have reviewed 57 cases with GIHM reported in literature and described two of their own patients with this disorder. The following has been summarized from their excellent review.

Clinical manifestation of GIHP were muscular weakness and flaccid quadriplegia in all cases. Weakness usually manifested at serum potassium level of 2.0 mEq/l or less. Pathological findings included necrotic fibers, sporadic vacuolar degeneration and cellular infiltration around necrotic fibers as well as blood vessels. Pathomechanism is based on mineralocorticoid-like effect of glycyrrhetinic acid, the active form of GL. The effect is, at first, directly on the kidneys or indirectly increases the aldosterone-like effect resulting in mineralocorticoid effect. As a result of this K^+ excretion is elevated following increased Na^+ absorption in distal tubules leading to hypokalemia. A risk factor for the development of GIHM is the use of concomitant medications such as hypotensive diuretics which aggravate hypokalemia.

Treatment is immediate discontinuation of licorice consumption, hospitalization, and correction of hypokalemia. Complete cure was obtained in all of the reported cases.

Gold Salts

Gold salts may produce a myokymic syndrome as reported by Caldron et al (1987). EMG showed myokymic discharges and muscle biopsy showed small angular fibers of type 1 and 2, some degeneration, disturbances of glycogen content and increased ACh esterase but no inflammatory changes; these changes suggest neurogenic atrophy. Treatment with carbamazepine and discontinuation of gold therapy usually results in remission.

Growth Hormone

Myositis has been reported in two patients after treatment with growth hormone somatotropin for growth hormone deficiency (Yordam et al 1994). These patients had myalgia as well as muscle weakness with elevation of serum creatine kinase levels. Muscle biopsy specimens of both patients showed focal infiltrates of mononuclear cells along with increased number of central nuclei with light microscopy. Somatotropin was discontinued and the symptoms resolved with normalization of serum creatine kinase levels in both patients. The growth hormone injections in these patients contained a diluent, m-cresol, which might have caused myositis and further investigations are necessary to determine if the adverse reaction is caused by the diluent or the growth hormone.

Interferon

A case of myopathy has been reported in a patient given interferon-α-2b for hepatitis C infection. After 19 weeks of treatment the patient had muscle pain and weakness with rise of serum creatine kinase. These adverse reactions subsided after discontinuation of interferon therapy. (Arai et al 1995).

Ipecac (see also above "Emetine")

This is the dried root of plant used as a syrup for expectorant, emetic, and antidysenteric properties. It is available as an over-the-counter preparation. The principal alkaloid is emetine hydrochloride. A case of ipecac-induced myopathy has been reported after long-term abuse of ipecac (Bennett et al 1982). Progressive muscle weakness and skin lesions suggested dermatomyositis. Muscle biopsy showed inflammatory changes and muscle enzymes were normal. Strength returned after cessation of ipecac abuse. Myopathy has been reported following use of ipecac syrup by young women with eating disorders (Dresser et al 1993, Thyagarajan et al 1993). Muscle biopsy findings were vacuolar degeneration and myosinolysis of muscle fibers with loss of sarcoplasm and small cytoplasmic bodies. Myopathy cleared up in these patients after cessation of ipecac abuse.

Labetalol

Willis et al (1990) reported severe generalized myopathy in two children treated with labetalol. There was proximal muscle weakness and markedly elevated CK. Improvement occurred immediately after withdrawal of the drug. Muscle biopsies were consistent with diagnosis of necrotic myopathy.

Leuprolide Acetate

This is a synthetic nonapeptide analog of gonadotrophin releasing hormone and is used for the palliative treatment of advanced prostatic carcinoma. Crayton et al (1991) reported a patient treated with leuprolide acetate who developed biopsy-proven myositis. Drug withdrawal and steroid therapy resulted in clinical remission of myositis within two months. Although malignant disease may be associated with myositis, the causal relation of the drug to the adverse effect was considered probable in this case for the following reasons:

- Temporal relationship. Reaction followed soon after the first dose of the drug.
- Treatment of the underlying malignancy usually improves myositis rather than aggravates it.
- Myositis of the malignancy usually does not respond to steroids.
- Myositis improved after discontinuation of the drug even though there was no change in the malignant condition.

Phenylbutazone

Curran and Jamieson (1987) described one case of dermatomyositis-like syndrome with myalgia and proximal muscle weakness which developed one week after administration of this drug. CK was elevated and EMG findings of prolonged distal latency, increased insertional activity were consistent with the diagnosis of inflammatory myopathy. Improvement occurred after steroid therapy.

Phenytoin

Myopathy has been reported as a hypersensitivity reaction to phenytoin (Barclay et al 1992). Five cases reported in literature were considered to occur on an immunologic basis. In one case muscle biopsy demonstrated necrosis and regeneration of muscle fibers without evidence of inflammation (Harney and Glasberg 1983).

Propylthiouracil

Shergy and Caldwell (1988) reported a case of polymyositis with raised CK in a patient with hyperthyroidism following treatment with propylthiouracil. Muscle biopsy showed atrophic fibers undergoing degeneration and regeneration as well as inflammatory cells. Although polymyositis may occur in hyperthyroidism, CK levels are usually normal or decreased. Therefore, polymyositis was considered to be drug-induced in this case.

Retinoids

Three patients have been reported to have developed painful myopathy after receiving etiretinate therapy (Hodak et al 1987). Serum CK was elevated, EMG showed myopathic changes, and muscle biopsy showed necrotic fibers with accumulation of glycogen. Withdrawal of the drug led to a rapid recovery. Myositis has been reported in a patient on tretinoin therapy for acute promyelocytic leukemia (Miranda et al 1994). a muscle biopsy specimen showed focal necrosis of the muscle fibers, infiltration with inflammatory cells of the endomysium and the perimysium without changes in the skin, vasculitis, or leukemic involvement. the patient improved after discontinuation of tretinoin.

Tranilast

This is an antiasthmatic agent used in Japan and eosinophilic polymyositis following its administration has been reported by Arase et al (1990).

There was eosinophilia and elevation of serum CK. Muscle biopsy showed infiltration with eosinophils and lymphocytes. The patient recovered but the reaction recurred after rechallenge with tranilast. This may have been a hypersensitivity reaction.

Vincristine

This antineoplastic agent is known to produce peripheral neuropathy (see Chapter 11) but proximal myopathy occurs in some patients (Bradley et al 1970). Electronmicroscopic studies have shown that the drug has an effect on the membrane systems leading to the formation of complex spheromembranous bodies thought to be derived from the sarcoplasmic reticulum and autophagous degeneration of muscle fibers.

Zidovudine (Azothymidine, AZT)

This is a dideoxynucleoside analog of thymidine used in the treatment of AIDS patients. It acts by interfering with viral reverse transcriptase, thereby inhibiting HIV replication. Panegyres et al (1990) described a myopathy with vesicular changes in AIDS patients on AZT therapy. The muscle symptoms resolved on discontinuation of the drug and repeat muscle biopsy in one of the patients showed no abnormality. Mhiri et al (1991) identified this myopathy to be a result of AZT-induced mitochondrial dysfunction in AIDS patients.

Characteristic Features. Chalmers et al (1991) described the characteristics of AZT-induced myopathy as follows:
- There is progressive proximal muscle weakness.
- There is exercise-exacerbated myalgia in thighs and calves.
- It occurs only in AIDS patients.
- Usually occurs in patients on full dose of AZT for more than 9 months.
- Elevated CK.
- EMG showing fibrillations and positive waves in proximal muscles. Changes consistent with myopathy.

- The histological appearance of muscle biopsies at light microscopic level is that of a necrotizing myopathy with vacuolar degenerating fibers corresponding to mitochondrial alterations and ultrastructural level.
- Improvement in myalgia and muscle strength within 6–12 months after cessation of AZT therapy.

Clinical and biochemical evidence of myopathy was seen in 17% of the AIDS patients who had been receiving zidovudine for more than 260 days and in none of those on short-term therapy (Peters et al 1993). Serum creatine kinase levels rose before the onset of clinical signs and returned to normal within 4 weeks of cessation of therapy. Ultrastructural abnormalities also improved after discontinuation of the drug.

Histopathology. Numerous "ragged red fibers" (also called AZT fibers), indicative of abnormal mitochondria were found in the biopsy specimens from zidovudine-treated patients (Dalakas et al 1990) and are considered to be unique to AZT-induced myopathy (Pezeshkpour et al 1991). These mitochondrial abnormalities consist of sarcolemmal or central accumulation of red granular material and longitudinal or circumferential "red rimmed cracks" as well as increased neutral fat that is attributed to impaired mitochondrial control of fatty acid use. It is possible to distinguish AZT-induced myopathy from the inflammatory myopathy of AIDS (Chen et al 1992). It is not certain if AZT can induce myopathy in humans in the absence of AIDS. AZT injected into thigh muscles of hamsters produces a mitochondrial myopathy but it differs from the AZT myopathy in that there are no ragged red fibers or ultrastructural changes in the mitochondria (Reyes et al 1992). Lamperth et al (1991) found that normal human myocytes in culture, following 19 days of exposure to AZT, exhibited abnormal mitochondria characterized by proliferation, enlargement, abnormal cristae, and electron-dense deposits in matrix.

Pathomechanism. Arnaudo et al (1991) found that, in AZT-induced myopathy, mitochondrial DNA was reduced by as much as 78% in muscle biopsy specimens. This was reversible with discontinuation of the drug and was considered to be due to zidovudine-induced inhibition of mitochondrial DNA replication by DNA polymerase γ T. Although an individual predisposition to AZT-induced myopathy cannot be excluded, long duration of treatment with AZT is a significant factor (Spadaro et al 1993). AZT myopathy is part of a wider disorder affecting cellular function in other tissues as well (Peters et al 1993).

AZT is now recognized to be a unique muscle mitochondrial toxin, causing depletion of muscle mtDNA, which result in myopathy. Some myopathies of childhood are also characterized by depletion of mtDNA (Moraes et al 1991) and AZT may serve as a model toxin for the study of molecular events in some mitochondrial encephalomyopathies.

Management. Biopsy proven zidovudine myopathy have also been reported to remain stable up to 6 months without dosage reduction or discontinuation of AZT (Cupler et al 1994). Muscle biopsy in patients with AIDS who had zidovudine-induced myopathy have been found to have a reduction in muscle carnitine levels (Dalakas et al 1994). L-carnitine used concurrently with AZT in patients with AIDS has been shown to rescue the myotubules and their mitochondria from the AZT-associated destruction and lipid storage (Semino-Mora et al 1994). This finding may have therapeutic implications.

Prevention of Drug-Induced Myopathy

The following measures are suggested for preventing drug-induced myopathy:
- Monitoring of patients receiving drugs known to produce myopathy for earlier detection and discontinuation of medication.
- Avoidance of known risk factors such as alcohol consumption.
- Avoidance of depolarizing muscle relaxants such as suxamethonium during general anesthesia in patients susceptible to myotonia. These should be substituted by non-depolarizing relaxants. Some of the non-depolarizing neuromuscular blocking agents such as doxacurium chloride and steroid-based and if

combined with high dose steroids, can also lead to myopathy (Marik 1996).
- Overdosage of suspected drugs should be avoided.
- Avoidance of combination of simultaneous use of two drugs known to cause myopathy. Combination of colchicine with cyclosporin in renal transplant patients increases the risk of development of myopathy (Tapal 1996; Jagose and Bailey 1997; Ducloux et al 1997).
- Avoidance of the use of combination of neuromuscular blocking agents with corticosteroids as this increases the risk of myopathy (Fischer and Baer 1996).
- Identification of patients with genetic susceptibility to adverse effects of certain drugs might help to avoid the use of drugs which are prone to induce myopathy in such patients. Further advances in pharmacogenetics should enable this.

Rhabdomyolysis

Rhabdomyolysis or acute muscle necrosis is the most serious form of toxic myopathy encountered in clinical practice. The condition is characterized by widespread muscle pain, weakness and dark urine. Myoglobinuria is an early feature and may lead to the following complications:
- Hyperuricemia
- Rapidly rising serum creatinine
- Metabolic acidosis
- Disseminated intravascular coagulation
- Acute renal failure
- Electrolyte disturbances: K, Ca, and Mg.
- Cardiomyopathy
- Respiratory failure
- Compartment syndromes due to swelling of muscles of extremities.

Death may result from acute metabolic disturbances but the prognosis of renal, muscular, and neurologic dysfunction is good (Koppel 1989).

Causes. The main causes of rhabdomyolysis are shown in Table 13.8.

Drugs Reported to Induce Rhabdomyolysis. Drugs including alcohol have been implicated in up to 81% of the cases in published reports (Ga-

Table 13.8. Causes of rhabdomyolysis (modified from Chichmanian et al 1991).

Traumatic and physical causes
  – crush injuries
  – excessive muscular exercise
  – convulsive crises
  – hyperthermia
Toxic causes
  – drugs
  – alcohol
Hereditary myopathies
  – congenital myopathy
  – muscular dystrophy
  – metabolic myopathy
Infections
  – viral
  – bacterial
Metabolic and electrolyte disturbances
  – metabolic acidosis
  – hypokalemia
  – hyponatremia
  – hypomagnesemia
Immunologic disorders: polymyositis
Genetic: carnitine palmitoyltransferase II deficiency

bow et al 1982). Several drugs have been reported to induce rhabdomyolysis but the causal relation has not been established in all of them. Drugs which have been reported to induce rhabdomyolysis are listed in Table 13.9.

Pathomechanism of Drug-Induced Rhabdomyolysis. Drugs may have a direct toxic effect on the myocytes. The suggested mechanisms include the following (Haller and Knochel 1984):
– Inhibition of calcium metabolism by sarcoplasmic reticulum.
– Disruption of muscle cell membrane.
– Inhibition of Na-K ATPase and alterations in carbohydrate metabolism.

Several drugs can cause muscle damage by inducing hypokalemia. These include thiazide diuretics, chlorthalidone, amphotericin B, laxatives, carbenoxolone and licorice (Mastaglia 1982). Rhabdomylolysis occurring with hypokalemia is usually associated with potassium levels 2 mmol/L or less. Hyponatremia has been asso-

Table 13.9. Drugs reported to induce rhabdomyolysis.

Alcohol	Interferon-α (Greenfield et al 1994; Reinhold et al 1997)
Amiodarone (Itoh et al 1998)	Interleukin-2 (Anderlini et al 1995)
Aminocaproic acid	Isoniazid (Wattel et al 1978)
Amoxapine (Jennigs et al 1983)	Licorice
Amphetamines (Gabow et al 1982)	Lithium (Unger et al 1982)
Amphotericin (Gabow et al 1982)	Neuroleptics (Jermain and Crismon 1992)
Antineoplastics	Opioids (Nicolls et al 1982; Gibbs and Shaw 1985)
– Cytarabine (Margolis et al 1987)	Pentamidine (Sensakovic et al 1985)
– Cyclophosphamide (Tabata et al 1996)	Phencyclidine (Cogan et al 1978)
Anesthetics*	Phenylpropanolamine (Blewitt and Siegel 1983)
Barbiturates (Penn et al 1972)	Phenmetrazine (Black and Murphy 1984)
Carbenoxolone (Gabow et al 1982)	Phenothiazines
Chlorpromazine (Lazarus and Toglia 1985)	Pindolol (Aihara et al 1990)
Cholesterol-lowering agents*	Retinoids: acitretin (Lister et al 1996)
– Benzafibrate (Kantrowicz et al 1992)	Rohypnol (Briner et al 1986)
– Pravastatin (Hino et al 1996)	Salicylates (Leventhal et al 1989; Nawata et al 1994)
– Lovastatin (Tobart et al 1988; Wallace and Mueller 1992)	Sodium valproate
– Simvastatin (Van Puijenbroek et al 1996)	Streptomycin (Nakahara et al 1992b)
Cimetidine	Streptokinase
Cocaine (Flaque-Coma 1990)	Succinylcholine
Colchicine (Dawson and Starkebaum 1997)	Suxamethonium (Book et al 1994)
Corticosteroids (De Smet et al 1991)	Tacrolismus (Hibi et al 1995)
Cotrimoxazol	Terbutaline
Cyclosporine	Theophylline
Diazepam (Briner et al 1986; Fernandez-Real et al 1994)	Tricyclic antidepressants
Diuretics* (Shintani et al 1991)	Vasopressin (de Cuenca Moron et al 1993;
Fenoverine (Chariot et al 1995)	Moreno-Sanchez et al 1991; Pierce and Nickl 1993)
Furosemide (Brucato et al 1993)	
Glutethimide (Penn et al 1972)	

*Well documented (see text). The rest of the list is based on isolated case reports.

ciated with rhabdomyolysis in acute water intoxication. Drugs which produce hyponatremia. One case of raised creatine kinase level due to a non-thiazide antihypertensive agent indapamide-induced hyponatremia has been reported by Read et al (1994). Two cases of rhabdomyolysis due to hyponatremia possibly due to benzodiazepine use were reported by Fernandez-Real et al (1994). Hyponatremia and depression of membrane potential induced by benzodiazepines could have had a synergistic effect in disrupting the cell membrane in these cases.

Drugs which induce involuntary muscle contractions or hypokalemia contribute to development of rhabdomyolysis. Two drug-induced conditions, malignant hyperthermia and neuroleptic malignant syndrome are associated with rhabdomyolysis.

Malignant Hyperthermia

In humans genetically predisposed to malignant hyperthermia (MH), anesthetics can induce muscular rigidity, hypermetabolism and fever. MH occurs in 1 out of 20,000 anesthetized adults. Various inhalation anesthetic agents and depolarizing muscle-relaxing agents have been implicated. MH has also been reported to be caused by intravenous lidocaine used for ventricular arrhythmias (Tatsukawa et al 1992).

Pathophysiology. The pathomechanism of MH is not well understood but the following explanations have been offered:
- Some abnormalities in the regulation of intracellular concentration of calcium in the skeletal muscles are considered to contribute to the pathophysiology of this syndrome (Endo et al 1983).
- There is evidence that free radicals are involved in the pathogenesis of MH (Duthie and Arthur 1993).
- The basic defect is an autosomal dominantly inherited dysregulation of intracellular calcium and the gene has been located on the long arm of chromosome 19. In pigs the susceptibility to MH is caused by a single mutation in the ryanodine receptor (RYR) in skeletal muscle but the human genetics is more complex

and currently known mutations in human RYR account for no more than 20% of the susceptible families.
- Exercise, alcohol, anesthetics and drugs may trigger rhabdomyolysis in patients with genetic susceptibility to MH (Denborough 1998). Heytens et al (1991) reported a child with susceptibility to MH who developed extensive rhabdomyolysis with cardiac arrest during anesthesia. If untreated these patients may die within minutes of ventricular fibrillation, within hours from pulmonary edema or coagulopathy, or within days from neurological damage or renal failure (MacLennan and Phillips 1992).

Myopathy and MH. Three clinical myopathies that predispose to MH have been defined (Denborough 1998).
- *Evan's myopathy*. It is named after the first family in which it was discovered and is the most common type also referred to referred to as MH myopathy. It is usually subclinical but some muscle wasting may occur. Serum CK may be raised but is usually normal. Structural changes in the muscle are non-specific.
- *King-Denborough syndrome*. This was identified in Australia in 1970 and is rare. It is inherited as a recessive trait and is usually found in boys.
- *Central core disease*. Association between this and MH has been recognized since 1973. All members of the family in which central core disease is diagnosed should be considered susceptible to MH unless proven otherwise.

Clinical Presentation. The commonest clinical presentation is a hypermetabolic state characterized by fever on exposure to general anesthetics. Rhabdomyolysis with its complications is an important feature oft he syndrome. It may also present as a myopathy or a a form of neuroleptic malignant syndrome with genetic susceptibility.

Management. Dantrolene sodium, a hydantoin derivative has been found to be effective for the treatment of MH (Britt 1987; Blank and Boggs 1993) and has lowered the mortality from this condition considerably. This drug relaxes the skeletal muscle by inhibiting the release of calcium from sarcoplasmic reticulum.

Prevention. Detection of individuals susceptible to MH is important for prevention. New genetic tests should be helpful (Ellis 1992). Caffein-halothane contracture test used currently needs to be standardized (Larach et al 1992). Treves et al (1994) have shown that the presence of arginine-to-cystine point mutation in the recombinant ryanodine receptor expressed in COS-7 transfected cells causes abnormal transient release of cytosolic Ca^{2+} in response to 4-chloro-m-cresol, an agent capable of eliciting in vitro contracture of MH-susceptible muscles.

Neuroleptic Malignant Syndrome (NMS)

This syndrome is described in Chapter 23. Association of NMS with rhabdomyolysis has been reported by Kleinknecht et al (1982). Some of the risk factors such as immobilization, use of neuroleptics, and elderly psychiatric patients are common in both conditions and NMS should be considered in the differential diagnosis of rhabdomyolysis (O'Neill et al 1992).

Factors Contributing to Drug-Induced Rhabdomyolysis

Drug Overdose. In case of drug-overdose, the following factors contribute to rhabdomyolysis (Penn et al 1972):
- Seizures
- Muscle compression and/or occlusion of regional blood supply
- Metabolic acidosis
- Hypoxia
- Prolonged coma with immobilization

Psychiatric Patients. These patients are at risk for development of rhabdomyolysis for the following reasons (Jermain and Crismon 1992):
- Motor hyperactivity, catatonia or physical agitation. CK values can rise to 2–3 times normal values in acute psychotic states.
- Overdosage of psychotropic drugs.

- Physical restraints used to immobilize agitated patients.
- Seizures, hyponatremia, and dehydration are seen more commonly in psychiatric patients.
- Neuroleptic malignant syndrome as an adverse effect of neuroleptics is seen more commonly in psychiatric patients.

Anesthetics

Anesthetics may act as a trigger for the onset of rhabdomyolysis in patients with pre-existing occult causes. Acute rhabdomyolysis has been reported after halothane (Rubiano et al 1987). Tang et al (1992) reported anesthesia-induced rhabdomyolysis in infants with unsuspected Duchenne dystrophy. The authors recommended a dystrophin test in addition to CK determination for detection of this condition in patients undergoing anesthesia.

Diuretics

Hypokalemic myopathy with rhabdomyolysis has been reported during treatment with diuretics (Shintani et al 1991). In addition to hypokalemia, diuretics may also induce hypocalcemia and hypomagnesemia which lead to tetany and muscle spasms with further predisposition to rhabdomyolysis. A case of tetany and rhabdomyolysis has been reported with furosemide (Brucato et al 1993).

Cholesterol-Lowering Agents

Myopathy due to cholesterol-lowering agents has already been described earlier in this chapter. This adverse effect may proceed on to rhabdomyolysis which has been reported in association with lovastatin, simvastatin, clofibrate, benzafibrate and gemfibrozil. No case of rhabdomyolysis was observed in over 1800 patients treated with fluvastatin (Jokubaitis 1994). In 1995, the Committee on Safety of Medicines of UK, reported that the incidence of rhabdomyolysis with cholesterol-lowering agents is 1/100,000 treatment years. Clinical trials with atrovastatin, a new

HMG-CoA inhibitor, have shown that only 0.7% of the patients had confirmed serum transaminase levels higher than three times the normal values but none of them had conclusive characterization of drug-induced myopathy (Black et al 1998).

Lovastatin. Rhabdomyolysis is an uncommon adverse effect associated with lovastatin therapy alone. In most of the reported cases lovastatin was used in combination with other agents such as cholestyramine (Chrysanthopoulos and Kounis 1992), gemfibrozil (Pierce et al 1990; Kogan and Orenstein 1990), and cyclosporine (Norman et al 1988). However, Wallace and Mueller (1992) have reported a case of lovastatin-induced rhabdomyolysis in the absence of other medications known to potentiate this adverse effect. Tobart (1988) reported 17 cases (0.04%) of lovastatin-associated rhabdomyolysis out of 4000 patients participating in several clinical trials with this drug. Some of these patients were receiving concomitant drugs. The relative risk of developing rhabdomyolysis was calculated to be 0.15% for patients receiving no concomitant therapy and 5% for those receiving lovastatin and gemfibrozil. In another study the incidence of rhabdomyolysis was found to be 0.1% in a population receiving a dose of 40 mg lovastatin daily whereas it was 0.2% in those receiving a dose of 80 mg daily (Bradford et al 1991).

Simvastatin. The action of this drug is similar to that of lovastatin as an inhibitor of HMG-CoA reductase and a case is reported where its use was followed by MELAS (mitochondrial myopathy, encephalopathy, lactic acidosis, and stroke-like episodes) syndrome (Chariot et al 1993). This patient developed rhabdomyolysis and low muscle concentration of enzyme CoQ10. After drug withdrawal and CoQ10 therapy, myopathy improved and muscle CoQ10 concentration returned to normal. These findings are consistent with the hypothesis that simvastatin complications are due to mitochondrial dysfunction through CoQ10 deficiency (Folkers et al 1990).

Rhabdomyolysis caused by simvastatin is increased by concomitant therapy with drugs such as cyclosporin that interfere with pharmacokinetics of HMG-CoA reductase inhibitor (Blaison et al 1992).

The risk of rhabdomyolysis is increased with pravastatin-fenofibrate combination and it is recommended that these two drugs should not be combined (Raimondeau et al 1992).

Pathomechanism Rhabdomyolysis Associated with Cholesterol-Lowering Agents. The pathomechanism of myopathic changes is poorly understood but various mechanisms have been considered under the section of myopathy. Mechanisms relevant to rhabdomyolysis are:

- The mechanism of lovastatin-induced rhabdomyolysis is not well understood but it is speculated that this may be due to inadequate synthesis of CoQ and heme A in the inner mitochondrial membrane with subsequent derangement of cellular energy production and cell death (Manoukian et al 1990). Statin therapy can be associated with high blood lactate/pyruvate ratio suggestive of mitochondrial dysfunction (De-Pinieux et al 1996).
- Benzafibrate and fibric acid derivatives related to clofibrate have been reported to induce rhabdomyolysis (Kanterwiecz et al 1992). The pathomechanism is not clear. Direct muscle toxicity has been suggested to be related to chlorine molecule present in all fibric acid derivatives with the exception of gemfibrozil (Haubenstock et al 1984).
- Depletion of metabolites of geranylgeranyl pyrophosphate, and not inhibition of cholesterol synthesis, is considered to be the primary cause of HMG CoA reductase-induced myotoxicity (Flint et al 1997).

Cyclosporine

Rhabdomyolysis has been reported in 7 transplant patients treated with cyclosporine as an interaction with comedications such as lovastatin which are known to produce rhabdomyolysis (Arellano and Krupp 1991). Rhadomyolysis caused by cyclosporine alone was reported in one case (Grezard et al 1990) and another such case was observed during postmarketing surveillance of 3017 patients for one year, indicating an incidence rate of less than 0.05%. Caution should be exercised if cyclosporine is used concomitantly with a drug known to induce rhabdomyolysis.

Alejandro and Petersen (1994) reported one case of acute renal failure in a cardiac transplant patient taking lovastatin and cyclosporine and reviewed four similar cases from the literature. Rhabdomyolysis with combined lovastatin and cyclosporin appears to be dose-related interaction during these episodes associated with impaired hepatic metabolism associated with lovastatin intake. These authors have recommended the following guidelines for transplant patients taking lovastatin and cyclosporine:

- Maintain lovastatin dose at 20 to 40 mg/day
- Advise patients to report any muscle symptoms as soon as possible
- Monitor blood levels of creatine kinase, cyclosporine, and liver function tests when either drug is started or increased.
- Withdraw or decrease dose of lovastatin if there is an elevated CK even if the patient is asymptomatic.
- Avoid combination therapy with other antilipidemic drugs such gemfibrozil, niacin, and clofibrate.

Management of Drug-Induced Rhabdomyolysis

Guidelines recommended for the management of rhabdomyolysis are shown in Table 13.10.

Table 13.10. Guidelines recommended for management of rhabdomyolysis.

Early detection
- routine estimation of serum CK and urinary myoglobin
- detection of localized areas of myonecrosis by CT scan
Fluid replacement
Bicarbonate infusion
- to alkalinize urine and to prevent dissociation of myoglobin to its nephrotoxic metabolite ferrihemate
Promotion of diuresis: mannitol
- to dilute nephrotoxic substances
- to flush through blocked renal tubules
Treatment of complications of rhabdomyolysis
- hyperphosphatemia: oral phosphate-binding antacids
- hyperkalemia: usually corrects itself
- renal failure: dialysis
- disseminated intravascular coagulation: heparin useless
- compartment syndromes: decompressive fasciotomy
- seizures: anticonvulsants
- hyperthermia: cooling

References

Aberfeld DC, Bienestock H, Shapiro MS, et al: Diffuse myopathy related to meperidine addiction in a mother and daughter. Arch Neurol 1968; 19: 384–388.

Adams EM, Horowitz HW, Sundstrom WR: Fibrous myopathy in association with pentazocine. Arch Int Med 1983; 143: 2203–2204.

Aguayo AJ, Hudgson P: Observations on the short-term effects of chloroquine on skeletal muscle. J Neurol Sci 1970; 11: 301–325.

Aihara M, Takahashi R, Ohtake T, et al: Pindolol-induced rhabdomyolysis in sarcoid myopathy. Rinsho Shinkei-gaku 1990; 30: 103–106.

Alejandro DSJ, Petersen J: Myoglobinuric acute renal failure in a cardiac transplant patient taking lovastatin and cyclosporine. J Am Soc Nephrology 1994; 5: 153–160.

Anderlini P, Buzaid AC, Legha SS, et al: Acute rhabdomyolysis after concurrent administration of interleukin-2, interferon-α and chemotherapy for metastatic melanoma. Cancer 1995; 76: 678–679.

Arai H, Tanaka M, Ohta K, et al: Symptomatic myopathy associated with interferon therapy for chronic hepatitis C. Lancet 1995; 345: 582.

Arase S, Kato S, Nakanishi H, et al: Eosinophilic polymyositis induced by tranilast. J Dermatology 1990; 17: 182–186.

Arellano F, Krupp P: Muscular disorders associated with cyclosporin (letter). Lancet 1991; 337: 915.

Arnadottir M, Eriksson LO, Germershausen JI, et al: Low dose simvastatin is a well tolerated and efficacious cholesterol-lowering agent in ciclosporin-treated kidney transplant recipients: double-blind, randomized, placebo-controlled study in 40 patients. Nephron 1994; 68: 57–62.

Arnaudo E, Dalakas M, Shanske S, et al: Depletion of muscle mitochondrial DNA in AIDS patients with zidovudine-induced myopathy. Lancet 1991; 337: 508–510.

Askari A, Vignos PJ, Moskowitz RW: Steroid myopathy in connective tissue disease. Am J Med 1976; 61: 485–492.

Avina-Zubieta JA, Johnson ES, Suarez-Almazor ME, et al: Incidence of myopathy in patients treated with antimalarials. A report of three cases and a review of the literature. Brit J Rheumatol 1995; 34: 166–170.

Aydintug AO, Cevera R, D'Cruz D, et al: Polymyositis complicating D-Penicillamine treatment. Postgrad Med J 1991; 67: 1018–1020.

Barclay CL, McLean M, Hagan N, et al: Severe phenytoin hypersensitivity with myopathy. Neurology 1992; 42: 2303.

Batchelor TT, Taylor LP, Thaler HT, et al: Steroid myopathy in cancer patients. 1997; 48: 1234–1238.

Bennett HS, Spiro AJ, Pollack MA, et al: Ipecac-induced myopathy simulating dermatomyositis. Neurology 1982; 32: 91–94.

Berger O, Zifko U, Jellinger K, et al: Nekrotisierende Myopathie bei Lipidsenkern. Nervenarzt 1993; 64: 539–544.

Black DM, Bakker Arkema RG, Nawrocki JW: An overview of the clinical safety profile of atorvastatin (lipitor), a new HMG-CoA reductase inhibitor. Arch Intern Med 1998; 158: 577–584.

Black WD, Murphy WM: Non-traumatic rhabdomyolysis and acute renal failure associated with oral phenmetrazine hydrochloride. J Tenn Med Assoc 1984; 77: 80–81.

Blaison G, Weber JC, Sachs D, et al: Rhabdomyolysis caused by simvastatin in a patient following heart transplantation and cyclosporine therapy. Rev Med Interne(Paris) 1992; 13: 61–63.

Blank LW, Boggs SD: Successful treatment of an episode of malignant hyperthermia using a large dose of dantrolene. J Clin Anesth 1993; 5: 69–72.

Blewitt GA, Siegel EB: Renal failure, rhabdomyolysis, and phenylpropanolamine. JAMA 1983; 249: 3017–3018.

Bonnet C, Zabraniecki L, Bertin P, et al: Amiodarone-induced neuromyopathy mimicking polymyositis. Rev Rheum 1995; 62: 468.

Book WJ, Abel M, Eisenkraft JB: Adverse effects of depolarizing neuromuscular blocking agents. Drug Safety 1994; 10: 331–349.

Bradford RH, Shear CL, Chremos AN, et al: Expanded clinical evaluation of lovastatin (EXCEL) study results. I. Efficacy in modifying plasma proteins and adverse event profile in 8245 patients with moderate hypercholesterolemia. Arch Int Med 1991; 151: 43–49.

Bradley WG: The neuromyopathy of vincristine in the guinea pig. an electrophysiological and pathological study. J Neurol Sci 1970; 10: 133–162.

Briner VA, Colombi a, Brunner W, et al: Die akute Rhabdomyolyse. Schweiz Med Wochenschr 1986; 116: 198–208.

Britt B: Dantrolene—an update. In Britt B (Ed.): Malignant hyperthermia, Boston, Martinus Nijhoff Publishing, 1987, pp 326–367.

Britt CW, Light RR, Peters BH, et al: Rhabdomyolysis during treatment with epsilon-aminocaproic acid. Arch Neurol 1980; 37: 187–188.

Brucato A, Bonati M, Gaspari F, et al: Tetany and rhabdomyolysis due to surreptitious furosemide— importance of magnesium supplementation. Clin Toxicol 1993; 31: 341–344.

Caldron PH, Wilbourn AJ, Bravo EE: Gold myokymia syndrome. A rare toxic manifestation of chrysotherapy. Cleve Clin J Med 1987; 54: 225–228.

Cayley FEW: Potassium deficiency in p-amino-salicylic acid therapy. Cardiac and paralytic effects. Lancet 1950; 1: 447–448.

Carroll GJ, Will RK, Peter JB, et al: Penicillamine-induced polymyositis and dermatomyositis. J Rheumatol 1987; 14: 995–1001.

Chalmers AG, Greco CM, Miller RG: Prognosis in AZT myopathy. Neurology 1991; 41: 1181–1184.

Chappel R, Willems J: D-Penicillamine-induced myositis in rheumatoid arthritis. Clinical Rheumatology 1996; 15: 86–87.

Chariot P, Abadia R, Danan C, et al: Simvastatin-induced rhabdomyolysis followed by a MELAS syndrome. Am J Med 1993; 94: 109–110.

Chariot P, Ratiney R, Le Maguet F, et al: Fenoverine-induced rhabdomyolysis. Human and Experimental Toxicology 1995; : 14: 654–656.

Chen SC, Barker SM, Mitchell DH, et al: Concurrent zidovudine-induced myopathy and hepatotoxicity in patients treated for human immunodeficiency virus (HIV) infection. Pathology 1992; 24: 109–111.

Chichmanian RM, Mignot G, Spreux A: Rhabdomyolses mediamenteuses. Ann Med Interne (Paris) 1991; 142: 587–591.

Chow LTC, Chow W: Acute compartment syndrome: an unusual presentation of gemfibrozil-induced myositis. Med J Aust 1993; 158: 48–49.

Chrysanthopoulos C, Kounis N: Rhabdomyolysis due to combined treatment with lovastatin and cholestyramine. BMJ 1992; 304: 1225.

Chucrallah A, Girolami UD, Freeman R, et al: Lovastatin/gemfibrozil myopathy: A clinical, histochemical, and ultrastructural study. Eur Neurol 1992; 32: 293–296.

Clouston PD, Donnelly PE: Acute necrotizing myopathy associated with amiodarone therapy. BMJ 1984; 288: 1878.

Cogen FC, Rigg F, Simmons JL, et al: Phencyclidine-associated acute rhabdomyolysis. Ann Int Med 1978; 88: 210–212.

Cohen LJ: CPK Test—Effect of intramuscular injection in myocardial infarction. JAMA 1972; 219: 625–626.

Crayton H, Bohlmann T, Suft R, et al: Drug-induced polymyositis secondary to leuprolide acetate (Lupron) therapy for prostatic carcinoma. Clin Exp Rheumatol 1991; 9: 525–528.

Cupler EJ, Hench K, Jay CA, et al: The natural history of zidovudine-induced mitochondrial myopathy (abstract). Neurology 1994; 44(suppl 2): A132.

Curran JR, Jamieson TW: Dermatomyositis-like syndrome associated with phenylbutazolidine therapy. J Rheumatol 1987; 14: 397–398.

Dalakas MC, Leon-Monzon M, Bernardini I, et al: Zidovudine-induced mitochondrial myopathy is associated with muscle carnitine deficiency and lipid storage. Ann Neurol 1994; 35: 482–487.

Dalakas MC, Illa I, Pezeshkpour GH, et al: Mitochondrial myopathy caused by long-term zidovudine myopathy. NEJM 1990; 322: 1098–1105.

Danon MJ, Carpenter S: Myopathy with thick filament (myosin) loss following prolonged paralysis with vercuronium during steroid treatment. Muscle & Nerve 1991; 14: 1131–1139.

Dawson TM, Starkebaum G: Colchicine-induced rhabdomyolysis. Journal of Rheumatology 1997; 24: 2045–2046.

de Cuenca Moron, Canga F, Moreno D, et al: Necrosis cutanea y rabdomiolisis tras infusion intravenosa de vasopresina. Rev Clin Esp 1993; 192: 79–82.

De Smet Y, Jaminet M, Jaeger U, et al: Acute corticosteroid myopathy in patient with asthma. Rev Neurol (Paris) 1991; 147: 682–685.

Decramer M, Stas KJ: Corticosteroid-induced myopathy involving respiratory muscles in patients with chronic obstructive pulmonary disease or asthma. Am Rev Respir Dis 1992; 146: 800–802.

Dekhuijzen PNR, Decramer M: Steroid-induced myopathy and its significance to respiratory disease: a known disease rediscovered. Eur Respir J 1992; 5: 997–1003.

Denborough M: Malignant hyperthermia. Lancet 1998; 352: 1131–1136.

De-Pinieux G, Chariot P, Ammi-Said M, et al: Lipid-lowering drugs and mitochondrial function: effects of HMG-CoA reductase inhibitors on serum ubiquinone and blood lactate/pyruvate ratio. Br J Clin Pharmacol 1996; 42: 333–337.

Dippel E, Zouboulis CC, Tebbe B, et al: Myopathies associated with long-term interferon α treatment in 4 patients with skin disorders. Arch Dermatol 1998; 134: 880–881.

Dresser LP, Massey EW, Johson EE, et al: Ipecac myopathy and cardiomyopathy. JNNP 1993; 56: 560–562.

Dropcho EJ, Soong S: Steroid-induced weakness in patients with primary brain tumors. Neurology 1991; 41: 1235–1239.

Duane DD, Engel AG: Emetine myopathy. Neurology 1970; 20: 733–739.

Dubois EL: Triamcinolone in the treatment of systemic lupus erythematosus. JAMA 1958; 167: 1590.

Ducloux D, Schuller V, Bresson-Vautrin C, et al: Colchicine myopathy in renal transplant recipients on cyclosporin. Nephrol Dial Transplant 1997; 12: 2389–2392.

Dunenci J, Chodosh J, Segal MS: Dexamethasone therapy in bronchial asthma. Ann Allerg 1959; 17: 695.

Duthie GG, Arthur JR: Free radicals and calcium homeostasis: relevance to malignant hyperthermia? Free Rad Biol Med 1993; 14: 435–442.

Ellis F: Detecting susceptibility to malignant hyperthermia. BMJ 1992; 304: 791–792.

Endo M, Yagi S, Ishizuka T, et al: Changes in the calcium-induced Ca release mechanism in the sarcoplasmic reticulum of the muscle from a patient with malignant hyperthermia. Biomed Res 1983; 4: 83.

Estes ML, Ewing-Wilson D, Chou SM, et al: Chloroquine neuromyotoxicity. Am J Med 1987; 82: 447–455.

Fernandez-Real JM, Ricart-Engel W, Camafort-Babkowski M: Hyponatremia and benzodiazepines result in rhabdomyolysis. Ann Pharmacother 1994; 28: 1200–1201.

Fernandez-Sola J, Campistol J, Casademont J, et al: Reversible cyclosporin myopathy. Lancet 1990; 335: 362–363.

Fiallo P, Taglapietra AG: Severe acute myopathy induced by isoretinoin. Archives of Dermatology 1996; 132: 1521–1522.

Finger DR, Plotz PH, Heywood G: Myositis following treatment with high-dose interleukin-2 for malignancy. Journal of Rheumatology 1995; 22: 2188.

Fischer JR, Baer RK: Acute myopathy associated with combined use of corticosteroids and neuromuscular blocking agents. Ann Pharmacother 1996; 30): 1437–1445.

Flaque-Coma J: Cocaine and rhabdomyolysis: report of a case and review of literature. Bol Asoc Med PR 1990; 82: 423–424.

Flint OP, Masters BA, Gregg RE, et al: Inhibition of cholesterol synthesis by squalene synthase inhibitors does not induce myotoxicity in vitro. Toxicol Appl Pharmacol 1997; 145: 91–98.

Folkers K, Langsjoen P, Willis R, et al: Lovastatin decreases coenzyme Q levels in humans. Proc Natl Acad Sci U S A 1990; 87: 8931–4.

Fryberg RH, Bernstein CA, Helmlan L: Further experience with triamcinolone in treatment of patients with rheumatoid arthritis. Arthritis Rheum 1958; 1: 215.

Gabow PA, Kaehny WD, Kelleher SP: The spectrum of rhabdomyolysis. Medicine 1982; 61: 141–152.

Gibb WRG, Shaw IC: Myoglobinuria due to heroin abuse. J Roy Soc Med 1985; 78: 862–863.

Glueck C, Oakes N, Speirs J, et al: Gemfibrozil-lovastatin therapy for primary hyperlipoproteinemias. Am J Cardiol 1992; 70: 1–9.

Goy JJ, Stauffer JC, Deruaz JP, et al: Myopathy as possible side-effect of cyclosporin. Lancet 1989 Jun 24; 1(8652): 1446–7.

Greenfield SM, Harvey RS, Thompson RPH: Rhabdomyolysis after treatment with interferon α. BMJ 1994; 309: 512.

Grezard O, Lebranchu Y, Birneke, et al: Cyclosporin-induced muscular toxicity. Lancet 1990; 335: 177.

Griffin D, Fairman N, Coursin D, et al: Acute myopathy during treatment of status asthmaticus with corticosteroids and steroidal muscle relaxants. Chest 1992; 102: 510–514.

Gutmann L, Gutmann L: Critical illness neuropathy and myopathy. Arch Neurol 1999; 56: 527–528.

Haller RG, Knochel JP: skeletal muscle disease in alcoholism. Med Clin North Am 1984; 68: 91–103.

Harney J, Glasberg MR: Myopathy and hypersensitivity to phenytoin. Neurology 1983; 33: 790–791.

Hattori N, Shimatsu A, Murabo H, et al: Clofibrate-induced myopathy in a patient with primary hypothyroidism. Jpn J Med 1990; 29: 545–547.

Haubenstock A, Schrocksnadel W, Bauer K, et al: Predominance of lactic dehydrogenase isoenzyme in a patient with benzofibrate-induced rhabdomyolysis. Clin Chem 1984; 30: 1587–1588.

Heytens LG, Even B, Martin JJ, et al: Differential diaganosis of anesthesia induced rhabdomyolysis. A case report. Acta Neurol Belg 1991; 91: 303–307.

Hibi S, Misawa A, Tamai M, et al: Severe rhabdomyolysis associated with tacrolismus. Lancet 1995; 346: 702.

Higuchi I, Izumo S, Kuriyama M, et al: Germanium myopathy: clinical and experimental pathological studies. Acta Neuropathol 1989; 79: 300–304.

Himmelman E, Schröder JM: Colchicine myopathy in a case of familial mediterranean fever: immunohistochemical and ultrastructural study of accumulated tubulin-immunoreactive material. Acta Neuropathol 1992; 83: 440–444.

Hino I, Akama H, Furuya T, et al: Pravastatin-induced rhabdomyolysis in a patient with mixed connective tissue disease. Arthritis and Rheumatism 1996; 39: 1259–1260.

Hirano M, Ott BR, Raps EC, et al: Acute quadriplegic myopathy. Neurology 1992; 42: 2082–2087.

Hodak E, David M, Gadoth N, et al: Etiretinate-induced

skeletal muscle damage. Brit J Dermatol 1987; 116: 623–626.

Inoue M, Jimi T, Machida H, et al: Benzafibrate myopathy in two patients with chronic renal failure. Rinsho Shinkeigaku 1992; 32: 725–728.

Itoh KI, Kato R, Hotta N: A case report of myolysis during high-dose amiodarone therapy for uncontrolled ventricualr tachycardia. Japanese Circulation Journal 1998; 62: 305–308.

Jacobson TA, Chin MM, Fromell GJ, et al: Fluvastatin with and without niacin for hypercholesterolemia. Am J Cardiol 1994; 74: 149–154.

Jagose JT, Bailey RR: Muscle weakness due to colchicine in renal transplant recipients. New Zealand Medical Journal 1997; 110: 343.

Jennings AE, Levey AS, Harrington JT: Amoxapine-associated acute renal failure. Arch Int Med 1983; 143: 1525–1527.

Jensen K: Myopati under behandling med fibrater og lovastatin. Ugeskr Laeger 1991; 153: 862.

Jermain DM, Crismon ML: Psychotropic drug-related rhabdomyolysis. Ann Pharmcotherapy 1992; 26: 948–954.

Johnson KR, Hsueh WA, Glusman SM, et al: Fibrous myopathy. A rheumatic complication of drug abuse. Arthritis Rheum 1976; 19(5): 923–6.

Jokubaitis LA: Updated clinical safety experience with fluvastatin. Am J Cardiol 1994; 73: 18D–24D.

Jonsson J, Gelpi JR, Light JA, et al: Colchicine-induced myoneuropathy in a renal transplant patient. Transplantation 1992; 53: 1369–1371.

Kanterwiecz E, Sanmarti R, Riba J, et al: Benzofibrate induced rhabdomyolysis. Ann Rheum Dis 1992; 51: 536–538.

Karpati G: Denervation and disuse atrophy of skeletal muscles: involvement of endogenous glucocorticoid hormones? Trends Neurosci 1984; 7: 61–62.

Kim HA, Song YW: Polymyositis developing after prolonged injections of pentazocine. Journal of Rheumatology 1996; 23: 1644–1646.

Kinney MAO, Harrison BA: Propofol-induced myotonia in myotonic dystrophy. Anesthesia Analgesia 1996; 83: 665–666.

Kleinknecht D, Parent A, Blot P, et al: Rhabdomyolysis with acute renal failure and malignant neuroleptic syndrome. Ann Med Intern (Paris) 1982; 133: 549–552.

Kogan AD, Orenstein S: Lovastatin-induced acute rhabdomyolysis. Postgrad Med J 1990; 66: 294–296.

Koppel C: Clinical features, pathogenesis and management of drug-induced rhabdomyolysis. Med Toxicol Adverse Drug Exp 1989; 4: 108–126.

Kuncl RW, Duncan G, Watson D, et al: Colchicine myopathy and neuropathy. NEJM 1987; 316: 1562–1568.

Kwiencinski H: Myotonia induced by chemical agents. CRC Crit Rev Toxicol 1981; 8: 279–310.

Lamperth L, Dalakas MC, Dagani F, et al: Abnormal skeletal and cardiac muscle mitochondria induced by zidovudine (AZT) in human muscle *in vitro* and in an animal model. Lab Invest 1991; 65: 742–751.

Lane RJM, Mastaglia FL: Drug-induced myopathy in man. Lancet 1979; 2: 562–566.

Larach MG, Landis JR, Bunn JS, et al: Prediction of malignant hyperthermia susceptibility in low-risk subjects. Anesthsiology 1992; 76: 16–27.

Latronico N, Fenzi F, Recupero D, et al: Critical illness myopathy and neuropathy [see comments]. Lancet 1996; 347: 1579–1582.

Lazarus AL, Toglia JU: Fatal myoglobinuric renal failure in a patient with tardive dyskinesia. Neurology 1985; 35: 1055–1057.

Lee BI, Shin SJ, Yoon SN, et al: Acute myopathy induced by colchicine in a cyclosporin-treated renal transplant recipient: a case report and review of literature. Journal of Korean Medical Science 1997; 12: 160–161.

Leventhal LJ, Kuritsky L, Ginsberg R, et al: Salicylate-induced rhambdomyolysis. Am J Emerg Med 1989; 7: 409–410.

Litin SC, Anderson CF: Nicotinic acid-associated myopathy: a report of three cases. Am J Med 1989; 86: 481–483.

London SF, Gross KF, Ringel SP: Cholestrol-lowering agent myopathy (CLAM). Neurology 1991; 41: 1159–1160.

MacLennan DH, Phillips MS: Malignant hyperthermia. Science 1992; 256: 789–794.

Magarian GJ, Lucas LM, Colley C: Gemfibrozil-induced myopathy. Arch Int Med 1991; 151: 1873–1874.

Manoukian AA, Bhagwan NP, Hayashi T, et al: Rhabdomyolysis secondary to Lovastatin therapy. Clin Chem 1990; 36: 2145–2147.

Margolis D, Ross E, Miller KB: rhabdomyolysis associated with high-dose cytarabine. Cancer Treat Rep 1987; 71: 1325–1326.

Marik PE: Doxacurium-corticosteroid acute myopathy: another piece to the puzzle. Critical Care Medicine 1996; 24: 1266–1267.

Marolda M, Palma V, Camporeale M, et al: Steroid myopathy: clinical and immunological study of a case. Ital J Neurol Sci 1991; 12: 409–413.

Mastaglia FL: Adverse effects of drugs on muscles. Drugs 1982; 24: 304–321.

Mastaglia FL: Toxic myopathies. In Rowland LP, DiMauro S (Eds.): Handbook of clinical neurology, vol 18: Myopathies, Amsterdam, Elsevier Publishing Company, 1992, pp 595–622.

Mateer JE, Farrell BJ, Chou SSM, et al: Reversible ipecac myopathy. Arch Neurol 1985; 42: 188–190.

Mhiri C, Baudrimont M, Bonne G, et al: Zidovudine myopathy: a distinctive disorder associated with mitochondrial dysfunction. Ann Neurol 1991; 29: 606–614.

Miranda N, Oliveira P, Frade MJ, et al: Myosits with tretinoin (letter). Lancet 1994; 344: 1096.

Moraes CT, Shanske S, Tritschler HJ, et al: mtDNA depletion with variable tissue expression: a novel genetic abnormality in mitochondrial disease. Am J Hum Genet 1991; 48: 492–501.

Moreno-Sanchez D, Casis B, Martin A, et al: Rhabdomyolysis and cutaneous necrosis following intravenous vasopressin infusion. Gastroenterology 1991; 101: 529–532.

Muller R, Kugelberg E: Myopathy in Cushing's syndrome. JNNP 1959; 27: 314.

Nakahara K, Kuriyama M, Yoshidome H, et al: Experimental simvastatin-induced myopathy in rabbits. J Neurol Sci 1992a; 113: 114–117.

Nakahara Y, Katoh S, Yamada H, et al: A successfully treated case of acute renal failure due to acute immune hemolytic anemia and non-traumatic rhabdomyolysis induced by streptomycin reinjection. Nippon Jinzo Gakkai Shi 1992b; 34: 1233–1236.

Nawata Y, Kagami M, Matsumara R, et al: Chronic salicylate intoxication and rhabdomyolysis in a patient with scleroderma and Sjögren's syndrome. J Rheumatol 1994; 21: 357–359.

Nicolls K, Niall JF, Moran JE: Rhabdomyolysis and renal failure. Complications of narcotic abuse. Med J Austral 1982; 2: 387–389.

Noppen M, Velkeniers B, Dierckx R, et al: Cyclosporin and myopathy. Ann Int Med 1987; 107: 945–946.

Norman H, Illingsworth D, Munson J, et al: Myolysis and acute renal failure in a heart transplant recipient receiving Lovastatin. NEJM 1988; 318: 46–47.

Older SA, Finbloom DS, Pezeshkpour GH: Colchicine myoneuropathy and renal dysfunction. Ann Rheum Dis 1992; 51: 1343–1344.

O'Neill D: Rhabdomyolysis and the neuroleptic malignant syndrome. JAGS 1992; 40: 1288–1289.

Page SR, Nussey SS: Myositis in association with carbimazole. Lancet 1989; 1: 964.

Panegyres PK, Papadimitriou JM, Hollingsworth PN, et al: Vesicular changes in the myopathies of AIDS. Ultrastructural observations and their relationship to zidovudine treatment. JNNP 1990; 53: 649–655.

Panegyres PK, Squier M, Mills KR, et al: Acute myopathy associated with large parenteral dose of corticosteroids in myasthenia gravis. JNNP 1993; 56: 702–704.

Penn AS, Rowland LP, Fraser DW: Drugs, coma, and myoglobinuria. Arch Neurol 1972; 26: 336–344.

Peppers MP: Myalgia and arthralgia associated with enalapril and ramipril. Am J Health System Pharmacy 1995; 52: 203–204.

Peters BS, Winer J, Landon DN, et al: Mitochondrial myopathy associated with chronic zidovudine therapy in AIDS. QJ Med 1993; 86: 5–15.

Pezeshkpour G, Illa I, Dalakas M: Ultrastructural characteristics and DNA immunocytochemistry in human immunodeficiency virus and zidovudine-associated myopathies. Hum Pathol 1991; 22: 1281–1288.

Pierce LR, Wysowski DK, Gross TP: Myopathy and rhabdomyolysis associated with lovastatin-gemfibrozil combination therapy. JAMA 1990; 264: 71–75.

Pierce ST, Nickl N: Rhabdomyolysis associated with use the of intravenous vasopressin. Am J Gastroenterol 1993; 88: 424–427.

Prendergast BD, George CF: Drug-induced rhabdomyolysis—mechanisms and management. Postgrad Med J 1993; 69: 333–336.

Pritchard JB: Toxic substances and cell membrane function. Fed Proc 1979; 38: 2220–2225.

Raimondeau J, Le Marec HL, Chevallier JC, et al: Myolyse biologique survenue à l'occasion d'un relais thérapeutique fénofibrate-pravastatine. La Presse Medicale 1992; 21: 663–664.

Read SJ, Trenerry HM, Whiting GF: Hyponatremia and raised creatine kinase level associated with indapamide: Hyponatremia and raised creatine kinase level associated with indapamide. Med J Australia 1994; 161: 607–608.

Reinhold U, Hart C, Hering R, et al: Fatal rhabdomyolysis and multiple organ failure associated with adjuvant high-dose interferon α in malignant melanoma. Lancet 1997; 349: 540–541.

Restrepo JF, Guzman R, Pena MA, et al: Fibrous myopathy induced by propoxiphene injection. J Rheumatol 1993; 20: 596–597.

Reyes MG, Casanova J, Varricchio F, et al: Zidovudine myopathy. Neurology 1992; 42: 1252.

Rieger EH, Halasz NA, Wahstrom HE: Colchicine neuromyopathy after renal transplantation. Transplantation 1990; 49: 1196–1198.

Riggs JE, Schochet SS, Gutmann L, et al: Chronic human colchicine neuropathy and myopathy. Arch Neurol 1986; 43: 521–523.

Rose SJ, Stokes TC, Patel S, et al: Carnitine deficiency associated with long-term pivampicillin treatment: effect of a replacement therapy regime. Postgrad Med J 1992; 68: 932–934.

Roth RF, Itabashi H, Louie J, et al: Amiodarone toxicity: myopathy and neuropathy. Am Heart J 1990; 119: 1223–1225.

Rubiano R, Chang JL, Carroll J, et al: Acute rhabdomyolysis following halothane anesthesia without succinylcholine. Anesthesiology 1987; 67: 856–857.

Sarrot-Reynauld F, Charras-De Matteis H, Massot C: Neuromyositis related to taking of omeprazole. Rev Med Int 1996; 17(suppl 3): 514.

Sauvaget F, Piette JC, Herson S, et al: Fenofibrate induced polymyositis. Rev Med Interne (Paris) 1991; 12: 52–54.

Scelsa SN, Simpson DM, McQuiston HL, et al: Clozapine-induced myotoxicity in patients with chronic psychotic disorders. Neurology 1996; 46: 1518–1523.

Schalke B, Schmidt B, Toyka K, et al: Pravastatin-associated inflammatory myopathy. NEJM 1992; 327: 649–650.

Schiff D, Drislane FW: Rapid-onset colchicine myoneuropathy. Arthr Rheum 1992; 35: 1535–1536.

Semino-Mora MC, Leon-Monzon M, Dalakas MC: L-carnitine prevents destructive effect of zidovudine on human muscle mitochondria and myotubules in culture (abstract). Neurology 1994; 44(suppl 2): A132.

Sensakovic JW, Suarez M, Perez J, et al: Pentamidine treatment of pneumocystis carinii pneumonia in the acquired immune deficiency syndrome. Association with acute renal failure and myoglobinuria. Arch Int Med 1985; 145: 2247.

Shee CD: Risk factors for the hydrocortisone myopathy in acute severe asthma. Respir Med 1990; 84: 510–511.

Shergy WG, Caldwell DS: Polymyositis after propylthiouracil treatment for hyperthyroidism. Ann Rheum Dis 1988; 47: 340–347.

Shintani S, Murase H, Tsugagoshi H, et al: Glycyrrhizin (licorice)-induced hypokalemic myopathy. Eur Neurol 1992; 32: 44–51.

Shintani S, Shiiga T, Tsukagoshi H: Marked hypokalemic rhabdomyolysis with myoglobinuria due to diuretic treatment. Eur Neurol 1991; 31: 396–398.

Sholl JS, Hughley MJ, Hirschmann RA: Myotonic muscular dystrophy associated with ritodrine tocolysis. Am J Obstet Gynecol 1985; 151: 83–86.

Sinsawaiwong S, Phanthumchinda K, Jogpiputvanich S, et al: Colchicine-induced myopathy in renal failure. J Med Assoc Thailand 1997; 80: 667–670.

Sitwell LD, Weinshenker BG, Monpetit V, et al: Complete ophthalmoplegia as complication of acute corticosteroid- and pancuronium-associated myopathy. Neurology 1991; 41: 921–922.

Smith PF, Eydelloth RS, Grossman SJ, et al: HMG-CoA reductase inhibitor-induced myopathy in the rat: cyclosporine A interaction and mechanism studies. J Pharmacol Exp Ther 1991; 257: 1225–35.

Solis RA, Pomales SY, Torres EA: Polymyositis induced by interferon α-2b in a patient with chronic hepatitis C. Am J Gastroenterol 1996; 91: 2041.

Spadaro M, Tilia G, Massara MC, et al: Myopathy in long-term AZT therapy: clinical, electrophysiological and biopsy studies in 67 HIV+ subjects. Ital J Neurosci 1993; 14: 369–374.

Steer JH, Mastaglia FL: Protein degradation in bupvacaine-treated muscles. The role of extracellular calcium. J Neurol Sci 1986; 75: 343–351.

Stoltenburg-Didinger G, Neuhaus GA: Toxische Ursachen von Muskelschmerzen. Internist 1987; 28: 596–605.

Tabata N, Tanaka R, Suga S, et al: Rhabdomyolysis following administration of cyclophosphamide: a case report in a BMT recipient. Bone Marrow Transplantation 1996; 17: 1167–1169.

Takahashi K, Ogita T, Okudaira H, et al: D-penicillamine-induced polymyositis in patients with rheumatoid arthritis. Arthritis Rheum 1986; 29: 560–564.

Tang TT, Oechler HW, Siker D, et al: Anesthesia-induced rhabdomyolysis in infants with unsuspected Duchenne dystrophy. Acta Pediatr 1992; 81: 716–719.

Tapal MF: Chronic colchicine myopathy. Scandinavian Journal of Rheumatology 1996; 25: 105–106.

Tatsukawa H, Okuda J, Kondoh M, et al: Malignant hyperthermia caused by intravenous lidocaine for ventricular arrhythmia. Int Med 1992; 31: 1069–1072.

Thyagarajan D, Day BJ, Wodak J, et al: Emetine myopathy in a ptient with eating disorder. Med J Australia 1993; 159: 757–760.

Tobart JA: Efficacy and long term adverse effect pattern of lovastatin. Am J Cardiol 1988; 62: 28J–34J.

Treves S, Larini F, Menegazzi P, et al: Alterations of intracellular Ca^{2+} transients in COS-7 cells transfected with the cDNA encoding skeletal muscle ryanodine receptor carrying a mutation associated with malignant hyperthermia. Biochem J 1994; 301(Pt 3): 661–665.

Unger J, Decaux G, L'Hermite M: Rhabdomyolysis, acute renal failure, endocrine alterations and neurological sequelae in a case of lithium self-poisoning. Acta Clin Belg 1982; 37: 216–223.

van den Berg AA, Iqbal S: Post suxamethonium myalgia —will we ever learn? Anesthesia and Intensive Care 1996; 24: 116–117.

van der Naalt J, Haaxma-Reiche H, van den Berg A, et al: Acute myoneuropathy after colchicine treatment. Ann Rheum Dis 1992; 51: 1267–1268.

Van Puijenbroek EP, Du Buf-Vereijken PWG, Spooren PFMJ, et al: Possible increased risk of rhabdomyolysis during concomitant use of simvastatin and gemfibrozil. Journal of Internal Medicine 1996; 240: 403–404.

Waclawik AJ, Sufit R, Beinlich BR, et al: Acute myopathy with selective degeneration of myosin filaments following status asthmaticus treated with methylprednisolone and vecuronium. Neuromuscul Disord 1992; 2: 19–26.

Wagner JM, Cohen S: Fibrous myopathy from butorphanol injections. Case report. J Rheumatol 1991; 18: 1934–1935.

Wallace CL, Mueller BA: Lovastatin-induced rhabdomyolysis in the absence of concomitant drugs. Ann Pharmacother 1992; 26: 190–192.

Watson AJS, Dalbow MH, Stachura I, et al: Immunologic studies in cimetidine-induced nephropathy and polymyositis. NEJM 1983; 308: 142–145.

Wattel F, Chopin lC, Durocher A, et al: Rhabdomyolyses au cours des intoxications aigues. Nouv Press Med 1978; 7: 2553–2560.

Willis JK, Tilton AH, Harkin JC, et al: Possible myopathy due to labetalol. Pediatr Neurol 1990; 6: 275–276.

Yordam N, Kandemir N, Topaloglu H, et al: Myositis associated with growth hormone therapy. J Pediatrics 1994; 125: 671.

Younger DS, Mayer SA, Weimer IH, et al: Colchicine-induced myopathy and neuropathy. Neurology 1991; 41: 943.

Chapter 14
Diseases of the Spine and Spinal Cord

Introduction

Drugs may affect the spinal column or the spinal cord. Various adverse effects will be discussed according to the classification shown in Table 14.1.

Clinical manifestations of spinal disorders are quite variable and may be reported as adverse effects without any mention of involvement of the spine or the spinal cord. A patient may report only backache or sensory disturbances below the level of lesion in the spinal cord or only impairment of bladder function. Motor impairment may be reported as paraplegia or quadriplegia or by the term "transverse myelitis." Very high cervical lesions may produce respiratory difficulties. Some processes such as steroid-induced epidural lipomatosis may produce the same clinical picture as an intraspinal neoplasm.

Backache

Backache is a nonspecific symptom. It may due to any drug producing generalized myositis or musculoskeletal pain. Filgrastim (recombinant granulocyte colony stimulating factor) is associ-ated with musculoskeletal pain in 20% of the cases and in some the only complaint is backache. The pathomechanism is not known but the bone pain may be associated with increased hematopoiesis induced by the drug. Backache may be the result of degenerative process in the intervertebral disc or it may also be a symptoms of serious intraspinal events such as hematomyelia.

Streptokinase infusion has been reported to produce severe low back pain which sometimes radiates down to the lower extremities and resolves promptly on discontinuation of the drug (Bourke 1992). The pathomechanism is not known but backache has not been reported with tissue plasminogen activator which is used for the same indication, i. e., for dissolving the clot in coronary artery thrombosis.

Drugs Affecting the Vertebral Column

Vertebral column is affected by all drugs affecting the skeletal system and the discussion of this topic is beyond the scope of this work. Drugs producing osteoporosis can lead to fractures of the vertebrae and compression of the spinal cord. Deformities of the spinal column may be due to muscular disorders induced by drugs.

A case of intractable backache secondary to vertebral compression has been reported after intravertebral alcohol injection for the treatment of vertebral hemangioma (Heiss et al 1996). This required surgical treatment involving removal of the vertebral body and spinal fusion. Histological examination of the vertebral tissue showed focal osteonecrosis.

Toxicity of Intrathecal Agents

Several drugs, introduced into the intrathecal space either for diagnostic or therapeutic purposes, or inadvertently, may produce undesirable effects on the spinal cord or its coverings (Table 14.2).

Table 14.2. Intrathecal drugs that may affect the spinal cord adversely.

Antineoplastic agents
Baclofen
Chymopapain
Cortic osteroids
Lidocaine for spinal anesthesia
Morphine
Radiologic contrast materials

Intrathecal Antineoplastic Agents

Leukoencephalopathy (see Chapter 3) and aseptic meningitis (see Chapter 16) have been reported as complication of this treatment. Two serious complications relevant to the spinal cord are ascending myelopathy and paraplegia. Over 40 such cases have been reported some of whom recovered partially or completely, some remained permanently paraplegic while there were deaths either due to complications associated with myeloencephalopathy or progression of malignancy.

Methotrexate (MTX). MTX is given intrathecally and usually combined with radiation therapy as prophylaxis against meningeal involvement in leukemias. Resar et al (1993) reported a case of ascending myelopathy leading to quadriplegia and respiratory difficulties following intrathecal methotrexate. In another case ascending spinal cord necrosis and polyradiculopathy following intrathecal MTX therapy led to respiratory failure and death (Bellon et al 1995).

Although there are several case reports of paraplegia following intrathecal MTX therapy (Garcia-Tena et al 1995; Beretta et al 1996), overall frequency of occurrence of paraplegia remains low. In one series, no case of paraplegia was observed among 57 patients where intrathecal methotrexate was used for the prophylaxis

of meningeal leukemia (Geiser et al 1975). Komp et al (1982) encountered only one case of paraplegia in 194 patients where intrathecal methotrexate was used for prophylaxis of acute lymphoblastic leukemia. A case of leukoencephalopathy with predominant involvement of the cervical spinal cord was reported following intrathecal methotrexate and radiotherapy (Case Records of the Massachusetts General Hospital 1984). In this case there was massive destruction of both the gray as well as the white matter of the spinal cord predominantly in the dorsal and lateral columns. Edema associated with necrosis extended down to the sacral region. Histological examination showed that the destruction involved both the myelin and the axons with formation of axon retraction balls, a finding previously reported in methotrexate leukoencephalopathy. Pathomechanism is not fully understood but it is similar to that of methotrexate-induced encephalopathy (see Chapter 3). The findings cannot be explained by the effect of radiotherapy alone.

Diagnosis and Management. If the onset of paraplegia is acute after intraspinal injection, in cancer patients with thrombocytopenia, the possibility of acute subdural or extradural hemorrhage should be considered. In the onset is subacute, the differential diagnosis includes the following:

– Infiltration of the nerve roots with tumor
– Metastatic lesions of the spinal cord
– Radiation myelopathy if radiotherapy has been used previously

Preservative-free solutions and diluents should be used for MTX injection. Steroids have been used for the treatment but the use of intrathecal steroids carries the risk of spinal arachnoiditis.

Cytosine Arabinoside (ARA-C). Resar et al (1992) have reviewed the literature and found 11 cases of myelopathy following intrathecal ARA-C. Kleinschmidt-DeMasters and Yeh (1992) reported a 22-year old male with malignant immunoblastic leukemia who developed a "locked-in" syndrome within 48 hours of receiving a single 100 mg intrathecal dose of ARA-C plus intravenous ARA-C, cisplatin and doxorubicin. He remained quadriplegic but alert until his death three weeks later. Autopsy showed infarction of the medulla and the spinal cord. Another case of myelopathy has been reported in a patient on a combination of ARA-C and fludarabine (Kornblau et al 1993).

Pathomechanism of ARA-C neurotoxicity has been reviewed in Chapter 3. ARA-C is detoxified in peripheral tissues by an ubiquitous enzyme, cytidine deaminase, but this enzyme is almost absent in the brain and the CSF. Intrathecal ARA-C, particularly when combined with intravenous ARA-C, can have additive toxic effects. No data is available to establish correlation between ARA-C metabolites in CSF and neurotoxicity and without routine monitoring of concentration of ARA-C in the CSF, it is difficult to ascertain the schedule of IT ARA-C which maximizes dose intensity and minimizes neurotoxicity. Therefore, an interval of at least 2–3 days should elapse between ARA-C treatments.

Baclofen

A case of myelopathy following intrathecal baclofen has been reported (Lee et al 1992). However, baclofen in concentrations of 2000 μg/ml (higher than those used in patients) have failed to show any adverse effect on meninges, nerve roots, or the spinal cords in toxicology studies using dogs (Sabbe et al 1993).

Chymopapain

This is a proteolytic enzyme derived from the fruit *Carica papaya*, and is used for chemonucleolysis, i. e., injection into the intervertebral disc space for treatment of herniated lumbar disc. Smith and Brown (1967) reported a case of paraplegia at 10th thoracic level which developed one week after chemonucleolysis of the last three lumbar discs. At surgery hemorrhagic arachnoiditis was found and the cause was not ascertained but postulated to be related to the hemorrhage from the procedure interacting with the retained oily contrast medium used for myelography. Further cases of paraplegia were reported by Sussman (1967) and Eguro (1983) but

the pathomechanism was not determined. Steinmeier and von Wild (1987) reported a case where chymopapain injection was considered to cause extrusion of a degenerated lumbar disc and surgery was required to remove it.

Corticosteroids

In the 1960s intrathecal methyprednisone was used for the treatment of arachnoiditis due to pantopaque myelography and other causes and was claimed to be safe (Sehgal et al 1963). Depot-medrol, the preparation used for this purpose, contains a carrier polyethyleneglycol which may produce arachnoiditis and myelitis. The intrathecal use of this product is contraindicated (Physician's Desk Reference 1998). Repeated epidural injections of steroids over long periods may also induce extradural lipomatosis. Bacterial meningitis and cauda equina syndrome has been reported after epidural steroid injection (Cooper and Sharpe 1996). Two case have been reported of intrinsic cervical spinal cord damage which occurred when cervical epidural steroid injections were administered while the patient were under sedation (Hodges et al 1998).

Lidocaine

Intrathecal lidocaine is used for spinal anesthesia. Neurological deficits following spinal anesthesia are rare. Schell et al (1991) reported two cases of persistent sacral nerve root deficits after continuous spinal anesthesia performed with high dose hyperbaric lidocaine using a micro catheter. In the immediate postoperative period there was lower extremity paresis, perianal anesthesia, and urinary retention. Perianal hypesthesia and difficulty with defecation persisted. Transient radicular irritation after hyperbaric lidocaine leading to backache has also been reported (Newman et al 1997).

Loo and Irestedt (1999) reported 6 cases of cauda equina syndrome in association with spinal anesthesia using hyperbaric 5% lidocaine. These effects were likely the result of direct neurotoxicity and persisted in all of the six patients at follow-up 5–17 months after spinal anesthesia. The authors recommended that hyperbaric lidocaine should not be administered in concentrations greater than 2% and the total dose should not exceed 60 mg.

Morphine

Epidural or intrathecal infusion of morphine and bupivacaine mixtures are presently used for treatment of refractory cancer pain. It is difficult to evaluate any involvement of the spinal cord in patients with advanced malignancy in some of whom there is extension to the spinal cord and several of whom have been treated with neurotoxic chemotherapy. In an autopsy study of patients who had received these treatment, several lesions of the spinal cord as well as thickening of the leptomeninges was noted (Sjöberg et al 1992). The role of intrathecal morphine in the pathogenesis of these lesions cannot be assessed.

Radiologic Contrast Materials

The older oily contrast materials such as pantopaque for myelography were considered to react with blood introduced into the CSF from a traumatic lumbar puncture and produce arachnoiditis (Howland and Curry 1966). In a review of 111 cases of myelography with pantopaque, Keogh (1974) found that 12.6% had pain in the sacrum and buttocks following the procedure. Newer water-soluble contrast media are considered to be safer but a case of transient paraplegia has been reported following metrizamide myelography (Peroutka et al 1982).

Drug-Induced Myelopathy

The term "myelopathy" means functional disturbances of the spinal cord or non-specific pathological processes involving the substance of the spinal cord. The term "myelitis" indicates an inflammatory process involving the spinal cord. Apart from drugs introduced intrathecally, systemically given drugs may cross the BBB and

have a direct toxic effect on the spinal cord. Myelopathy may also be caused indirectly by the drugs which impair the spinal cord circulation by hypotension or by inducing vasospasm or vasculitis of the spinal arteries.

Myelopathy is not always an isolated finding. It may be associated with involvement of the brain when the term "encephalomyelopathy" is used or may be accompanied by polyneuropathy when the term "myeloneuropathy" is used. Drugs associated with myelopathy are listed in Table 14.3.

Table 14.3. Drugs reported to be associated with myelopathy.

Antineoplastics*
Corticosteroids*
Cyclosporine
Folic acid
Germanium
Heroin*
Muzolimine
Nitrous oxide
Penicillin
Vaccines*: antirabies, hepatitis B, influenza, measles/
    mumps/rubella, tick-borne encephalitis

*Well documented. Other drugs have isolated case reports; causal relationship is not established.

Antineoplastics

Cytosine arabinoside, cisplatin, and methotrexate have been reported to induce myelopathy.

Cytosine arabinoside (ARA-C). Given as a low-dose intravenous infusion, ARA-C has been reported to produce myelopathy in a patient with leukemia. (Hoffman et al 1993). Their patient developed urinary retention, and decreased sensation below T7 dermatome on 23rd day of therapy when hematological recovery had already occurred. CT scan and myelography did not show any lesion but CSF examination showed pleocytosis and elevated protein. There was no evidence of involvement of the spinal cord by leukemia. This patient eventually developed an encephalopathy but recovered from it but the myelopathy remained unchanged. Adverse effect of combination of intravenous ARA-C with intrathecal ARA-C have already been discussed.

Cisplatin. Cisplatin is associated with several other manifestations of neurotoxicity such as ototoxicity, leukoencephalopathy, seizures, and peripheral neuropathy. Lhermitte's sign (sudden electric shock-like sensation travelling down the spine to the legs after flexion of neck) which indicates pathology of the spinal cord such as demyelinating disease, tumor or radiation myelopathy, has been reported after cisplatin therapy (Eales et al 1986; Dewar et al 1986; Walther et al 1987; List and Kummet 1990). This myelopathy usually resolves after discontinuation of cisplatin but sensory and motor deficits persist in some cases. Paraneoplastic myelopathy was ruled out in these case as it usually precedes the diagnosis of cancer and improves with treatment of cancer. Direct involvement of the spinal cord with malignancy was also ruled out in these cases.

Corticosteroids

Epidural lipomatosis or collection of unencapsulated fat in the extradural space can occur in Cushing's syndrome (Nöel et al 1992). It is a rare but well known complication of chronic corticosteroid therapy and over 31 cases have been reported in the literature (Kaneda et al 1984; Zampella et al 1987; Bischoff 1988; Roy-Camille et al 1991; Taborn 1991; Laroche et al 1993). The epidural mass can lead to compression of the spinal cord. Clinical manifestations include sensory and motor loss, weakness of the limbs, sphincter disturbances. These may progress to inability to walk and paraplegia. Diagnosis is established by CT scan (Buthiau et al 1988; Jungreis and Cohen 1987) and/or myelography. First line treatment is reduction of dose of corticosteroids. There may be some regression of the mass after discontinuation of steroids but surgical decompression with excision of extradural fat mass may be necessary (Haddad et al 1991). Eleven of the thirteen cases reviewed by Roy-Camille et al (1991) had surgical treatment with good results.

Cyclosporine

Spastic paraparesis developed in a man after he took cyclosporine following a liver transplant (Jalan et al 1994). The patient's cyclosporine levels ranged between 180–280 nmol/L (therapeutic range 170–240). The cyclosporine dose was reduced to maintain a trough level between 70–100 nmol/L and his paraparesis gradually improved. The reason for this patient's sensitivity to cyclosporine dose at the upper limit of therapeutic range is not clear. Other cases of reversible symmetrical polyneuropathy with paraplegia have been reported following use of cyclosporine in conjunction with transplantation (Terrovitis et al 1998; Jalan et al 1994). The patients recovered after tapering of the dose of cyclosporine.

Folic Acid

Folic acid when given to patients with vitamin B_{12} deficiency can aggravate subacute combined degeneration of the spinal cord.

Germanium

Kamijo et al (1991) reported the case of a girl who had been given preparations containing germanium compounds for 28 months and developed various symptoms of neurotoxicity. She died of renal failure and postmortem examination showed gliosis and degeneration of the dorsal columns of the spinal cord.

Heroin

There are several reports of transverse myelitis as a complication of intravenous heroin abuse (Goodhart et al 1982; Krause et al 1983; Grassa et al 1984; Guidotti et al 1985; Pascual-Calvet et al 1989). There is usually swelling of the spinal cord at the site of the lesion and in some cases there is evidence of vasculitis as a cause of these lesions. The pathomechanism is not known but it may be a hypersensitivity reaction to some of the diluents used in the preparation of the solution for injection.

Muzolimine

Pohlman-Eden et al (1991) described 7 patients with renal failure who developed fatal myeloencephalopathy after treatment with high doses of muzolimine, a new diuretic. The most severe deficits like severe tetraspastic paresis were seen in non-dialyzed renal insufficiency patients leading to the hypothesis that a partially dialyzable toxic metabolite of muzolimine may be responsible for this complication.

Nitrous Oxide

Myeloneuropathy has been described as a sequel of chronic exposure to nitrous oxide for recreational purposes (Layzer 1978; Blanco and Peters 1983; Lunsford et al 1983; Heyer et al 1986; Shimizu et al 1989). No evidence of impaired neurological function was found in dentists who utilized nitrous oxide in their practices (Dyck et al 1980). There are seven case reports of patients who developed paraplegia after nitrous oxide anesthesia. In three of these the risk factor was vitamin B_{12} deficiency which was corrected after the onset of neurological deficit. One of these recovered completely (King et al 1995), the second improved (Rösener et al 1996) whereas the third who also had phenylkenonuria did not improve (Lee et al 1999). Holloway and Alberico (1990) reported two patients with undiagnosed B_{12} deficiency who developed myelopathy after prolonged spinal surgery under nitrous oxide anesthesia. This was corrected by administration of vitamin B_{12} and the patients recovered.

Nitrous oxide produces multifocal reversible symptoms in the nervous system similar to those of vitamin B_{12} deficiency. Neurological dysfunction is due to progressive demyelination sometimes followed by axonal loss. It is similar to subacute combined degeneration of the spinal cord and may be accompanied polyneuropathy.

Pathomechanism. This has been reviewed by Louis-Ferdinand (1994). The mechanism responsible for neurotoxicity of and myelotoxicity of nitrous oxide involves the inhibition of methionine synthase (MetSyn) and resulting reduction in S-adenosyl methionine (SAM) and tetra-

hydrofolate (THF). Nitrous oxide inactivates vitamin B_{12} and prevents its utilization whereas in subacute combined degeneration of pernicious anemia there is problem with the absorption of B_{12}.

Management. The following methods have been used:
- Treatment is discontinuation of nitrous oxide and treatment with vitamin B_{12}. Partial to complete recovery followed in most of the cases reported.
- Folinic acid and methionine have been shown to protect against megaloblastosis and neurotoxicity occurring following nitrous oxide administration (Schilling 1986). Methionine is converted to SAM and elevates the methylation ration SAM:SAH thereby enhancing methylation of myelin (Weir et al 1988).

Penicillin

Tesio et al (1992) reviewed 6 cases from literature and presented two further cases of paraplegia following intramuscular injection of penicillin in the gluteal region. Another case was reported by Runge and Röder (1989). The hypothesized pathomechanism is inadvertent injection of penicillin into the superior gluteal artery with retrograde propulsion of the drug into he aorta and entry into the anterior spinal artery which may be obstructed or undergo spasm. The resulting paraplegia is usually irreversible and in one case of Tesio (1992), MRI some years later showed spinal cord atrophy which could be the sequel of spinal cord infarction.

Vaccines

Semple antirabies vaccine. This is a suspension of phenol inactivated rabies virus in the brains of sheep, is used in many developing countries. Neuroparalytic complications occur in about 1:2200 cases. Guillain-Barré syndrome has been reported in association with this virus (see Chapter 22). Swamy et al (1992) reported a case of Brown-Sequard syndrome due to Semple antirabies vaccine who recovered completely with immunosuppressive therapy. Bahri et al (1996) who also reported a case of myelitis are of the opinion that Semple-type adult animal nerve tissue vaccine produces an unacceptable rate of severe post-vaccinal neurological complications in adults and that human diploid cell rabies vaccine should be used for post-exposure rabies vaccination.

Hepatitis B Vaccine. This has been reported to be associated with myelitis in 3 case reports (Shaw et al 1988; Travisani et al 1993; Mahassin et al 1993). The causal link in these cases was based on the temporal relationship and exclusion of other causes of myelitis. Pathomechanism is not known but may be similar to that of vaccine-associated encephalomyelitis (see Chapter 3).

Vaccine Against Tick-Borne Encephalitis (TBE). This has been reported to be associated with various neurological complications including a case of subacute myelo-radiculopathy which recovered (Goerre et al 1993).

Measles, Mumps and Rubella Vaccine. A case of transverse myelitis with flaccid paraplegia and a sensory level at T1 level is reported in a 20-year old man following vaccination (Joyce and Rees 1995). The patient was treated with intravenous steroids with slight improvement but paralysis persisted below T6 level. There are three other cases of transverse myelitis associated with rubella vaccine.

Influenza Vaccine. One case of Brown-Sequard syndrome occurred in a patient following the administration of trivalent influenza vaccine (Antony et al 1995). The patient responded well to intravenous steroids and physical therapy. Another reversible paralytic syndrome was reported following influenza virus vaccination (Aggarwal et al 1995). It was considered to be possibly a postviral or postvaccinial autoimmune illness that was triggered by influenza vaccine.

Lesions of the Anterior Horn Cells and Anterior Nerve Roots

Anterior horn cells are usually resistant to neurotoxic effects of pharmaceutical agents. Leys

and Petit (1990) reported a case with lesions of the anterior horn cells as shown on EMG developing after polyradiculopathy following amitriptyline therapy.

Poliomyelitis developing as a result of vaccine to prevent it is an example of adverse reaction involving anterior horn cells. Mermel et al (1993) reported a case of vaccine-associated poliomyelitis in an immunocompetent man who had received a three dose primary series of oral polio vaccine as a child. MRI showed high signal abnormalities in the anterior horn cells. The overall risk of paralytic poliomyelitis associated with oral polio vaccine in the US is one case per 2.5 million doses (Prevot et al 1995). In Latin America, the overall risk of vaccine-associated paralytic poliomyelitis is 1 case per 1.5–2.2 million doses of oral poliovirus vaccine administered.

Provocation paralysis, may occur rarely in children who receive multiple intramuscular injections after oral polio vaccine. This may explain the high incidence of vaccine-associated paralytic poliomyelitis in Romania, where the use of intramuscular injections of antibiotics in children with febrile illness is common (Strebel et al 1995).

Drug-Induced Lhermitte Sign

This sign is elicited by flexion of the neck leading to sudden electric sensation traveling down the spine to the arms and legs. Neck flexion leads to stimulation of abnormally excited demyelinated nerve fibers and leads to the generation of ectopic sensory discharges in nerves. It was first reported as a symptom of multiple sclerosis (Lhermitte 1920). It is associated with a few other conditions which include the following:
- Cervical spondylosis
- Cervical spinal cord tumor
- Subacute combined degeneration of the spinal cord
- Radiation myelopathy
- Bone marrow transplantation
- Drugs: chemotherapy, nitrous oxide, withdrawal from selective serotonin reuptake inhibitors

Bone Marrow Transplantation (BMT). Wen et al (1992) reported four patients who developed Lhermitte's sign after BMT. The causes is not clear but multiple factors are involved in such patients which include the use of immunosuppressants such as cyclosporine and antineoplastic agents with potential for myelotoxicity.

Drugs. Lhermitte's sign has been reported in patients with myelopathy resulting from nitrous oxide abuse (Vishnubhakat and Beresford 1991). It is seen in cisplatin chemotherapy (Martinez Lopez et al 1995). Van den Bent (1998) observed a transient Lhermitte's sign in five of 87 patients treated with more than two cycles of docetaxel which developed either concurrently or after the onset of docetaxel-induced sensory neuropathy and disappeared after the discontinuation or dose reduction of chemotherapy.

Withdrawal from Selective Serotonin Reuptake Inhibitors (SSRIs). Brief electric shocks throughout the body, which last one or two seconds, have been reported during withdrawal from SSRIs (Bryois et al 1998). One patient with Lhermitte's sign was reported after withdrawal from paroxetine therapy (Reeves and Pinkofsky 1996).

Drug-Induced Spinal Hemorrhage

This is usually due to anticoagulants but thrombolytic therapy and aspirin may also cause it.

Anticoagulants. Intracranial hemorrhage as a complication of anticoagulant therapy has been discussed in Chapter 9. Intraspinal hemorrhage less frequently than intracranial hemorrhage and can be extradural, subdural, subarachnoid or intramedullary.

Unlike intracranial hemorrhage which is mostly subdural or intracerebral, intraspinal hemorrhage due to anticoagulants is mostly extradural and in the thoracic region (Dahlin and George 1984). The spinal extradural space is large and has profuse venous plexuses. Rupture of one of the delicate veins is followed by considerable bleeding in the extradural space. Trauma or lumbar puncture performed inadvertently

in a patient on anticoagulants may start such a bleeding. The patient may become paraplegic in a short time. The diagnosis can be confirmed by CT scan or MRI. Prompt surgical evacuation of the hematoma, which is usually located posteriorly, leads to recovery of function of the spinal cord. Less frequent anteriorly located hematomas may be more difficult to evacuate and require an anterior surgical approach to the spine.

Subarachnoid and subdural hemorrhage was found on surgery in a patient on anticoagulant therapy who experienced sudden excruciating back pain and became paraplegic (Bernsen and Hoogenraad 1992). Brown-Sequard syndrome (lesion of one half of spinal cord leading to ipsilateral paralysis and loss of position sense with contralateral loss of pain and temperature sense) has been reported in a patient with subarachnoid hemorrhage due to anticoagulants (Koehler and Kuiters 1986). After substitution of coagulation factors subdural hematoma can be managed by irrigation and suction drainage through a catheter placed in the subarachnoid space via lumbar puncture (Schwerdtfeger et al 1990).

Intramedullary hemorrhage due to anticoagulation is rare (Constantini et al 1992; Murphy and Nye 1991; Pisani et al 1985). The outlook for recovery from paraplegia is poor after evacuation of the hematoma.

Low molecular weight heparin (enoxaparin). From May 1993 to February 1998, the FDA received reports of 43 patients in the United States who had spinal or epidural bleeding after receiving enoxaparin mostly for prophylaxis of deep vein thrombosis associated with surgery (Wysowski et al 1998). Emergency laminectomy to evacuate the hematoma was performed in 28 of these patients and permanent paraplegia often due to delay in diagnosis occurred in 16 patients. The following risk factors were identified in these patients:

– Use of higher than recommended doses

– Administration to patients before establishing hemostasis in surgery

– Use of epidural catheters and spinal puncture

– Concomitant administrations of medications known to increase bleeding

– Vertebral column abnormalities

– Old age

The incidence of spinal hemorrhage is low considering that 33 million doses of enoxaparin were dispensed during 1993–1998 (Chaikin and Lim 1998). Currently, enoxaparin product labeling includes a warning about this potential complication.

Thrombolytic Therapy. A case of intramedullary spinal cord hemorrhage has also been reported after streptokinase treatment for myocardial infarction (Cruickshank et al 1992).

Aspirin. Several cases of spinal extradural hematoma have been reported in patients on use of aspirin as a low-dose prophylaxis or excessive intake (Heye 1995; Franscini et al 1994; Locke et al 1976). Because aspirin is widely used, its role in causing spinal epidural hematoma remains conjectural. However, coagulation abnormalities and improvement after discontinuation of aspirin point to a casual link.

References

Aggarwal A, Lacomis D, Guiliani MJ, et al: A reversible paralytic syndrome with anti-Gd 1b antibodies following influenza immunization. Muscle and Nerve 1995; 18: 1199–1201.

Andrus JK, Strebel PM, de Quandros CA, et al: Risk of vaccine-associated paralytic poliomyelitis in Latin America, 1989–1991. Bulletin of the World Health Organization 1995; 73: 33–40.

Antony SJ, Fleming DF, Bradley TK: Postvaccinial (influenza) disseminated encephalopathy (Brown-Sequard syndrome). J Natl Med Assoc 1995; 87(9): 705–708.

Bahri F, Letaief A, Ernez M, et al: Neurological complications in adults following rabies vaccine prepared from animal brains. Presse Med 1996; 25(10): 491–3.

Bellon JR, Smith AS, Cohen ML: Ascending cord necrosis. Complication of intrathecal chemotherapy with radiologic-pathologic correlation. Clin Pediatr (Phila) 1995; 34(9): 506–9.

Beretta F, Sanna P, Ghielmini M, et al: Paraplegia following intrathecal chemotherapy. Schweiz Med Wochenschr 1996; 126(25): 1107–11.

Bernsen RA, Hoogenraad TU: A spinal hematoma occurring in the subarachnoid as well as in the subdural space in a patient treated with anticoagulants. Clin Neurol Neurosurg 1992; 94: 35–37.

Bischoff Ch: Epidurale Lipomatose als Komplikation einer chronischen Glucocorticoidmedikation. DMW 1988; 113: 1964–1967.

Blanco G, Peters H: Myeloneuropathy and macrocytosis

associated with nitrous oxide abuse. Arch Neurol 1983; 40: 416–418..

Bourke J: Streptokinase and low back pain. NZ Med J 1992; 105: 482.

Bryois C, Rubin C, Zbinden JD, et al: Withdrawal syndrome caused by selective serotonin reuptake inhibitors: apropos of a case. Schweiz Rundsch Med Prax 1998; 87(10): 345–8.

Buthiau D, Piette JC, Ducerveau MN, et al: Steroid-induced epidermal lipomatosis: CT survey. J Computer Assist Tomogr 1988; 12: 501–503.

Case Records of the Massachusetts General Hospital: Case 36–1984. NEJM 1984; 311: 653–662.

Chaikin P, Lim J, Wysowski DK, Talarico L, Bacsanyi J, et al: Spinal and epidural hematoma and low molecular weight heparin. NEJM 1998; 338: 1774–1775 (letter).

Constantini S, Ashkenazi E, Shoshan Y, et al: Thoracic hematomyelia secondary to coumadin anticoagulant therapy: a case report. Eur Neurol 1992; 32: 109–111.

Cooper AB, Sharpe MD: Bacterial meningitis and cauda equina syndrome after epidural steroid injections. Can J Anaesth 1996; 43(5 Pt 1): 471–4.

Cruickshank GS, Duncan R, Hadley DM, et al: Intrinsic spinal cord hemorrhage due to streptokinase treatment for myocardial infarction. JNNP 1992; 55: 740.

Dahlin PA, George J: Intraspinal hematoma as a complication of anticoagualnt therapy. Clin Pharm 1984; 3: 656–661.

Dewar J, Lunt H, Abernethy DA, et al: Cisplatin neuropathy with Lhermitte's sign. JNNP 1986; 49: 96–99.

Dyck PJ, Grina LA, Lambert EH, et al: Nitrous oxide neurotoxicity studies in man and rat. Anesthesiology 1980; 53: 205–209.

Eales R, Tait DM, Peckham MJ: Lhermitte's sign as a complication of cisplatin-containing chemotherapy for testicular cancer. Cancer Treat Rep 1986; 70: 905–907.

Eguro H: Transverse myelitis following chemonucleolysis. J Bone Joint Surg (Am) 1983; 65: 1328–1330.

Franscini L, Ballmer PE, Sturzenegger M: Evaluation of back pain secondary to spinal epidural hematoma associated with aspirin intake and a partial platelet glycoprotein Ia/IIa deficiency. Arch Intern Med 1994; 154(23): 2769–71.

Garcia-Tena J, Lopez-Andreu JA, Ferris J, et al: Intrathecal chemotherapy-related myeloencephalopathy in a young child with acute lymphoblastic leukemia. Pediatr Hematol Oncol 1995; 12(4): 377–85.

Geiser CF, Bishop Y, Jaffe N, et al: Adverse effects of intrathecal methotrexate in children with acute leukemia in remission. Blood 1975; 45: 189–195.

Goerre S, Kesselring J, Hartmann K, et al: Neurologische Nebenwirkungen nach Impfung gegen Frühsommer-Meningo-Enzephalitis. Schweiz Med Wschr 1993; 123: 654–657.

Goodhart LC, Loizou LA, Anderson M: Heroin myelopathy. JNNP 1982; 45: 562–563.

Grassa C, Montanari E, Scaglioni A, et al: Acute heroin myelopathy: case report. Ital J Neurol Sci 1984; 5: 63–66.

Guidotti M, Passerini D, Brambilla M, et al: Heroin myelopathy: a case report. Ital J Neurosci 1985; 6: 99–100.

Haddad SF, Hitchon PW, Godersky JC: Idiopathic and

corticosteroid-induced spinal epidural lipomatosis. N Neurosurg 1991; 74: 38–42.

Heiss JD, Doppman JL, Oldfield EH: Treatment of vertebral hemangioma by intralesional injection of absolute ethanol. N Engl J Med 1996; 334(20): 1340.

Heye N: Is there a link between acute spinal epidural hematoma and aspirin? Spine 1995; 20: 1931–2.

Heyer EJ, Simpson DM, Bodis-Wollner I, et al: Nitrous oxide: clinical and electrophysiologic investigation of neurologic complications. Neurology 1986; 36: 1618–1622.

Hodges SD, Castleberg RL, Miller T, et al: Cervical epidural steroid injection with intrinsic spinal cord damage. Two case reports. Spine 1998; 23(19): 2137–2142.

Hoffman DJ, Howard JR, Sarma R, et al: Encephalopathy, myelopathy, optic neuropathy, and anosmia associated with intravenous cytosine arabinoside. Clin Neuropharmacology 1993; 16: 258–262.

Holloway KL, Alberico M: Postoperative myeloneuropathy: A preventable complication in patients with B_{12} deficiency. J Neurosurg 1990; 72: 732–736.

Jalan R, Plevris JN, MacGilchrist A, et al: Reversible spastic paraparesis due to cyclosporin toxicity. Am J Gastroenterol 1994; 89: 645–646.

Joyce KA, Rees JE: Transverse myelitis after measles, mumps, and rubella vaccine. BMJ 1995; 311: 422.

Jungreis CA, Cohen WA: Spinal cord compression induced by steroid therapy: CT findings. J Computer Assist Tomography 1987; 11: 245–247.

Kamijo M, Yagihashi S, Kida K, et al: An autopsy case of chronic germanium intoxication presenting as peripheral neuropathy; spinal ataxia; and chronic renal failure. Rinsho Shinkeigaku 1991; 31: 191–196.

Kaneda A, Yamaura I, Kamikozuru M, et al: Paraplegia as a complication of corticosteroid therapy. A case report. J Bone Joint Surg (Am) 1984; 66: 783–785.

Keogh AJ: Meningeal reactions seen with myelography. Clin Radiol 1974; 25: 361.

King M, Coulter C, Boyle RS, et al: Neurotoxicity from overuse of nitrous oxide. Med J Australia 1995; 163: 50–51.

Kleinschmidt-DeMasters BK, Yeh M: "Locked-in Syndrome" after intrathecal cytosine arabinoside therapy for malignant immunoblastic lymphoma. Cancer 1992; 70: 2504–2507.

Koehler PJ, Kuiters RR: Brown-Sequard syndrome caused by a spinal subarachnoid hematoma due to anticoagulant therapy. Surg Neurol 1986; 25: 191–193.

Komp DM, Fernandez CH, Falletta JM, et al: CNS prophylaxis in acute lymphoblastic leukemia. Comparison of two methods. A Southwest Oncology Group Study. Cancer 1982; 50: 1031–1036.

Kornblau SM, Cortes-Franco J, Estey E: Neurotoxicity associated with fludarabine and cytosine arabinoside chemotherapy for acute leukemia and myelodysplasia. Leukemia 1993; 7: 378–383.

Krause GS: Brown-Sequard syndrome following heroin injection. Ann Emerg Med 1983; 12: 581–583.

Laroche F, Chemouilli P, Carlier R, et al: Efficacy of conservative treatment in a patient with spinal cord compression due to corticosteroid-induced epidural lipomatosis. Rev Rhumatisme 1993; 60: 729–731.

Layzer RB: Myelopathy after prolonged exposure to nitrous oxide. Lancet 1978; 2: 1227–1230.

Lear J, Rajapakse R, Pohl J: Low back pain associated with streptokinase. Lancet 1992; 340: 851.

Lee P, Smith I, Piesowicz A, et al: Spastic paraparesis after anaesthesia. Lancet 1999; 353(9152): 554.

Lee TH, Chen SS, Su SL, et al: Baclofen intoxication: report of four cases and review of literature. Clin Neuropharmacol 1992; 15: 56–62.

Leys D, Petit H: Clinical signs of amyotrophic lateral sclerosis developing after polyradiculoneuropathy associated with amitriptyline. BMJ 1990; 300: 614.

Lhermitte J: Les formes douloureuses de la commotion de la moelle epiniere. Rev Neurol 1920; 36: 257–262.

List AF, Kummet TD: Spinal cord toxicity complicating treatment with cisplatin and etoposide. Am J Clin Oncol 1990; 13: 256–258.

Locke GE, Giorgio AJ, Biggers SL Jr, et al: Acute spinal epidural hematoma secondary to aspirin-induced prolonged bleeding. Surg Neurol 1976; 5(5): 293–6.

Loo CC, Irestedt L: Cauda equina syndrome after spinal anaesthesia with hyperbaric 5% lignocaine: a review of six cases of cauda equina syndrome reported to the Swedish Pharmaceutical Insurance 1993–1997. Acta Anaesthesiol Scand 1999; 43(4): 371–379.

Louis-Ferdinand RT: Myelotoxic, neurotoxic and reproductive adverse effects of nitrous oxide. Adverse Drug React Toxicol Rev 1994; 13: 193–206.

Lunsford JM, Wynn MH, Kwan WH: Nitrous oxide-induced myeloneuropathy. J Foot Surg 1983; 22: 222–225.

Mahassin F, Algayres JP, Valmary J, et al: Acute myelitis following hepatitis B vaccination. Presse Med 1993; 22: 1997–1998.

Martinez Lopez E, Gallego Cullere J, Illarramendi Manas JJ, et al: Lhermitte's sign as a complication of cisplatin treatment. Med Clin (Barc) 1995 4; 104(8): 317–8.

Mermel L, de Mora DS, Sutter RW: Vaccine-associated paralytic poliomyelitis. NEJM 1993; 329: 810–811.

Murphy MA, Nye DH: Thoracic intramedullary hematoma as a complication of warfarin: case report and literature review. Aust NZ J Surg 1991; 61: 789–792.

Newman LM, Iyeer NR, Truman KJ: Transient radicular irritation after hyperbaric lidocaine spinal anesthesia in parturients. International Journal of Obstetric Anesthesia 1997; 6: 132–134.

Nöel P, Pepersack T, Vanbinst A, et al: Spinal epidural lipomatosis in Cushings's syndrome secondary to an adrenal tumor. Neurology 1992; 42: 1250–1251.

Pascual-Calvet J, Pou A, Pedro-Botet J, et al: Non-infective neurological complications associated with heroin use. Arch Neurobiol (Madrid) 1989; 52 (suppl 1): 155–161.

Peroutka SJ, Ullrich C, Fisher RS, et al: Transient arreflexia and quadriplegia following metrizamide myelography (letter). Ann Neurol 1982; 12: 406–407.

Physician's Desk Reference, Oradell, NJ, Medical Economics Company, 1998.

Pisani R, Carta F, Guiducci G, et al: Hematomyelia during

anticoagulant therapy. Surg Neurol 1985; 24: 578–580.

Pohlman-Eden B, Berli P, Maibach EA: Muzolimine-induced severe neuromyeloencephalopathy: report of seven cases. Act Neurol Scand 1991; 83: 41–44.

Prevots DR, et al: Completeness of reporting for paralytic poliomyelitis, United States, 1980 through 1991: implications for estimating the risk of vaccine-associated disease. Arch Pediatr Adolescent Med 1994; 148: 479–485.

Reeves RR, Pinkofsky HB: Lhermitte's sign in paroxetine withdrawal. J Clin Psychopharmacol 1996; 16(5): 411–412.

Resar LMS, Phillips PC, Kastan MB, et al: Acute neurotoxicity after intrathecal cytosine arabinoside in two adolescents with acute lymphoblastic leukemia of B-cell type. Cancer 1993; 71: 117–123.

Rosener M, Dichgans J: Severe combined degeneration of the spinal cord after nitrous oxide anaesthesia in a vegetarian. J Neurol Neurosurg Psychiatry 1996; 60(3): 354.

Roy-Camille R, Mazel C, Husson JL, et al: Symptomatic spinal epidural lipomatosis induced by long-term steroid treatment. Spine 1991; 16: 1365–1371.

Runge U, Röder H: Querschnittssyndrom nach intramuskulärer Penicillininjektion. Z Ärztl Fortbild 1989; 83: 537–538.

Sabbe MB, Grafe MR, Pfeifer BL, et al: Toxicology of baclofen continuously infused into the spinal intrathecal space of the dog. Neurotoxicology 1993; 14: 397–410.

Schell RM, Brauer FS, Cole DJ, et al: Persistent sacral nerve root deficits after continuous spinal anesthesia. Canad J Anesth 1991; 38: 908–911.

Schilling RF: Is nitrous oxide a dangerous anesthetic for vitamin B12-deficient subjects? JAMA 1986; 255: 1605–1606.

Schwerdtfeger K, Caspar W, Alloussi S, et al: Acute spinal intradural extramedullary hematoma: a non-surgical approach for spinal cord compression. Neurosurgery 1990; 27: 312–314.

Sehgal AD, Tweed DC, Gardner WJ, et al: Laboratory studies after intrathecal corticosteroids. Arch Neurol 1963; 9: 74–78.

Shaw FE, Graham DJ, Guess HA, et al: Post-marketing surveillance for neurological adverse events reported after hepatitis B vaccination. Am J Epidemiol 1988; 127: 337–352.

Shimizu T, Nishimura Y, Fujishima Y, et al: Subacute myeloneuropathy after abuse of nitrous oxide: an electronmicroscopic study on the peripheral nerve. Rinsho Shinkeigaku 1989; 29: 1129–1135.

Sjöberg M, Karlsson PA, Nordborg C, et al: Neuropathologic findings after a long-term intrathecal infusion of morphine and bupivacaine for pain treatment in cancer patients. Anesthesiology 1992; 76: 173–186.

Smith L, Brown JE: Treatment of lumbar intervertebral disc lesions by direct injection of chymopapain. J Bone Joint Surg 1967; 49-B: 502–517.

Steinmeier R, von Wild K: Klinische Erfahrungen mit intradiskaler Chymopapain-Applikation bei lumbalen Bandscheibenvorfall. Nervenarzt 1987; 58: 450–455.

Strebel PM, Ion-Nedelcu N, Baughman AL, et al: Intramuscular injections within 30 days of immunization with oral poliovirus vaccine—a risk factor for vaccine-associated paralytic poliomyelitis. NEJM 1995; 332: 500–506.

Sussman BJ: Inadequacies and hazards of chymopapain injections as treatment for intervertebral disc disease. J Neurosurg 1975; 42: 389–396.

Swamy HS, Vasanth A, Sasikumar: Brown-Sequard syndrome due to Semple antirabies vaccine: case report. Paraplegia 1992; 30: 181–183.

Taborn J: Epidural lipomatosis as a cause of spinal cord compression in polymyalgia rheumatica. J Rheumatol 1991; 18: 286–288.

Terrovitis IV, Nanas SN, Rombos AK, et al: Reversible symmetric polyneuropathy with paraplegia after heart transplantation. Transplantation 1998; 65(10): 1394–1395.

Tesio L, Bassi L, Strada L: Spinal cord lesion after penicillin gluteal injection. Paraplegia 1992; 30: 442–444.

Travisani F, Gattinara GC, Caraceni P, et al: Transverse myelitis following hepatitis B vaccination. J Hepatology 1993; 19: 317–318.

van den Bent MJ, Hilkens PH, Sillevis Smitt PA, et al: Lhermitte's sign following chemotherapy with docetaxel. Neurology 1998 Feb; 50(2): 563–564

Vishnubhakat SM, Beresford HR: Reversible myeloneuropathy of nitrous oxide abuse: serial electrophysiological studies. Muscle Nerve 1991; 14(1): 22–26.

Walther PJ, Rossitch E, Bullard DE: The development of Lhermitte's sign during cisplatin chemotherapy. Cancer 1987; 60: 2170–2172.

Weir DG, Keating S, Molloy A, et al: Methylation deficiency causes vitamin B12-associated neuropathy in the pig. J Neurochem 1988; 51: 1949–1952.

Wen PY, Blanchard KL, Block CC, et al: Development of Lhermitte's sign after bone marrow transplantation. Cancer 1992; 69: 2262–2266.

Wysowski DK, Talarico L, Bacsanyi J, et al: Spinal and epidural hematoma and low molecular weight heparin. NEJM 1998; 338: 1774–1775 (letter).

Yapa RS: Folic acid therapy dangers. Practitioner 1988; 232: 987.

Zampella JK, Duvall ER, Sekar BC, et al: Symptomatic spinal epidural lipomatosis as complication of steroid immunosuppression in cardiac transplant patients. Report of two cases. J Neurosurg 1987; 67: 760–764.

Chapter 15
Drug-Induced Cerebellar Disorders

Introduction

Several drugs produce cerebellar dysfunction as a part of encephalopathy (see Chapter 3). Cerebellar hemorrhage may occur following use of anticoagulants or thrombolytics (see Chapter 9). This chapter includes discussion of those drug-induced adverse effects where cerebellar disorder is either mentioned specifically or is a prominent feature. The main clinical manifestations of cerebellar disorders with anatomical correlations are as follows:
- *Dyssynergia, dysmetria*, and *dysarthria* are usually due to lesions of the lateral parts of posterior cerebellar hemispheres.
- *Ataxia* of stance and gait is usually due to damage to the cerebellar vermis and anterior lobe.

The present understanding of the physiologic mechanism of cerebellar dysfunction is based mostly on animal experiments. Precise clinico-pathological correlations in humans are limited because cerebellar atrophies result in diffuse loss of Purkinje cells and deterioration of both afferent and efferent cerebellar pathways (Diener and Dichgans (1992). Patients presenting with cerebellar symptoms may have any of the several causes shown in Table 15.1.

Table 15.1. Various causes of cerebellar symptoms.

Initial manifestations of multisystem atrophies such as olivopontocerebellar atrophy
Idiopathic late-onset cerebellar ataxia
Tumors: these lesions have a space occupying effect leading to rise of intracranial pressure.
Infections: cerebellar abscess
Vascular lesions of the cerebellum involving the neighboring structures such as the brainstem
Metabolic disorders
Adverse effect of drugs and toxins

Drug-induced disorders of the cerebellum can be distinguished from the naturally occurring diseases of the cerebellum are characterized by the following three features:
- They are not progressive
- They are not usually associated with rise of intracranial pressure
- They may regress after discontinuation of the offending drug.

Table 15.2. Drugs associated with cerebellar disorders.

Alcohol*
Antidepressants
Antineoplastic drugs
  Cytosine arabinoside*
  DABIS
  Docetaxel
  Doxyfluridine
  Fluorouracil
  Procarbazine
  Vincristine
Aprindine (Bouget et al 1980)
Bromisovalum
Cimetidine
Cyclosporine*
Drug interactions
  Amiodarone and phenytoin (Ahmad 1995)
  Carbamazepine and clarithromycin (Yasui et al 1997)
  Carbamazepine and lithium (Marcoux 1996)
Histamine H_2 receptor antagonists
Isoniazid
Lithium*
Metronidazole
Nefazodone (Puzantian and Shaw 1996)
Omeprazole (Varona et al 1996)
Phenytoin*
Procainamide (Schwartz et al 1984)
Tretinoin
Vaccines

*Causal relationship is well established and these are described in more detail in the text. For the others there are isolated case reports, but causal relationship is not established.

It is well known that cerebellum is particularly sensitive to a variety of metabolic insults such as hypoxia, hypoglycemia, heavy metals and other intoxications, nutritional deficiencies and metabolic disorders. The reason for this selective cerebellar vulnerability has not been fully understood. Plaitakis (1993) has described a thiamin deficiency-induced model of cerebellar ataxia where there is a selective involvement of 5-HT fibers.

Drugs associated with cerebellar disorders are listed in Table 15.2.

Alcohol

Alcoholic cerebellar degeneration is well recognized. Long-standing alcoholics may develop ataxia due to degeneration of the Purkinje cells of the cerebellar cortex. This cell loss is particularly severe in those who have Wernicke-Korsakoff syndrome. This indicates that cerebellar degeneration does not result only from the direct toxic effect of alcohol but other factors such as thiamine deficiency also play a part. Abstinence from alcohol and thiamine replacement may lead to some improvement in these cases. History of alcoholism should be obtained in all patients presenting with cerebellar degeneration, particularly those where a drug-induced cause is suspected.

Antidepressants

Cerebellar disorders including dysmetria, ataxia, and intention tremor have been reported during treatment with antidepressants (Bartels et al 1989). These authors have reported 9 cases and reviewed the literature on this subject. Pathomechanism is explained by the effect of neurotransmitter alterations on the noradrenergic afferents of the cerebellar cortex. Ataxia resulting from high dose antidepressant therapy is also considered to due to reversible intoxication of the cerebellar structures. Dosage reduction is usually enough to reverse the symptoms of cerebellar toxicity and there are no permanent sequelae (Schied and Bartels 1983).

Antineoplastic Drugs

Signs of cerebellar dysfunction are common among cancer patients and various causes include those shown in Table 15.3.

Table 15.3. Some causes of cerebellar disorders in cancer patients.

Paraneoplastic syndromes: remote effects of cancer
Cancer metastases
Metabolic disorders in cancer patients
– Hypoxia-ischemia
– Hypoglycemia
– Electrolyte disturbances
– Rapid correction of hyponatremia
– Hyperthermia
Antineoplastic drugs

Evaluation of a cancer patient with cerebellar signs is not always easy because of the multiplicity of factors involved. These patients usually have metabolic and nutritional deficiencies and patients with severe cancer cachexia may develop Wenicke's encephalopathy with resulting loss of Purkinje's cells in the cerebellum and difficulty with gait (Victor et al 1989). Rapid correction of hyponatremia is well known to cause the syndrome of central pontine myelinolysis and also causes degenerative lesions of the superior vermis of the cerebellum in experimental animals (Kleinschmidt-DeMasters and Norenberg 1981). Paraneoplastic syndromes often involve the cerebellum. Peripheral neuropathies associated with cancer and/or antineoplastic therapy may produce gait disturbances that may resemble cerebellar ataxia. Neuroimaging techniques such as CT scan and MRI help to identify metastatic lesions and cerebellar atrophy. Among the various drugs reported, only cytosine arabinoside is well documented.

Cytosine Arabinoside. Cytosine arabinoside (ARA-C) has been used widely in the treatment of acute non-lymphatic leukemia (ANLL) for years without any report of significant neurotoxicity. Since 1979, high doses of ARA-C (up to 30 times the usual dose) have been shown to induce remissions in patients with ANNL refractory to conventional treatment. Reports of neurotoxicity with this regimen have included aseptic meningitis, myelopathy and encephalopathy with prominent cerebellar dysfunction (Sylvester et al 1987; Herzig et al 1987; Salinsky et al 1983; Beaudreuil et al 1995). Risk factors for the development of neurotoxicity are age (over 50 years) and renal dysfunction (Hasle 1990; Vogel and Horoupian 1993); Jolson et al 1992). Symptoms are usually reversible but persistent cerebellar dysfunction has been reported has been reported and attributed to cumulative effect of the drug rather than high plasma levels of the drug (Boesen et al 1988). Such cumulative effects may occur even with low dose ARA-C (Benger et al 1985).

Clinicopathological Features. Cerebellar neurotoxicity due to ARA-C is manifested by ataxia of gait, limb movements, dysarthria, and nystagmus. Pathological examination shows loss of Purkinje cells in cerebellar hemispheres (Winkelman and Hines 1983; Dworkin et al 1985). Cerebellar atrophy has been demonstrated by CT and MRI (Miller et al 1989).

Pathomechanism. ARA-C neurotoxicity is mediated primarily through inhibition of DNA synthesis; accordingly cytotoxicity to tumor cells is restricted to cells in S-phase. Experimental studies in mice have shown that neonatal administration of ARA-C causes necrosis of proliferating cells in the external granular layer of the mouse cerebellum and the mice thus treated develop severe cerebellar abnormalities (Shimada et al 1975).

DABIS. This is an alkylating quaternary nitrogen compound used as an antineoplastic agent. Cerebellar ataxia has been reported as a complication of its use (van der Burg et al 1991).

Docetaxel. One case of ataxia has been reported following docetaxeltherapy and it resolved after discontinuation of therapy (Hofstra et al 1997).

Doxyfluridine. This is an antineoplastic agent of fluropyrimidine group related to 5-FU. One patient with acute reversible cerebellar syndrome has been reported after second course of therapy with doxyfluridine and developed encephalopathy after the next two cycles (Heier and Fossa 1985).

5-Fluorouracil (5-FU). High doses of 5-FU have been associated with cerebellar syndromes (Riehl and Brown 1964). This syndrome is rarely seen with the doses used these days. Acute cerebellar syndrome has also been reported with flucytosine, the active metabolite of which is 5-fluorouracil (Cubo Delgado et al 1997). This subsided after replacement of flucytosine by flucanazole.

Bromisovalum

Encephalopathy due to chronic bromide use has been described in Chapter 3. Two patients with cerebellar atrophy documented by CT scan following chronic bromisovalum abuse have been reported (van Balkom et al 1985).

Cyclosporine

Cyclosporine is an immunosuppressant used primarily in conjunction with organ transplant. Leucoencephalopathy related to this drug is described in Chapter 3. Some of the neurological complications associated with the use of this drug are attributed to liver disease and liver transplantation. Poor liver function before transplantation may damage the blood brain barrier and facilitate cyclosporine neurotoxicity. Cerebellar ataxia and tremor has been reported in patients treated with cyclosporine after bone marrow transplantation (Atkinson et al 1985). A case of cyclosporine-associated leukoencephalopathy presenting with cerebellar ataxia and dysarthria was reported by Belli et al (1993). This complication presented 6 months after liver transplantation and 3 months after steroid withdrawal, whereas the neurological complications are usually seen within the first month after transplantation. Hyperintensities of the white matter in the cerebellum were shown on MRI and these resolved on withdrawal of cyclosporine. Resumption of cyclosporine at a low dose was associated with a rapid, recurrent neurotoxicity. This patient did not suffer from hypertension and cyclosporine levels were always found to be within normal limits. The late occurrence as well as association with acute hepatitis suggests the possibility of graft dysfunction as a contributing factor.

One patient developed cerebellar edema with brainstem compression following use of cyclosporine as an immunosuppressant for lung transplant (Nussbaum et al 1995). Replacement of cyclosporine by FK506 was accompanied by a rapid recovery. Cyclosporine precipitated cerebellar syndrome and psychiatric symptoms in another patient with rejection of renal allograft (Sharma et al 1995). The symptoms resolved 8 hours after discontinuation of cyclosporine but recurred when cyclosporine was resumed. After the final withdrawal of cyclosporine, the patient recovered completely from neurotoxic effects.

Cimetidine

This is a histamine H_2-receptor antagonist is used for gastritis. One case of cerebellar ataxia has been reported following use of this medication at therapeutic doses for 4 days (Hamano et al 1998). Drugs of this category pass through the blood-brain barrier and possibly block the H_2 receptors in the brain producing CNS adverse effects.

Isoniazid

A case of cerebellar syndrome has been reported following isoniazid treatment of a patient with tuberculosis on hemodialysis (Blumberg and Gil 1990). MRI showed cerebellar atrophy but the patient improved following discontinuation of isoniazid. Pathomechanism is considered to involve pyridoxine deficiency. A case has been reported of cerebellar ataxia in a 10-year old child on isoniazid therapy who recovered following discontinuation of the drug and treatment with pyridoxine (Lewin and McGreal 1993).

Lithium

Lithium has been used widely for the treatment of manic depressive illness over the past two de-

cades. Neurological sequelae of acute lithium intoxication including, cerebellar disorders, are common and well known (Reisberg and Gershon 1979). Chronic sequelae are less common and less known. In a report of 23 cases and review of 100 cases from literature, 10% of the patients were found to have permanent neurological sequelae and 14% died (Hansen and Amdisen 1978). There are several other reports and reviews of neurological sequelae of chronic lithium intoxication (Schou 1984; Nagaraja 1987). Cerebellar ataxia with scanning speech are usual manifestations. Although there are multiple lesions in the brain, the major involvement is of the cerebellum (Ferbert and Czernik 1987). Adityanjee (1989) mentioned 55 cases of long-lasting neurological sequelae of lithium intoxication and suggested the acronym SILENT (syndrome of irreversible lithium-affectuated neurotoxicity) to describe this condition. The most persistent signs in these patients were cerebellar. Cerebellar atrophy has been demonstrated by CT scan (Jacome 1987) and cerebellar degeneration with vacuolization and loss of Purkinje cells has been demonstrated on autopsy (Naramoto et al 1993; Schneider and Mirra 1994).

Pathomechanism of lithium neurotoxicity is not known but the risk factors are shown in Table 15.4.

Table 15.4. Risk factors for lithium neurotoxicity.

Somatic illnesses with fever, e. g., Q fever (Modestin and Foglia 1988; Pfadenhauer and Stapf 1994)
Concomitant treatment with other antipsychotic drugs such as haloperidol
Concomitant treatment with diuretics
Renal insufficiency
High serum levels of lithium
Individual susceptibility in the absence of the above risk factors

Management. There is no specific antidote for lithium toxicity. Initial management is the same as for any overdose. Recovery usually occurs if lithium neurotoxicity is detected early and lithium is discontinued. Techniques aimed at lowering high serum levels result in brisk recovery from acute toxic effects but do not prevent long term neurotoxicity. In serious cases with plasma lithium levels above 3.5 mmol/L, dialysis is required to enhance elimination. With the exception of use of lithium for suicide, acute as well as chronic toxicity can be prevented in most cases by careful use of lithium and recognition that this drug has a narrow therapeutic window.

Metronidazole

Metronidazole, a 5-nitroimidazole, is widely used for the treatment of trichomoniasis, giardiasis, amebiasis, and anaerobic infections. It produces a number of neurological adverse effects including peripheral neuropathy, encephalopathy, cerebellar dysfunction and seizures. Cerebellar toxicity, manifesting by ataxia and dysarthria, has been reported with high doses of metronidazole therapy for amoebiasis (Dubois et al 1983; Kusumi et al 1980; Ferroir et al 1985). Ahmed et al (1995) have reported a case with metrinidazole toxicity who presented with ataxia, dizziness, confusion, and vertigo. MRI showed abnormal increased signal within the cerebellum as well as supratentorial white matter. The patient improved after withdrawal of the drug and MRI lesions resolved.

Phenytoin

Phenytoin is used for partial and generalized seizures. The most characteristic feature of phenytoin neurotoxicity is cerebellar dysfunction; nystagmus, tremor, and ataxia. There is some controversy regarding the role of phenytoin in producing cerebellar disorders. In the past cerebellar degeneration has been attributed mostly to hypoxia caused by seizures. Spielmeyer (1930) observed degeneration of Purkinje cells in the brains of epileptic patients long before phenytoin was introduced as an anticonvulsant in 1930. This finding as well as cerebellar atrophy found in epileptic patients due to perinatal anoxic-ischemic damage can be differentiated from phenytoin-induced cerebellar disease (Gessaga and Ulrich 1985). Cerebellar degeneration has been reported in a patient with tubercular meningitis who received phenytoin as prophylactic therapy

but never had a seizure (Rapport and Shaw 1977). Subacute phenytoin neurotoxicity has also been reported in non-epileptic patients where the indication for use is cardiac arrhythmia (Tindall and Willerson 1978). Neurotoxicity (including cerebellar signs) has been reported in five patients abusing cocaine adulterated with phenytoin (Katz et al 1993; Koppel et al 1995).

Most of the cerebellar disorders following phenytoin therapy are transient but persistent cerebellar deficits have also been described. Progressive irreversible ataxia has been documented in patients on long-term phenytoin treatment with levels not generally considered excessive. Unlike that found in cute toxicity, this type of ataxia is permanent (Benabou et al 1995). Cerebellar degeneration following long-term therapy with phenytoin has been documented by several authors (Ghatak et al 1976; Koller et al 1980; McLain et al 1980; Rosich 1980). Cases of cerebellar atrophy with persisting neurological deficits provide for the chronic irreversible damage with phenytoin (Pumar et al 1995; Pulliainen et al 1998).

Pathology. In the pre-CT era, pneumoencephalography in cases of phenytoin-induced cerebellar toxicity showed enlargement of fourth ventricle, enlarged cerebellopontine angle cistern, and widened interfolial sulci indicating cerebellar atrophy (Selhorst et al 1972). Cerebellar atrophy as demonstrated by MRI has been reported following acute intoxication with phenytoin (Masur et al 1989). This case was followed up for more than four years and no change was seen in cerebellar atrophy thus ruling out cerebellar degenerative disorders (Masur et al 1990). Cerebellar atrophy documented by CT scan has also been reported in irreversible cases of cerebellar ataxia following overdose of phenytoin (Imamura et al 1992; Kim et al 1991; Lindwall and Nilsson 1984; Baier et al 1984; McCrea et al 1980). Atrophy has also been demonstrated by MRI scan (Luef et al 1993) and at autopsy (Abe and Yagishita 1991) in cases of chronic phenytoin toxicity. In a case control study, cerebellar atrophy was seen in patients with epilepsy exposed to phenytoin in the absence of seizures and preexisting cerebellar damage (Ney et al 1994). Neuropathological examination in phenytoin-induced cerebellar atrophy shows loss of Purkinje cells with multilamellar structures within the degenerating Purkinje cells (Breiden-Arends et al 1981). Similar loss of Purkinje cells was observed in biopsies in patients with epilepsy on phenytoin therapy (Salcman et al 1978).

Pathomechanism. This is not well understood but the following explanations have been considered:
- Folic acid deficiency associated with use of phenytoin has been suggested as an explanation of cerebellar atrophy (Meyer-Wahl 1980).
- Experimental studies on mature mice have demonstrated degeneration of granular cell layer of the cerebellum caused by phenytoin (Volk et al 1986). The terminal stage is characterized by three axonal events as seen on electron microscopy: rarefaction, coagulation necrosis, and phagocytosis of spheroidal cells by glial elements (Takeichi 1983).
- Administration of phenytoin to newborn mice has been shown to induce damage to the developing cerebellum (Ohmori et al 1992). One experimental study failed to show any changes in cerebellar cortex after phenytoin intoxication (Garcia et al 1984).
- Focal seizures in humans mediate cell injury in the cerebellum by inducing concomitant aberrant discharges with resulting neuroexcitatory-mediated damage. A specific site for binding phenytoin has been identified in the vicinity of Purkinje cells (Hammond and Wilder 1983) and phenytoin has been shown to induce increased firing rates in cerebellar neurons (Julien and Halpern 1972). Seizure-induced neuronal excitability and phenytoin-induced neuronal excitability may act in combination to cause cerebellar atrophy (Ney et al 1994). The question whether phenytoin seizures play a part in the pathogenesis of cerebellar atrophy remains unanswered. Large prospective studies are required to settle this issue.

Management. The following are important considerations in management:
- Early detection of cerebellar disturbances in patients on phenytoin therapy is important because the manifestations such as ataxia reverse

when the drug is stopped whereas in chronic toxicity, cerebellar ataxia is usually considered irreversible (Botez et al 1985). SPECT scan has been shown to detect early abnormalities of rCBF in the cerebellum in epileptic patients on long-term phenytoin therapy and this abnormality is reversed by reduction of dose or discontinuation of the drug (Jibiki et al 1993).
- Periodic monitoring of phenytoin serum levels is important as a guide to prevent neurotoxicity due to high concentrations of the drug.
- Phenytoin should be used with caution in epileptic patients who have evidence of cerebellar atrophy even though they have no clinical manifestations of cerebellar dysfunction.
- Carbamazepine can be considered as an alternative medication in these cases because it has been shown that cerebellar atrophy does not increase susceptibility to carbamazepine neurotoxicity (Specht et al 1994). Although therapeutic blood levels of carbamazepine are not associated with cerebellar toxicity, cerebellar dysfunction has been reported with toxic levels of carbamazepine (Haefeli et al 1994) and as a drug interaction with dextropropoxyphene (Allen 1994).

Tretinoin

Cerebellar hemorrhage has been reported in a patient with acute myelocytic leukemia after treatment with tretinoin (Parma et al 1996). Other cases have been reported indicating the tendency of tretinoin to induce late adverse effects such as thrombohemorrhagic occurrences.

Vaccine

A 5-year old child has been reported to develop an acute cerebellar syndrome 8 days after receiving influenza vaccine (Saito and Yanagisawa 1989). CT scan was normal and CSF examination showed moderate pleocytosis. Symptoms disappeared after 4 months but recurred 33 months later without any obvious precipitating factor and persisted. Cerebellar atrophy was documented by CT and MRI.

The incidence of gait disturbances after measles, mumps and rubella virus vaccine in Denmark since 1987 has been estimated to be 6 per 100,000. There were 24 such cases reported by physicians of which a cerebellar disorder was diagnosed in 3 (Plesner 1995).

References

Abe H, Yagishita S: Chronic phenytoin intoxication occurred below the toxic concentration in serum and its pathological findings. No To Shinkei 1991; 43: 89–94.

Adityanjee: The syndrome of irreversible lithium-effectuated neurotoxicity (SILENT). Pharmacopsychiatry 1989; 22: 81–83.

Ahmed A, Loes DJ, Bressler EL: Reversible magnetic resonance imaging findings in metronidazole-induced encephalopathy. Neurology 1995; 45: 588–589.

Ahnad S: Amiadarone and phenytoin interaction. J Am Geriatr Soc 1995; 43: 1449–1450.

Allen S: Cerebellar dysfunction following dextropropoxyphene-induced carbamazepine toxicity. Postgraduate Medical Journal 1994; 70: 764.

Atkinson K, Biggs J, Darveniza P, et al: Spinal cord and cerebellar-like syndromes associated with the use of cyclosporine in human recipients of allogeneic human bone marrow. Transplant Proc 1985; 17: 1673–1675.

Baier WK, Beck U, Doose H: Cerebellar atrophy following diphenyhydantoin intoxication. Neuropediatrics 1984; 15: 76–81.

Bartels M, Hornung K, Schied HW: Zerebelläre Nebenwirkungen während der Behandlung mit Antidepressiva. Psychiat Prax 1989; 16: 109–112.

Beaudreuil J, Lortholary O, Jarrousse B, et al: Cerebellar toxicity of cytosine-arabinoside in a young man following cerebral anoxia. Ann Med Interne (Paris) 1995; 146(8): 597–8.

Belli LS, De Carlis L, Romani F, et al: Dysarthria and cerebellar ataxia: late occurrence of severe neurotoxicity in a liver transplant recipient. Transpl Int 1993; 6: 176–178.

Benabou R, Carpenter S, Andermann F: Progressive irreversible ataxia after long-term phenytoin therapy (abstract). Neurology 1995; 45(suppl 4): A368.

Benger A, Browman GP, Walker IR: Clinical evidence of a cumulative effect of high dose cytarabine on cerebellum in patients with acute leukemia: a leukemia intergroup report. Cancer Treat Rep 1985; 69: 240–241.

Blumberg EA, Gil RA: Cerebellar syndrome caused by isoniazid. DICP Ann Pharmacother 1990; 24: 829–831.

Boesen P, Fallenborg J, Spaun E: Severe persistent cerebellar dysfunction complicating cytosine arabinoside therapy. Acta Med Scand 1988; 224: 189–191.

Botez MI, Gravel J, Attig E, et al: Reversible chronic cerebellar ataxia after phenytoin intoxication. Neurology 1985; 35: 1152–1157.

Bouget J, Revillon L, Almange C, et al: Syndrome neurologique grave au cours d'un traitement par l'aprindine. Sem Hop Paris 1980; 56: 682–684.

Breiden-Arends C, Gullota F: Diphenylhydantoin, epilepsy, cerebellar atrophy: histological and electron microscopical examinations (German). Fortschr Neurol Psychiatr 1981; 49: 406–414.

Cubo Delgado E, Sanz Boza R, Garcia Urra D, et al: Acute cerebellopathy as a probable toxic effect of flucytosine. Eur J Clin Pharmacol 1997; 51: 505–506.

Diener HC, Dichgans J: Pathophysiology of cerebellar ataxia. Movement Disorders 1992; 7: 95–109.

Dubois A, Raffanel C, Pignodel C, et al: Syndrome cerebelleux aigu associe a une neuropathie sensitive chez un maladie traite par le metronidazole. La Presse Med 1983; 12: 1547–1548.

Dworkin LA, Goldman RD, Zivin LS, et al: Cerebellar toxicity following high dose cytosine arabinoside. J Clin Oncol 1985; 3: 613–616.

Ferbert A, Czernik A: Persistierndes Kleinhirnsyndrom nach Lithium-Intoxikation. Nervenarzt 1987; 58: 764–770.

Ferroir JP, Roger V, Mahieux F, et al: Polyneuritis, convulsive crises, and cerebellar syndrome; complications of treatment with metronidazole (letter in French). Presse Med 1985; 14: 2108.

Garcia HF, Crespo JV, Otero SO, et al: Experimental study of the cerebellar cortex about diphenylhydantoin administration. Arch de Neurobiol 1984; 6: 353–362.

Gessaga E, Ulrich H: The cerebellum of epileptics. Clin Neuropathol 1985; 4: 235–245.

Ghatak NR, Santoso RA, McKinney WM: Cerebellar degeneration following long-term phenytoin therapy. Neurology 1976; 26: 818–820.

Haefeli WE, Meyer PG, Lüscher TF: Circadian carbamazepine toxicity. Epilepsia 1994; 35: 400–402.

Hamano T, Takano A, Miyao S: Reversible adverse effects on the CNS induced by histamine H_2 receptor antagonists. Eur Neurol 1998; 39: 242.

Hammond EJ, Wilder BJ: Immunofluorescent evidence for the specific binding site for phenytoin in the cerebellum. Epilepsia 1983; 24: 269–274.

Hansen HE, Amdisen A: Lithium intoxication. (Report of 23 cases and review of 100 cases from the literature). Q J Med 1978; 47: 123–44.

Hasle H: Cerebellar toxicity during cytarabine therapy associated with renal insufficiency. Cancer Chemother Pharmacol 1990; 27: 76–78.

Heier M, Fossa SD: Neurological manifestations in a phase 2 study of 13 patients treated with doxyfluridine. Acta Neurol Scand 1985; 72: 171–175.

Herzig RH, Hines JD, Herzig GP, et al: Cerebellar toxicity with high dose cytosine arabinoside. J Clin Oncol 1987; 5: 927–932.

Hofstra LS, van der Graaf WT, de Vries EG, et al: Ataxia following docetaxel infusion. Ann Oncol 1997; 8(8): 812–813.

Imamura T, Ejima A, Sahara M, et al: Cerebellar atrophy and persistent cerebellar ataxia after acute intoxication with phenytoin. No To Shinkei 1992; 44(2): 149–153.

Jacome DE: Cerebellar syndrome in lithium poisoning. JNNP 1987; 50: 1722–1724.

Jibiki I, Kido H, Yamaguchi N, et al: Probable cerebellar

abnormality on N-isopropyl-(iodine-123)- p-iodoam-phetamine single photon emission computed tomography scans in an epileptic patient receiving long-term high-dose phenytoin therapy. Neuropsychobiology 1993; 27: 204–209.

Jolson HM, Bosco L, Burt B, et al: Clustering of adverse drug events: analysis of risk factors for cerebellar toxicity with high-dose cytarabine. J Natl Cancer Inst 1992; 84: 500–505.

Julien RM, Halpern LM: Effects of diphenylhydantoin and other antiepileptic drugs on epileptiform activity and Purkinje cell discharge rates. Epilepsia 1972; 13: 387–400.

Katz AA, Hoffman RS, Silverman RA, et al: Phenytoin toxicity from smoking crack cocaine adulterated with phenytoin. Annals of Emergency Medicine 1993; 22: 1485–1487.

Kim JH, Kwon SH, Lee MS, et al: Cerebellar atrophy following long-term anticonvulsant therapy—three cases. J Korean Med Assoc 1991; 34: 1251–1256.

Kleinschmidt-DeMasters BK, Norenberg MD: Cerebellar degeneration in a rat following rapid correction of hyponatremia. Ann Neurol 1981; 10: 561–565.

Koller WC, Glatt SL, Fox JH: Phenytoin-induced cerebellar degeneration. Ann Neurol 1980; 8: 203–204.

Koppel BS, Daras M, Samkoff L: Phenytoin toxicity from illicit use (letter). Neurology 1995; 45: 198.

Kusumi RK, Plouffe JF, Wyatt RH: Central nervous system toxicity associated with metridazole therapy. Ann Int Med 1980; 93: 59–60.

Lewin PK, McGreal D: Isoniazid toxicity with cerebellar ataxia in a child. Can Med Assoc J 1993; 148: 49–50.

Lindwall O, Nilsson B: Cerebellar atrophy following phenytoin intoxication. Ann Neurol 1984; 16: 258–260.

Lopez JA, Agarwal RP: Acute cerebellar toxicity after high dose cytarabine associated with CNS accumulation of its metabolite uracil arabinoside. Cancer Treat Rep 1984; 68: 1309–1310.

Luef G, Marosi M, Felber S, et al: Kleinhirnatrophie und Phenytoinintoxikation. Nervenarzt 1993; 64: 548–551.

Marcoux AW: Carbamazepine-lithium drug interaction. Ann Pharmacother 1996; 30: 547.

Masur H, Fahrendorf G, Oberwittler C, et al: Cerebellar atrophy following acute intoxication with phenytoin. Neurology 1990; 40: 1800.

Masur H, Ludolph AC, Galanski M: Cerebellar atrophy following acute intoxication with phenytoin. Neurology 1989; 39: 432–433.

McCrea ES, Rao CV, Diaconis JN: Roentgenographic changes during long-term diphenylhydantoin therapy. South Med J 1980; 73: 312–317.

McLain LW, Martin JT, Allen JH: Cerebellar degeneration due to chronic phenytoin therapy. Ann Neurol 1980; 7: 18–23.

Meyer-Wahl L: Folensäuremangel als Mitursache für Kleinhirnatrophien. Nervenarzt 1980; 51: 619–622.

Miller L, Link MP, Bologna S, et al: Cerebellar atrophy caused by high-dose cytosine arabinoside; CT and MR findings. AJR 1989; 152: 343–344.

Modestin J, Foglia A: Lithiumintoxikation mit persistier-

enden neurologischen Störungen. Schweiz Med Wschr 1988; 118: 173–176.

Nagaraja D, Taly AB, Sahu RN, et al: Permanent neurological sequelae due to lithium toxicity. Clin Neurol Neurosurg 1987; 89: 31–34.

Naramoto A, Koizumi N, Itoh N, et al: An autopsy case of cerebellar degeneration following lithium intoxication with neuroleptic malignant syndrome. Acta Pathol Japonica 1993; 43: 55–58.

Ney GC, Lantos G, Barr WB, et al: Cerebellar atrophy in patients with long-term phenytoin exposure and epilepsy. Arch Neurol 1994; 51: 767–771.

Nussbaum ES, Maxwell RE, Bitterman PB, et al: Cyclosporine A toxicity presenting with acute cerebellar edema and brainstem compression. J Neurosurg 1995; 82: 1068–1070.

Ohmori H, Kobahashi T, Yasuda M: Neurotoxicity of phenytoin administered to newborn mice on developing cerebellum. Neurotoxicology and Teratology 1992; 14: 159–165.

Parma M, Casaroli I, Pogliani EM: Occurrence of cerebellar thrombohemorrhage during all-trans retinoic acid (ATRA) therapy in case of acute promyelocytic leukemia. Hematologica 1996; 81: 379–380.

Pfadenhauer K, Stapf U: Acute cerebellar syndrome associated with lithium therapy and Q-fever-pneumonia. Lithium 1994; 5: 59–62.

Phillips PC, Reinhard CS: Antipyrimidine neurotoxicity: cytosine arabinoside and 5-fluorouracil. In Rottenberg DA (Ed.): Neurological complications of cancer treatment, Boston, Butterworth, 1991, pp 97–114.

Plaitakis A: 3-acetylpyridine and thiamine deficiency-induced cerebellar models and the pathophysiology of ataxia. In Truillas P, Fuxe K (Eds.): Serotonin, the cerebellum, and ataxia, New York, Raven Press, 1993, pp 269–290.

Plesner A: Gait disturbances after measles, mumps and rubella vaccine. Lancet 1995; 345: 316.

Pulliainen V, Jokelainen M, Hedman C, et al: A case of cerebellar atrophy after phenytoin intoxication: neurologic, neuroradiologic and neuropsychological findings. J Epilepsy 1998; 11: 241–247.

Pumar JM, Villalun J, Martinez de Alegria A, et al: Cerebellar atrophy after protracted phenytoin treatment. Revista Espanola de Neurologia 1995; 10: 201–202.

Puzantian T, Shaw RJ: Nefazadone and symptoms suggesting neurotoxicity. A case report. J Clin Psychiatry 1996; 57: 595.

Rapport RL, Shaw CM: Phenytoin-related cerebellar degeneration without seizures. Ann Neurol 1977; 2(5): 437–439.

Reisberg G, Gershon S: Toxicology and side effects of lithium therapy. In Cooper TB, Gershon S, Kline NS, et al (Eds.): Lithium controversies and unresolved issues. International Congress Series 478, Proceedings of International Lithium Conference, New York, 1978, Amsterdam, Excerpta Medical Publications, 1979, pp 449–478.

Riehl JL, Brown WJ: Acute cerebellar syndrome secondary to 5-fluorouracil therapy. Neurology 1964; 14: 961–967.

Rosich A: Degeneration cerebelosa permanente secundaria a la difenil hidantoina. Med Clin (Barcelona) 1980; 75: 387–390.

Saito H, Yanagisawa T: Acute cerebellar ataxia after influenza vaccination with recurrence and marked cerebellar atrophy. Tohoku J Exp Med 1989; 158: 95–103.

Salcman M, Defendi R, Correll J, et al: Neuropathological changes in cerebellar biopsies of epileptic patients. Ann Neurol 1978; 3: 10–19.

Salinsky MC, Llevine RL, Aubuchon JP, et al: Acute cerebellar dysfunction with high dose ARA-C therapy. Cancer 1983; 51: 426–429.

Schied HW, Bartels M: Transitory cerebellar ataxia from high dosage combination thymoleptic therapy (German). Pharmacopsychiatria 1983; 16: 64–67.

Schneider JA, Mirra SS: Neuropathologic correlates of persistent neurologic deficit in lithium intoxication Ann Neurol 1994; 36: 928–931.

Schou M: Long-lasting neurological sequelae with lithium intoxication. Acta Psychiatr Scand 1984; 70: 594–602.

Schwartz AB, Klausner SC, Yee S, et al: Cerebellar ataxia due to procainamide toxicity. Arch Int Med 1984; 144: 2260–2261.

Selhorst JB, Kaugman B, Horwitz SJ: Diphenylhydantoin-induced cerebellar degeneration. Arch Neurol 1972; 453–455.

Sharma RK, Kumar P, Rai P, et al: Cyclosporin neurotoxicity in a renal transplant recipient. Nephron 1995; 70: 269.

Shimada M, Wakaizumi S, Kasubuchi Y, et al: Cytarabine and its effect on cerebellum of suckling mouse. Arch Neurol 1975; 32: 555–559.

Specht U, Rohde M, Schmidt T, et al: Cerebellar atrophy does not increase susceptibility to carbamazepine toxicity. Acta Neurol Scand 1994; 89: 1–4.

Spielmeyer W: The anatomical substrate of the convulsive state. Arch Neurol Psychiatry 1930; 23: 869–875.

Sylvester RK, Fisher AJ, Lobell L: Cytarabine-induced cerebellar syndrome: case report and literature review. Drug Intell Clin Pharm 1987; 21: 177–180.

Takeichi M: Neurobiological studies of experimental diphenyhydantoin intoxication—III. Electron microscopic studies on development and disintegration mechanism of altered axon terminals and synaptic endings in rat cerebellum with chronic diphenylhydantoin intoxication. Folia Psychiatr Neurol Jpn 1983; 37: 455–464.

Tindall RS, Willerson J: Subacute phenytoin intoxication syndromes. Arch Int Med 1978; 138: 1168–1169.

van Balkom A, van de Wetering BJM, Tavy DLJ, et al: Cerebellar atrophy due to bromisovalum abuse demonstrated by computed tomography. JNNP 1985; 48: 342–347.

van der Burg MEL, Planting AST, Stoter G, et al: Phase I study of DABIS maleate given once every 3 weeks. Eur J Cancer 1991; 27: 1635–1637.

Varona L, Ruiz J, Zarranz JJ: Gait ataxia during omeprazole therapy. Ann Pharmacother 1996; 30: 192.

Victor M, Adams RD, Collins GH: The Wernicke-Korsakoff syndrome and related neurologic disorders due to alcoholism and malnutrition, Philadelphia, FA Davis Co, 1989.

Vogel H, Horoupian DS: Filamentous degeneration of Neurons: a possible feature of cytosine arabinoside neurotoxicity. Cancer 1993; 71: 1303–1308.

Volk B, Kirchgässer N, Detmar N: Degeneration of granule cells following chronic phenytoin administration: an electronmicroscopic investigation of the mouse cerebellum. Exp Neurol 1986; 91: 60–70.

Winkelman MD, Hines JD: Cerebellar degeneration caused by high-dose cytosine arabinoside: a clinicopathological study. Ann Neurol 1983; 14: 520–527.

Yasui N, Otani K, Kanecko S, et al: Carbamazepine toxicity induced by clarithromycin coadministration in psychiatric patients. Int Clin Psychopharmacol 1997; 12: 225–229.

Chapter 16
Drug-Induced Aseptic Meningitis

Introduction

Drug-induced aseptic meningitis (DIAM) is a form of aseptic meningitis—a self-limiting inflammatory disorder involving the leptomeninges without evidence of bacterial or fungal etiology. Viral infection is the usual cause although chemical agents such as drugs may produce the same clinical syndrome. Criteria for diagnosis of aseptic meningitis as a syndrome by Wallgren, the first person who described it, are as follows (Wallgren 1925):

- An acute onset of signs and symptoms of meningeal involvement such as headache, fever, and stiff neck.
- Changes in CSF typical of meningitis, e. g., pleocytosis.
- Absence of bacteria in CSF as demonstrated by culture.
- Short and benign course of the illness; the patient recovers within a matter of days.
- Absence of local parameningeal infection, e. g., otitis media.
- Absence from the community of epidemic diseases of which meningitis is a feature

The etiology of Mollaret's meningitis, a recurrent form of aseptic meningitis, is not clear (Mollaret 1944) (see Neurobase article on this topic). The criteria for the diagnosis of this form of meningitis are similar to those of Wallgren except that Mollaret's meningitis is recurrent and, in the interval between the attacks, the patient is free from symptoms and signs (Frederiks and Bruyn 1989). A case of Mollaret's meningitis has been published where two of the five attacks were drug-induced (Thilmann et al 1991).

The term "hypersensitivity meningitis" was used in the literature, before the term aseptic meningitis was introduced, to describe the meningeal reaction accompanying serum sickness and allergic reactions in a patient following first dose of the second course of sulfathiazole (Longcope 1943). Some of these cases fulfill the present criteria of DIAM. With the increasing recognition of DIAM, several reports and reviews have appeared in the recent literature (Moris and Garcia-Monco 1999).

Causes of Aseptic Meningitis

Causes of aseptic meningitis are shown in Table 16.1.

Table 16.1. Causes of aseptic meningitis.

Viral infections
Neoplastic disease: brain tumors, meningeal carcinomatosis
Systemic diseases
– Immunodeficiency states, e. g., AIDS
– Systemic lupus erythematosus
– Sarcoidosis
– Behcet's disease
– Vogt-Koyanagi-Harada syndrome
– Sjögren's syndrome
– Mixed connective tissue diseases
Defects at base of skull, e. g., posttraumatic CSF fistula
Iatrogenic
– Neurosurgical procedures
– Intrathecal injections of drugs and diagnostic agents
– Drugs

Clinical Features of Aseptic Meningitis

The classical signs of meningitis—headache neck stiffness and fever—are the classical features of aseptic meningitis as well. Other symptoms include photophobia, myalgia, nausea and vomiting. If aseptic meningitis is a part of a neurotoxic reaction to the drug, there may be manifestations other than meningitis. In aseptic meningitis following vaccination, there is evidence of viral infection with associated signs such as parotid swelling in case of MMR vaccine. Convulsions may occur in some children probably associated with viral encephalitis. Some of the variations in clinical presentation will be described along with different categories of drugs inducing aseptic meningitis.

Pathomechanism of Drug-Induced Aseptic Meningitis

The proposed mechanisms of drug-induced aseptic meningitis (DIAM) fall into two categories: hypersensitivity reactions and direct irritation of the meninges. The latter usually involves direct instillation of an agent into the meninges. The circumstantial evidence in favor of a hypersensitivity reaction is the rapid development of symptoms following drug ingestion, progressively shorter periods in recurrent cases, and development of classic features (facial edema, conjunctivitis, pruritus) in some cases. Elevated levels of immune complexes in CSF of patients with DIAM would support the hypersensitivity reaction theory (Chez et al 1989; Gordon et al 1990). Some patients may be able to tolerate a drug initially but develop DIAM on subsequent administration. One explanation is that the drug may behave as a hapten that binds to intravascular proteins, prompting the body's immune system to subsequently recognize those proteins as foreign antigens (Ballas and Donta 1982).

Unlike the hypersensitivity reactions, DIAM due to direct irritation may be delayed up to several weeks following the administration of the drug. The toxicity of the drug or the chemical in the CSF is related to he following criteria:
- Concentration of the drug or the chemical
- Lipid solubility
- Particle size
- Ability to ionize the CSF
- Duration of contact with CSF

Predisposing Factors

The following risk factors can be identified from studying DIAM case reports:
- Patients suffering from autoimmune disorders may be at greater risk for developing DIAM. SLE-like diseased mice have been shown to develop meningitis when treated with ibuprofen whereas disease-free mice did not develop this complication (Berliner et al 1985).
- Patients with deficiency of regulatory protein factor I usually present with pyogenic bacterial infections. This results from the reduced complement-dependent ability of the serum to opsonize and kill bacteria. A case has been reported where deficiency of this factor led to recurrent aseptic meningitis (Bonin et al 1993).
- Patients with AIDS.

Laboratory Findings and Diagnosis

Drug-induced aseptic meningitis (DIAM) should be considered in the differential diagnosis of acute and recurrent aseptic meningitis (Chaudury and Cunha 1991). The peripheral white blood count may be normal or elevated. The following laboratory investigations are recommended:
- The peripheral white blood count may be normal or elevated. A predominance of mononuclear cells in the CSF is characteristic of chronic recurrent meningitis (Wilhelm and Ellner 1986).
- Lumbar puncture usually reveals a high opening pressure. CSF examination shows pleocytosis ranging from a hundred to several thousand cells. The predominant cells are polymorphonuclears but rarely lymphocytic and eosinophilic forms of DIAM have also been reported. Eosinophils in the CSF are characteristic of aseptic meningitis associated with IVIG.
- CSF proteins are usually elevated. CSF culture results are always negative.
- CSF lactic acid levels differentiate aseptic from early purulent meningitis (Bailey et al 1990). DIAM should be suspected in patients

who have a normal CSF lactic acid level and a predominance of polymorphonuclear cells.

In a patient with headache, fever, meningeal signs and CSF results consistent with meningitis, infections should be ruled out as a cause. Diagnosis of DIAM is made by exclusion unless there is clear cut evidence of relationship to the drug.

Magnetic Resonance Imaging. Pathologic meningeal enhancement has been reported in patients with bacterial and viral meningitis. Eustace and Buff (1994) described a 52-year-old woman with drug-induced aseptic meningitis in whom diffuse meningeal enhancement was observed with MRI after administration of gadolinium diethylenediaminepenta-acetic acid. MRI was done in the two cases of trimethoprim-induced aseptic meningitis reported by Blumenfeld et al (1996) which showed diffuse supratentorial white matter abnormalities that cleared up after recovery from meningitis. MRI could be a valuable adjunct diagnostic procedure in DIAM.

Drugs and Chemicals Associated with Aseptic Meningitis

A list of drugs and chemicals reported to be associated with aseptic meningitis is shown in Table 16.2.

Antimicrobial Drug

A complicating factor in antibiotic-associated aseptic meningitis is that some of these patients may have a partially treated bacterial meningitis with negative CSF culture. Trimethoprim/sulfamethoxazole combination is the most frequently reported cause of DIAM.

Sulfonamides. Barrett and Thier (1963) reported a case of aseptic meningitis in a patient receiving sulfamethoxazole. This episode recurred twice after rechallenge. Two other cases were reported by Fisher and Sydney (1939) who experienced headache, stiff neck and fever following administration of sulfanilamide and later devel-

Table 16.2. Drugs and chemicals associated with aseptic meningitis.

Antimicrobial drugs
 – sulfonamides
  • trimethoprim
  • trimethoprim/sulfamethoxazole*
  • sulfasalazine (Alloway and Mitchell 1993; Merrin and Williams 1991)
 – cephalosporin (Creel and Hurtt 1995)
 – ciprofloxacin (Asperilla et al 1989)
 – isoniazid
 – penicillin (River et al 1994)
Antineoplastics (systemic use):cytosine arabinoside
Corticosteroids
 – methylprednisolone acetate
 – hydrocortisone sodium succinate
Non-steroidal anti-inflammatory drugs
 – diclofenac (Codding et al 1991)
 – ibuprofen*
 – naproxen (Sylvia et al 1988)
 – sulindac (Yasuda et al 1989)
 – tolmetin
 – ketoprofen (Roel et al 1991)
 – aspirin overdose (Nair & Stacey 1993)
Intrathecal drugs
 – antineoplastics: cytosine arabinoside and methotrexate
 – antimicrobials
 – baclofen
 – steroids
 – spinal anesthesia
Intrathecal diagnostic agents
 – radiologic contrast media
  • iophendylate
  • metrizamide
 – radiolabelled albumin
Miscellaneous drugs
 – azathioprine
 – carbamazepine (Dang and Riley 1996; Simon et al 1990; Hemet et al 1994)
 – intravenous immunoglobulin*
 – muromonab-CD3*
 – phenazopyridine
 – pyrazinamide
 – ranitidine (Durand and Suchet 1996)
 – vaccines
  • poliomyelitis
  • measles, mumps, and rubella
  • hepatitis B (Heinzlef et al 1997)

* Well documented.

oped encephalomyelitis. A serum sickness-like reaction was described in a patient following first dose of the second course of sulfathiazole (Longcope 1943).

Trimethoprim/Sulfamethoxazole (TMP/SMX). Review of the publications reveals 35 patients

Table 16.3. Aseptic meningitis following trimethoprim and trimethoprim/sulfamethoxazole.

Author and Year	Background Disease	Rechallenge
Auxier 1990	None	yes
Binrdorf & Kaufman 1991	None	yes
Biosca et al 1986	None	yes
Blumenfeld et al 1996, 2 cases	None	no
Carlson & Wiholm 1987, Patient 4	Sjögren's syndrome	yes
Carlson & Wiholm 1987, Patient 1	None	yes
Carlson & Wiholm 1987, Patient 2	SLE	yes
Carlson & Wiholm 1987, Patient 3	Positive rheumatoid factor	yes
Carlson & Wiholm 1987, Patient 5	Multiple allergies	no
Davis et al 1994*	None	yes
de la Monte et al 1985	Sjögren's syndrome	yes
Derbes 1984	Sjögren's syndrome	yes
Escalante & Stimmler 1992	SLE	no
Gilroy et al 1997	None	no
Gordon and Allon 1990	Crohn's disease, migraine	yes
Haas 1984	None	yes
Harrison et al 1994	HIV infection	yes
Hedlund et al 1990	None	yes
Joffe et al 1989, Patient 1	Rheumatoid arthritis	yes
Joffe et al 1989, Patient 2	None	no
Joffe et al 1989, Patient 3	None	no
Jurado et al 1996, 2 patients	None	no
Karlsson M 1986	None	yes
Kremer et al 1983	None	yes
Pashankar et al 1995	Insulin-dependent diabetes mellitus	no
Patey et al 1998	HIV	no
Poles and Theodor 1996	None	yes
River et al 1994 Patient 1	SLE	yes
River et al 1994 Patient 2	None	yes
Rudy and Rutstein 1997	Pneumocystis carinii/AIDS	no
Streifer 1986	None	yes
Tunkel and Starr 1990	None	no
Wahlström et al 1982	None	yes

*This patient had previously developed aseptic meningitis after use of ibuprofen (see Table 16.4).

who developed aseptic meningitis after administration of TMP/SMX or TMP-containing drugs (Table 16.3). This is a fraction of the cases which are reported to various manufacturers of these drugs. Rechallenge was done in 22 of these cases with recurrence of aseptic meningitis. There was a past history of similar reaction to TMP/SMX in a few cases which was not recognized as drug-induced aseptic meningitis. Known risk factors such as autoimmune diseases and HIV infection was present in 13 of these cases.

Sulfasalazine. It is used for the treatment of rheumatoid arthritis and has several CNS adverse effects including aseptic meningitis. In a case reported by Alloway and Mitchell (1993), the reaction occurred 12 days after start of therapy and

subsided the day following discontinuation of sulfasalazine. The patient described by Merrin and Williams (1991) suffered from Sjögren's syndrome and aseptic meningitis developed 3 weeks after start of sulfasalazine therapy. Recovery after discontinuation of drug was followed by recurrence of reaction after rechallenge.

Ciprofloxacin. A case of eosinophilic meningitis has been described following use of ciprofloxacin in a young woman (Asperilla and Smego 1989). Eosinophilic meningitis is quite rare and this subject has been reviewed by Weingarten et al (1985). The pathomechanism of drug-induced eosinophilic meningitis is uncertain but it is presumably an idiosyncratic reaction.

Table 16.4. Cases of ibuprofen-induced aseptic meningitis.

Author and year	Background disease	Rechallenge
Agus et al 1990 – Case 1	Mixed CTD	no
Agus et al 1990 – Case 2	Undifferentiated CTD	yes
Bar Sela et al 1980	Degenerative joint	yes
Bernstein 1980	Mixed CTD	yes
Bouland et al 1986	Osteoarthritis	yes
Chez et al 1989	None	yes
Conoso and Cohen 1975	Migratory polyarthritis	no
Davis et al 1984*	HIV infection	no
Durback et al 1988	Undifferentiated CTD	yes
Ewert 1989	Positive rheumatoid factor	yes
Finch and Strottman 1979	SLE	yes
Giansiracusa et al 1980	SLE	no
Gilbert & Eichenbaum 1989	SLE	no
Grimm and Wolf 1989	SLE	yes
Hoffmann and Gray 1982	Mixed CTD	–
Jensen et al 1987	SLE	yes
Katona et al 1988	SLE	yes
Kindmark et al 1987	None	yes
Lawson and Grady 1985	None	yes
Lee et al 1983	None	no
Mandell et al 1976*	SLE	yes
Mifsud 1988	None	yes
Parera et al 1984	Osteoarthritis	yes
Peck and Joyner 1982	Mixed CTD	–
Quinn et al 1984	None	no
Ruppert and Barth 1981	SLE	yes
Samuelson & Williams 1979	SLE	yes
Treves et al 1983	SLE	yes
van der Zwan & Dam 1992	None	no
Wasner 1978	SLE	yes
Widener and Littman 1978	SLE	yes

SLE = systemic lupus erythematosus, CTD = connective tissue disease.
* This patient also developed aseptic meningitis on a subsequent occasion after administration of trimethoprim/sulfamethoxazole (see Table 16.3).

Cephalosporins. Creel et al (1993) reported a patient with penicillin allergy who had three episodes of aseptic meningitis over a five-year period, each following exposure to a different cephalosporin antibiotic. There was no local or systemic allergic reaction but intrathecal synthesis of specific anti-ceftazidime IgG was demonstrated. River et al (1994) reported a case that had 7 episodes of aseptic meningitis over a period of 7 years and each was preceded by the use of amoxicillin or penicillin. There are other case reports of aseptic meningitis with amoxicillin (Czerwenka et al 1999; Jacobsson and Elowson 1999).

Isoniazid. One case of aseptic meningitis has been described in patient who was given isonia-

zid because of a positive purified protein derivative test for tuberculosis. The patient experienced fever and malaise with nausea and vomiting. The patient recovered after discontinuation of isoniazid but became sick again after resumption of isoniazid with fever and neck stiffness. Lumber puncture showed an elevated CSF pressure, increased neutrophil count, but no pathogenic organisms. The patient was treated with oral steroids and recovered.

Non-Steroidal Anti-Inflammatory Drugs

Non-steroidal anti-inflammatory drugs (NSAID) are used for a large list of indications including rheumatic disorders, chronic pain syndromes, and acute musculoskeletal injuries. The principal mechanism of action of NSAIDs is decreased synthesis of prostaglandins by inhibition of enzyme cyclo-oxygenase. These drugs have anti-inflammatory, analgesic, and antipyretic properties but can also produce adverse effects of which gastric ulceration and renal insufficiency are well known but CNS effects such as aseptic meningitis are less known. Five NSAIDs have been implicated in causing DIAM. This reaction appears to be unrelated to the NSAID chemical class or NSAID-mediated effects. There does not appear to be cross-reactivity of the NSAIDs, because with a few exceptions, many of these patients who develop aseptic meningitis after exposure to one NSAID have been previously and subsequently treated with other NSAIDs without any reaction (Hoppmann et al 1991). Patients with SLE appear to be at greater risk for developing NSAID-induced aseptic meningitis.

Ibuprofen. This is one of the most frequently implicated drug in DIAM. There are 33 cases reported in medical literature and these are listed in Table 16.4. The most common background disease among these patients was SLE (13 cases). Meningitis mostly occurred within weeks of start of therapy but cases have been reported as late as two years after initiation of therapy. The CSF findings in these cases varied greatly. In general there was polymorphonuclear pleocytosis, an elevation in protein concentration, and normal glucose content. Staining and culture of CSF for microorganisms were negative in all cases.

Ibuprofen has been shown to induce aseptic meningitis in a strain of mice which is a model of SLE, whereas none of the unexposed mice showed this reaction (Berliner et al 1985).

Sulindac. Four cases of sulindac-induced aseptic meningitis have been reported. One of these patients had SLE (Ballas and Donta 1982). The symptoms cleared up after discontinuation of the drug and did not recur when aspirin was administered. Another patient with connective tissue disorder tolerated other NSAIDs including ibuprofen but developed recurrent DIAM following sulindac (Greenberg 1988). Yasuda et al (1989) reported a patient with mixed connective tissue disorder who developed aseptic meningitis three days after intake of sulindac. CT scan in the acute stage showed contrast enhancement in the cerebral hemispheres indicating that the BBB was breached due to an acute hypersensitivity reaction with inflammation of the meninges. In the fourth case recurrent DIAM developed in a patient without any evidence of SLE or connective tissue disorder (Von Reyn 1983). In all of these cases any role of prostaglandins in the pathogenesis of DIAM was excluded.

Naproxen. Two cases of DIAM have been reported following use of naproxen. In the first case a healthy young man developed this reaction after use of naproxen for spasm of neck muscles and recovered after discontinuation of naproxen (Sylvia et al 1988). The second case is that of a patients with SLE who experienced three episodes of DIAM after intermittent use of naproxen for two years.

Tolmetin. One case of DIAM following tolmetin has been reported in a young woman with SLE who had a similar reaction previously following ibuprofen (Ruppert and Barth 1981).

Diclofenac. There is one case reported of DIAM in association with diclofenac in a patient with SLE (Codding et al 1991). This patient refused a lumbar puncture as well as a rechallenge. The diagnosis of DIAM was based on temporal association as well as recovery after discontinuation of the drug. Two similar cases (unpublished) have been reported to the manufacturer (Ciba-Geigy Ltd, Basel, personal communication) in patients with rheumatic disorders.

Ketoprofen. There is only one case of aseptic meningitis reported in association with ketoprofen (Roel et al 1991).

Aspirin Overdose. A case of aseptic meningitis due to aspirin overdose has been reported by Nair and Stacy (1993).

Antineoplastics (Systemic Use)

Neurotoxic effects of antineoplastic agents when administered systemically are described in Chapter 3. Cases of DIAM have been reported with systemic use of cytarabine.

Cytarabine. Neurotoxicity of cytarabine is well known. The usual manifestations are cerebellar syndromes, leucoencephalopathy, and peripheral neuropathy. A case of acute cerebellar dysfunction and aseptic meningitis has been described following high-dose systemic Ara-C therapy (Thordarson and Talstad 1986). Another patient has been reported to suffer from recurrent episodes of aseptic meningitis without other signs of neurotoxicity following repeated intravenous infusions of cytarabine for acute lymphoblastic leukemia (Flasshove et al 1992).

Intrathecal Drugs

Antineoplastics. Aseptic meningitis has been described following use of intrathecal methotrexate (Weiss et al 1974). Clinical manifestations occur 2 to 4 hours after intrathecal injection of methotrexate (MTX). Meningism is rarely seen after the first injection but incidence increases with the number of intrathecal injections and is dose-related (Mott et al 1972). Incidence varies from 9.8% (Sullivan et al 1969) to 90% (Naiman et al 1970). No neurological complications were observed in a series of 300 patients where low doses of MTX (10 mg/kg ere used (Mollica et al 1971). Presence of chemical preservatives in the solution for intrathecal injection may contribute to the meningeal reaction.

Intrathecal administration of cytarabine for meningeal leukemia has been associated with CNS toxicity including aseptic meningitis (Band et al 1973). It is usually used in cases where the tumor is resistant to MTX. The symptoms and signs are similar to the aseptic meningitis induced by methotrexate and because its use follows that of MTX, the incidence and predisposing factors are difficult to determine.

Antibiotics. Intrathecal aminoglycosides have been given without significant local reactions although there are reports of neurotoxicity involving loss of hearing and polyradiculitis. A case of aseptic meningitis has been reported following gentamicin (Buckley et al 1977).

Corticosteroids. Intrathecal injections of methylprednisolone acetate have been associated with aseptic meningitis (Sehgal et al 1963; Plumb and Dismukes 1977). Epidural injection of steroids is considered safer but cases of aseptic meningitis have also been reported following this procedure (Gutknecht 1987; Karmochkine et al 1993). It is likely that in these cases subarachnoid space was entered inadvertently.

Spinal Anesthesia. Gibbons (1969) reported three cases of aseptic meningitis in postpartum women following low spinal anesthesia and attributed it to a contamination from use of a detergent to clean the syringes. Papaceit-Vidal et al (1990) reported a case of aseptic meningitis following intradural anesthesia. No cause was found and the symptoms cleared up within 48 hours without treatment.

Intrathecal Baclofen. There is one reported case of aseptic meningitis following intrathecal baclofen; the patient recovered spontaneously (Naveira et al 1996).

Intrathecal Diagnostic Agents

Radiologic Contrast Media. Neurotoxicity of radiological contrast media includes transient encephalopathy, seizures and meningeal reactions (Junck and Marshall 1983). Aseptic meningitis has been reported as a complication of metrizamide myelography (Sand et al 1986; DiMario 1985; Gelmers 1984; Baker et al 1982; Kelley et al 1980). Eosinophilic meningitis has been reported after repeated iophendylate injection myelography (Kalyanaraman 1980). This was considered to be a hypersensitivity reaction and the patient recovered after removal of the residual iophendylate and large doses of corticosteroids.

Radiolabelled Albumin. Aseptic meningitis has also been described following use of intrathecal isotopes for diagnostic purposes. Aseptic meningitis has been described as a complication of scinticisternography utilizing [111]-indium-DTPA (Forster et al 1975) and intrathecal injection of radioiodinated serum albumin (Oldham and Staab 1970; Nicol 1967). Both iodine and albumin might be implicated as causing an "allergic" reaction when injected into the subarachnoid space.

Intraventricular Chemotherapy. Chamberlain and colleagues studied the complications associated with intraventricular chemotherapy via an Ommaya reservoir and intraventricular catheter system in 120 patients with leptomeningeal metastases (Chamberlain et al 1997). Aseptic/chemical meningitis occurred in 52 of the patients.

Miscellaneous Agents

Azathioprine

Patients with SLE have been reported to manifest aseptic meningitis following azathioprine therapy (Sergent and Lockshin 1978).

Carbamazepine

There are three case reports of aseptic meningitis associated with carbamazepine therapy. One of these patients had trigeminal neuralgia and Sjögren's syndrome with recurrent attacks of aseptic meningitis which resolved after discontinuation of carbamazepine (Hilton and Stroh 1989). Two patients received carbamazepine for a bipolar disorder and aseptic meningitis was temporally related to carbamazepine and did not recur after discontinuation of this drug (Simon et al 1990; Hemet et al 1994).

Intravenous Immunoglobulin

In recent years intravenous immunoglobulin (IVIG) has been employed in the treatment of a variety of medical conditions such as idiopathic thrombocytopenic purpura, Guillain-Barré syndrome, dermatomyositis, and Kawasaki's disease. There are 16 published case reports of aseptic meningitis following IVIG (Kato et al 1988; Casteels-Van Daele et al 1990; Watson et al 1991; Vera-Ramirez et al 1992; Pallares and Marshall 1992; Mselati et al 1992; Meiner et al 1993; Rao et al 1993; Mitterer et al 1993; Oddou

et al 1995; Sirvent et al 1996; Shorr and Kester 1996; Gabor 1997; Lafferty et al 1997; Picton and Chisholm 1997; Warrier et al 1997).

Epidemiology. Sekul et al (1994) carried out a retrospective analysis of a prospective cohort study to determine the incidence of aseptic meningitis in patients treated with high dose intravenous immunoglobulin. Six (11%) of 54 patients developed aseptic meningitis within 24 hours after completion of the infusions and lasted 3 to 5 days. In addition to this MEDWatch program of FDA in the USA received 22 reports of aseptic meningitis associated with six different intravenous immunoglobulin products (Scribner et al 1994).

Course. Aseptic meningitis usually appears on the second or the third day of therapy except in the case reported by Kato et al (1988) where the reaction appeared two days after the discontinuation of combined IVIG and steroid therapy. In most of the reported cases IVIG therapy was discontinued after onset of aseptic meningitis but in the case of Mitterer et al (1993), IVIG could not be discontinued because of the low platelet count and risk of life-threatening hemorrhage. Despite continuation of therapy, the symptoms of meningitis cleared up on the 4th day of treatment with IVIG.

Pathomechanism. The mechanism is not well understood but the following hypotheses have been proposed:

– Serum immunoglobulins, particularly IgG, can cross the blood brain barrier (Cutler et al 1970). Breech of blood brain barrier in patients with autoimmune disorders of the CNS may allow entry of the even the high molecular weight IgM into the CSF compartment (Dalakas and Papadopoulos 1984). One of the cardinal features of Guillain-Barré syndrome is the high concentration of protein in the lumbar CSF. The endothelial barriers of the dorsal root ganglia and ventral roots, which already leak more than under normal conditions, become severely damaged and permit the passage of plasma proteins including IVIG (Wurster and Haas 1994).

– The infused IgG is derived from a pool of multiple donors (Newland et al 1991) and is allogenic. Within the CSF, it may react with antigenic determinants on the endothelial cells of the meningeal vasculature, release cytokines, and lead to an inflammatory reaction as evidenced by the pleocytosis in the CSF.

- IVIG-associated aseptic meningitis is presumed to be an acute hypersensitivity reaction limited to the leptomeninges without systemic anaphylaxis.
- Patients with a history of migraine are more likely to develop aseptic meningitis while receiving IVIM and this may be due to increased cerebrovascular sensitivity in migraineurs (Sekul et al 1994).

Muromonoab-CD3 (OKT3)

This monoclonal murine IgG immunoglobulin directed at the T3 receptors of the T-lymphocyte and has been reported to be effective in the treatment of steroid resistant kidney allograft rejection (Thistlewaite et al 1987). Aseptic meningitis was reported in 10 patients following use of OKT3 in a cardiac transplantation program (Adair et al 1991). Emmons et al (1986) reported 4 patients with aseptic meningitis following use of OKT3 after renal transplantation. Marks et al (1991) reported 2 cases one of which developed bilateral optic nerve blindness in addition to aseptic meningitis. Nosocomial aseptic meningitis was described in another 4 patients associated with administration of OKT3 (Martin et al 1988). Other cases of aseptic meningitis in association with OKT3 therapy have been reported by (Rello 1990; Roden et al 1987; Sutton 1989; Thomas et al 1999). Approximately 200 cases of aseptic meningitis have been reported in patients who received OKT3. Patients on this drug should be monitored for symptoms suggestive of meningeal irritation and therapy should be discontinued if such symptoms develop.

Pathogenesis. First dose reaction to OKT3 was originally considered to be idiosyncratic but recurrence with subsequent administration is against this theory. Serum levels of various cytokines are elevated during this reaction and tumor necrosis factor-α (TNF-α) is considered to be the prime mediator (Abramowicz et al 1989).

Phenazopyridine

Herlihy (1987) reported a case of aseptic meningitis in a patient with cancer of prostate following treatment with phenazopyridine. This recurred on rechallenge.

Pyrazinamide

Bodokh et al (1993) have reported a case of aseptic meningitis in a patient with history of SLE who received pyrazinamide for pulmonary tuberculosis. Neurological complication of SLE was ruled out and this reaction was attributed to the drug.

Vaccines

Vaccine-associated poliovirus meningitis has been reported in children with ventriculoperitoneal shunts (Gutriez and Abzug 1990). Aseptic meningitis occurs in 1% of persons infected with wild type of poliovirus but the isolation of vaccine strains of poliovirus from the CSF of the patients reported is unclear. Hypoglobulinemia in one of the patients might have predisposed to the virus-infection of the CNS following oral polio vaccine or the vaccine poliovirus may have exited from the intestinal tract into the peritoneal cavity and ascended via the ventriculoperitoneal shunt into the CSF.

Aseptic meningitis has also been reported after measles, mumps and rubella vaccine (Tesovic et al 1993). A US survey showed the risk of meningitis after mumps vaccination to be 0.4 cases/million doses within 30 days (Anonymous 1984). The incidence in Japan was reported to be higher (Fujinaga et al 1991; Sugiura and Yamada 1991). The differences may be due to methods used to ascertain and define cases. Using active case ascertainment method for adverse event surveillance in the UK, Miller et al (1993) estimated the risk to be 1 /11000 doses. In evaluating the risk, it should be noted that frequency of meningitis in mumps is 1/1000 cases and the risk may be higher during epidemics (Peltola 1993). Fifty-four cases of aseptic meningitis following mumps vaccine were reported to the regional pharmacovigilance centers in France during a 9-year period; this represents a mean incidence of 0.82 cases per 100,000 doses of vaccine (Jonville-Bera et al 1996). Japan introduced the measles-mumps-rubella vaccine in 1989 but withdrew it in 1993 due to a case of aseptic meningitis. This occurred in 1 out of 905 children inoculated (Ueda et al 1995). The rates of virologically confirmed aseptic meningitis in Kimura and colleagues study were 16.6, 11.6, 3.2, and 0 per 10,000 recipients for the standard measles-mumps-rubella, Takeda measles-mumps-rubella, Kitasato measles-mumps-rubella, and Biken measles-mumps-rubella vaccines, respectively (Kimura et al 1996).

The immense benefit of the vaccine should offset a few cases of vaccine-associated meningitis.

Concluding Remarks

Drug-induced aseptic meningitis can occur as an adverse reaction to a wide variety of pharmaceuticals. The course is usually benign and the reaction subsides after discontinuation of the offending agent. There is one case report where DIAM occurred in the same patient in response to two different medications: trimethoprim/sulfamethoxazole and ibuprofen (Davis et al 1994).

Possible pathomechanisms of DIAM are:
– Hypersensitivity reaction
– Mechanical irritation of the meninges.
– Cytokine-mediated reaction.

Patients with underlying collagen vascular or rheumatic disorders are more susceptible to the hypersensitivity type of DIAM. Drugs most often associated with DIAM are:
– Triamethroprim/sulfamethoxazole
– Ibuprofen
– Azathioprine
– Intravenous immunoglobulin
– Muromonoab-CD3

References

Abramowicz D, Schandane L, Goldman M, et al: Release of tumor necrosis factor α, interleukin-2, and interfer-on γ in serum after injection of OKT3 monoclonal antibody in kidney transplant recipients. Transplantation 1989; 47: 606–608.

Adair JC, Woodley SI, O'Connell JB, et al: Aseptic meningitis following cardiac transplantation: clinical characteristics and relationship to immunosuppressive regimes. Neurology 1991; 41: 249–252.

Agus B, Nelson J, Kramer N, et al: Acute central nervous system symptoms caused by ibuprofen in connective tissue disorders. J Rheumatol 1990; 17: 1094–1096.

Alloway JA, Mitchell SR: Sulfasalazine neurotoxicity: a report of aseptic meningitis and a review of literature. J Rheumatol 1993; 20: 409–11.

Alloway JA, Mitchell SR: Sulfasalazine neurotoxicity: a report of aseptic meningitis and a review of literature. J Rheumatol 1993; 20: 409–411.

Anonymous: Mumps prevention. Recommendations of the Immunization Practices Advisory Committee. MMWR 1989; 38: 388–340.

Asperilla MO, Smego R: Eosinophilic meningitis associated with ciprofloxacin. Am J Med 1989; 87: 589.

Auxier GG: Aseptic meningitis associated with administration of tremthroprim and sulfamethoxazole. AJDC 1990; 144: 144–145.

Bailey EM, Domenico P, Cunha BA: Bacterial or viral meningitis? Measuring lactate in CSF can help you know quickly. Postgrad Med 1990; 88: 217–223.

Baker FJ, Gossen G, Bertoni JM: Aseptic meningitis complicating metrizamide myelography. AJNR 1982; 3: 662–663.

Ballas ZK, Donta ST: Sulindac-induced aseptic meningitis. Arch Int Med 1982; 142: 165–166.

Band PR, Holland JF, Bernard J, et al: Treatment of central nervous system leukemia with intrathecal cytocine arabinoside. Cancer 1973; 72: 744–748.

Barrett PVD, Thier SO: Meningitis and pancreatitis associated with sulfamethizole. NEJM 1963; 268: 36–37.

Bar-Sela S, Levo Y, Zeevi D, et al: A lupus-like syndrome due to ibuprofen hypersensitivity. J Rheumatol 1980; 7: 379–380.

Berliner S, Weinberger A, Shoenfeld Y, et al: Ibuprofen may induce meningitis in (NZB X NZW)F_1 mice. Arthr Rheum 1985; 28: 104–107.

Bernstein RF: Ibuprofen-related meningitis in mixed connective tissue disease. Ann Int Med 1980; 92: 206–207.

Biosca M, de la Figuera M, Garcia-Bragado F, et al: Aseptic meningitis due to trimethoprim-sulfamethoxazole. JNNP 1986; 49: 332–333.

Birndorf LB, Kaufman DI: Aseptic meningitis with retinal lischemia due to trimethoprim.sulfamethoxazole. Neuro-ophthalmology 1991; 11: 215–222.

Blumenfeld H, Cha JH, Cudkowicz ME: Trimethoprim and sulfonamide-associated meningoencephalitis with MRI correlates. Neurology 1996; 46: 556–8.

Bodokh I, Lacour JP, Costa I, et al: Meningite aseptique sous pyrazinamide lors de lupus erythemateux. La Presse Med 1993; 22: 595–596.

Bonin AJ, Zeitz HJ, Gewurz A: Complement Factor I deficiency with recurrent aseptic meningitis. Arch Int Med 1993; 153: 1380–1383.

Bouland DL, Specht NL, Hegstad DR: Ibuprofen and aseptic meningitis. Ann Int med 1986; 104: 731.

Buckley RM, Watters W, MacGregor RR: Persistent meningeal inflammation associated with intrathecal gentamycin. Am J Med Sc 1977; 274: 207–209.

Canoso JJ, Cohen AS: Aseptic meningitis in systemic lupus erythematosus. Arthr Rheum 1975; 18: 369–374.

Carlson J, Wiholm B: Trimethoprim associated with menaingitis. Scand J Infect Dis 1987; 19: 687–691.

Casteels-Van Daele M, Wijndaele L, Hunnick K: Intravenous immune globulin and acute aseptic meningitis. NEJM 1990; 323: 614–615.

Chamberlain MC, Kormanik PA, Barba D: Complications associated with intraventricular chemotherapy in patients with leptomeningeal metastases. J Neurosurg 1997; 87: 694–9.

Chaudury HJ, Cunha BA: Drug-induced aseptic meningitis. Postgrad Med 1991; 90: 65–70.

Chez M, Sila CA, Ransohoff RRM, et al: Ibuprofen-induced meningitis. Neurology 1989; 39: 1578–1580.

Codding C, Targoff IN, McCarty GA: Aseptic meningitis in associationl with diclofenac treatment in a patient with systemic lupus erythematosus. Athr Rheum 1991; 34: 1340–1341.

Creel GB, Hurtt M: Cephalosporin-induced recurrent aseptic meningitis. Ann Neurol 1995; 37: 815–7.

Creel JB, Sullican T, Hurtt M: Cryptogenic aseptic meningitis due to cephalosporin allergy (abstract). Neurology 1993; 43: A253.

Cutler RW, Watters GV, Hammerstad JP: The origin and turnover rates of cerebrospinal fluid albumin and γ globulin in man. J Neurol Sci 1970; 10: 259–268.

Czerwenka W, Gruenwald C, Conen D: Aseptic meningitis after treatment with amoxicillin. BMJ 1999; 318(7197): 1521.

Dalakas MC, Papadopoulos NM: Paraproteins in the spinal fluid of patients with paraproteinemic polyneuropathies. Ann Neurol 1984; 15: 590–593.

Dang CT, Riley DK: Aseptic meningitis secondary to carbamazepine therapy. Clin Infect Dis 1996; 22: 729–730.

Davis BJ, Thompson J, Peimann A, et al: Drug-induced aseptic meningitis caused by two medications. Neurology 1994; 44: 984–985.

de la Monte SM, Hutchins GM, Gupta PK: Aseptic meningitis, trimethoprim, and Sjögren's syndrome. JAMA 1985; 253: 2192.

Derbes SJ: Trimethoprim-induced aseptic meningitis. JAMA 1984; 252: 2865.

DiMario FJ: Aseptic meningitis secondary to metrizamide lumbar myelography in a 4 1/2-month-old infant. Pediatrics 1985; 76: 259–262.

Durand JM, Suchet L: Ranitidine and aseptic meningitis. BMJ 1996; 312: 886.

Durback MA, Freeman J: Recurrent ibuprofen-induced aseptic meningitis. Arthrit Rheum 1988; 31: 813–815.

Einarsson O, Andersson J, Sigstedt B: Upprepad meningit och perimyokardit efter intag av trimethoprim. Läkartidningen 1982; 79: 4854.

Emmons C, Smith J, Flanagan M: Cerebrospinal fluid inflammation during OKT3 therapy. Lancet 1986; 2: 510–511.

Escalante A, Stimmler MM: Trimethoprim-sulfamethoxazole induced meningitis in Systemic Lupus Erythematosus. J Rheumatol 1992; 19: 800–802.

Eustace S, Buff B: Magnetic resonance imaging in drug-induced meningitis. Can Assoc Radiol J 1994; 45(6): 463–465.

Ewert BH: Ibiprofen-associated meningitis in a woman with only serologic evidence of a rheumatologic disorder. Am J Med Sci 1989; 297: 326–327.

Finch WR, Strottman MP: Acute adverse reactions to ibuprofen in systemic lupus erythematosus. JAMA 1979; 241: 2616–2618.

Fisher JH, Sydney MB: Encephalomyelitis following administration of sulfanilamide. Lancet 1939; 1: 301–305.

Flasshove M, Schütte HJ, Kellner R, et al: Meningeal fluid granulocytosis after cytarabine. Eur J Cancer 1992; 28: 243.

Forster G, Sacks S, Christoff N: Aseptic meningitis as a complication of scinticysternography utilising [111]indium-DTPA. Clin Neurol Neurosurg 1975; 4: 289–292.

Frederiks JAM, Bruyn GW: Mollaret's meningitis. In McKendall RR (Ed.): Viral disease. Vol 12(56) of Handbook of Clinical Neurology, Amsterdam, Elsevier Science Publishers, 1989, pp 627–635.

Fujinaga T, Motegi Y, Tamura H, et al: A perfecture-wide survey of mumps meningitis associated with measles, mumps, and rubella vaccine. J Pediatr Infect Dis 1991; 10: 204–209.

Gabor EP: Meningitis and skin reaction after intravenous immune globulin therapy (letter). Ann Intern Med 1997; 127: 1130.

Garagusi VF, Neefe LI, Mann O: Acute meningoencephalitis: association with isoniazid administration. JAMA 1976; 235: 1141–1142.

Gelmers HJ: Exacerbation of systemic lupus erythematosus, aseptic meningitis and acute mental symptoms, following metrizamide lumbar myelography. Neuroradiology 1984; 26: 65–66.

Giansiracusa DF, Blumber S, Kantrowitz FG: Aseptic meningitis associated with ibuprofen. Arch Int Med 1980: 140: 1553.

Gibbons RB: Chemical meningitis following spinal anesthesia. JAMA 1969; 210: 900–902.

Gilbert GJ, Eichenbaum HW: Ibuprofen-induced meningitis in an elderly patient with systemic lupus erythematosus. South Med J 1989; 82: 514–515.

Gordon MF, Allon M, Coyle PK: Drug-induced meningitis. Neurology 1990; 40: 163–164.

Greenberg GN: Recurrent sulindac-induced aseptic meningitis in a patient tolerant to other non-steroidal anti-inflammatory drugs. South J med 1988; 81: 1463–1464.

Grimm AM: Aseptic meningitis associated with non-prescription ibuprofen use. Ann Pharmacother 1989; 23: 712.

Gutknecht DR: Chemical meningitis following epidural injection of corticosteroids. Am J Med 1987; 82: 570.

Gutriez K, Abzug MJ: Vaccine-associated poliovirus meningitis in children with ventriculoperitoneal shunts. J Pediatr 1990; 117: 424–427.

Haas EJ: Trimethoprim-sulfamethoxazole: another cause of recurrent meningitis. JAMA 1984; 252: 346.

Hedlund J, Aurelius E, Andersson J: Recurrent encephalitis due to trimthroprim intake. Scand J Infect Dis 1990; 22: 109–112.

Heinzlef O, Moguilewski A, Roullet E: Acute aseptic meningitis after hepatitis B vaccination (letter). Presse Med 1997; 26: 328.

Hemet C, Chassagne P, Levade MH, et al: Aseptic meningitis secondary to carbamazepine treatment of manic-depressive illness. Am J Psychiatry 1994; 151: 1393.

Herlihy TE: Phenazopyridine and aseptic meningitis. Ann Int Med 1987; 106: 172–173.

Hilton E, Stroh EM: Aseptic meningitis associated with administration of carbamazepine. J Infect Dis 1989; 159: 363–364.

Hoffman M, Gray RG: Ibuprofen-induced meningitis in mixed connective tissue disease. Clin Rheumatol 1982; 1: 128–130.

Hoppmann RA, Peden JG, Ober SK: Central nervous system side effects of nonsteroidal anti-inflammatory drugs. Aseptic meningitis, psychosis, and cognitive dysfunction. Arch Intern Med 1991; 151: 1309–13.

Horn AC, Jarrett SW: Ibuprofen-induced aseptic meningitis in rheumatoid arthritis. Ann Pharmacother 1997 Sep; 31(9): 1009–11.

Jacobsson G, Elowson S: Amoxicillin caused aseptic meningoencephalitis. Lakartidningen 1999; 96(3): 201–202

Jensen S, Glud TK, Bacher T, et al: Ibuprofen-induced meningitis in a male with systemic lupus erythematosus. Acta Med Scand 1987; 221: 509–511.

Joffe AM, Farley JD, Linden D, et al: Trimethoprim-sulfamethoxazole-associated aseptic meningitis: case reports and review of the literature. Am J Med 1989; 87: 322–338.

Jonville-Bera AP, Autret E, Galy-Eyraud C, et al: Aseptic meningitis following mumps vaccine. Pharmacoepidemiol Drug Safety 1996; 5: 33–37.

Junck L, Marshall WH: Neurotoxicity of radiological contrast agents. Ann Neurol 1983; 13: 469–484.

Kalyanaraman K: Eosinophilic meningitis after repeated iophendylate injection myelography. Arch neurol 1980; 37: 602.

Karlsson M: Meningitsymptom efter medicinering med trimethoprim. Läkartidningen 1986; 83: 2666–2667.

Karmochkine M, Chaibi P, Rogeux O, et al: Meningite chimique simulant une meningite infectieuse apres infiltration intradurale de corticoides. La Presse Med 1993; 22: 82.

Kato E, Shindo S, Eto Y, et al: Administration of immune globulin associated with aseptic meningitis. JAMA 1988; 259: 3269–3271.

Katona BG, Wigley FM, Walters JK, et al: Aseptic meningitis from over-the-counter ibuprofen. Lancet 1988; 1: 59.

Kelley RE, Daroff RB, Sheremata WA, et al: Unusual effects of metrizamide lumbar myelography. Arch Neurol 1980; 37: 588–589.

Kimura M, Kuno-Sakai H, Yamazaki S, et al: Adverse events associated with MMR vaccines in Japan. Acta Paediatr Jpn 1996; 38: 205–11.

Kindmark CO, Carlsson IU, Hedbäck B, et al: Aseptik meningit efter behandling med ibuprofen. Läkartidningen 1987; 84: 2782–2783.

Kremer I: Aseptic meningitis as an adverse effect of cotrimoxazole. NEJM 1983; 308: 1481.

Lafferty TE, DeHoratius RJ, Smith JB: Aseptic meningitis as a side effect of intravenous immune γ globulin (letter). J Rheumatol 1997; 24: 2491–2492.

Lawson JM, Grady MJ: Ibuprofen-induced aseptic meningitis in a previously healthy patient. West J Med 1985; 143: 386–387.

Lee RP, King EG, Russel AS: Ibuprofen: a severe systemic reaction. Canad Med Assoc J 1983; 129: 854–855.

Longcope WT: Serum sickness and analogous reactions from certain drugs particularly the sulfonamides. Medicine 1943; 22: 251–286.

Mandell B, Slen HS, Hepburn B: Fever from ibuprofen in a patient with lupus erythematosus. Ann Int Med 1976; 85: 209–210.

Mandell BF, Raps EC: Severe systemic hypersensitivity reaction to ibuprofen occurring after prolonged therapy. Am J Med Sci 1987; 82: 817–820.

Marks WH, Perkel M, Lorber MI: Aseptic encephalitis and blindness complicating OKT3 therapy. Clin transplantation 1991; 5: 435–438.

Martin MA, Massanari M, Nghiem DD, et al: Nosocomial aseptic meningitis associated with administration of OKT3. JAMA 1988; 259: 2002–2005.

Meiner Z, Ben-Hur T, River Y, et al: Aseptic meningitis as a complication of intravenous immunoglobulin therapy for myasthenia gravis. JNNP 1993; 56: 830–831.

Merrin P, Williams IA: Meningitis associated with sulfasalazine in a patient with Sjögren's syndrome and polyarthritis. Ann Rheum Dis 1991; 50: 645–646.

Mifsud AJ: Drug-related recurrent meningitis. J Infect 1988; 17: 151–153.

Miller E, Goldacre M, Pugh S, et al: Risk of aseptic meningitis after measles, mumps, and rubella vaccine in UK children. Lancet 1993; 341: 979–982.

Mitterer M, Pescosta N, Vogelseder W, et al: Two episodes of aseptic meningitis during intravenous immunoglobulin therapy of idiopathic thrombocytopenic purpura. Ann Hematol 1993; 67: 151–152.

Mollaret MP: La meningite endothelio-leucocytaire multirecurrente benigne syndrome nouveau ou maladie nouvelle. Rev Neurol 1944; 76: 57–76.

Mollica F, Drake JC, Chabner BA: Neurotoxicity and elevated cerebrospinal fluid methotrexate concentration in meningeal leukemia. Lancet 1971; ii: 771.

Moris G, Garcia-Monco JC: The challenge of drug-induced aseptic meningitis. Arch Intern Med 1999; 159(11): 1185–1194

Mott MG, Stevenson P, Wood CBS: Methotrexate meningitis. Lancet 1972; 2: 656.

Mselati JC, Carlier JC, Routon MC, et al: Immunoglobulines intraveineuses et meningite aseptique. Arch Fr Pediatr 1992; 49: 215.

Naiman JN, Rupprecht LM, Tanyeri G, et al: Intrathecal methotrexate. Lancet 1970; i: 571.

Nair J, Stacy M: Aseptic meningitis associated with salicylate abuse. Psychosomatics 1993; 34: 372.

Naveira FA, Speight KL, Rauck RL, et al: Meningitis after injection of intrathecal baclofen. Anesth Analg 1996; 82: 1297–1299.

Newland AC, Macy MG, Veys PA: Intravenous immunoglobulin mechanisms of action and their clinical application. In Imbach P (Ed.): Immunotherapy with intravenous immunoglobulins, London, Academic Press, 1991, pp 15–25.

Nicol CF: A second case of aseptic meningitis following isotope cisternography using I[131] human serum albumin. Neurology 1967; 17: 199–200.

Oddou S, Molinier S, Coso D, Boulet JM, et al: Aseptic meningitis following treatment with immunoglobulins: physiopathological and prognostic value of screening. Presse Med 1995; 24(19): 916.

Oldham RK, Staab EV: Aseptic meningitis following intrathecal injection of radioiodinated serum albumin. Radiology 1970; 97: 317–321.

Pallares DE, Marshall GS: Acute aseptic meningitis associated with administration of intravenous immune globulin. Am J Pediatr Hematol Oncol 1992; 14: 279–281.

Papaceit-Vidal JP, Linares Gil MJ, del Morai MV: Meningitis aseptica tras anestesia intradural. Rev Esp Anestesiol Reanim 1990; 37: 153–155.

Patey O, Lacheheb A, Dellion S, et al: A rare case of cotrimoxazole-induced eosinophilic aseptic meningitis in an HIV-infected patient. Scand J Infect Dis 1998; 30(5): 530–531.

Peck MG, Joyner PU: Ibuprofen-associated aseptic meningitis. Clin Pharm 1982; 1: 561–565.

Peltola H: Pumps vaccination and meningitis (commentary). Lancet 1993; 341: 994–995.

Perera DR, Seifert AK, Greely HM: Ibuprofen and meningoencephalitis. Ann Int Med 1984; 100: 619.

Picton P, Chisholm M: Aseptic meningitis associated with high dose immunoglobulin: case report. BMJ 1997; 315: 1203–1204.

Plumb VJ, Dismukes WE: Chemical meningitis related to intrathecal corticosteroid therapy. South Med J 1977; 70: 1241–1243.

Quinn JP, Weinstein RA, Caplan LR: Eosinophilic meningitis and ibuprofen therapy. Neurology 1984; 34: 108–109.

Rao SP, Teitlbaum J, Miller ST: Intravenous immune globulin land aseptic meningitis. AJDC 1992; 146: 539–540.

Rello J: Aseptic meningitis associated with muromonab-CD3. DICP Ann Pharmacother 1990; 34: 1233.

River Y, Averbuch-Heller, Weinberger M, et al: Antibiotic-induced meningitis. JNNP 1994; 57: 705–708.

Roden J, Klintmalm GB, Husberg BS, et al: Cerebrospinal fluid inflammation during OKT3 therapy. Lancet 1987; 2: 272.

Roel JE, Gadano AC, Falcon JL: Ketoprofeno y meningitis aseptica. Medicina 1991; 51: 186.

Ruppert GB, Barth WF: Ibuprofen hypersensitivity in systemic lupus erythematosus. South Med J 1981: 74: 241–243.

Ruppert GB, Barth WF: Tolmetin-induced aseptic meningitis. JAMA 1981a: 245: 67–68.

Samuelson CO, Williams HJ: Ibuprofen-associated meningitis in systemic lupus erythematosus. West J Med 1979; 131: 57–59.

Sand T, Anda S, Hellum K, et al: Chemical meningitis in metrizamide myelography. Neuroradiology 1986; 28: 69–71.

Scribner CL, Kapit RM, Phillips ET, et al: Aseptic meningitis and intravenous immunoglobulin therapy. Annals of Internal Medicine 1994; 121: 305–306.

Sehgal AD, Tweed DC, Gardner WJ, et al: Laboratory studies after intrathecal corticosteroids. Arch Neurol 1963; 9: 74–78.

Sekul EA, Cupler EJ, Dalakas MC: Aseptic meningitis associated with high-dose intravenous immunoglobulin therapy: frequency and risk factors. Annals of Internal Medicine 1994; 121: 259–262.

Sergent J, Lockshin M: Azathioprine-induced meningitis in systemic lupus erythematosus. JAMA 1978; 240: 529.

Shorr AF, Kester KE: Meningitis and hepatitis complicating intravenous immunoglobulin therapy. Ann Pharmacother 1996; 30: 1115–6.

Simon LT, Hsu B, Adornato BT: Carbamazepine-induced aseptic meningitis. Ann Int Med 1990; 112: 627–628.

Sirvent N, Monpoux F, Benet L, et al: Aseptic meningitis during treatment with immunoglobulins (letter). Arch Pediatr 1996; 3: 830–1.

Sonnenblick M, Abraham AS: Ibuprofen hypersensitivity in systemic lupus erythematosus. BMJ 1978; 1: 619–620.

Streiffer RH, Hudson JG: Aseptic meningitis and trimethoprim-sulfamethoxazole. J Family Practice 1986; 23: 314.

Sugiura A, Yamada A: Aseptic meningitis as a complication of mumps vaccination. J Pediatr Infect Dis 1991; 10: 209–213.

Sullivan MP, Vieti TJ, Fernbach DJ, et al: Clinical investigations in the treatment of meningeal leukemia: radiation therapy regime versus conventional intrathecal methotrexate. Blood 1969; 45: 189–194.

Sutton JD: Aseptic meningitis associated with CD3 administration. DICP Ann Pharmacother 1989; 23: 257.

Sylvia LM, Forlenza SW, Brocavich JM: Aseptic meningitis associated with naproxen. Drug Intell Clin Pharm 1988; 22: 399–401.

Tesovic G, Begovac J, Bace A: Aseptic meningitis after measles, mumps, and rubella vaccine. Lancet 1993; 341: 1541.

Thilman AF, Möbius E, Thilmann RR, et al: Rezidivierende aseptische Meningitis (Mollaret-Meningitis) spontanes und Medikamentös induziertes Auftreten. Fortschr Neurol Psychiat 1991; 59: 493–497.

Thistlewaite JR, Gaber AO, Haag BW, et al: OKT3 treatment of steroid resistant renal allograft rejection. Transplantation 1987; 43: 176–183.

Thomas MC, Walker R, Wright A: HaNDL syndrome after "benign" OKT3-induced meningitis. Transplantation 1999; 67(10): 1384–5.

Thordarson H, Talstad I: Acute meningitis and cerebellar dysfunction complicating high-dose cytosine arabinoside therapy. Acta Med Scand 1986; 220: 493–495.

Treves R, Gastine H, Richard A, et al: *Responsabillite de l'ibuprofen dans une meningite aseptique et une insuffisance renale aigue au cours d'un lupus erythemateux dissemine. Rev Rhum 1983; 50: 75–76.

Tunkel AR, Starr K: Trimethoprim-sulfamethoxazole-associated aseptic meningitis. Am J Med 1990; 88: 696.

Ueda K, Miyazaki C, Hidaka Y, et al: Aseptic meningitis caused by measles-mumps-rubella vaccine in Japan. Lancet 1995; 346: 701–2.

van der Zwan A, van Dam JG: Ibuprofen meningitis. Ned Tijdschr Geneeskd 1992; 136: 1613–1614.

Vera-Ramirez M, Charlet M, Parry GJ: Recurrent aseptic meningitis complicating intravenous immunoglobulin therapy for chronic inflammatory demyelinating polyradiculoneuropathy. Neurology 1992; 42: 1636–1637.

von Reyn CF: Recurrent aseptic meningitis due to sulindac. Ann Int Med 1983; 99: 343–344.

Wahlström B, Nyström-Rosander C, Aberg H, et al: Recurrent meningitis and perimyocarditis after trimethoprim. Läkartidningen 1982; 79: 4854–4855 (in Swedish).

Wallgren A: Die Ätiologie der Enkephalomeningitis bei Kindern besonders des Syndromes der akuten abakteriellen (aseptischen) Meningitis. Acta Paediatrica 1951; 40: 541–565.

Wallgren A: Une nouvelle maladie infectieuse du systeme nerveux central? Acta Pediatr Scand 1925; suppl 14: 158–182.

Warrier I, Bussel JB, Valdez L, et al: Safety and efficacy of low-dose intravenous immune globulin (IVIG) treatment for infants and children with immune thrombocytopenic purpura. Low-Dose IVIG Study Group. J Pediatr Hematol Oncol 1997; 19: 197–201.

Wasner CK: Ibuprofen meningitis and systemic lupus erythematosus. J Rheumatol 1978: 5: 162–164.

Watson JD, Ginson J, Joshua DE, et al: Aseptic meningitis with high-dose intravenous immunoglobulin therapy. JNNP 1991; 54: 275–276.

Weingarten JS, O'Sheal SF, Margolis WS: Eosinophilic meningitis with hypereosinophilic syndrome. Am J Med 1985; 78: 674–676.

Weiss HD, Walker MD, Wiernik PGH: Neurotoxicity of commonly used antineoplastic drugs. NEJM 1974; 291: 75–81.

Weksler BB, Lehany AM: Naloxen-induced recurrent aseptic meningitis. DICP Ann Pharmacother 1991; 25: 1183–1184.

Widener HJ, Littman BH: Ibuprofen-induced meningitis in systemic lupus erythematosus. JAMA 1978; 239: 1062–1064.

Wilhelm C, Ellner JJ: Chronic meningitis. Neurol Clin 1986; 4: 115–141.

Wurster U, Haas J: Passage of intravenous immunoglobulin and interaction with the CNS. JNNP 1994; 57 (suppl): 21–25.

Yasuda Y, Akiguchi I, Kameyama M: Sulindac-induced aseptic meningitis in mixed connective tissue disease. Clin Neurol Neurosurg 1989; 91: 257–260.

Chapter 17
Drug-Induced Benign Intracranial Hypertension

Introduction

The clinical syndrome of benign raised intracranial pressure without a space-occupying lesion was first recognized in 1897 by Quincke who had already discovered lumbar puncture. Subsequently various terms have been used for this condition:
- Otitic hydrocephalus
- Pseudotumor cerebri (Nonne 1904)
- Benign intracranial hypertension (Foley 1955)
- Idiopathic intracranial hypertension (Buchheit et al 1969)

The term benign intracranial hypertension (BIH) is the most frequently used of the above. The syndrome as defined by Foley (1955) is one of prolonged raised intracranial pressure without ventricular enlargement or focal neurological signs or disturbances of consciousness and intellect. Sorensen et al (1986) have pointed out that the term "benign" may be misleading as five of their series of 20 patients with BIH had persistent intellectual impairment. The most frequent symptoms are headaches and diplopia, and impairment of visual acuity. Papilledema and bilat-

Table 17.1. Diagnostic criteria of benign intracranial hypertension (from Radakrishnan et al 1994).

Signs and symptoms of raised intracranial pressure
No localizing neurological signs in an awake and
  alert patient except for abducent palsy
Documented elevation of intracranial pressure
  (> 250 mm H$_2$O)
Normal CSF composition
Normal neuroimaging studies except for small
  ventricles and empty sella turcica

---

eral abducent nerve palsies are the only signs. BIH may occur without headache (Smith 1985) and papilledema (Marcelis and Silberstein 1991). Diagnostic criteria of BIH are as shown in Table 17.1.

The incidence of BIH is 1 to 2 per 100,000 per year in the general population (Durcan et al 1988). It is more common in the females than in the males by a factor of 3:1. In the high risk group of obese females in the reproductive age group, the annual incidence rises to 19 to 21 per 100,000 (Radakrishnan et al 1993).

Pathophysiology of Benign Intracranial Hypertension

Obese women in the childbearing period are at risk for developing BIH. Factors associated with causation of BIH are shown in Table 17.2.

Obesity is considered to be an important cause. Increased intraabdominal pressure associated with central obesity is the probable etiology of benign intracranial hypertension. This concept is the basis for gastric plication to educe obesity which has been shown to have a much higher rate of success than CSF-peritoneal shunting procedure (Sugerman et al 1999).

The syndrome may appear de novo in otherwise healthy persons. Several explanations have been considered for the pathophysiology of BIH. These include the following (Fishman 1992):
- An increased rate of CSF formation
- Sustained increase in intracranial venous pressure
- A decreased rate of CSF absorption by arachnoid villi apart from venous occlusive disease

Table 17.2. Factors associated with the causation of BIH.

Cranial venous outflow disturbances
  – intracranial: lateral or superior sagittal sinus throm-
    bosis
  – extracranial: head and neck surgery
  – venous hypertension: cardiac failure, respiratory
    disease
Endocrine disorders
  – menstrual irregularities with obesity
  – adrenal insufficiency (Addison's disease)
  – corticosteroid excess (Cushing's syndrome)
  – pituitary disorders
  – hypothyroidism
Hematological disorders
  – iron deficiency anemia
  – pernicious anemia
  – polycythemia rubra vera
  – thrombocytopenia
  – paroxysmal nocturnal hemoglobinuria
  – myeloma
Obesity
Drugs
Miscellaneous
  – HIV infection
  – systemic lupus erythematosus
  – antiphospholipid antibodies

Table 17.3. Drug-related acute intracranial hypertension.

Ketamine as an anesthetic (Fontana et al 1980)
Nalidixic acid for urinary infection (Granström 1984)
Intravenous nitroglycerine for hypertension
  (Ohar et al 1985)
Suxamethonium in patients with brain tumors
  (Stirt et al 1987)
Sodium nitroprusside for hypertension
  (Grisvold et al 1981)
Urapadil for hypertension in head injury
  (Singbartl et al 1990)

– Increase in brain volume because of an increase in cerebral blood volume or interstitial
fluid.

Histological evidence for cerebral edema in
brain biopsy specimens taken at time of surgical
decompression for BIH was provided by Sahs
and Joynt (1956). This is not a constant finding
because Wall et al (1995) have reported two
patients with BIH who died unexpectedly and
no evidence of cerebral edema was seen at autopsy.

Drug-Induced Benign
Intracranial Hypertension
(BIH)

BIH is not always diagnosed as such in adverse
drug reaction reports. Often the presenting
symptom headache and the presenting sign papilledema are reported. Acute rise of intracranial
pressure following drug therapy has been reported in situations listed in Table 17.3.

The mechanism of rise of intracranial pressure
in the above cases is not known. Some of the
drugs used for lowering blood pressure by vasodilatation may have contributed to the rise of intracranial pressure. Only one of the above,
nalidixic acid, is associated with BIH as well.

Suxamethonium has been considered to be
contraindicated in neurosurgical anesthesia because of its potential of increasing intracranial
pressure. However, a recent study demonstrated
that suxamethonium did not alter cerebral blood
flow velocity, cortical activity, or intracranial
pressure in patients with brain injury (Kovarik et
al 1994).

Griffin (1992) published an exhaustive review
of the subject including unpublished case reports
from the data banks of Hoffmann La Roche, Basel and the Committee for Safety of Medicines
of UK. Askmark et al (1989) reviewed the data
of WHO and found 162 cases of drug-related
BIH reported during a period from 1972 to 1987.
The ten most frequently reported drugs were:
– minocycline
– isoretinoin
– nalidixic acid
– tetracycline
– trimethoprim-sulfamethoxazole
– cimetidine
– prednisolone
– methylprednisolone
– tamoxifen
– beclomethasone

This list does not correspond with the results of
review of the literature on this subject as shown
in Table 17.4.

Table 17.4. Drugs reported to be associated with BIH.

Amiadarone*
Amphotericin
Aspirin
Chorionic gonadotrophins
Ciprofloxacin
Corticosteroids* (withdrawal)
Cyclosporine
Cytosine arabinoside
Danazol*
Growth hormone*
Insulin-like growth factor-1
Lithium*
Minocycline*
Nalidixic acid*
Nitrofurantoin
Non-steroidal anti-inflammatory drugs (NSAID)*
Oral contraceptives
Perhexiline
Phenytoin
Quinagolide
Retinoids*
Sulfonamides
Tetracycline*
Thyroid preparations
Vaccination: DPT
Vitamin A (excess and deficiency)*

*Well documented. Evidence for the other drugs consists of isolated case reports, and a causal relationship has not been established.

Pathogenesis of Drug-Induced Benign Intracranial Hypertension

In addition to the general factors in the etiology of BIH, the following drug-related factors have been considered:

- Hypovitaminosis can reduce CSF absorption due to interstitial fibrosis of the meninges
- Hypervitaminosis A through increase of CSF production
- Lithium-induced inhibition of Na$^+$, K$^+$, and AT-Pase pump at arachnoid villi interferes with vitamin A transport leading to hypervitaminosis A
- Effect on cyclic AMP at arachnoid villi: lithium and tetracycline
- Intracranial infusion of arginine vasopressin leads to rise of intracranial pressure and reduces CSF absorption and may be a factor in the etiology of BIH (Seckl and Lightman 1991)

- Genetic susceptibility may predispose to development of drug-induced BIH

Amiodarone

Amiodarone has been reported to induce BIH (Fikkers et al 1986; Van Zandijcke and Dewachter 1986; Grogan and Narkun 1987). Acute intracranial hypertension has also been reported during amiodarone infusion which may be explained by the vasodilator effect of the drug (Lopez et al 1985).

Amphotericin

Intravenous amphotericin given for cryptococcal infection has been reported to induce BIH in an AIDS patient without any neuromeningeal involvement (Heudier et al 1992). BIH regressed after withdrawal of the drug and treatment for cerebral edema.

Aspirin

Two cases of BIH related to aspirin therapy have been reported in children (Falcini et al 1989). Both regressed after discontinuation of the drug. The pathomechanism is not known.

Chorionic Gonadotrophin

Haller et al (1993) have reported a case of BIH associated with β human chorionic gonadotrophin (β-hCC) therapy in a child with undescended testes. BIH manifested three weeks after completion of a 5-week treatment. The child recovered completely after treatment with acetazolamide. BIH has been reported previously in a case with high serum levels of endogenous β-hCC due to a testicular tumor. BIH developed after treatment of the tumor with chemotherapy and return of β-hCC levels to normal (March et al 1988). The patient recovered from BIH. Both these cases indicate that BIH may be a withdrawal effect from β-hCC.

Ciprofloxacin

Winrow and Supramaniam (1990) have reported a case of BIH after the use of ciprofloxacin in a teenager with cystic fibrosis. This patient improved after discontinuation of the drug and treatment with repeated lumbar punctures to lower the intracranial pressure.

Corticosteroids

Walker and Adamkiewicz (1964) reported 4 cases and reviewed another 24 reports from literature regarding BIH associated with prolonged corticosteroid therapy. The syndrome was seen during the withdrawal phase of the steroids. The authors considered the general effect of adrenal suppression from corticosteroids as a factor in the pathogenesis of this syndrome although the cause is not known. BIH has been reported in corticosteroid deficient states (Aanderud and Jorde 1988) and following removal of ACTH-secreting pituitary tumors (Martin et al 1981; Weisman et al 1983). Corticosteroids are also used in the treatment of cerebral edema and gradual tapering of the steroids reduces the chances of developing BIH. Rarely BIH develops with increase in corticosteroid dose (Vyas et al 1981).

Little has been added to our understanding of this problem and similar cases continue to be reported (Fardal 1982; Lipnick et al 1990; Cardinale et al 1991; Liu et al 1994; Lorrot et al 1999).

Cyclosporine

Asymptomatic optic disc edema and elevated intracranial pressure, resolving after discontinuation or lowering of the cyclosporine dose, has been reported in six allogeneic bone marrow transplant patients (Avery et al 1991). Pseudotumor cerebri developed in an 11-year old boy on cyclosporine therapy after undergoing allogeneic bone marrow transplantation complicated by graft versus host disease. The opening pressure of the lumbar puncture was 500 mm of water. The patient improved within five days of

discontinuing his cyclosporine (Cruz et al 1996). Another case of pseudotumor cerebri was reported in a child maintained on cyclosporine following successful renal transplantation (Katz 1997).

Cytosine Arabinoside (ARA-C)

One case of BIH has been reported following high dose ARA-C therapy for promyelocytic leukemia (Evers et al 1992). The patient recovered after lumbar punctures to reduce the intracranial pressure. One theoretically possible mechanism in this case is the ARA-C-induced local phosphorus depletion and disruption of the ATPase dependent choroidal secretion of CSF.

Danazol

Danazol is a synthetic ethisterone derivative, which inhibits the secretion and production of pituitary gonadotrophin hormones. It has anabolic and androgenic effects and is used in the treatment of endometriosis, benign cystic breast disease, and some hematologic disorders. Several cases of BIH have been reported in patients on danazol therapy (Shah et al 1987; Vernay et al 1988; Hamed et al 1989; Loukili et al 1990; Schmitz et al 1991). Cessation of danazol led to improvement in most of the cases. The mechanism is unknown but it may be related to danazol-induced fluid retention and weight gain. One case has been reported after withdrawal of danazol therapy (Fanous et al 1991). One possible explanation is that some metabolites of danazol with a long half-life may continue to play a role in raising intracranial pressure after the drug is withdrawn.

Growth Hormone

Twenty-three cases of BIH have been reported worldwide between 1986 and 1993 in association with the use of recombinant growth hormone (Malozowski et al 1993). Three additional cases were reported after treatment with insulin growth factor I, the primary mediator of action of growth hormone. Some of these patients had the risk factors for BIH such as obesity, renal failure, and endocrine disorders. Price et al (1995) have reported a case of BIH in an 11-year old girl where the diagnosis was delayed because the initial symptoms was only headaches which are reported commonly in children on growth hormone therapy and usually resolve spontaneously. BIH has been reported in three children from Australia and one from New Zealand, who were being treated with recombinant human growth hormone (Crock et al 1998). The incidence of BIH in children treated with growth hormone is small (1.2 per 1000 cases overall).

The following measures are recommended for improved detection of BIH:

- Headaches in a patient on growth hormone therapy should be reported to the physician
- Fundoscopy should be done on these patients prior to start of growth hormone therapy and during routine reviews.

Insulin-Like Growth Factor (IGF)-1

Transient bilateral papilledema with BIH has been reported in a 10-year old boy treated with IDF-1 therapy for growth hormone receptor deficiency (Lordereau-Richard et al 1994). This occurred after increasing the dose. Recovery was complete after interruption of IGF-1 therapy and the treatment was resumed 9 months later at a lower dose without recurrence of BIH.

Lithium

BIH is known as a complication of long-term lithium therapy in patients with bipolar affective disorders and several cases have been reported in the literature (Lobo et al 1978; Pesando et al 1980; Chatillon et al 1989; Ames et al 1994). It has also been reported in patients on short-term lithium therapy (Alvarez-Cermeno et al 1989). In most of the cases BIH resolved on discontinuation of lithium therapy. In those patients where the lithium therapy could not be discontinued, BIH did not resolve.

Pathomechanism of lithium-induced BIH is not known. Patients treated with lithium whose antidiuretic hormone-cyclic adenosine monophosphate mechanism is disturbed are most likely to develop pseudotumor cerebri via dysregulation of sodium balance, thyroid hormone production, and glucose metabolism (Levine and Puchalski 1990). Lithium-induced inhibition of vitamin A transport in the choroid plexus can lead to hypervitaminosis A (Saul et al 1985).

Minocycline

This is a semisynthetic tetracycline with greater lipid solubility than tetracycline itself and permeates the BBB more readily (see also the section on tetracycline). Several cases of minocycline-induced BIH have been reported (Weller and Klockgether 1997; Boyd 1995; Wandstrat and Phillips 1995; Donnet et al 1992; Delaney et al 1990; Lubetzki et al 1988; Lander 1989; Le Bris et al 1988; Castot et al 1983; Beran 1980). Most of these patients had taken minocycline for treatment of acne and some had taken retinoids concomitantly which are also known to be associated with BIH. Pathomechanism is not known. The treatment is discontinuation of minocycline. Some of the cases required other measures for lowering intracranial pressure.

Nalidixic Acid

Nalidixic acid, the quinolone frequently used in the treatment of acute dysentery, is now emerging as an important cause of BIH in infants and young children. Since Boreus and Sundström (1967) reported the first case of BIH in a child on treatment with nalidixic acid, several other cases have been reported. Mukherjee et al (1990) have reported 12 cases following nalidixic acid overdose. A study of 20 such cases from India showed that all the patients had received a higher than recommended dose of nalidixic acid and that 85% of them were given the drug unnecessarily, i. e., for acute watery diarrhea (Riyaz et al 1998). A high concentration of the drug in the commercial preparations as well as the lack of awareness about this among physicians were considered to be possible contributory factor leading to this situation.

Nitrofurantoin

Three case reports have been published of BIH following nitrofurantoin therapy of urinary infections (Sharma and James 1974; Mushet 1977; Korzets et al 1988). Pathomechanism is not known.

Non-Steroidal Anti-Inflammatory Drugs (NSAID)

NSAIDs have been reported to cause BIH. Twenty-four new cases of papilledema with or without BIH associated with NSAID therapy were reported to the National Registry of Drug-induced Ocular effects in the USA (Fraunfelder et al 1994). More than half of these cases were related to the use of propionic acid derivatives (ibuprofen and naproxen) and no cases were seen with pyrazolone derivatives.

There are reports of indomethacin (Konomi et al 1978) and ketoprofen (Larizza et al 1979) producing BIH in patients with Bartter's syndrome. BIH subsided in both cases after discontinuation of the offending drugs. Inhibition of prostaglandins by these drugs may lead to the retention of sodium and fluids, thus precipitating BIH.

Oral Contraceptives (OC)

BIH has been reported following the use of OCs (Arbenz and Wormser 1965; Cosnet 1969; Vespignani et al 1984). This appears to be related to the estrogen and progesterone content of these pills which leads to water retention and weight gain which are risk factors for BIH. BIH has been reported after replacement therapy with mestranol and norethisterone (Sheehan 1982).

Levonorgestrel implants. Two cases of BIH have been reported in young women with levonorgestrel implants (Alder et al 1995). In one of these the symptoms resolved whereas in the other, there was recurrence of symptoms

which was controlled by acetazolamide. Although the causal relation is not certain, the authors recommend periodic examination of ocular fundus in patients with such implants who complain of headaches and visual problems. Sunku et al (1993) have reported two patients who developed BIH after levonergestrel implants for contraception. The patients recovered after removal of implants and treatment with diuretics.

Perhexiline

BIH following perhexiline therapy has been reported by Stephens et al (1978), Mandelcorn et al (1982), and Vespignani et al (1984). Its profile in this respect is similar to that of amiodarone—a drug in the same therapeutic category.

Phenytoin

BIH has been reported in a patient with seizure disorder treated with phenytoin (Kalanie et al 1986). This was confirmed by positive rechallenge in this case.

Quinagolide (CV 205 502)

This is a novel non-ergot derived dopamine agonist which is used for the treatment of hyperprolactinemia in patients intolerant of bromocriptine. Two cases have been reported where withdrawal of this drug has led to development of BIH (Atkin et al 1994). These patients had other risk factors: one had an empty sella secondary to an operation and the other patient was on oral contraceptives. Both of these patients had migraine headaches. The headaches improved in intensity during treatment and increased in intensity after withdrawal. The relationship to quinagolide is indicated by appearance of BIH in both patients 2 weeks after discontinuation of the drug and disappearance a month after restarting quinagolide therapy. Vascular basis of migraine as well as BIH suggests that quinagolide may have an effect on the cerebral vasculature.

Retinoids

Isoretinoin and etiretinate are used for the treatment of acne and other skin conditions. There are several published reports of association of these retinoids with BIH (Bonnetblanc et al 1983; Spector and Carlisle 1984; Viraben et al 1985; Fraunfelder et al 1985; Roytman et al 1988; Lebowitz et al 1988; Smith-Whitley and Lange 1993). Griffin (1992) reviewed 64 unpublished cases of BIH associated with retinoids manufactured by Hoffmann La Roche, Basel. The pathomechanism of this adverse effect is not known. In some cases tetracycline and minocycline (both of which are known to cause BIH) were used concomitantly with retinoids. In other cases there was no concomitant medication.

Tretinoin. This is a retinoid that induces maturation and decreased proliferation of acute promyelocytic leukemia (APL) cells. Although BIH is known as a complication of APL, cases of tretinoin-induced BIH have been reported (Sano et al 1998; Chen et al 1998; Selleri et al 1996). The symptoms usually resolve after discontinuation of therapy.

Sulfonamides

Trimethoprim-sulfamethoxazole has been reported to be associated with BIH (Jain and Rosner 1992; Askmark et al 1989). Another case has been reported with use of sulfenazone (Murgia et al 1989). These drugs are also known to be associated with aseptic meningitis (see Chapter 16).

Tetracycline

Association between BIH and tetracycline was first reported by Gellis (1956) and later by Millichap (1959). Since then several case reports of BIH associated with tetracycline therapy have appeared (Maroon and Mely 1971; Meacock and Hewer 1981; Pearson et al 1981; Pierog et al 1986; Minutello et al 1988). Walters et al (1981) presented five such cases. Over 50 cases have been reported in the literature to date. Symptoms

disappeared in most of the cases after discontinuation of tetracycline although papilledema persisted for several months in two of the cases. Combination with vitamin A in young women was recognized to be risk factor.

One retrospective study (Ireland et al 1990) and one prospective case-control study (Guiseffi et al 1991) involving a total of 90 patients found no statistical association between tetracycline-induced and other types of BIH. Gardner et al (1995) described two fraternal twin sisters who developed BIH after beginning treatment with tetracycline. The authors reviewed 19 familial cases of BIH from the literature and suggested genetic susceptibility may be a factor in the development of drug-induced BIH. Effect of tetracycline on cyclic AMP (second messenger to ADH) has been proposed as a mechanism for tetracycline-induced BIH (Walter and Gubbay 1981).

Most of the previously reported cases are in the adults. Quinn et al (1999) reported six young patients BIH ranging in age from 12 to 17 years who were being treated for acne vulgaris. All patients responded to treatment, with recovery in one day to 4 weeks.

Thyroid Preparations

BIH has been associated with initiation of levothyroxine therapy for hypothyroidism (Van Dop et al 1983; McVie 1983; Rohn 1985; Williams 1997). Huseman and Torkelson (1984) described the first case of BIH following T_4 replacement for hypothalamic hypothyroidism. The cause of increased intracranial pressure following T_4 remains unclear. BIH has been reported with different kinds of thyroid replacement therapies: T_3, and combinations of T_3 and T_4. Careful and frequent neurologic and fundoscopic assessment is recommended during the initiation of thyroid replacement therapy in hypothyroid states.

Vaccination

BIH has been reported following DPT vaccination in 10 cases (Salinas et al 1990). There are other reports of bulging anterior fontanella in infants after vaccination when vitamin A supplementation is given (de Franciso et al 1993).

Vitamin A

Taken in the form of retinol or retinyl esters vitamin A appears to be safe at doses of 5,000 to 10,000 IU/ day. Beta-carotene has not reported to have any ocular toxicity (Gross and Helfgott 1992). Toxic reactions are common when vitamin A is taken in megadoses. Marie and See (1954) were the first to describe a case of benign hydrocephalus following hypervitaminosis A in a 17 month old child. In a series of 17 cases of vitamin A toxicity, nearly half of patients has signs and symptoms of BIH (Muenter et al 1971). Headaches were reported after 10 weeks of daily intake of 50,000 IU of vitamin A. Several reports of BIH due to hypervitaminosis A have been described in the literature since then and have been reviewed by Griffin (1992). There are other single case reports (Gangemi et al 1985; Bhettay and Bakst 1988; Bousser 1998; Sharieff and Hanten 1996; Wettstein and O'Neill 1998; Drouet and Valance 1998).

Pathomechanism. Mechanisms by which vitamin A alters CSF circulation are still controversial but it may involve the following:
- An obstruction in the CSF pathways
- An increase in CSF secretion (Siegel and Spacjman 1972; Fishman 1992) may occur via the following:
  - interaction with transthyretin (Herbert et al 1986)
  - impaired vitamin A transport in the choroid plexus
- It is also possible that alterations in vitamin A metabolism modify the functions of arachnoid villi and reduce the absorption of CSF.

Management of BIH due to hypervitaminosis A involves withdrawal of this vitamin under medical observation. The symptoms usually resolve spontaneously. BIH has also been reported to be caused by vitamin A deficiency during infancy (Kasarskis and Bass 1982). This may lead to thickening of the meninges with interstitial fibrosis and reduced CSF absorption (Kasarkis et al 1978). Prevention of this would obviously be adequate vitamin A intake.

Management of Drug-Induced BIH

Various methods for the management of BIH are listed in Table 17.5.

Recognition of association of BIH with drugs is important. There is no specific diagnostic method for ascertaining the specific contributing factors. Improvement following discontinuation of the suspected drug is one piece of the evidence. If the elevated intracranial pressure is being treated at the same time, the value of dechallenge in linking the drug to the adverse reaction is questionable. Various methods are used for lowering the intracranial pressure; lumbar punctures, dehydrating agents such as mannitol, loop diuretics such as furosemide, corticosteroids, etc. Such a decision is made by the physician treating the patient according to the severity of the situation. A case of BIH due to tetracycline was treated successfully by using acetazolamide without discontinuing tetracycline therapy (Wandstrat and Phillips 1995).

The old method of surgical subtemporal decompression is rarely performed now-a-days but a reassessment has shown it to be quite effective in patients where medical measures have failed to control the symptoms (Kessler et al 1998). Ventriculo-peritoneal shunts have been performed more frequently and afford good relief from headaches but the small ventricles present a technical difficulty in inserting catheters into this space.

Table 17.5. Management of benign intracranial hypertension.

Recognition and treatment of contributing diseases
Discontinuation of the offending drug
Reduction of intracranial pressure
  – Medical measures
    • Lumbar punctures
    • Dehydrating agents
  – Surgical procedures
    • Subtemporal decompression
    • Ventriculoperitoneal shunt
    • Optic nerve fenestration

Further visual loss may be precipitated by the late failure of shunt. The main concern is preservation of vision and the preferred operation is optic nerve sheath fenestration (Sergott et al 1988). In this procedure a window is made through the dura and arachnoid which enclose the optic nerve and contain CSF. Improvement of optic nerve head has been shown after optic nerve sheath fenestration (Berman and Wirtschafter 1992) in those patients who do not respond to oral medications to decrease intracranial pressure.

References

Aanderud S, Jorde R: ACTH deficiency associated with increased intracranial hypertension: a case report. Acta Endocrinol (Copenhagen) 1988; 118: 346.

Alder JB, Fraunfelder FT, Edwards R: Levonorgestrel implants and intracranial hypertension. N Engl J Med 1995; 332(25): 1720–1721.

Alvarez-Cermeno JC, Fernandez JM, O'Neill A, et al: Lithium-induced headache. Headache 1989; 29: 245–246.

Ames D, Wirshing WC, Cokey HT, et al: The natural course of pseudotumor cerebri in lithium-treated patients. J Clin Psychopharmacol 1994; 14: 286–287.

Arbenz JP, Wormser P: Pseudotumor cerebri durch Sexualhormone. Schweiz Med Wochenschr 1965; 95: 1654.

Arber N, Shirin H, Fadila R, et al: Pseudotumor cerebri associated with leuprorelin acetate. Lancet 1990; 335: 668.

Askmark H, Lundberg PO, Olsson S: Drug-related headache. Headache 1989; 29: 441–444.

Atkin SL, Masson EA, Blumhardt LD, et al: Benign intracranial hypertension associated with the withdrawal of a non-ergot dopamine agonist. JNNP 1994; 57: 371–372.

Avery R, Jabs DA, Wingard JR, et al: Optic disc edema after bone marrow transplantation. Possible role of cyclosporine toxicity. Ophthalmology 1991; 98: 1294–1301.

Beran RG: Pseudotumor cerebri associated with minocycline therapy for acne. Med J Australia 1980; 1: 323–324.

Berman EL, Wirtschafter JD: Improvement of optic nerve head appearance after surgery for pseudotumor cerebri. JAMA 1992; 267: 1130.

Bhettay EM, Bakst CM: Hypervitaminosis A causing benign intracranial hypertension. S Afr Med J 1988; 74: 584–585.

Bonnetblanc JM, Hugon J, Dumas M: Intracranial hypertension with etiretinate. Lancet 1983; ii: 974.

Boreus LO, Sundström B: Intracranial hypertension in a child during treatment with nalidixic acid. BMJ 1967; 2: 744–745.

Bousser MG: Benign intracranial hypertension and chronic hypervitaminosis A. Rev Neurol (Paris) 1998; 154(11): 784–5

Boyd I: Benign intracranial hypertension induced by minocycline. Current Therapeutics 1995; 36: 70–71.

Buchheit W, Burton C, Haag B, et al: Papilledema and idiopathic intracranial hypertension: report of familial occurrence. NEJM 1969; 280: 938–942.

Cardinale A, Rosati C, Giani I, et al: Pseudotumor cerebri da sospensioni di corticosteroidi. Minerva Pediatr 1991; 43: 457–460.

Castot A, Vincens M, Garnier R, et al: Hypertension intracranniene aigue probable apres prise de minocycline chez la nourisson. Therapie 1983; 38: 93–99.

Chatillon JD, Schaison M, Berche M, et al: Deux complication neuro-ophthalmiques rares d'un traitement au long cours par les sels de lithium. L'encephale 1989; 15: 415–417.

Chen HY, Tsai RK, Huang SM: ATRA-induced pseudotumour cerebri—one case report. Kao Hsiung I Hsueh Ko Hsueh Tsa Chih 1998; 14(1): 58–60.

Cosnet JE: Stroke and the pill. BMJ 1969; 2: 450.

Crock PA, McKenzie JD, Nicoll AM, et al: Benign intracranial hypertension and recombinant growth hormone therapy in Australia and New Zealand. Acta Paediatr 1998; 87(4): 381–386.

Cruz OA, Fogg SG, Roper-Hall G: Pseudotumor cerebri associated with cyclosporine use. Am J Ophthalmol 1996; 122(3): 436–7.

de Francisco A, Chakraborty J, Chowdhury HR, et al: Acute toxicity of vitamin A given with vaccines in infancy. Lancet 1993; 342: 526–527.

Delaney RA, Wee D, Naraynaswamy TR: Pseudotumor cerebri and acne. Mil Med 1990; 155: 511.

Donnet A, Dufour H, Graziani N, et al: Minocycline and benign intracranial hypertension. Biomed Pharmacother 1992; 46: 171–172.

Drouet A, Valance J: Benign intracranial hypertension and chronic hypervitaminosis A. Rev Neurol (Paris) 1998; 154(3): 253–256.

Durcan FJ, Corbett JJ, Wall M: The incidence of pseudotumor cerebri. Arch Neurol 1988; 45: 875–877.

Evers JP, Jacobson RJ, Pincus J, et al: Pseudotumor cerebri following high-dose cytosine arabinoside. Brit J Hematol 1992; 80: 559–560.

Falcini F, Taccetti G, Montanelli F, et al: Benign intracranial hypertension during treatment with acetylsalicylic acid: presentation of 12 cases in children. Pediatr Med Chir 1989; 11: 319–321.

Fanous M, Hamed LM, Margo CE, et al: Pseudotumor cerebri associated with danazol withdrawal. JAMA 1991; 266: 1218–1219.

Fardal RW: Pseudotumor cerebri following steroid injections. Hawaii Med J 1982; 41: 414.

Fikkers BG, Bogousslavsky J, Regli F, et al: Pseudotumor cerebrai with amiodarone. JNNP 1986; 49: 606.

Fishman RA: Disorders of intracranial pressure. In Cerebrospinal fluid in diseases of the nervous system, 2nd ed, Philadelphia, WB Saunders, 1992, pp 103–155.

Foley J: Benign forms of intracranial hypertension

—"Toxic" and "Otitic" hydrocephalus. Brain 1955; 78: 1–41.

Fontana M, Mastrostefano R, Pietrangeli A, et al: Acute intracranial hypertension due to ketamine in a patient with delayed radionecrosis simulating an expansive process. J Neurosurg Sci 1980; 24: 93–98.

Fraunfelder FT, LaBraico JM, Meyer SM: Adverse ocular reactions possibly associated with isoretinoin. Am J Ophthalmol 1985; 100: 534–537.

Fraunfelder FT, Samples JR, Fraunfelder FW: Possible optic nerve side effects associated with nonsteroidal anti-inflammatory drugs. J Toxicol Cut & Ocular Toxicol 1994; 13: 311–316.

Gangemi M, Maiuri F, Di Martino L, et al: Intracranial hypertension due to acute vitamin A intoxication. Acta Neurol (Napoli) 1985; 7: 27–31.

Gardner K, Cox T, Digre KB: Idiopathic intracranial hypertension associated with tetracyclineuse in fraternal twins. Neurology 1995; 45: 6–10.

Gellis S: Editorial. In Gellis S (Ed.): Year book of pediatrics, Year Book Publishers, Chicago, 1956, p 40.

Gränstrom G: Benign intracranial hypertension: an unexpected side effect of nalidixic acid. Läkartidningen 1984; 81: 1837–1838.

Griffin JP: A review of the literature on benign intracranial hypertension associated with medication. Adv Drug React Toxicol Rev 1992; 11: 41–58.

Griswold W, Reznik V, Mendoza SA: Nitroprusside-induced intracranial hypertension. JAMA 1981; 246: 2679–2680.

Grogan WA, Narkun DM: Pseudotumór cerebri with amiodarone. JNNP 1987; 50: 651.

Gross EG, Helfgott MA: Retinoids and the eye. Dermatologic Clinics 1992; 10: 521–531.

Guiseffi V, Wall M, Siegel PZ, et al: Symptoms and disease association in idiopathic intracranial hypertension (pseudotumor cerebri): a case control study. Neurology 1991; 41: 239–244.

Haller JS, Meyer DR, Cromie W, et al: Pseudotumor cerebri following β human chorionic gonadotrophin hormone treatment for undescended testicles. Neurology 1993; 43: 448–449.

Hamed LM, Glaser JS, Schatz NJ, et al: Pseudotumor cerebri induced by danazol. Am J Ophthalmol 1989; 107: 105–110.

Herbert J, Wilcox JN, Pham KT et al: Transthyretin: a choroid plexus-specific transport protein in human brain. Neurology 1986; 36: 900–911.

Heudier P, Chichmanian RM, Taillan B, et al: Hypertension intracranienne bénigne médicamenteuse. Therapie 1992; 47: 403–407.

Huseman CA, Torkelson RD: Pseudotumor cerebri following treatment of hypothalamic and primary hypothyroidism. AJDC 1984; 138: 927–931.

Ireland B, Corbett J, Wallace R: The search for causes of idiopathic intracranial hypertension. Arch Neurol 1990; 47: 315–320.

Jain N, Rosner F: Idiopathic intracranial hypertension: report of seven cases. Am J Med 1992; 93: 391–395.

Kalanie H, Niakan E, Harati Y, et al: Phenytoin-induced benign intracranial hypertension. Neurology 1986; 36: 443.

Kasarskis EJ, Bass NH: Benign intracranial hypertension induced by deficiency of vitamin A during infancy. Neurology 1982; 32: 1292–1295.

Kasarskis EJ, Maffeo CJ, Johnson RN, et al: Intracranial hypertension in vitamin a deficient rats: reversible metabolic derangement of cerebrospinal fluid absorption (abstract). Neurology 1978; 28: 349.

Katz B: Disk edema subsequent to renal transplantation. Surv Ophthalmol 1997; 41: 315–20.

Kessler LA, Novelli PM, Reigel DH: Surgical treatment of benign intracranial hypertension—subtemporal decompression revisited. Surg Neurol 1998; 50(1): 73–76.

Konomi H, Imai M, Nihei K, et al: Indomethacin causing pseudotumor cerebri in Bartter's syndrome. NEJM 1978; 298: 855.

Korzets A, Rathaus M, Chen B, et al: Pseudotumor cerebri and nitrofurantoin. Drug Intell Clin Pharm 1988; 22: 345.

Kovarik WD, Mayberg TS, Lam AM, et al: Succinylcholine does not change intracranial pressure, cerebral blood flow velocity, or the electroencephalogram in patients with neurologic injury. Anesthesia and Analgesia 1994; 78: 469–473.

Lander CM: Minocycline-induced benign intracranial hypertension. Clin Exp Neurol 1989; 26: 161–167.

Larizza D, Colombo A, Lorini R, et al: Ketoprofen causing pseudotumor cerebri in Bartter's syndrome. NEJM 1979; 300: 976.

Le Bris P, Glacet Bernard A, Coscas G, et al: Papilledema caused by minocycline: apropos of one case. J Fr Ophtamol 1988; 11: 681–684.

Lebowitz MA, Berson DS: Ocular effects of oral retinoids. J Am Acad Dermatol 1988; 19: 209–211.

Levine SH, Puchalski C: Pseudotumor cerebri associated with lithium therapy in two patients. J Clin Psychiatry 1990; 51: 251–253.

Lipnick RN, Tsokos GC, Bray GL, et al: Autoimmune thrombocytopenia in pediatric systemic lupus erythematosus: alternative therapeutic modalities. Clin Exptl Rheumatol 1990; 8: 315–319.

Liu GT, Kay MD, Bienfang DC, et al: Pseudotumor cerebri associated with corticosteroid withdrawal in inflammatory bowel disease. Am J Ophthalmology 1994; 117: 352–357.

Lobo A, Pilek E, Stokes PE: Papilledema following therapeutic dosages of lithium carbonate. J Nerv Ment Dis 1978; 166: 526–529.

Lopez AC, Lopez AM, Jimenez SF, et al: Acute intracranial hypertension during amiodarone infusion. Crit Care Med 1985; 13: 688–689.

Lordereau-Richard I, Roger M, Chaussain JL: Transient bilateral papilloedema in a 10-year old boy treated with recombinant insulin-like growth factor 1 for growth hormone receptor deficiency. Acta Paediatr 1994; suppl 399: 152.

Lorrot M, Bader-Meunier B, Sebire G, et al: Benign intracranial hypertension: an unrecognized complication of corticosteroid therapy. Arch Pediatr 1999; 6(1): 40–42.

Loukili M, Cordonnier M, Capelluto E, et al: Pseudotumor cerebri induit par danazol. Bull Soc Belge Ophtalmol 1990; 239: 139–144.

Lubetzki C, Sanson M, Cohen D, et al: Benign intracranial hypertension and minocycline. Rev Neurol 1988; 144: 218–220.

Malozowski S, Tanner LA, Wysowski D, et al: Growth hormone, insulin-like growth factor I, and benign intracranial hypertension. NEJM 1993; 329: 665–666.

Mandelcorn M, Murphy J, Coleman J: Papilledema without peripheral neuropathy in a patient taking perhexiline maleate. Canad J Ophthalmol 1982; 17: 173.

Marcelis J, Silberstein SD: Idiopathic intracranial hypertension without papilledema. Arch Neurol 1991; 48: 392–399.

March LF, Morgan DAL, Jefferson D: Benign intracranial hypertension during chemotherapy for testicular teratoma. Br J Radiol 1988; 61: 692.

Marie J, See G: Acute hypervitaminosis A of the infant. Am J Dis Child 1954; 87: 731.

Maroon JC, Mealy J: Benign intracranial hypertension: sequel to tetracycline therapy in a child. JAMA 1971; 216: 1479–1480.

Martin NA, Linfoot J, Wilson CB: Development of pseudotumor cerebri after removal of adrenocorticotropic hormone-secreting pituitary adenoma. A case report. Neurosurgery 1981; 8: 699.

McVie R: Pseudotumor cerebri and thyroid replacement therapy. NEJM 1983; 309: 731732 (letter).

Meacock DJ, Hewer RL: Tetracycline and benign intracranial hypertension. BMJ 1982; 282: 1240.

Millichap JG: Benign intracranial hypertension and otitic hydrocephalus. Pediatrics 1959; 23: 257–259.

Minutello JS, Dimayuga RG, Carter J: Pseudotumor cerebri, a rare reaction to tetracycline therapy. J Periodontology 1988; 59: 848–851.

Muenter MD, Perry HO, Judwig J: Chronic vitamin A intoxication in adults. Am J Med 1971; 50: 129–136.

Mukherjee A, Dutta P, Lahiri M, et al: Benign intracranial hypertension after nalidixic acid overdose in infants. Lancet 1990; 335: 1602.

Murgia S, Del Curto E, Zecca G: Benign intracranial hypertension caused by sulfenazone. Pediatr Med Chir 1989; 11: 541–542.

Mushet GR: Pseudotumor and nitrofurantoin therapy. Arch Neurol 1977; 34: 257.

Nonne M: Über Fälle von Symptomenkomplex "Tumor cerebri" mit Ausgang in Heilung (Pseudotumor cerebri). Z Nervenheilkunde 1904; 27: 169–216.

Ohar JM, Fowler AA, Selhorst JB, et al: Intravenous nitroglycerine-induced intracranial hypertension. Critical Care Med 1985; 13: 867–868.

Pearson MG, Littlewood SM, Bowdon AN: Tetracycline and benign intracranial hypertension. BMJ 1981; 282: 568–569.

Pesando P, Nuzzi G, Maraini G: Bilateral papilledema in long term therapy with lithium carbonate. Pharmakopsychiatr Neuropsychopharmacol 1980; 13: 235–239.

Pierog SH, Al Salihi FL, Cinotti D: Pseudotumor cerebri —a complication of tetracycline treatment of acne. J Adolesc HealthCare 1986; 7: 139–140.

Price DA, Clayton PC, Lloyd IC: Benign intracranial hypertension induced by growth hormone treatment. Lancet 1995; 345: 458–459.

Quinn AG, Singer SB, Buncic JR: Pediatric tetracycline-induced pseudotumor cerebri. J Aapos 1999; 3(1): 53–57.

Radakrishnan K, Ahlskog E, Cross SA, et al: Idiopathic intracranial hypertension (pseudotumor cerebri). Arch Neurol 1993; 50: 78–80.

Radhakrishnan K, Ahlskog E, Garrity JA, et al: Idiopathic intracranial hypertension. Mayo Clin Proc 1994; 69: 169–180.

Riyaz A, Aboobacker CM, Sreelatha PR: Nalidixic acid induced pseudotumour cerebri in children. J Indian Med Assoc 1998; 96(10): 308, 314.

Rohn R: Pseudotumor cerebri following treatment of hypothyroidism. AJDC 1985; 139: 752.

Roytman M, Frumkin A, Bohn TG: Pseudotumor cerebri caused by isoretinoin. Cutis 1988; 42: 399–400.

Sahs AL, Joynt RJ: Brain swelling of unknown cause. Neurology 1956; 6: 791–802.

Salinas EC, Mir ES, Comalat AF, et al: Hipertension endocraneal benigna tras immunizacion con DTP y polio. Ann Esp Pediatr 1990; 32: 466–467.

Sano F, Tsuji K, Kunika N, et al: Pseudotumor cerebri in a patient with acute promyelocytic leukemia during treatment with all-trans retinoic acid. Internal medicine 1998; 37: 546–549.

Saul RF, Hamburger HA, Selhorst JB: Pseudotumor cerebri secondary to lithium therapy. JAMA 1985; 253: 2869–2870.

Schmitz U, Honisch C, Zierz S: Pseudotumor cerebri and carpal tunnel syndrome associated with danazol therapy. J Neurol 1991; 238: 355–357.

Seckl J, Lightman S: Intracerebroventricular vasopressin reduced CSF absorption rate in conscious goat. Exp Brain Res 1991; 84: 173–176.

Selleri C, Pane F, Notaro R, et al: All-trans-retinoic acid (ATRA) responsive skin relapses of acute promyelocytic leukemia followed by ATRA-induced pseudotumor cerebri. Brit J Haematol 1996; 92: 937–940.

Sergott RC, Savino PJ, Bosley TM, et al: Modified optic nerve sheath decompression provides long-term visual improvement for pseudotumor cerebri. Arch Ophthalmol 1988; 106: 1391–1397.

Shah A, Roberts T, McQueen INF, et al: Danazol and benign intracranial hypertension. BMJ 1987; 294: 1323.

Sharieff GC, Hanten K: Pseudotumor cerebri and hypercalcemia resulting from vitamin A toxicity. Annals of Emergency Medicine 1996; 27: 518–521.

Sharma DB, James A: Benign intracranial hypertension associated with nitrofurnatoin therapy. BMJ 1974; 4: 771.

Sheehan JP: Hormone replacement treatment and benign intracranial hypertension. BMJ 1982; 284: 1675–1676.

Siegel NJ, Spacjman TJ: Chronic hypervitaminosis A with intracranial hypertension and low cerebrospinal fluid concentration of protein. Clin Pediatr 1972; 11: 580–584.

Singbartl G, Metzger G: Urapadil-induced increase of intracranial pressure in head trauma patients. Intensive Care Med 1990; 16: 272–274.

Smith JL: Whence pseudotumor cerebri? J Clin Neuroophthalmol 1985; 5: 55–56.

Smith-Whitley K, Lange B: Fatal all-trans retinoic acid pneumonitis. Ann Int Med 1993; 118: 472–473.

Sorensen PS, Thomsen AM, Gjerris F: Persistent disturbances of cognitive functions in patients with pseudotumor cerebri. Acta Neurol Scand 1986; 73: 264–268.

Spector RH, Carlisle J: Pseudotumor cerebri caused by a synthetic vitamin A preparation. Neurology 1984; 34: 1509–1511.

Stephens WP, et al: Raised intracranial pressure due to perhexiline maleate. BMJ 1978; 1: 21.

Stirt JA, Grosslight KR, Bedford RF, et al: Defasciculation with metocurine prevents succinylcholine-induced increases in intracranial pressure. Anesthesiology 1987; 67: 50–53.

Sugerman HJ, Felton WL 3rd, Sismanis A, et al: Gastric surgery for pseudotumor cerebri associated with severe obesity. Ann Surg 1999; 229(5): 634–642.

Sunku AJ, O'Duffy AE, Swanson JW: Benign intracranial hypertension associated with levonorgestrel (abstract). Ann Neurol 1993; 34: 299.

Van Dop C, Conte FA, Koch TK, et al: Pseudotumor cerebri associated with initiation of levothyroxine therapy for juvenile hypothyroidism. NEJM 1983; 308: 1076–1080.

Van Zandijcke M, Dewachter A: Pseudotumor cerebri with amiodarone. JNNP 1986; 49: 1463–1464.

Vernay D, Thevenet JP, Tournilhac M: Encephalopathie iatrogéne au danazol. Therapie 1988; 43: 501.

Vespignani H, Lepori JC, Gehin P, et al: L'hypertension intracranienne bènigne: a propos de 4 observations d'étiologie médicamenteuse. Rev Otoneuroophtalmol 1984; 56: 277–286.

Viraben R, Mahieu C, Fontan B: Benign intracranial hypertension during etiretinate therapy for mycosis fungoides. J Am Acad Dermatol 1985; 13: 515–517.

Vyas CK, Talwar KK, Bhatnagar V, et al: Steroid-induced benign intracranial hypertension. Postgrad Med J 1981; 57: 181–182.

Walker AE, Adamkiewicz JJ: Pseudotumor cerebri associated with prolonged corticosteroid therapy. JAMA 1964; 188: 779–784.

Wall M, Dollar JD, Sadun AA, et al: Idiopathic intracranial hypertension. Arch Neurol 1995; 52: 141–145.

Walters B, Gubbay S: Reply to enquiries (letter). Br Med J 1981; 282: 1240.

Walters BNJ, Gubbay SS: Tetracycline and benign intracranial hypertension: report of five cases. BMJ 1981; 282: 19–20.

Wandstrat TJ, Phillips J: Pseudotumor cerebri responds to acetazolamide. Ann Pharmacother 1995; 29: 318.

Wandstrat TL, Phillips J: Pseudotumor cerebri treated with acetazolamide: case report. Ann Pharmacother 1995; 29: 318.

Weissman MN, Page LK, Bejar RL: Benign intracranial hypertension after transsphenoidal adenomectomy. Neurosurgery 1983; 13: 195.

Weller M, Klockgether T: Minocycline-induced benign intracranial hypertension. J Neurol 1998; 245: 55.

Wettstein A, O'Neill J: Benign intracranial hypertension associated with hypervitaminosis A. Australian Family Physician 1998; 27(suppl 1): 55–56.

Williams JB: Adverse effects of thyroid hormones. Drugs & Aging 1997; 11: 460–469.

Winrow AP, Supramaniam G: Benign intracranial hypertension after ciprofloxacin administration. Arch Dis Child 1990; 65: 1165–1166.

Chapter 18
Disorders of the Autonomic Nervous System

Introduction

The autonomic nervous system (ANS) supplies and influences virtually every organ in the body. The ANS is affected by afferent signals from different parts of the body as well as neurons in the spinal cord and in the brain, mainly in the hypothalamus and brainstem. The efferent component of the ANS has two divisions: sympathetic and parasympathetic.

Disorders of the ANS are also referred to by the term "autonomic failure". A detailed description of these is given in the book by Bannister and Mathias (1992). These disorders can be primary or secondary. Drug-induced disorders belong to the second category.

Classification of Drug-Induced Disorders of the ANS

Drugs may act by stimulating or inhibiting either of the two divisions of the ANS. This is only a partial dissociation of the effect. The agonists and antagonists are often close cousins and share each other's properties to some extent. Drugs not normally acting on the ANS may have side effects involving the ANS. A minor side effect may aggravate or unmask an autonomic deficiency, e. g., hypotension in Shy-Drager's syndrome is enhanced by levodopa. Autonomic disorders are not always discreet. Some of them are part of other neurological syndrome such as neuroleptic malignant syndrome. Some of the autonomic side effects of drugs are mentioned along with other drug-induced syndromes but in this chapter the emphasis will be placed on the autonomic

Table 18.1. A practical classification of drug-induced autonomic disorders.

Decrease of sympathetic activity (Mathias 1991)
 – Centrally acting drugs
   Anesthetics
   Barbiturates
   Clonidine
   Methyldopa
 – Peripherally acting drugs
   Sympathetic neuron: guanethidine
   Alpha adrenoceptor blockade: phenoxybenzamine
   Beta adrenoceptor blockade: propranolol
Increase of sympathetic activity: sympathomimetic syndromes
Decrease of parasympathetic activity: anticholinergic syndromes
Increase of parasympathetic activity: cholinergic syndromes)
As part of other drug-induced neurological disorders
 – Drug-induced transverse myelitis (see Chapter 14)
 – Drug-induced Guillain-Barré syndrome (see Chapter 22)
 – Lambert-Eaton syndrome (see Chapter 13)
Autonomic neuropathy
Postural hypotension (see Chapter 4)
Autonomic disturbances associated with drug withdrawal
Reflex sympathetic dystrophy

effects. A practical classification of drug-induced autonomic disorders is shown in Table 18.1.

Anticholinergic Syndrome

Anticholinergic intoxication has been described since early written history. Datura stramonium (a toxic anticholinergic plant) is described as a poison by Homer in *The Odyssey*. It occurs during the postoperative period in about 1% of the cases following general anesthesia and 4% following regional anesthesia. It may occur as a result of drugs used during this period or as a result of insufficient release of acetylcholine (Johnson et al 1981).

Clinical Manifestations

The anticholinergic syndrome has both physical signs and neuropsychological manifestations:
- *General systemic effects*. Tachycardia, dilated and unreactive pupils, blurred vision, flushed face, warm and dry skin, dry mouth and throat, hyperpyrexia.
- *Neuropsychiatric effects*. Anxiety, agitation, confusion, delirium, hallucinations, delusions, fluctuating level of consciousness, impairment of memory, seizures.

Drug-Induced Anticholinergic Syndrome.
Anticholinergic syndrome can occur as a side effect of drugs listed in Table 18.2. Acetylcholine has an important function in modulating the interaction between several other central neurotransmitters. The effect of most of the drugs is easy to explain because of their known effect in decreasing parasympathetic activity. The post important of these are drugs used in anesthesia and perioperative period and antidepressants which will be considered separately.

Differential Diagnosis

Conditions from which the central anticholinergic syndrome should be differentiated are shown in Table 18.3.

Table 18.3. Differential diagnosis of central anticholinergic syndrome.

Overdose of anesthetic drugs
Altered hydration
Electrolyte disturbances
Hypoglycemia
Hypoxia
Hypercapnia, hyperthermia
Endocrine disorders
Neurological damage resulting from surgery

Table 18.2. Drugs that can produce anticholinergic syndrome.

Anesthesia, analgesia, and postoperative medications
- Atropine sulfate
- Benzodiazepines
- Halothane
- Hyoscine
- Influrane
- Ketamine
- Opioids
- Transdermal scopolamine
Antiarrhythmics: Propafenone, quinidine
Antiasthmatic: Ipratropium bromide
Antiemetics: cyclizine and meclizine
Antihistaminics with anticholinergic activity
- Brompheniramine
- Chlorpheniramine
- Cyclizine
- Diphenylhydramine
- Promethazine
Antiincontinence agents
- Oxybutynin
- Propantheline bromide
Antiparkinsonian medications
- Amantadine
- Benzatropine
- Biperiden
- Ethopropaine
- Procyclidine
- Trihexyphenidyl
Antipsychotics
- Clozapine
- Chlorpromazine
- Chlorprothixene
- Thioridazine
Antispasmodics for the gastrointestinal tract
- Hexocyclium
- Hyoscyamine
- Isopropamide
- Oxyphenonium
- Propantheline
- Tridihexethyl
Baclofen
Ophthalmic preparations
- Atropine 1% Ophthalmic solution
- Cyclopentolate
- Eucatropine
- Tropicamide
Tricyclic antidepressants
- Amitriptyline
- Imipramine
- Clomipramine
Drug interactions
- Desipramine and venlafaxine (Benazzi 1998)
- Venlafaxine-fluoxetine (Benazzi et al 1997)
- Paroxetine and clozapine (Joos et al 1997)

Anticholinergic Syndrome in Anesthesia. Many of the drugs used in anesthesia and intensive care may cause blockade of the central cholinergic transmission and produce a central cholinergic syndrome (Schneck and Rupreht 1989). This may also result when the central cholinergic sites are occupied by specific drugs and there is insufficient release of acetylcholine (Rupreht and Dworacek 1990). The etiology of central anticholinergic syndrome is multi-factorial, but the diagnosis should be considered in all patients who demonstrate abnormal post-anesthetic awakening. Central anticholinergic syndrome may follow general anesthesia where premedication with hyoscine has been carried out. In one study 18 of the 962 anesthesized patients developed the syndrome (Link et al 1997). The findings of this study indicate that the diagnosis of central anticholinergic syndrome should be considered when there is delayed recovery from anesthesia, and if other causes for that condition have been excluded.

Treatment

The first priority in treatment of severe cholinergic syndrome is the support of vital functions. In addition to neurological manifestations, there may be respiratory or cardiac arrest. The most important drug for treatment of central anticholinergic syndrome is physostigmine. A 1 mg dose of intravenous physostigmine produces a rapid return to a normal level of consciousness (Martin and Howell 1997). Efficacy of bethanechol, a parasympathomimetic agent, to counteract the adverse effects of nortriptyline has been shown in a double-blind study (Rosen et al 1993). Thiamine has been shown to reduce the scopolamine-induced cognitive deficits by its cholemimetic action (Meador et al 1993).

Anticholinergic Effects of Antidepressants. The anticholinergic effects of antidepressants are most marked with some tricyclic antidepressants and can be peripheral or central. The most frequently occurring are sedation and memory impairment (central effects) as well as dry mouth and blurred vision (peripheral effects). Selective serotonin reuptake inhibitors have much less an-ticholinergic side effects and selective monoamine oxidase A inhibitors such as moclobemide do not have such side effects at all. The elderly are more susceptible to the anticholinergic effects of antidepressants and, because of polypharmacy, they are more likely to have drug interactions which accentuate anticholinergic effects. Anticholinergic properties of amitriptyline may have a euphoric effect leading to abuse potential and toxicity (Wohlreich and Welch 1993).

Management of anticholinergic effects of antidepressants has been discussed by Riedel and van Praag (1995). Important points of management and prevention are:

– Use antidepressants with the least anticholinergic effects and reduce the dose
– Caffeine attenuates the anticholinergic effects
– Avoid use of comedications which increase the anticholinergic effect

Anticholinergic Syndrome after Topical Applications. Systemic absorption of topical ophthalmic anticholinergic drugs may lead to systemic toxicity. This subject has been reviewed by Rengstorff and Doughty (1982). Anticholinergic toxicity has been confirmed by anticholinergic radioreceptor assay after application of homatropine ophthalmic solution (Tune et al 1992). Central anticholinergic syndrome may also occur after transdermal application of scopolamine patch (Holland 1992).

Cholinergic Syndrome

Drugs which produce this syndrome are:
– Cholinomimetics such as carbachol
– Anticholinesterases such as physostigmine and neostigmine.

Signs of Excessive Cholinergic Stimulation. These are as follows (Cook et al 1992):

– *Muscarinic.* Increased bronchial, salivary, ocular, and intestinal secretions; sweating; miosis; bronchospasm; intestinal hypermobility and bradycardia.
– *Nicotinic.* Muscle twitching; fasciculations; weakness and paralysis.
– *CNS.* Loss of consciousness; convulsions; respiratory depression.

Sympathomimetic Syndromes

Drugs that produce these syndromes are listed in Table 18.4. Common signs are:
- Delusions
- Paranoia
- Hypertension
- Hyperreflexia
- Seizures
- Dysrhythmias

Table 18.4. Drugs producing sympathomimetic syndromes.

Amphetamine
Beta-adrenoceptor stimulants (isoprenaline)
Caffeine overdose
Cocaine
Ephedrine
Phenylpropanolamine
Theophylline

Autonomic Neuropathy

Autonomic dysfunction is well recognized as a complication of peripheral neuropathy. This subject has been reviewed by McDoughall and McLeod (1996). Most of the nerve fibers in both divisions of the ANS are small myelinated (2–6 Fm) and unmyelinated fibers. Diseases such as diabetes mellitus and amyloidosis that primarily affect small nerve fibers in peripheral neuropathy, or Guillain-Barré syndrome which causes demyelination of small myelinated fibers are most likely to cause autonomic dysfunction. Hyperhidrosis of the extremities is very common in peripheral neuropathy and is usually caused by the degeneration and impaired function of the cholinergic postganglionic sympathetic unmyelinated fibers that travel with peripheral nerves to innervate the sweat glands. Orthostatic hypotension is most likely to occur when autonomic fibers in the splanchnic bed are damaged.

The term acute autonomic neuropathy was first used by Thomashefsky et al (1972) to describe a case with acute onset of pupillotonia, dry mouth, urinary and fecal retention, and hypohidrosis with gradual and incomplete recovers. No cause could be identified but the features were consistent with diffuse abnormality of postgan-glionic cholinergic function. Categories of various causes of peripheral autonomic disorders are listed in Table 18.5.

Table 18.5. Categories of causes of peripheral autonomic disorders.

Acute dysautotonia
Hereditary
Inflammatory
Infections
Metabolic and nutritional disorders
Paraneoplastic syndromes
Immunologic disorders
Drugs and toxins

Drug-Induced Autonomic Neuropathy

Drugs which have been reported to cause autonomic neuropathy are listed in Table 18.6.

Table 18.6. Drug reported to cause autonomic neuropathy.

Amiodarone
Antineoplastics
  ARA-C
  Cisplatin
  Gemcitabine
  Taxol
  Vincristine
Ergot compounds
Perhexiline maleate

Antineoplastic Drugs

Antineoplastic drugs produce a peripheral neuropathy of the "dying back" type which affects both the large as well as the small fibers (see Chapter 11). Hansen (1990) observed autonomic dysfunction in 10 of the 28 patients with lasting remissions following treatment of cancer with chemotherapy and no obvious signs of peripheral neuropathy. None of the subjects had postural hypotension. The incidence of cardiovascular autonomic neuropathies was found to be higher in cancer patients treated with vinca alkaloids as compared with control cancer patients not treated with chemotherapy (Roca et al 1985).

ARA-C (Cytosine Arabinoside). Nevill et al (1989) described a patient with acute leukemia who developed Horner's syndrome and a severe demyelinating peripheral neuropathy leading to death after receiving high-dose cytosine arabinoside therapy.

Cisplatin. A case of cisplatin-induced severe autonomic neuropathy associated with postural hypotension was reported by Rosenfeld and Broder (1984). This adverse reaction resolved after discontinuation of cisplatin.

Gemcitabine. One patient with non-small-cell lung cancer was reported to develop autonomic neuropathy following treatment with gemcitabine (Dormann et al 1998). The symptoms were acid regurgitation, difficulty in swallowing and constipation. The patient was given parenteral nutrition and cisapride. He recovered four weeks after the completion of chemotherapy.

Taxol. Autonomic neuropathy with severe orthostatic hypotension has been reported in two women following treatment with taxol for ovarian cancer (Jerian et al 1993). Diabetes mellitus was considered to be a risk factor in one of these cases.

Vincristine. Autonomic complications of treatment with vincristine manifest as constipation, abdominal pain, paralytic ileus and urinary retention.

Amiodarone. Amiodarone usually produces a sensori-motor neuropathy (see Chapter 11) but autonomic failure with postural hypotension has also been reported (Manolis et al 1987).

Ergot. A case of autonomic dysesthesias due to ergot toxicity has been reported by Evans et al (1980). It was determined that pain was not due to vasoconstrictor effect of ergotamine. The pain was relieved by sympathetic block.

Perhexiline Maleate. This drug can cause peripheral neuropathy as well as autonomic neuropathy manifested by postural hypotension and abnormal valsalva ratio (Fraser et al 1977).

Autonomic Disturbances Associated with Drug Withdrawal

Withdrawal of drugs such as alcohol, opiates, and clonidine may result in reverse sympathetic overactivity, with increased sweating, hypertension and piloerection. A withdrawal syndrome has been reported after intrathecal administration of morphine (Tung et al 1980) and withdrawal of clonidine used for treatment of hypertension (Ropiquet et al 1984).

Reflex Sympathetic Dystrophy (RSD)

Various names are given to this syndrome; Sudeck's atrophy in German-speaking and algodystrophy in French-speaking countries. The term causalgia has almost become synonymous with RSD. The pathophysiology of this disorder is not known. At present there is some agreement that RSD may be caused by an abnormal sympathetic nervous reflex. Veldman et al (1993) have studied 829 patients with this disorder and proposed that RSD should be considered an exaggerated regional response to an injury rather than a disturbance of sympathetic nervous system.

Clinical Features. Reflex sympathetic dystrophy (RSD) affects one or more extremities and is characterized by distal pain, tenderness, swelling, and vasomotor instability. Pain and sensory disturbances are the most frequent early symptoms. Tissue atrophy involving skin, muscles, and bone (osteoporosis) bone develops later. Sympathetic signs such as hyperhidrosis are frequent but are not considered to be of diagnostic value.

Causes. It is usually a complication observed after an injury (e. g., fracture) or an operation on a limb. Changes similar to RSD may appear with a myocardial infarction (shoulder-hand syndrome), after peripheral nerve injury (causalgia), after local cold injury (trench foot), revascularization of an ischemic extremity (reperfusion syndrome), or may be drug-induced. In 10–26%

Table 18.7. Drugs associated with reflex sympathetic dystrophy.

Antitubercular drugs (isoniazid)
Antiepileptic drugs: phenobarbital
Cyclosporine
Ergotamine

of cases no precipitating factor can be found. RSD has been reported in association with the drugs shown in Table 18.7.

Diagnosis. The clinical diagnosis is suggested by the presence of at least 2 symptoms and signs from each of the categories of neuropathic pain and autonomic dysfunction.

Neuropathic pain: Burning, dysesthesia, paresthesia, mechanical allodynia, hyperalgesia to cold

Autonomic dysfunction: cynanosis, skin mottling, hyperhidrosis, edema, temperature difference of $> 3°C$ between limbs.

NMR spectroscopy shows impairment of high energy phosphate metabolism and electron microscopic studies of skeletal muscles show signs of oxidative stress.

Management. The aggravating cause such as a medication should be removed. Other measures are:
- Treatment with oral vasodilators abolishes or reduces the pain.
- Physiotherapy prevents muscle contractures
- Sympathetic block has been very popular but its efficacy has not been proven by controlled studies. The block may be surgical or chemical.
- Spinal cord stimulation has been shown to be effective in relief of pain (Kumar et al 1997).

Antitubercular Drugs

Gemperli (1969) described isoniazid-induced algodystrophy or fibrosing arthropathy which cleared up on discontinuation of the medication. Twenty-two cases due to various antitubercular drugs were reported by Deshayes et al (1969). The most frequent form was shoulder-hand syndrome. The pathomechanism is not known. Vitamin B_6 deficiency and serotonin disturbances have been ruled out as causes.

Antiepileptic Drugs

The symptoms of RSD in association with barbiturate therapy were first described by Beriel and Barbier (1934). Horton and Gerster (1984) reported that among 149 cases of RSD, 25 (16.8%) were treated with barbiturates at the time of onset of symptoms. In one-third of the cases, other provocating factors for RSD were absent. Joints were involved bilaterally in 76% of the cases, upper limbs in 76%, and Dupuytren's contracture was found in 20% of the cases. Recovery was prompt after discontinuation of the medication. Recurrence of RSD occurred in 6 cases after rechallenge with barbiturates.

Several other reports support the relation of phenobarbital to RSD (Mattson et al 1989). Taylor and Posner (1989) noted shoulder-hand syndrome in 12% of patients with brain tumor treated with phenobarbital as compared with 5% in patients not so treated. Van der Korst (1966) reported that one third of patients with shoulder-hand syndrome had been receiving phenobarbital. Sanchez-Navarro et al (1987) have reported a case treated with phenobarbital where the diagnosis was made by bone scintography before radiological signs of osteoporosis appeared. In other cases reviewed by them, the outcome was favorable only in those where phenobarbital was discontinued.

Phenobarbital is associated with other connective tissue disorders as well. The pathomechanism of RSD with phenobarbital is not known. Barbiturates produce hyperalgesia at low doses by disinhibition of lower level pain control neurons and also have an effect at the level of sympathetic ganglia. These properties may have a bearing on the pathomechanism of RSD.

The association of RSD with AEDs other than phenobarbital is less well established. No definite relationship has been identified with phenytoin and carbamazepine. Falasca et al (1994) have reported a case in association with valproic acid. This patient recovered after discontinuation of valproic acid and treatment with prednisone despite continuation of barbiturate.

There is no consensus regarding management of AED-associated RSD. Discontinuation of the medication, corticosteroids, and physical therapy are the usual treatments. If instituted early, the response may be rapid but some cases have significant residual disability.

Cyclosporine

Munoz-Gomez et al (1991) reported 7 patients who developed RSD in the lower extremities among 240 renal transplant patients who received cyclosporine as an immunosuppressant. The manifestations were severe pain, periarticular soft tissue swelling and vasomotor changes in affected areas. A patchy osteoporotic pattern was seen radiographically with increase uptake of [99m]technicium. The manifestations occurred at plasma cyclosporine levels of > 200 ng/ml and improved when the plasma levels of cyclosporine declined to < 200 ng/ml.

The pathomechanism is not known. RSD is not reported in renal transplant patients who do not receive cyclosporine. Steroids may have a protective effect and have been reported to be effective for the treatment of RSD when used early in the course of the disease. However, Petit et al (1993) reported RSD in a patient receiving cyclosporine along with prednisone following liver transplant. They found calcitonin therapy to be effective in treating this complication.

Ergotamine

RSD with transient dystonia has been reported in a patient on long-term migraine treatment with ergotamine (Merello et al 1991). This patient met the diagnostic criteria of RSD, including burning pain, hyperesthesia and swelling, as well as radiographic changes (osteopenia) and increased [99m]technicium. Transient dystonia was considered to be component of RSD because it disappeared after treatment of RSD by discontinuation of ergotamine, administration of methylprednisone and calcitonin. The pathomechanism in this case was considered to be related to ischemia as the patient had intermittent claudication in lower extremities prior to onset of RSD.

References

Bannister R, Mathias CJ: Autonomic failure, 3rd ed, Oxford, Oxford University Press, 1992.

Benazzi F: anticholinergic toxic syndrome with venlafaxine-desipramine combination. Pharmacopsychiatry 1998; 31: 36–37.

Benazzi F: Severe anticholinergic side effects with venlafaxine-fluoxetine combination. Canad J Psychiatry 1997; 42: 980–981.

Beriel L, Barbier J: Le rhumatisme gardenalique. Lyon Med 1934; 153: 77–83.

Cook JE, Wenger CB, Kolka MA: Chronic pyridostigmine bromide administration: side effects among soldiers working in a desert environment. Military Medicine 1992; 157: 250–254.

Deshayes P, Houdent G, Morere P: Algo-Dystrophie de la chimiotherapie anti-tuberculeuse: a propos de 22 observations. Rev Rhum Mal Osteoartic 1969; 36: 316–322.

Dormann AJ, Grunewald T, Wigginghaus B, et al: Gemcitabine-associated autonomic neuropathy. Lancet 1998; 351: 644.

Evans PJD, Lloyd JW, Peet KMS: Autonomic dysaethesia due to ergot toxicity. BMJ 1980; 281: 1621.

Falasca GF, Toly TM, Reginato AJ, et al: Reflex sympathetic dystrophy associated with antiepileptic drugs. Epilepsia 1994; 35: 394–399.

Fraser DM, Cambell IW, Miller HC: Peripheral and autonomic neuropathy after treatment with perhexiline maleate. BMJ 1977; 3: 675–676.

Gemperli R: Beitrag zur isoniazid-induzierten fibrosierenden Arrthropathie (Algodystrophie). Schweiz Med Wschr 1969; 99: 1762–1765.

Hansen SW: autonomic neuropathy after treatment with cisplain, vinblastine, and bleomycin for germ cell cancer. BMJ 1990; 300: 511–512.

Holland MS: Central anticholinergic syndrome in a pediatric patient following transdermal scopolamine patch placement. Nurse Anesthesia 1992; 3: 121–124.

Horton P, Gerster JC: Reflex sympathetic dystrophy syndrome and barbiturates. A study of 25 cases treated with barbiturates compared with 124 cases treated without barbiturates. Clin Rheumatol 1984; 3: 493–500.

Jerian SM, Sarosy GA, Link CJ, et al: Incapacitating autonomic neuropathy precipitated by taxol. Gynecologic Oncology 1993; 51: 277–280.

Johnson AL, Hollister LE, Berger PA: The anticholinergic intoxication syndrome: diagnosis and treatment. J Clin Psychiatry 1981; 42: 313–317.

Joos AA, Konig F, Frank UG, et al: Dose-dependent pharmacokinetic interaction of clozapine and paroxetine in an extensive metabolizer. Pharmacopsychiatry 1997; 30(6): 266–70.

Kumar K, Nath RK, Toth C: Spinal cord stimulation is effective in the management of reflex sympathetic dystrophy. Neurosurgery 1997; 40(3): 503–508; discussion 508–509 .

Link J, Papadopoulos G, Dopjans D, et al: Distinct central anticholinergic syndrome following general anaesthesia. Eur J Anaesthesiol 1997; 14(1): 15–23.

Manolis AS, Tordjman T, Mack KD, et al: Atypical pulmonry and neurologic complications of amiadarone in the same patient. Arch Int Med 1987; 147: 1805–1809.

Martin B, Howell PR: Physostigmine: going . . . going . . . gone? Two cases of central anticholinergic syndrome following anaesthesia and its treatment with physostigmine. Eur J Anaesthesiol 1997; 14(4): 467–70.

Mathias CJ: Disorders of the autonomic nervous system. In Bradley WG, et al (Eds.): Neurology in clinical practice, Butterworth-Heinemann, Boston, 1991, pp 1661–1685.

Mattson RH, Cramer JA, McCutchen CB, et al: Barbiturate-related connective tissue disorders. Arch Int Med 1989; 149: 911–914.

McDougall AJ, McLeod JG: Autonomic neuropathy, I. Clinical features, investigation, pathophysiology, and treatment. J Neurol Sci 1996; 137(2): 79–88.

Meador KJ, Nichols ME, Franke P, et al: Evidence for central cholinergic effect of high dose thiamine. Ann Neurol 1993; 34: 724–726.

Merello MJ, Noguess MA, Leiguarda RC, et al: Dystonia and reflex sympathetic dystrophy induced by ergotamine. Mov Dis 1991; 6: 263–264.

Munoz-Gomez J, Collado A, Gratacos J, et al: Reflex sympathetic dystrophy syndrome of the lower limbs in renal transplant patients treated with cyclosporin A. Arthr Rheum 1991; 34: 625–630.

Nevill TJ, Benstead TJ, McCormick CW, et al: Horner's syndrome and demyelinating peripheral neuropathy caused by high-dose cytosine arabinoside. Am J Hematol 1989; 32: 314–315.

Petit H, Schaeverbeke T, Malavialle P, et al: Reflex sympathetic dystrophy syndrome of the foot in liver transplant patients treated with ciclosporin A (abstract). Rev Rheum 1993; 60: 616.

Rengstorff RH, Doughty CB: Mydriatric and cycloplegic drugs: a review of ocular and systemic complications. Am J Optometry & Physiol Optics 1982; 59: 162–177.

Riedel WJ, van Praag HM: Avoiding and managing anticholinergic effects of antidepressants. CNS Drugs 1995; 3: 245–259.

Roca E, Bruera E, Politi PM, et al: Vinca alkaloid-induced cardiovascular autonomic neuropathy. Cancer Treat Rep 1985; 69: 149–151.

Ropiquet S, Petit J, Oksenhendler G, et al: Syndrome de sevrage lors d'une administration péridurale de morphine après interruption d'un traitment par la clonidine. Ann Fr Anesth Reanim 1984; 3: 380–382.

Rosen J, Pollock BG, Altieri LP, et al: Treatment of nortriptyline's side effects in elderly patients: a double-blind study of bethanechol. Am J Psychiatry 1993; 150: 1249–1251.

Rosenfeld CS, Broder LE: Cisplatin-induced autonomic neuropathy. Cancer Treat Rep 1984; 68: 659–660.

Rupreht J, Dworacek B: Central anticholinergic syndrome during anesthesia. Ann Fr Anesth Reanim 1990; 9: 295–304.

Sanchez-Navarro JJ, del Pino Montes J, Cardero Sanchez M: Sindrome de distrofia simpatico refleja por fenobarbital. Rev Clin Esp 1987; 181: 203–205.

Schneck HJ, Rupreht J: Central anticholinergic syndrome (CAS) in anesthesia and intensive care. Acta Anesthesiol Belg 1989; 40: 219–228.

Taylor LP, Posner JB: Phenobarbital rheumatism in patients with brain tumor. Ann Neurol 1989; 25: 92–94.

Thomashefsky AJ, Horwitz SJ, Feingold MH: Acute autonomic neuropathy. Neurology 1972; 22: 251–255.

Tune LE, Balsma FW, Hilt DC: Anticholinergic delirium caused by topical homatropine ophthalmologic solution: confirmation by anticholinergic radioreceptor assay in two cases. J Neuropsychiatry 1992; 4: 195–197.

Tung AS, Tenicela R, Winter PM: Opiate withdrawal syndrome following intrathecal administration of morphine. Anesthesiology 1980; 53: 340.

Van der Korst JK, Colenbrander H, Cats A: Phenobarbital and the shoulder-hand syndrome. Ann Rheum Dis 1966; 25: 553–555.

Veldman PHJM, Reynen HM, Arntz IE, et al: Signs and symptoms of reflex sympathetic dystrophy: prospective study of 829 patients. Lancet 1993; 342: 1012–1016.

Wohlreich MM, Welch W: Amitriptyline abuse presenting as acute toxicity. Psychosomatics 1993; 34: 191–193.

Chapter 19
Drug-Induced Sleep Disorders

Introduction

Sleep disorders are frequently reported as adverse reactions to drugs yet most of these are subjective complaints and very few of these patients have sleep laboratory studies. Sleep disorders are associated with several medical conditions and may occur as a part of other adverse drug reactions. For example, patients with movement disorders may have difficulty sleeping and patients on diuretics may have to get up frequently at night to urinate. An attempt is made to discuss those drug-related sleep disorders which are reported independent of other adverse reactions. Some of the information in this chapter is quoted from an excellent review of this subject by Novak and Shapiro (1997). Some of the basics of sleep physiology that are relevant to a discussion of drug-induced sleep disorders are discussed here.

Basics of Sleep Physiology

Sleep is an essential biological process that is required for physical and psychological restoration. Sleep is divided in rapid eye movement (REM) and non-REM sleep with cycling between the two types. There are age-related changes in sleep physiology with infants requiring longer hours of sleep and the requirement decreases with age. Various factors which influence sleep include circadian rhythms, exposure to light, noise, psychological stress, temperature of the environment and partial or complete sleep deprivation.

Sleep architecture is altered by medical conditions and their treatment. Psychotropic drugs, coffee and alcohol markedly influence sleep while non-psychotropic drugs may affect sleep as a side effect.

Several neurotransmitters play a role in the regulation of sleep and wakefulness including serotonin, noradrenaline, acetylcholine, dopamine and gamma amino butyric acid (GABA). Several drugs interact with one or more of these neurotransmitters which are also involved in the pathogenesis of CNS disorders.

A proper assessment of sleep disorders requires an overnight polysomnographic study which is usually done in a sleep laboratory. Changes in sleep stages, number of arousals, sleep-related breathing disorders and movements during sleep. This is not only important for evaluation of sleep disorders but also for investigations of action of drugs on sleep.

Classification of Drug-Related Sleep Disorders

there are several ways to classify the large number of sleep disorders. For the practical purposes of evaluation of adverse effects of drugs on sleep a simplified clinical classification is shown in Table 19.1.

Table 19.1. Classification of drug-induced sleep disorders.

Excessive sleepiness: sleep attacks
Drug-induced insomnia
Rebound and withdrawal insomnia
Drug-induced sleep disordered breathing: sleep apnoe
Movement disorders during sleep
Drug-induced parasomnias: sleep behavioral disorders
    Vivid dreams and nightmares
    Sleep walking
    Sleep paralysis
    Enuresis
    Bruxism

Excessive Sleepiness

This term should be differentiated from somnolence which literally means sleepiness but in a medical context it is abnormal drowsiness and is discussed in Chapter 4. However, the terms sleepiness and drowsiness often overlaps and are used interchangeably in various reports. Excessive sleepiness may be an extension of the effect of hypnotic drugs either due to excess dosage or an idiosyncratic response of the patient. Elderly patients with liver or kidney disorders may not metabolize or excrete some of these drugs adequately. Excessive sleepiness can also be an unintended side effect of several drugs given for other indications (Table 19.2). Excessive daytime sleepiness may be due to the effect of drugs on the sleep-wake cycle. Stimulant drugs may lead to disruption of sleep and subsequent excessive daytime sleepiness.

Table 19.2. Drugs that may have excessive drowsiness as a side effect.

Anticonvulsants
 – Phenobarbital
 – Phenytoin
 – Valproic acid
Antidepressants: tricyclic
Antiemetic drugs
 – Hyoscine
 – Prochlorperazine
 – Perphenazine
Antihistaminics
Antihypertensive drugs
 – Methyldopa
 – Reserpine
 – α-Antagonists
Antiparkinsonian drugs: pramipexole (Frucht et al 1999)

β-blockers
 – Propranolol
 – Labetalol
 – Timolol
 – Metaprolol

Anticonvulsants

Phenobarbital is known to have excessive sleepiness as an adverse effect. All of the other anticonvulsants have also been reported to be associated with occasional drowsiness and in some cases the reverse of it—insomnia.

Antidepressants

Tricyclic antidepressants (TCAs) promote sleep in patients with insomnia due to depression and are the most to cause drowsiness whereas SSRIs and MAO inhibitors are more likely to cause insomnia.

Antiemetic Drugs

Most antiemetic drugs penetrate the BBB and produce sleepiness by their action on the dopaminergic, histaminergic, or cholinergic systems. Hyoscine is a short acting but powerful anticholinergic agent which reduces the REM sleep but increases light (stage 2) sleep. REM sleep is increased on withdrawal of the drug. Prochlorperazine, perphenazine, trifluoperazine, and thiethylperazine may also produce sleepiness. Domperidone is an exception because it acts on the chemoreceptor trigger zone outside the BBB, and is unlikely to cause sleepiness.

Antihistaminics

Histamine, as a neurotransmitter, takes part in the regulation of sleep. Therefore, sleep is affected by antihistaminics. The older antihistaminics such as triprolidine cause daytime sleepiness. The newer H_1-antagonists such as terfandine do not penetrate the BBB or enter the brain slowly and do not induce sleep except in high doses. Among H_2-antagonists, cimetidine increases the duration of slow wave sleep but ranitidine does not.

Antihypertensive Drugs

Methyldopa can cause excessive sleep as well as nightmares. It increases the duration of REM sleep and reduces the amount of slow wave sleep. Possible pathomechanism of this adverse reaction is inhibition of synthesis of noradrenaline and serotonin. Reserpine increases REM sleep by blocking the synthesis of amines in the brain and by depleting the stores of catecholamines. α-antagonists such as prazosin may cause transient sleepiness at the start of treatment.

Antipsychotics

Most of the antipsychotics including classical as well as atypical agents frequently produce some drowsiness as a side effect.

β-Blockers

Sleep disruption and excessive daytime sleepiness caused by β-blockers depends on the lipid solubility of the drugs. Propranolol which is the most lipid soluble drug of this group is most liable to cause sleep disruption whereas atenolol, the least lipid soluble drug is the least likely to cause sleep disruption.

Drug-Induced Insomnia

This is a difficult symptom to evaluate. Patients with pre-existing insomnia are at greater risk for developing aggravation of this symptom as an adverse effect of drugs. Drugs which have been reported to be associated with insomnia are listed in Table 19.3.

Antidepressants

Monoamine Oxidase Inhibitors (MAOIs). Tranylcypromine, phenelzine, and isocarboxazid are effective antidepressants they can cause or exacerbate insomnia while ameliorating most other symptoms. The evaluation of this adverse reaction is difficult because insomnia may be one of the symptoms of depression. Three of 39 patients (4%) were reported to have discontinued treatment of major depression because of phenelzine-associated insomnia even though they sustained an excellent antidepressant response

Table 19.3. Drugs associated with insomnia.

Antidepressants
 – Monoamine oxidase inhibitors
 – Selective serotonin reuptake inhibitors: fluoxetine
 – MAO inhibitors
Antiepileptic drugs
 – Phenytoin
Antimalarials
 – Mefloquine
 – Chloroquine
Antineoplastics
 – Daunorubicin
 – Interferon-α
 – Medroxyprogesterone
Antiparkinsonian drugs: dopaminergic
Anxiolytic drugs: buspirone
Bismuth, chronic toxicity
Bronchodilators
 – Albutral
 – Ipratropium bromide
 – Metaproterenol
 – Salmeterol
 – Terbutaline
 – Theophylline
Cardiovascular drugs:
 – Antidiuretic: acetazolamide
 – Antiarrhythmic drugs: lorcainide, quinidine
 – Antihypertensives
  • β-blockers
  • Clonidine
  • Methyldopa
  • Reserpine
 – Calcium channel blockers: flunarizine
Cholesterol-lowering drugs: lovastatin
CNS stimulants
 – Amphetamine
 – Caffeine
 – Ephedrine
 – Methylphenidate
 – Nicotine
Drug withdrawal: opioids
Endocrine preparations
 – Corticosteroids
 – Oral contraceptives
 – Progesterone
 – Thyroid preparations

(Robinson and Zwillich 1991). Isocarboxazid-associated insomnia has been reported in 10% of patients pooled from three double-blind, placebo-controlled studies of this drug in the treatment of atypical depression (Zisook 1984). Nierenberg and Keck (1989) presented 13 cases of MAOI-associated insomnia managed with the addition of trazodone and nine (69%) were able to continue on combination of MAOI and trazodone without further problems. In three clinical trials of 72 depressed patients with sleep disturbances, brofaromine (selective MAOI) treatment had a clinically significant deteriorating effect on sleep (Haffmans and Knegtering 1993). Higher level of brofaromine in the plasma was associated with increase in the number and duration of intermittent awakenings. Non-responders experienced more frequent increase in sleep problems than responders. Moclobemide, a reversible MAOI, is associated with an incidence of insomnia of 7.9% compared to 5.4% in the placebo group in clinical trials (Chen and Ruch 1993). The same authors reported an incidence of insomnia of 9.8% with moclobemide in clinical trials comparing it with tricyclic antidepressants which were associated with insomnia in 8%. In a recent report from New Zealand, insomnia was found in 12 (19%) of 62 blindly treated depressed patients (Williams et al 1993).

Selective Serotonin Reuptake Inhibitors. Insomnia is a frequently reported side effect of fluoxetine, affecting 7% to 22% of the patients in a dose-related manner (Cooper 1988). A polysomnographic study has shown an unusually large number of eye movements in non-REM sleep (Keck et al 1991). The mechanism responsible for these is not known but it may be due to a general increase in central arousal.

Antimalarials

Mefloquine. This drug is associated with disturbances of sleep-wake rhythm including insomnia (Weinke et al 1991). Insomnia has been reported during the treatment of lupus erythematosus with chloroquine (Reis 1991).

Antiparkinsonian Drugs

Parkinson's disease patients treated with *dopaminergic* agents have abnormal sleep patterns and 30% of these have hallucinations. These patients have significantly greater REM aberrations than non-hallucinating patients and have more episodes of waking up during the night (Comella et al 1993).

Bismuth Toxicity

Chronic use of bismuth is associated with bismuth encephalopathy (see Chapter 3). Insomnia is a striking feature of bismuth encephalopathy.

Buspirone

This is an antianxiety drug with structure and pharmacology different from other anxiolytic agents. It lacks sedative effect but may have stimulant properties as there is a delayed and mild increase in sleep difficulty (Manfredi et al 1991).

Cardiovascular Drugs

Acetazolamide. This is a diuretic which is used prophylactically for mountain sickness and central apnea. Masuyama et al (1989) described the case of a mountaineer who took triazolam and acetazolamide together and had insomnia and respiratory depression. The authors pointed out that acetazolamide is not an antidote against benzodiazepines but rather potentiates their action.

Lorcainide. This is an antiarrhythmic agent, is associated with sleep disturbances in up to 45% of cases (Keefe et al 1982). The main types of disturbance are difficulty in falling asleep, nightmares and vivid dreams.

Clonidine (α-Agonist). This is associated with insomnia and vivid dreams.

β-blockers. Since their introduction β-blockers have been reported to cause sleep disturbances involving increased waking and vivid dreams. This effect is more marked with the three lipophilic drugs of this class: propranolol, metoprolol, and pindolol. However, complex factors other than lipophilicity, e. g., intrinsic sympathetic activity and serotonin-blocking properties, may be involved.

Hydrophilic β-blockers such as atenolol with known poor CNS penetration also cause some REM suppression and two explanations for this have been offered by Betts and Alford (1985): (1) the minimum amount of atenolol that enters the brain is sufficient to cause REM suppression or (2) effective peripheral β-blockade during sleep may reduce REM periods slightly.

Calcium Channel Blocker

Flunarizine therapy for migraine has been reported to be associated with insomnia in 3.4% of patients (Volta et al 1990). In some of the cases the relationship with the drug has been shown by improvement after discontinuation of the therapy and recurrence with resumption of therapy. The exact pathomechanism of this adverse effect is not known but it may be related to interference with the dopaminergic system which is the explanation for the extrapyramidal effects of this drug.

Cholesterol-Lowering Drugs

Sleep disturbances are associated with lipophilic HMG-CoA reductase inhibitor agent lovastatin (Vgontzas et al 1991; Rosenson and Goranson 1993; Sinzinger et al 1994). The self-reported disturbances include frequent awakenings, shorter sleep duration and early morning awakening. These disturbances clear up on discontinuation of the medication. The proposed pathomechanism is related to the differential penetration of these agents across the BBB, a property related to lipophilicity. In one study, neither lovastatin nor pravastatin, was shown to produce sleep disturbance or daytime sleepiness in patients with hypercholesterolemia (Kostis et al 1994). Simvastatin, another drug of this class, has been reported to produce less sleep disturbances indicating that lipophilicity alone is not responsible for these side effects.

CNS Stimulants

Amphetamine. Amphetamine is well known for inducing insomnia.

Caffeine. The effect of caffeine on sleep has been reviewed by Snell (1993). At high levels of arousal, caffeine in moderate doses may induce over-arousal, leading to prolonged wakefulness and impaired sleep.

Methylphenidate. This is used for the treatment of children with attention-deficit hyperactivity disorder (ADHD). Sleep disturbances are common in children with ADHD. Insomnia has been widely reported as a side effect of methylphenidate (Barkley 1977). Ahmann et al (1993) used Barkley Side Effects Questionnaire to assess the frequency of side effects of methylphenidate therapy for children with ADHD. Insomnia was found to be significantly increased in the treatment group as compared to the placebo group.

Laboratory sleep studies are controversial. Some investigators have found no alterations in sleep patterns following treatment of ADHD with psychostimulants whereas others have demonstrated disruption of REM sleep compared with normal controls. Variable adaptation of children to laboratory conditions is a confounding factor in the evaluation of these studies. An activity-based monitor known as Actigraph is more suitable for ambulatory assessment of sleep-wake cycles in children (Sadeh et al 1991). In a double-blind cross-over design study utilizing Actigraph, Tirosh et al (1993) found that methylphenidate does not appear to affect sleep patterns adversely and possibly normalizes them.

Nicotine. Transdermal nicotine is used for the management of smoking cessation. A review of the side effects of this treatment is insomnia and nightmares (Palmer et al 1992). Disruption of the sleep architecture was observed in a trial of transdermal nicotine for snoring in non-smokers (Devila et al 1994). This effect is consistent with increased catecholamine release following nicotine administration as a result of stimulation of the central nicotinic cholinergic pathways (Benowitz 1986).

Hormone Preparations

Patients receiving high dose corticosteroids complain of insomnia, vivid dreams, and nightmares (Turner and Elson 1993). Nightmares resolve by dosage reduction and insomnia can be avoided by changing the dosage schedule and confining the administration of steroids to earlier part of the day.

Rebound and Withdrawal Insomnia

The term "rebound insomnia" was first used by Kales et al (1978) to describe sleep disturbance characterized by increase in wakefulness above the previous baseline level. It is usually seen following the use of short-acting benzodiazepines (Roehrs et al 1990). It is not quite synonymous with "withdrawal insomnia" which implies drug dependence and is usually seen with long-term use of hypnotics. Other hypnotic drugs such as chloral hydrate can also lead to withdrawal problems. Barbiturates have no place in the treatment of insomnia. Tyrer (1993) defines withdrawal from sedative/hypnotic drugs as a temporary increase in the severity of insomnia within seven days of stopping treatment and lasts for one to three weeks before it returns to prewithdrawal levels. He considers the term "rebound insomnia" appropriate only if insomnia is not as pronounced as it was before the treatment started. If insomnia is worse than it was before the treatment started, he prefers the use of the term "recoil" or "overshoot" insomnia.

Gillin et al (1989) have reviewed various studies on this topic and concluded that rebound insomnia is a distinct possibility after discontinuation of triazolam in both insomniac patients and normal controls. The risk of insomnia after temazepam was low, while flurazepam with a long half-life caused only minimal rebound insomnia. In the study by Merlotti et al (1991), the subjects did not develop tolerance to triazolam but individuals with poor baseline sleep were found to be more susceptible to insomnia.

Pathomechanism. It is generally believed that rebound insomnia is related to rapid elimination of benzodiazepines which results in a CNS deficiency of inhibitor mechanisms (Kales et al 1983). Hypnotics suppress REM movements and there is compensatory excess of REMs after withdrawal.

Benzodiazepines are known to facilitate GABA receptor function which is a major inhibitory system in the CNS and withdrawal symptoms can be regarded as that of GABA deficiency. It may be presumed that during the period of drug administration, the production of endogenous benzodiazepines is suppressed by exogenous diazepines. This concept is compatible with lack of rebound effect with long-acting benzodiazepines (slow elimination) or gradual reduction of the dose of short-acting benzodiazepines which attenuates the rebound effect (Greenblatt et al 1987).

Another hypothesis is that the rebound insomnia is related to tolerance and decreased receptor density. The point against this hypothesis is that tolerance is related to the duration of administration which does not alter the intensity of rebound insomnia.

A clinical explanation is that rebound insomnia is related to oversedation (Roehrs et al 1990), i. e., increase doses which do not produce hypnotic effect. Another explanation is that sleep satiation, i. e., after the sleep need (induced by hypnotics) has been satisfied, there is lessening of sleep need following the discontinuation of the hypnotic. In support of this hypothesis is the data that subjects with insomnia receiving hypnotics show reduced daytime sleepiness.

Kales et al (1991) have shown that even under conditions of brief intermittent use and withdrawal, triazolam and to a lesser extent temazepam, produce rebound insomnia which predisposes to drug-taking behavior and increases the potential for drug-dependence.

Vivid Dreams and Nightmares

Most people experience vivid dreams and nightmares at some time during their life. These may be associated with sleep disturbances, psychiatric disorders, or may be reported as isolated events. Vivid dreams are often associated with insomnia which appears to be paradoxical. The explanation for this lies in the fact that waking appears to be necessary if the dreams are to be remembered. The increase in subjective dreaming with β-blockers may be an artefact of increased incidence of awakenings that they cause (Betts and Alford 1985). A β-blockers agent applied topically to the eye has been reported to produce severe nightmares (Mort 1992). Drugs which have been reported to be associated with these phenomena are listed in Table 19.4. The literature on this topic has been reviewed by Thompson and Pierce (1999) who have presented a causality assessment of the published cases.

Table 19.4. Drugs associated with vivid dreams and nightmares.

ACE inhibitor: captopril (Haffner et al 1993)
Antianxiety agent: bupropion (Balon 1996)
Antibiotics
  – Erythromycin (Black and Dawson 1988; Williams 1988)
  – Fluoroquinolone
    • Fleroxacin (Bowie et al 1989)
    • Ciprofloxacin (Dey 1995)
Antidepressants: selective serotonin reuptake inhibitors: fluoxetine (Lepkifker et al 1995)
Antiepileptics: valproic acid (Solomen and Bonsack 1993)
Antiparkinsonian drugs
  – Amantadine (Ing et al 1974)
  – Cabergoline (Webster et al 1992)
  – Levodopa (Miller and Nieberg 1974)
Antipsychotics
  – Chlorpromazine (DeHart (1969)
  – Thiothixene (Solomen 1983)
Benzodiazepines: nitrazepam (Girdwood 1973; Taylor 1973)
β-blockers: bisoprolol (Kuriyama 1994)
Corticosteroids, high dose
Cholinesterase inhibitor: donepezil (Ross and Shua-Haim 1998)
CNS stimulants
  – Amphetamine
  – Fenfluramine (used for weight reduction but withdrawn from the market in 1997)
  – Methylphenidate
  – Phenmetrazine
Calcium channel blocker: verapamil (Kumar and Hodges 1988)
Digoxin (Brezis et al 1980)
Ganciclovir (Chen et al 1992)
Hypnotic withdrawal
Non-steroidal anti-inflammatory drugs: Naproxen (Bacht and Miller 1991)
Opioids
Oxybutynin (Valsecia et al 1998)

Effect of Drugs on Breathing During Sleep

There is increasing clinical awareness of sleep disordered breathing (SDB), particularly obstructive sleep apnea which is a risk factor for cardiovascular diseases and cognitive decline. Sleep apnea may even manifest as insomnia. Several drugs affect respiration during sleep producing obstructive sleep apnea and nocturnal oxygen desaturation. Jain (1989) has reviewed the of control of breathing and pathomechanism of SDB. Sleep in normal persons predisposes to hypoventilation but reflex muscular dilatation of the pharynx occurs to prevent narrowing and increase of respiratory effort. This reflex is depressed by some drugs leading to pharyngeal narrowing and obstructive sleep apnea. Drugs have been reported to have an adverse effects on sleep during breathing are listed in Table 19.5.

Table 19.5. Drugs associated with sleep disordered breathing (from Robinson and Zwillich 1991).

Alcohol
Anesthetics
Antihypertensives
Narcotics
Sedative-hypnotics
Testosterone

Alcohol

Alcohol is well recognized as a respiratory depressant. Most normal persons will not experience significant SDB following alcohol ingestion prior to bedtime. However obesity, old age and chronic obstructive pulmonary disease (COPD) are risk factors for the development of obstructive sleep apnea and the use of alcohol in these conditions should be avoided.

Anesthetics

These agents, like other CNS depressants, decrease neural output to upper airway muscles to a greater extent than they depress the phrenic nerve activity. It is a common observation that normal persons develop upper airway obstruction during light general anesthesia if proper position of the head and neck is not maintained. Severe central apnea can develop following general anesthesia.

Antihypertensives

There is a high prevalence of sleep apnea among hypertensives and sleep apnea can also lead to daytime hypertension. The role of antihypertensive drugs on breathing during sleep has not been studied adequately. Methyldopa has been shown to depress upper airway function (Fletcher et al 1985) and propranolol has been reported to aggravate sleep apnea (Boudoulas et al 1983).

Narcotics

Narcotics such as morphine are powerful respiratory depressants. The effect of these agents on sleep apnea has not been fully investigated but their use should be avoided in patients with SDB.

Sedative-Hypnotics

Most agents of this type have a detrimental influence on breathing during sleep in patients with sleep apnea. SDB due to these drugs may be one explanation of excessive daytime sleepiness following their use. Benzodiazepines have a depressant effect on upper airway muscles and given as preanesthetics to patients with sleep apnea can lead to severe airway obstruction even while awake (Guilleminault 1980). Elderly patients are more susceptible to develop SDB as an effect of benzodiazepines as hypnotics.

Testosterone

Obstructive sleep apnea is more common in men except those who are hypogonadal indicating that sex hormones may have some influence on breathing during sleep. There are reports of patients who developed obstructive sleep apnea during testosterone replacement therapy (Johnson et al 1984; Sandbloom et al 1983). The

pathomechanism is not known but development of sleep apnea is recognized as a potential complication of androgen therapy.

Sleep Walking

Sleep walking occurs out of stage 4 of sleep and apparently represents a disorder of arousal and can be considered to be one form of parasomnia (Thorpy 1990). Subjects with epilepsy and those with a past or family history of sleep walking are more liable to manifest this as an adverse reaction to drugs (Monfort et al 1992). Sleep walking has been reported in association with the use of the following drugs:
- Lithium and neuroleptics (Charney et al 1979)
- Chloral hydrate derivatives (Luchins et al 1978)
- Benzodiazepines (Poitras 1980; Huapaya 1979)
- Zolpidem, an imidazopyridine hypnotic agent (Mendelson 1994)

Movement Disorders During Sleep

Various drug-induced disorders of movements such as myoclonic jerks and restless legs syndrome have been reported to occur during sleep. It is difficult to document or investigate most of these. Restless legs syndrome has been described in Chapter 8.

Sleep Paralysis

Sleep paralysis is a common condition with a prevalence of 5–50% (at least one episode during life time). Sleep paralysis (SP) is often associated with a mental disorder. Users of anxiolytic medication were nearly five times as likely to report SP, even after controlling for possible effects of mental and sleep disorders (Ohayon et al 1999). One case is reported of sleep paralysis in a patient on treatment with moclobemide for depression (Benazzi 1998). This resolved on discontinuing the drug but recurred on rechallenge thus proving the relation of the drug to the adverse event.

References

Ahmann PA, Waltonen SJ, Olson KA, et al: Placebo-controlled evaluation of ritalin side-effects. Pediatrics 1993; 91: 1101–1106.

Bakht FR, Miller LG: Naproxen-associated nightmares. South Med J 1991; 84: 1271–1273.

Balon R: Bupropion and nightmares. Am J Psychiatry 1996; 153: 579–580.

Barkley R: A review of stimulant drug research with hyperactive children. J Child Psychol Psychiatry 1977; 18: 137–165.

Benazzi F: Moclobemide-associated sleep paralysis. Human Psychopharmacology Clinical and Experimental 1998; 13: 377.

Benowitz NL: The human pharmacology of nicotine. Res Adv Alcohol Drug Probl 1986; 9: 1–52.

Betts TA, Alford C: β-blockers and sleep: a controlled trial. Eur J Clin Pharmacol 1985; 28(suppl): 65–68.

Black RJ, Dawson TA: Erythromycin and nightmares. Br Med J (Clin Res Ed) 1988; 296: 1070.

Boudoulas H, Schmidt H, Geleris P, et al: Case reports on deterioration of sleep apnea during therapy with propranolol—preliminary studies. Res Commun Chem Pathol Pharmacol 1983; 39: 3–10.

Bowie WR, Willetts V, Jewesson PJ: Adverse reactions in a dose-ranging study with a new long-acting fluoroquinolone, fleroxacin. Antimicrob Agents Chemother 1989; 33: 1778–1782.

Brezis M, Michaeli J, Hamburger R: Nightmares from digoxin. Ann Intern Med 1980; 93: 639–640.

Charney DS, Kales A, Soldatos CR, et al: Somnambulistic-like episodes secondary to combined lithium-neuroleptic treatment. Brit J Psychiatry 1979; 135: 418–424.

Chen DT, Ruch R: Safety of moclobemide in clinical use. Clin Neuropharmacol 1993; 16: S63-S68.

Chen JL, Brocavich JM, Lin AY: Psychiatric disturbances associated with ganciclovir therapy. Ann Pharmacother 1992; 26: 193–195.

Comella CL, Tanner CM, Ristanovic RK: Polysomnographic sleep measures in Parkinson's disease patients with treatment-induced hallucinations. Ann Neurol 1993; 34: 710–714.

Cooper GL: The safety of fluoxetine—an update. Br J Psychiatry 1988; 153(suppl 3): 77–86.

DeHart C: Adverse behavioral effects as manifestations of the major and minor tranquilizers. J Maine Med Assoc 1969; 60: 29–31.

Devila DG, Hurt RD, Offord KP, et al: The acute effects of transdermal nicotine on sleep architecture, snoring, and sleep-disordered breathing in non-smokers. Am J Res Crit Care Med 1994; 150: 469–474.

Dey SK: Nightmare due to ciprofloxacin in young patients. Indian Pediatr 1995; 32: 918–920.

Fletcher E, Lovoi M, Miller J, et al: Propranolol and sleep apnea (abstract). Am Rev Resp Dis 1985; 131(suppl): A103.

Frucht S, Rogers JD, Greene PE, et al: Falling asleep at the wheel: motor vehicle mishaps in persons taking pramipexole and ropinirole. Neurology 1999; 52: 1908–1910.

Gillin JC, Spinweber CL, Johnson LC: Rebound insomnia: a critical review. J Clin Psychopharmacol 1989; 9: 161–172.

Girdwood RH: Nitrazepam nightmares. BMJ 1973; 13: 353.

Greenblatt DJ, Harmatz JS, Zinny MA, et al: Effect of gradual withdrawal on the rebound sleep disorder after discontinuation of triazolam. NEJM 1987; 317: 722–728.

Guilleminault C, Cumminsky J, Dement WC: Sleep apnea syndrome. Adv Int Med 1980; 26: 347–372.

Haffmans J, Knegtering R: The selective reversible monoamine oxidase-A inhibitor brofaromine and sleep. J Clin Psychopharmacol 1993; 13: 291–292.

Haffner CA, Smith BS, Pepper C: Hallucinations as an adverse effect of angiotensin converting enzyme inhibition. Postgrad Med J 1993; 69(809): 240.

Huapaya LVM: Seven cases of sleepwalking induced by drugs. Am J Psychiatry 1979; 136: 985–986.

Ing TS, Rahn AC, Armbruster KF, et al: Letter: Accumulation of amantadine hydrochloride in renal insufficiency. N Engl J Med 1974; 291: 1257.

Jain KK: Oxygen in physiology and medicine, Springfield, Illinois, Charles C Thomas, 1989.

Johnson MW, Anch AM, Remmers JE: Induction of sleep apnea syndrome in a woman by exogenous androgen administration. Am Rev Resp Dis 1984; 129: 1023–1025.

Kales A, Manfredi RL, Vgontzas A, et al: Rebound insomnia after only brief and intermittent use of rapidly eliminated benzodiazepines. Clin Pharmacol Ther 1991; 49: 468–476.

Kales A, Scharf M, Kales J: Rebound insomnia: a new clinical syndrome. Science 1978; 201: 1039–1040.

Kales A, Soldatos CR, Bixler EO, et al: Rebound insomnia and rebound anxiety: a review. Pharmacology 1983; 26: 121–137.

Keck PE, Hudson lLJI, Dorsey CM: Effect of fluoxetine on sleep. Biol Psychiatry 1991; 29: 618–619.

Keefe DL, Peters F, Winkle RA: Randomized double-blind placebo-controlled crossover trial documenting oral lorcainide efficacy in suppression of symptomatic ventricular tachyarrhythmias. Am Heart J 1982; 103: 511–518.

Kostis JB, Rosen RC, Wilson AC: Central nervous system effects of HMG CoA reductase inhibitors: lovastatin and pravastatin on sleep and cognitive performance in patients with hypercholesterolemia. J Clin Pharmacol 1994; 34(10): 989–996.

Kumar KL, Hodges M: Disturbing dreams with long-acting verapamil. NEJM 1988; 318: 929–930.

Kuriyama S: Bisoprolol-induced nightmares. J Hum Hypertens 1994; 8: 730.

Lepkifker E, Dannon PN, Iancu I, et al: Nightmares related to fluoxetine treatment. Clin Neuropharmacol 1995; 18: 90–94.

Luchins DJ, Sherwood PM, Gillin JC, et al: A case of somnambulistic fillicide associated with psychotropic medication. Am J Psychiatry 1978; 135: 1404–1405.

Manfredi RL, Kales A, Vgontzas AN, et al: Buspirone:

sedative or stimulant effect? Am J Psychiatry 1991; 148: 1213–1217.

Masuyama S, Hirata K, Saito A: "Ondine's curse": side effect of acetazolamide? Am J Med 1989; 86: 637.

Mendelson WB: Sleep walking associated with Zolpidem. J Clin Psychopharmacol 1994; 14: 150.

Merlotti L, Roehrs T, Zorick F, et al: Rebound insomnia: duration of use and individual differences. J Clin Psychopharmacol 1991; 11: 368–373.

Miller EM, Nieburg HA: L-tryptophan in the treatment of levodopa-induced psychiatric disorders. Dis Nerv Sys 1974; 35: 20–23.

Monfort JC, Manus A, Levy-Soussan P: Activites automatiques avec amnesie induites par la prise de medicaments hypnotiques association a un passe personnel et familial de somnabulisme et d'epilepsie. Ann Med Psychol (Paris) 1992; 150: 371–374.

Mort JR: Nightmare cessation following alteration of ophthalmic administration of a cholinergic and a β blocking agent. Ann Pharmacother 1992; 26: 914–916.

Nierenberg AA, Keck PE: Management of monoamine oxidase inhibitor-associated insomnia with trazodone. J Clin Psychopharmlacol 1989; 9: 42–45.

Novak M, Shapiro CM: Drug-induced sleep disturbances. Drug Safety 1997; 16: 133–149.

Ohayon MM, Zulley J, Guilleminault C, et al: Prevalence and pathologic associations of sleep paralysis in the general population. Neurology 1999; 52(6): 1194–1200.

Palmer KJ, Buckley MM, Faulds D: Transdermal nicotine: a review of its pharmacodynamic and pharmacokinetic properties, and therapeutic efficacy as an aid to smoking cessation. Drugs 1992; 44: 498–529.

Poitras R: A propos d'episodes d'amnesias anterogrades associes a l'utilisation du triazolam. Union Med Can 1980; 109: 427–429.

Reis J: Insomnia induced by chloroquine in the treatment of lupus erythematosus disseminatus (letter in French). Presse Med 1991; 20: 659.

Robinson RW, Zwillich CW: The effect of drugs on breathing during sleep. In, Kryger MH, Roth T, Dement WC (Eds.): Principles and practice of sleep medicine, Philadelphia, Saunders, 1991, pp 501–512.

Roehrs T, Vogel G, Roth T: Rebound insomnia: its determinants and significance. Am J Med 1990; 88 (suppl 3A); 39S-42S.

Rosenson RS, Goranson NL: Lovastatin-associated sleep and mood disturbances. Am J Med 1993; 95: 548–549.

Ross JS, Shua-Haim JR: Aricept-induced nightmare in alzheimer's disease: 2 case reports. J Am Geriatr Soc 1998; 46: 119–120.

Sadeh A, Lavie P, Scher A, et al: Actigraph home monitoring of sleep-disturbed and control infants and young children: a new method for pediatric assessment of sleep-wake patterns. Pediatrics 1991; 87: 494–499.

Sandbloom RE, Matsumoto AM, Schoene RB, et al: Obstructive sleep apnea syndrome induced by testosterone administration. NEJM 1983; 308: 508–510.

Sinzinger H, Mayr F, Schmidt P, et al: Sleep disturbances and appetite after lovastatin. Lancet 1994; 343: 973.

Snell J: Coffee and caffeine: sleep and wakefulness. In, Garattini S (Ed.): Caffeine, coffee and health, New York, Raven Press, 1993, pp 255–290.

Solomen K, Bonsack BA: Bizarre nightmares associated with valproic acid: a rare side effect in the elderly. Clin Gerontol 1993; 14: 31–36.

Taylor F: Nitrazepam in the elderly. BMJ 1973; 13: 113–114.

Thompson DF, Pierce DR: Drug-induced nightmares. Ann Pharmacotherap 1999; 33: 93–98.

Thorpy MJ: Disorders of arousal. In Thorpy MJ (Ed.): Handbook of sleep disorders, New York, Marcel-Dekker Inc, 1990, pp 531–550.

Tirosh E, Sadeh A, Munvez R, et al: Effect of methylphenidate on sleep in children with attention-deficit hyperactivity disorder. AJDC 1993; 147: 1313–1315.

Turner R, Elson E: Steroids cause sleep disturbance. BMJ 1993; 306: 1477–1478.

Tyrer P: Withdrawal from hypnotic drugs. BMJ 1993; 306: 706–707.

Valsecia ME, Malgor LA, Espfindola JH, et al: New adverse effects of oxybutinin-night terror. Ann Pharmacother 1998; 32: 506.

Vgontzas AN, Kales A, Bixler EO, et al: Effects of provastatin and lovastatin on sleep efficiency and sleep stages. Clin Pharmacol Ther 1991; 50: 730–737.

Volta GD, Magoni M, Cappa S, et al: Insomnia and perceptual disturbances during flunarizine treatment. Headache 1990; 30: 62–63.

Webster J, Piscitelli G, Polli A, et al: Dose-dependent suppression of serum prolactin by cabergoline in hyperprolactinaemia: a placebo controlled, double blind, multicentre study. European Multicentre Cabergoline Dose-finding Study Group. Clin Endocrinol (Oxf) 1992; 37: 534–541.

Weinke T, Trautmann M, Held T, et al: Neuropsychiatric side effects after the use of mefloquine. Am J Trop Med Hyg 1991; 45: 86–91.

Williams NR: Erythromycin: a case of nightmares. Br Med J (Clin Res Ed) 1988; 296: 214.

Williams R, Edwards RA, Newburn GM, et al: A double-blind comparison of moclobemide and fluoxetine in the treatment of depressive disorders. Int Clin Psychopharmacol 1993; 7(3–4): 155–158.

Zisook S: Side effects of isocarboxazid. J Clin Psychiatry 1984; 45: 53–58.

Chapter 20
Eosinophilia Myalgia Syndrome

Introduction

Eosinophilia myalgia syndrome (EMS) was first recognized in 1989 by physicians in New Mexico in patients who had consumed tryptophan prior to the onset of illness (CDC 1989; Hertzman et al 1990; Eidson et al 1990). Tryptophan, the agent involved, is an essential amino acid. Based on reports in the literature during the past 20 years, tryptophan has been recommended for treatment of depression, insomnia, schizophrenia, and behavioral disorders. This was based on the assumption that serotonin content of the brain could be altered by exogenously administered tryptophan.

A warning was issued by FDA in November 1989 advising consumers to discontinue the use of tryptophan as a food supplement and self medication. Several other cases were uncovered later and over 1,000 cases had been reported to CDC (Center for Disease Control, Atlanta, Georgia) by mid-1990. Following the general discontinuation of tryptophan use, the number of new cases dropped remarkably. The case definition developed by the CDC on review of initial cases included the following criteria:

- Eosinophil count greater than 1000/mm³
- Incapacitating myalgia
- No evidence of infection or neoplasm that could explain the findings.

Investigations on this topic are still going on and a considerable amount of literature has accumulated on this topic including excellent reviews (Belongia et al 1992; Kaufman and Philen 1993; Harati 1994). Cases have been reported from outside the United States including 2 in Belgium (Van Garsse and Boeykens 1990) and 5 in Scotland (Douglas et al 1990) and 5 in Japan (Tsutsui

et al 1996). Tryptophan was also withdrawn from the market in the UK in 1989.

Epidemiology

There were 1531 cases of EMS reported to CDC by mid 1992, including 36 deaths. There are estimated to be twice as many cases which did not meet the criteria of CDC. The prevalence was higher in the Western states possibly because of the higher rate of consumption of tryptophan in those states. High prevalence was also reported in South Carolina, New Mexico, Minnesota, and Oregon because of active surveillance in these states.

Epidemiological studies have been reviewed by Belongia et al (1992; Belongia et al 1990; Slutsker et al 1990). These investigations demonstrated that EMS was not triggered by tryptophan *per se* but rather by exposure to a contaminant in tryptophan manufactured by one company (Showa Denko, K.K., Tokyo, Japan). This company used a fermentation process to synthesize tryptophan from its precursor using *Bacillus amyloliquefaciens*. In December 1988, this company introduced a new strain (strain V) of this bacillus which had been genetically modified to increase the synthesis of intermediates in tryptophan biosynthetic pathway and thus increase the yield of tryptophan. Chromatographic analysis of tryptophan manufactures this way showed the presence of peak E, the chemical structure of which was subsequently determined to be 1,1-ethylidenebis-tryptophan (EBT). This chemical is later hydrolyzed under acidic conditions and preliminary studies suggested that it may cause abnormalities of the fascia and microvasculature (Love et al 1991). Tryptophan consumed by EMS patients was traced back to Showa Denko and chromatographic analysis of tryptophan from rest of the cases showed no convincing evidence that it was manufactured by companies other than Showa Denko. The pooled attack rate among persons exposed to contaminated tryptophan may have been as high as 52%. Further investigations by Philen et al (1993) have raised the possibility that other chemical contaminants in tryptophan may modify the effect of EBT or that the cause may be an entirely different compound. One of these compounds is 3-(Phenylamino)-alanine which is very similar to the contaminant that caused the onset of EMS-like toxic oil syndrome in Spain in 1981. An epidemiologic study in Germany supports the role of a contaminant in L-tryptophan in the occurrence of EMS (Carr et al 1994).

Risk Factors

Few risk factors for EMS have been identified other than the consumption of contaminated tryptophan. There is a dose response relationship between the amount of contaminated tryptophan consumed and the risk of EMS. Other risk factors are:

- *Old age.* The risk of EMS may be increased in older patients independent of dose. Physiologic changes in hepatic and renal functions with aging may delay the clearance of the toxic substance.
- *Female sex.* This has been considered to be a possible risk factor. Another explanation is the greater use of tryptophan by females.
- *Asthma.* Underlying asthma has been noted in 25% of patients who are also females (Henning et al 1993). There are increased levels of eosinophils and eosinophil-derived toxins, markers of eosinophil activation, in the sera of these patients. This suggests that eosinophil activation prior to exposure to contaminated tryptophan may potentiate the pathogenic effect of such a contaminant.
- *Psychotropic drugs.* Concomitant use of psychotropic drugs such as antidepressants is suspected to be a risk factor.

Clinical and Pathological Features

These have been reviewed by Kilbourne (1992). Major manifestations are shown in Table 20.1.

Table 20.1. Distribution of major manifestations of EMS among the first 1000 cases (from Swygert et al 1990).

Myalgia	100%
Arthralgia	73%
Rash	60%
Peripheral edema	59%
Cough or dyspnea	59%
Fever	36%
Scleroderma	32%
Periorbital edema	28%
Alopecia	28%
Neuropathy	27%

Late symptoms and signs differ from the initial presentation and the proportion of various manifestations in later studies differs. This broad range of clinical signs and symptoms reported in patients with EMS indicates that a strict case definition may identify only about half the cases (Kamb et al 1992).

Differential Diagnosis. EMS should be differentiated from conditions with eosinophilia and inflammatory peripheral neuromuscular diseases shown in Table 20.2.

Table 20.2. Conditions to be considered in the differential diagnosis of EMS.

Toxic oil syndrome
Vasculitic conditions such as Churg-Strauss syndrome
Parasitic infections such as trichinosis
Idiopathic eosinophilic fascitis
Paraneoplastic myositis
Sarcoidosis

Toxic Oil Syndrome. This multisystem disease appeared as an epidemic in Spain in 1981 in relation to the intake of rapeseed cooking oil. Eosinophilia, myalgia, and rash are the presenting features in the first four months. The pathology of this syndrome is marked by chronic interstitial infiltrates, non-necrotizing angitis, endothelial proliferation, and fibrotic changes (Alonso-Ruiz et al 1993).

Myalgia. Muscle pain is a constant feature but serum creatinine kinase is rarely elevated and there is no evidence of myofibrillary degeneration. Myalgia may result from damage to the peripheral sensory nerves, rather than from myopathy. Muscle biopsies may show cellular infiltrates within the muscle fascia but these are mostly macrophages and T-lymphocytes and rarely eosinophils.

Peripheral Neuropathy. A diffuse sensory or sensorimotor neuropathy, identified by clinical examination or EMG, has been reported in one- to two-third of patients seen in various clinical centers (Thacker 1991; Varga et al 1993). These may be the initial presentation of the disease and may be accompanied by Guillain-Barré like ascending paralysis (Heiman-Patterson et al 1990). Smith and Dyck (1990) described 10 patients with EMS who presented with one of the following three patterns:
– Myopathy and neuropathy with connective tissue involvement
– Painful predominantly sensory neuropathy
– Sensori-motor neuropathy

EMG examination showed that sensory fibers were involved more than the motor ones and sural nerve biopsy findings were:
– Axonal degeneration of various degrees
– Epineural and perivascular inflammation with mononuclear or eosinophil cells
– Inflammatory vasculopathy

The term neuromyopathy is used for the lymphocytic perineuritis and neuritis along with EMS (Turi et al 1990).

Natural History of EMS

There is a median latency period of 127 days from exposure to tryptophan and manifestations of EMS. EMS is considered to be a long-term illness characterized by improvement during the first 25 weeks followed by a protracted period of symptom resolution (Culpepper et al 1991). Most of the patients in population-based cohort were still symptomatic one year after the onset of illness (Hedberg et al 1992). No method of treatment has been shown to reduce the long-term sequelae or the duration of the disease.

Pathomechanism

Although the bulk of the available evidence links contamination of tryptophan to EMS, Clauw et all (1990) supported the speculation that pathogenesis of EMS may be related to abnormalities of tryptophan metabolism. Normal metabolic pathways of tryptophan are shown in Figure 20.1.

The reasons given in support of EMS being an adverse reaction to tryptophan itself, rather than to a contaminant are as follows:
– Clinical similarity of EMS to eosinophilic fascitis which may have mononuclear cells as predominant cellular infiltrate rather than eosinophils.

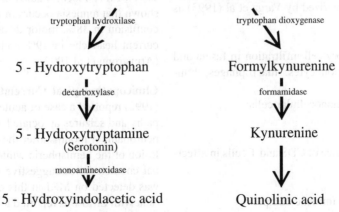

Figure 20.1. Major metabolic pathways of tryptophan.

- Hypereosinophilic rash and pulmonary disease seen in patients with EMS suggests that a hypersensitivity reaction may be responsible for some features of the syndrome.
- Patients who develop toxic reaction to tryptophan may have errors in tryptophan metabolism with abnormal enzyme activity that functions adequately with normal daily intake of tryptophan but shunt metabolites to kynurenine pathway in the presence of large amounts of the substance. An abnormal accumulation of metabolites of tryptophan may lead to EMS. Abnormal serotonin (5-HT) metabolism has been implicated in the pathogenesis of scleroderma (Stachow et al 1977). Scleroderma-like changes and myositis occur in carcinoid syndrome characterized by excessive production of serotonin and its metabolites.
- Concomitant use of antidepressants which inhibit uptake of serotonin may result in accumulation of metabolites of tryptophan.
- Pyridoxine deficiency has been reported in some patients with EMS may lead to abnormal metabolism of tryptophan because 5-HT decarboxylase is very sensitive to deficiency of this cofactor.

The etiological agent, e. g., contaminant, may trigger the onset of immunologically mediated inflammatory response. Varga et al (1992) have demonstrated autoantibodies to nuclear lamin C in the serum of a patient with EMS. The antibody titer declined dramatically after discontinuation of tryptophan and treatment with prednisone. This is evidence for autoimmune response in EMS. Immunological abnormalities in EMS have been summarized by Varga et al (1993) as follows:
- Cellular
  · Inflammatory cell infiltration in fascia and muscles: monocytes, macrophages, lymphocytes
  · Activated monocellular cells:
    – in tissues
    – in blood
  · Preponderance of CD8 and T cells in affected tissues
- Humoral
  · Circulating immune complex
  · Antinuclear antibodies

Eosinophils. These play a role in the pathogenesis of EMS as effector cells. The growth and maturation of eosinophils, their migration to the site of action and their viability and function are regulated by three cytokines: GM-CSF, IL-3, and IL-5 which are produced by activated T lymphocytes, mast cells, neutrophils, and eosinophils themselves. Cytokine-induced stimulation of eosinophils is an important feature of EMS. Patients with EMS have increased levels of IL-5 (Owen et al 1990). An EMS-like syndrome has been described in a patient without tryptophan use and increased level of serum GM-CSF (Bochner et al 1991).

Activated eosinophils release toxic granules which appear to be an important feature of EMS. An eosinophil-derived neurotoxin is postulated to be responsible for producing neuropathy in EMS. Eosinophil-derived granular proteins induce secretion of platelet-à-granule component of fibrogenic cytokines including TGF-α. Fibrosis of connective tissue is a consistent finding in late in the course of EMS. EMS fibroblasts in situ display elevated expression of transforming growth factors (TGF)-α_1 which plays a crucial role in the physiologic regulation of connective tissue metabolism and appears to participate in the pathogenesis of several experimentally induced and spontaneously occurring fibrotic conditions.

CNS Involvement in EMS: Clinical Features. In initial studies, symptoms such as loss of memory and difficulty in concentration were reported in 15% of patients with EMS (Culpepper et al 1991). More recent studies of CNS-EMS have shown that amnesia occurs in 88%, intermittent confusion in 38%, motor disorders in 31%, recurrent headache in 19% and dementia in 6% (Armstrong et al 1997).

Clinicopathological Correlations. Adair et al (1992) reported a case of acute leucoencephalopathy and seizures associated with axonal polyneuropathy 4 months after the onset of EMS. A lesion of the hemispheric white matter with signal characteristics suggestive of demyelination was detected on MRI in this case. Another patient with EMS was reported to develop progressive CNS involvement that did not improve despite discontinuation of tryptophan (Lynn et al 1992). Initially there was spastic monoparesis and ataxia but cognitive deficits suggestive of subcortical dementia developed later. MRI showed multiple white matter lesions in the cerebral hemispheres. Krupp et al (1992) carried out a small survey for the detection of cognitive deficits in EMS patients by questionnaires and neuropsychological testing and found that cognitive abnormalities suggestive of CNS involvement were frequent among EMS patients. Comprehensive neuropsychological testing revealed neurocognitive impairment in a series of patients and these were correlated with changes in white matter shown on MRI scans of these patients

Another series of patients with EMS and CNS abnormalities shown by proton MR spectroscopy and MRI included subcortical focal lesions, focal lesions in deep white matter, cortical atrophy, ventricular dilatation, and diffuse and periventricular white matter abnormalities (Armstrong et al 1997). MR spectroscopic findings established two distinct spectral patterns:

- Increased choline-containing compounds, decreased N-acetylaspartate, and increased lipid-macromolecules, consistent with inflammatory cerebrovascular disease
- Increased glutamine, decreased myo-inositol, and decreased choline, consistent with acute CNS injury or metabolic encephalopathy.

The pattern of cerebral lesions and neurometabolites is consistent with widespread inflammatory cerebrovascular disease. However, a subgroup of patients with CNS-EMS have neurometabolic changes consistent with a metabolic encephalopathy identical or similar to hepatic encephalopathy.

Pathomechanism. Cognitive deficits may be related to excessive production of quinolic acid, a known neurotoxin, in patients with EMS. This seems to be mediated by interferon-γ (Byrne et al 1986). Quinilic acid binds to NMDA receptors on brain cell surfaces. NMDA receptors in the basal ganglia, hippocampus, and cerebral cortex mediate cognitive functions such as memory and learning as well as synaptic plasticity. Levels of quinolic acid rise 1000-fold in patients with AIDS-dementia complex.

Animal Models of EMS. Lewis rat has been proposed as an animal model of EMS (Crofford et al 1990). Although the animals do not develop eosinophilia, the animals treated with contaminated tryptophan developed significant fascial thickening as compared to rats that received pure tryptophan.

Treatment

There is no generally accepted effective treatment for EMS. Corticosteroids may provide symptomatic relief of myalgia but they do not prevent the development of neuromuscular disease. Use of immunosuppressive therapy and plasmapheresis has been disappointing but methotrexate has been reported to be helpful (Martinez-Osuna et al 1991). Reduced severity of EMS has been reported to be associated with consumption of vitamin supplements including ascorbic acid before the onset of illness (Hatch and Goldman 1993).

Concluding Remarks

EMS is a striking example of how a presumably harmless food supplement and over-the-counter self-medication can produce a serious illness. Finding the etiologic factor is medical detective work. More research is needed to determine how the etiological agent is synthesized during the manufacturing process. Monitoring procedures are required to ensure that similar contamination does not occur in other biotechnology products. Investigation of pathomechanism of EMS will increase our understanding of eosinophilic and immunologic disorders and help in devising new therapies for these. Two lessons learned from this tragedy have been pointed out by Benjamin (1992). The first is the dubious advisability of allowing tryptophan to be sold without a physician's prescription. The second lesson is that FDA, without power to approve alterations of manufacturing process of a substance, cannot protect the consumers from such episodes. Mayeno and Gleich (1994) have pointed out that we had two epidemics related to food contamination (EMS and TOS) during the past decade. Neither the mechanism nor the specific contaminant have been demonstrated unequivocally. They are concerned that unless such agents are identified and proper preventive measures are taken, another food-related epidemic similar to TOS and EMS can still occur.

References

Adair JC, Rose JW, Digre KB: Acute encephalopathy associated with the eosinophilia-myalgia syndrome. Neurology 1992; 42: 461–462.

Alonso-Ruiz A, Calabozo M, Perez-Ruiz F, et al: Toxic Oil Syndrome. Medicine 1993; 72: 285–295.

Armstrong C, Lewis T, D'Esposito M, et al: Eosinophilia-myalgia syndrome: selective cognitive impairment, longitudinal effects, and neuroimaging findings. J Neurol Neurosurg Psychiatry 1997; 63(5): 633–641.

Belongia EA, Hedberg CW, Gleich GJ, et al: An investigation of the cause of eosinophilia-myalgia syndrome associated with tryptophane use. NEJM 1990; 323: 357–365.

Belongia EA, Mayeno AN, Osterholm MLT: The eosinophilia-myalgia syndrome and tryptophan. Ann Rev Nutr 1992; 12: 235–256.

Benjamin DM: When is a drug not a drug? The L-tryptophan tragedy: lessons to be learned. Drug Information Journal 1992; 26: 231–236.

Bochner BS, Friedman B, Krosjnaswamy B, et al: Episodic eosinophilia-myalgia-like syndrome in a patient without L-tryptophan use: association with eosinophil activation and increased serum levels of granulocyte-macrophage colony-stimulating factor. J Allergy Clin Immunol 1991; 88: 629–636.

Byrne GI, Lee CM, Kohler P, et al: Induction of tryptophan degradation in vitro and in vivo: a γ interferon-stimulated activity. J Interferon Res 1986; 6: 389–396.

Carr L, Rüther E, Berg PA, et al: Eosinophilia malgia syndrome in Germany: an epidemiologic review. Mayo Clin Proc 1994; 69: 620–625.

Center for Disease Control: Eosinophilia myalgia syndrome – New Mexico. MMWR 1989; 38: 765–767.

Clauw DJ, Nashel DJ, Umhau A, et al: Tryptophan-associated eosinophilic connective-tissue disease. JAMA 1990; 263: 1502–1506.

Crofford LJ, Rader JI, Dalakas MC, et al: L-tryptophan implicated in human eosinophilia-myalgia syndrome causes fascitis and perimyositis in the Lewis rat. J Clin Investigations 1990; 86: 1757–1763.

Culpepper RC, Williams RG, Mease PJ, et al: Natural history of eosinophilia-myalgia syndrome. Ann Int Med 1991; 115: 437–442.

Douglas AS, Eaglesd JM, Mowat NAG: Eosinophilia-myalgia syndrome associated with tryptophan. BMJ 1990; 301: 387.

Eidson M, Philen RM, Sewell CM, et al: L-tryptophan and eosinophilia myalgia syndrome in New Mexico. Lancet 1990; 335: 645–648.

Ephraim EE, Henning KJ, Kallenbach LR, et al: Risk factors for developing myalgia syndrome among L-tryptophan users in New York. J Rheumatology 1993; 20: 666–672.

Harati Y: Eosinophilia-myalgia syndrome and its relation to toxic oil syndrome. In de Wolff FA (Ed.) Handbook of clinical neurology, vol 20, Amsterdam, Elsevier, 1994, pp 249–271.

Haseler LJ, Sibbitt WL Jr, Sibbitt RR, et al: Neurologic, MR imaging, and MR spectroscopic findings in eosinophilia myalgia syndrome. AJNR Am J Neuroradiol 1998; 19(9): 1687–1694.

Hatch DL, Goldman LR: Reduced severity of eosinophilia-myalgia syndrome associated with the consumption of vitamin-containing supplements before illness. Arch Int Med 1993; 153: 2368–2373.

Hedberg K, Urbach D, Slutsker L, et al: Eosinophilia-myalgia syndrome: natural history in a population-based cohort. Arch Int Med 1992; 152: 1889–1892.

Heiman-Patterson TD, Bird SJ, Parry GJ, et al: Peripheral neuropathy associated with eosinophilia myalgia syndrome. Ann Neurol 1990; 28: 522–528.

Henning KJ, Jean-Baptiste E, Singh T, et al: Eosinophilia-myalgia syndrome in patients ingesting a single source of L-tryptophan. J Rheumatol 1993; 20: 273–278.

Hertzman PA, Blevilns IWWL, Mayer J, et al: Association of the eosinophilia-myalgia syndrome with the ingestion of tryptophan. NEJM 1990; 322: 869–873.

Kamb ML, Murphy JL, Jones JL, et al: Eosinophilia-myalgia syndrome in L-tryptophan exposed patients. JAMA 1992; 267: 77–82.

Kaufman LD, Philen RM: Tryptophan: current status and future trends for oral application. Drug Safety 1993; 8: 89–98.

Kilbourne EM: Eosinophilia-myalgia syndrome: coming to grips with a new illness. Epidemiologic Reviews 1992; 14: 16–36.

Krupp LB, Pepper C, Jandorf L, et al: Central nervous system involvement in eosinophilia-myalgia syndrome. Neurology 1992; 42(suppl 3): 294.

Love LA, Rader JI, Crofford L, et al: L-tryptophan (L-TRP) and 1,1'-ethylidenebis-tryptophan (EBT), a contaminant in eosinophilia myalgia syndrome (EMS) case-associated L-TRP, causes myofascial thickening and pancreatic fibrosis. Arthr Rheum 1991; 34(suppl): S131.

Lynn J, Rammohan KW, Bornstein RA, et al: Central nervous system involvement in the eosinophilia-myalgia syndrome. Arch Neurol 1992; 49: 1082–1085.

Martinez-Osuna P, Wallach PM, Seleznick MJ, et al: Treatment of eosinophilia myalgia syndrome. Sem Arthr Rheum 1991; 21: 110–121.

Mayeno AN, Gleich GJ: The eosinophilia-Myalgia syndrome: lessons from Germany. Mayo Clin Proc 1994; 69: 702–704.

Owen Jr WF, Petersen F, Sheff DM, et al: Hypodense eosinophils and interleukin 5 activity in the blood of patients with the eosinophilia myalgia syndrome. Proc Natl Acad Sci USA 1990; 87: 8647–8651.

Philen RM, Hill RH, Flanders WD, et al: Tryptophan contaminant associated with eosinophilia-myalgia syndrome. Am J Epidemiology 1993; 138: 154–159.

Slutsker L, Hoesley FC, Miller L, et al: Eosinophilia-myalgia syndrome associated with exposure to tryptophan from a single manufacturer. JAMA 1990; 264: 213–217.

Smith BE, Dyck PJ: Peripheral neuropathy in the eosinophilia-myalgia syndrome associated with L-tryptophan ingestion. Neurology 1990; 40: 1035–1040.

Stachow A, Jablonska S, Skiendzielewska A: 5-hydroxytryptamine and tryptamine pathway in scleroderma. Br J Dermatol 1977; 97: 147–154.

Swygert LA, Maes EF, Sewell LE, et al: Eosinophilia myalgia syndrome. JAMA 1990; 264: 1698–1703.

Thacker HL: Eosinophilia-myalgia syndrome: the Cleveland Clinic experience. Cleve Clin J Med 1991; 58: 400–8.

Tsutsui K, Taniuchi K, Mori T, et al: Eosinophilia-myalgia syndrome: a report of two cases in Japan. European Journal of Dermatology 1996; 6: 113–115.

Turi GK, Solitare GB, James N, et al: Eosinophilia-myalgia syndrome associated with neuromyopathy. Neurology 1990; 40: 1793–1796.

Van Garsse LGMM, Boeykens PPH: Two patients with eosinophilia-myalgia associated with tryptophan. BMJ 1990; 301: 21.

Varga J, Jimenez SA, Uitto J: L-tryptophan and the eosinophilia-myalgia syndrome: current understanding of the etiology and pathogenesis. J Invest Dermatol 1993; 97S–105S.

Varga J, Maul GG, Jimenez SA: Autoantibodies to nuclear lamin C in the eosinophilia-myalgia syndrome associated with L-tryptophan ingestion. Arthr Rheum 1992; 35: 106–109.

Chapter 21
Serotonin Syndrome

Introduction

Serotonin (5-hydroxytryptamine) was discovered in 1948 (Rapport et al 1948) and has been shown to have a major role in several psychiatric as well as nonpsychiatric disorders (anxiety, depression, migraine, etc.). Coadministration of L-tryptophan (a precursor of serotonin) with monoamine oxidase inhibitors was reported to induce delirium in a patient and the clinical picture resembled that of what is today described as serotonin syndrome (Oates and Sjoerdsma 1960). Excess of serotonin activity may lead to serotonin syndrome. Initially, the serotonin syndrome was described in animals and the characteristic features were tremor, rigidity, hypertonicity, hind limb abduction, straub tail, lateral head shaking, hyperactivity to auditory stimuli, myoclonus, general seizures, and various autonomic responses such as salivation, penile erection, and ejaculation (Gerson and Baldessarini 1980). Subsequently, this syndrome was defined in humans in 1982 (Insel et al 1982) and followed by the publication of several case reports and reviews (Bodner et al 1995; Brown et al 1996; Sporer 1996).

Clinical Features and Diagnosis

Clinical features and diagnostic criteria of the serotonin syndrome are shown in Table 21.1.

In the older literature on adverse effects of antidepressants and their interactions with other drugs, serotonin syndrome was not recognized. Conditions to be considered in differential diagnosis of serotonin syndrome include the following:
- Neuroleptic malignant syndrome
- Tyramine "cheese reaction"

Table 21.1. Clinical features and diagnostic criteria of serotonin syndrome (Sternbach 1991).

Coincident with addition of or increase in a known serotonergic agent to an established medication regimen, and at least three of the following features are present:
Mental status change (confusion, hypomania)
- Agitation
- Myoclonus
- Hyperreflexia
- Diaphoresis
- Shivering
- Tremor
- Diarrhoea
- Incoordination
- Fever
Other causes (e.g., infections, metabolic, substance abuse or withdrawal) have been ruled out.
A neuroleptic had not been started or increased in dosage prior to the onset of signs and symptoms.

Neuroleptic Malignant Syndrome. Some of the cases of serotonin syndrome are difficult to differentiate from neuroleptic malignant syndrome. A comparison of the clinical features of neuroleptic malignant syndrome and serotonin syndrome is shown in Table 21.2.

Table 21.2. Comparison of the clinical features of neuroleptic malignant syndrome and serotonin syndrome.

Clinical Features	Neuroleptic malignant syndrome	Serotonin syndrome
Myoclonus		X
Muscular rigidity	X	
Hyperreflexia		X
Hyperthermia	X	X
Autonomic dysfunction	X	
Agitation		X
Diaphoresis	X	X
Incoordination		X
Altered consciousness	X	

A feature common to both the syndromes is hyperthermia. Serotonin and dopamine are both important neurotransmitters in temperature regulation and it is likely that hyperthermic reactions result from drug-induced changes in the levels of these neurotransmitters (Nimmo et al 1993). Toxic reactions to the designer drug ecstasy resemble both serotonin syndrome and neuroleptic malignant syndrome because it affects both serotonin- and dopamine-containing neurons (Ames and Wirshing 1993). The predominant manifestations, however, are those of serotonin syndrome (Friedman 1993).

Tyramine "Cheese Reaction" and Overdose of Monoamine Oxidase Inhibitor. This is well known following ingestion of cheese by patients on monoamine oxidase inhibitor. The distinguishing feature of this is hypertension, which is not a characteristic of serotonin syndrome.

Patients with an overdose of monoamine oxidase inhibitors may show symptoms similar to those of serotonin syndrome. In severe cases death may result from hyperthermia, cardiopulmonary arrest, or disseminated intravascular coagulation with renal failure (Tackley and Tregaskis 1987; Miller et al 1991; Henry 1994).

The diagnosis of serotonin syndrome may be overlooked in patients with Parkinson's disease who are on serotonin reuptake inhibitors because of depression.

The diagnosis is based on history and clinical features. Various EEG abnormalities that are noted in cases of serotonin syndrome are: delta range activity, slow waves, spikes and waves, and triphasic waves (Dike 1997). This may be an important test in the setting of concomitant neurologic disorders.

As a modification of Sternbach's criteria, a serotonin syndrome scale, based on correlation of symptoms with serum paroxetine levels, has been proposed as a tool for clinicians (Hegerl et al 1998).

The onset of serotonin syndrome ranges from minutes after receiving the second drug to weeks after a stable dosage. Most cases involve only minor symptoms that resolve over 12 to 24 hours, other cases may proceed on to more serious sequelae.

Epidemiology

The incidence of serotonin syndrome in humans is difficult to determine as there are no universally accepted criteria for its diagnosis. The syndrome may be underreported due to the lack of awareness of this syndrome among medical professionals. More than 100 cases have been reported in the literature so far. Considering the millions of patients who are exposed to a combination of drugs that can produce serotonin syndrome, the frequency of occurrence is considered to be rare.

There has never been a population-based prospective study on serotonin syndrome but other studies give some insight into the relative incidence of this disease. Some studies have used a combination of monoamine oxidase inhibitors and tryptophan in a prospective manner to measure clinical efficiency and adverse effects (Oates and Sjoerdsma 1960; Coppen et al 1963; Glasman and Platman 1969). The patients who showed improvement frequently experienced adverse symptoms such as the feeling of intoxication, ataxia, and drowsiness which were not seen in the control group receiving monoamine oxidase inhibitor and placebo. These symptoms did not quite fulfill the criteria of serotonin syndrome and were seldom the cause for withdrawal of therapy.

In a pooled population of 4,568 patients with Parkinson's disease who were treated with a combination of deprenyl and an antidepressant, 11 (0.24%) were reported to have developed serotonin syndrome (Richard et al 1997). The incidence of serotonin syndrome during clomipramine monotherapy was reported to be 12.1% (8 of 66 patients) as determined by Sternbach's criteria (Kudo et al 1997).

Pathomechanism

L-tryptophan is a precursor of 5-hydroxytryptamine. It has been shown in animals that the administration of L-tryptophan increases brain levels of tryptamine and 5-hydroxytryptamine (Bogdanski et al 1958; Hess et al 1959). The syndrome was blocked by pretreatment with a

5-hydroxytryptamine decarboxylase inhibitor suggesting that its occurrence is 5-hydroxytryptamine dependent. Ingestion of excessive amounts of pure L-tryptophan by normal subjects can, in itself, produce significant CNS signs and symptoms. The following manifestations have been recorded in well-designed experiments in human volunteers (Smith and Prockop 1962):
– Euphoria
– Headache and dizziness
– Hyperreflexia

These effects were considered to be due to raised levels of 5-hydroxytryptamine induced by L-Tryptophan ingestion. These symptoms may be present in serotonin syndrome but pure L-tryptophan has not been shown to induce the full-blown serotonin syndrome. The enzyme monoamine oxidase (monoamine oxidase inhibitor) is involved in the degradation of 5-hydroxytryptamine and concomitant use of monoamine oxidase inhibitors may lead to accumulation of 5-hydroxytryptamine and its neurologic effects (Oates and Sjoerdsma 1960). The syndrome can be blocked by using various 5-hydroxytryptamine precursors in combination with medications that increase their bioavailability (Marley and Wozniak 1984).

According to 5-hydroxytryptaminergic hypothesis of obsessive-compulsive disorders, there is hypersensitivity of 5-hydroxytryptamine receptors (Zohar and Insel 1987; Hollander et al 1988). This lends support to the use of 5-hydroxytryptamine uptake inhibitors in obsessive-compulsive disorders. Serotonin syndrome may be due to drug effects causing enhanced transmission at the 5-hydroxytryptamine 1A level or at the postsynaptic level.

The reports of serotonin syndrome due to drug interaction are mostly anecdotal but the evidence that symptoms are due to 5-hydroxytryptamine is based on animal experiments (Yamawaki et al 1986). 5-hydroxytryptamine 1A activation of serotonin receptors in the brainstem and spinal cord with overall enhancement of neurotransmission is a possible mechanism. Myoclonus induced by 5-hydroxytryptamine has been demonstrated in guinea pigs (Klawans et al 1973).

The mechanism underlying serotonin syndrome following interaction between a monoamine oxidase inhibitor and a serotonin reuptake inhibitor is that monoamine oxidase can no longer perform its function of degrading serotonin. Restoration of enzymes that perform the degradation takes about two weeks following cessation of therapy and serotonin syndrome can develop if a monoamine oxidase inhibitor is switched over to a serotonin reuptake inhibitor within less than two weeks after discontinuation of the monoamine oxidase inhibitor.

Serotonin syndrome bears a striking clinical resemblance to high pressure neurologic syndrome, which is a sequel of deep diving and is an additional support for the serotonin theory of high pressure neurologic syndrome (Jain 1994).

The central 5-hydroxytryptamine 1A receptor is not the only receptor subtype that is involved in the etiology of serotonin syndrome. Other factors that may contribute are the endogenous as well as iatrogenic deficits in the peripheral 5-hydroxytryptamine metabolism, the activation of several 5-hydroxytryptamine subtypes, and a stimulus for the release of 5-hydroxytryptamine.

Predisposing Factors. The following factors predispose to the development of serotonin syndrome (Brown et al 1996):
– Inherited disorders
  · low endogenous monoamine oxidase inhibitor activity
  · decreased metabolism of serotonergic drugs
  · cardiovascular diseases: hypertension and hyperlipidemia
– Acquired diseases
  · Liver diseases: hepatitis
  · pulmonary disease
  · cardiovascular disease

Serotonin Syndrome as Adverse Effect of Serotonomimetic Drugs

Serotonin syndrome is most commonly the result of the interaction between serotonergic agents and monoamine oxidase inhibitors. It may also result as adverse effect of serotomimetic drugs.

Tricyclic Antidepressant Monotherapy. Serotonin syndrome has been reported in patients treated with a tricyclic antidepressants that are known to increase synaptic serotonin level and serotonergic activity in the brain. Examples of this is clomipramine (Lejoyeux et al 1993; Rosebush et al 1999).

Monotherapy with Reversible Monoamine Oxidase Inhibitors. The syndrome has also been reported with moclobemide (Brodribb et al 1994; Fischer 1995; Butzkueven 1997) and tranylcypromine (Pennings et al 1997).

Monotherapy with Selective Serotonin Reuptake Inhibitors (SSRIs). This is considered to be extremely rare but one case has been reported following a single parenteral infusion of citalopram (Fischer 1995). Overdose of the following SSRIs has been reported to be associated with serotonin syndrome:
- fluvoxamine, (Lenzi et al 1993; Gill et al 1999).
- sertraline (Kaminski et al 1994)

Antimigraine Drugs. Six patients with migraine are reported to have developed symptoms suggestive of the serotonin syndrome (Mathew et al 1996). Five were taking one or more serotomimetic agents for migraine prophylaxis (sertraline, paroxetine, lithium, imipramine, amitriptyline). In each case the symptoms and signs developed in close temporal proximity with the use of a migraine abortive agent known to interact with serotonin receptors. In three instances the agent was subcutaneous sumatriptan and, in three, intravenous dihydroergotamine. In each instance the symptoms were transient and there was full recovery. Sumatriptan has agonist action on the presynaptic and postsynaptic 5-HT$_{ID}$ receptor (Humphrey and Fenuik 1991). Gardner and Lynd (1998) have made a comprehensive search of the reports dealing with serotonin syndrome associated with sumatriptan use but found no compelling evidence for the contraindication of use of sumatriptan with serotomimetic agents and suggested that sumatriptan can be used cautiously with SSRIs or lithium. These authors, however, did not recommend combining serotonin with MAO inhibitors unless reliable data becomes available to demonstrate the safety of this combination.

Overdosage with Antidepressants. Combined overdose of monoamine oxidase inhibitors and serotonergic drugs can result in serotonin syndrome with a fatal outcome. Symptoms and signs of the syndrome may not develop until 6 to 12 hours after the overdose (Power et al 1995).

Metachlorophenylpiperazine (mCPP). mCPP ImCPP[Metachlorophenylpiperazine] is a nonselective 5-HT-receptor agonist/antagonist that is used extensively in psychiatry to assess central serotonergic function. Serotonin syndrome has been reported as a result of this test (Klaassen et al 1998).

Drug Interactions Causing Serotonin Syndrome

These are the most important and most frequent causes of serotonin syndrome. A classification of these interactions according to drug category is shown in Table 21.3.

Interaction of two Serotonin Reuptake Inhibitors. The selective pharmacology of the SSRIs results in a lower potential for pharmacodynamic drug interactions relative to other antidepressants such as the tricyclic antidepressants (TCAs) and monoamine oxidase inhibitors (MAOIs). However, serotonin syndrome can be induced by synergistic effect of two drugs from this category such as venlafaxine and fluoxetine (Bhatara et al 1998).

There are important pharmacokinetic interactions between SSRIs and other serotonergic drugs due principally to their effects on the cytochrome P450 (CYP) isoenzymes, the potential for which varies widely amongst the SSRI group, which may increase the likelihood of a pharmacodynamic interaction (Lane and Baldwin 1997). The exceptionally long washout period required after fluoxetine discontinuation may cause additional problems and/or inconvenience.

Serotonin Reuptake Inhibitors and Monoamine Oxidase Inhibitors. The use of fluoxetine and monoamine oxidase inhibitors, either together or in close succession, has been reported to be

Table 21.3. Drug interactions associated with serotonin syndrome.

– Combination of two serotonin reuptake inhibitors
  Fluoxetine and sertraline
– Serotonin reuptake inhibitors and
  1. monoamine oxidase inhibitors: isocarboxazid, phenelzine, selegeline, tranylcypromine, nortriptyline, amitriptyline, moclobemide
  2. dopaminergic agents (serotomimetic effect)
  3. tryptophan
  4. dexfenfluramine
  5. carbamazepine
  6. lithium
  7. pentazocine
  8. cold remedy containing ephedrine
  9. drugs which block 5-HT$_{2A}$ receptors (nefazodone and trazodone)
  10. anesthetics
  11. clonazepam
  12. opioids
– Tricyclic antidepressant (clomipramine) and
  1. monoamine oxidase inhibitors
  2. serotonin reuptake inhibitors
  3. s-adenosylmethionine
  4. lithium
– Monoamine oxidase inhibitors and
  1. venlafaxine
  2. tryptophan
  3. lithium
  4. cold remedy containing dextromethorphan
  5. opioids: meperidine
  6. ecstasy
– Miscellaneous interactions
  levodopa and bromocriptine
  clozapine and lithium
  trazodone with buspirone
  trazodone with isocarboxazid and methylphenidate

accompanied by serotonin syndrome in several cases (Sternbach 1988; Feigner et al 1990; Beasley et al 1993; Coplan and Gorman 1993). A case of serotonin syndrome has also been reported to be induced by the interaction of moclobemide with the serotonin reuptake inhibitor, imipramine (Brodribb et al 1994). One case of serotonin syndrome was seen in a patient who was first treated with fluoxetine and then with selective monoamine oxidase inhibitor, moclobemide (Benazzi 1996). Serotonin syndrome due to the interaction of fluoxetine with selegiline has been described (Suchowersky and deVries 1990). Another SSRI, venlafaxine has been shown to interact with tranylcypromine to produce serotonin syndrome (Hodgman et al 1997).

Cases of serotonin syndrome have been de-scribed as an interaction between sertraline selective serotonin reuptake inhibitor and monoamine oxidase inhibitors: isocarboxazid (Brannan et al 1994), phenelzine (Graber et al 1994), and tranylcypromine (Bhatara and Bandetti 1993). Another case of this syndrome occurred when fluoxetine was started 2 weeks after dis-continuation of tranylcypromine, a monoamine oxidase inhibitor (Ruiz 1994).

Serotonin Reuptake Inhibitors and Trypto-phan. Fluoxetine, a specific inhibitor of seroto-nin reuptake into neurons, has been found to be effective in the treatment of obsessive-compul-sive disorders. Fluoxetine was combined with L-tryptophan in the treatment of five patients and all of them developed a toxic reaction resem-bling serotonin syndrome (Steiner and Fontaine 1986). None of these patients had any undesir-able effects while on treatment previously with fluoxetine alone. A possible mechanism of this adverse reaction is that tryptophan increases the central nervous system levels of serotonin.

Serotonin Reuptake Inhibitors and Dexfen-fluramine. Concern has been expressed that a combination of these two medications could pro-duce serotonin syndrome (Schenck and Ma-howald 1996). However, no such cases have been reported as yet. Fenfluramine was taken off the market because of the adverse effects of pul-monary hypertension and cardiac valve abnor-malities which might have been caused by ex-cess of serotonin. Fenfluramine raises serotonin levels by preventing absorption of serotonin into platelets.

Selective Serotonin Reuptake Inhibitors and Carbamazepine. Serotonin syndrome has been reported in a patient on carbamazepine and fluo-xetine therapy for affective disorder and the symptoms resolved after discontinuation of fluo-xetine (Dursun et al 1993). The pathomechanism of serotonin syndrome in this case is not clear. A fatal case of serotonin syndrome has been report-ed with concomitant use of paroxetine and car-bamazepine (Apelland et al 1999).

Serotonin Reuptake Inhibitors and Lithium. Serotonin syndrome was reported in a case where fluvoxamine was added to long-standing lithium therapy (Öhman and Spigset 1993). The patient recovered 2 weeks after fluvoxamine was replaced by nortriptyline. Another case of serotonin syndrome occurred when lithium was added to paroxetine in the management of a bipolar disorder (Sobanski et al 1997). Serum levels of paroxetine became elevated and the syndrome resolved after reduction of paroxetine dose.

Serotonin Reuptake Inhibitors and Pentazocine. Pentazocine, an opioid analgesic, blocks the neuronal uptake of 5-hydroxytryptamine and interaction with fluoxetine has been reported to result in serotonin syndrome (Hansen et al 1990).

Serotonin Reuptake Inhibitor (Paroxetine) and Cold Remedy. Serotonin syndrome has been described as an interaction between paroxetine and an over-the-counter cold remedy containing ephedrine and dextromethorphan (Skop et al 1994). Cold remedies containing ingredients such as pseudoephedrine and phenylpropanolamine also act as MAO inhibitors and can interact with serotonin reuptake inhibitors to produce serotonin syndrome.

Serotonin Reuptake Inhibitor (Paroxetine) and Drugs which Block 5-HT$_{2A}$ Receptors (Nefazodone and Trazodone). Serotonin syndrome was reported in a patient who had been on nefazodone for a bipolar affective disorder for 6 months when this was tapered and switched to paroxetine (John et al 1997). Subsequent readministration paroxetine 7 days later and did not produce any adverse effects. Another case report describes serotonin syndrome as an interaction between paroxetine and trazodone (Reeves and Bullen 1995).

Serotonin Reuptake Inhibitor (Sertraline) and Anesthetics. Serotonin syndrome has been described after ankle block in a patient who was on sertraline therapy (Jahn et al 1994). The likely explanation in this case is that that the medications used for anesthesia, lidocaine, midazolam and fentanyl, bind to plasma proteins and cause an increased free fraction of sertraline owing to displacement from plasma proteins.

Serotonin Reuptake Inhibitor (Paroxetine) and Clonazepam. There is one case report of serotonin syndrome following use of clonazepam in a patient who was on proxetine therapy for anxiety. Her symptoms resolved after treatment with intravenous lorazepam. This interaction is of clinical importance because patients with anxiety disorders may take these two medications together and may develop serotonin syndrome.

Serotonin Reuptake Inhibitor (Paroxetine) and Opioid (Tramadol). Serotonin syndrome occurred in a patient with depression who was on treatment with paroxetine and was given trazodol for relief of pain (Egberts et al 1997). This interaction was possibly caused by inhibitory action of tramadol on the metabolism of paroxetine. The patient recovered after tramadol was discontinued and the dose of paroxetine was reduced.

Serotonin Reuptake Inhibitor (Fluvoxamine) and Buspirone. One case of serotonin syndrome is reported in a patient during treatment with fluvoxamine for obsessive compulsive disorder and buspirone (a partial agonist at 5-HT$_{1A}$ receptors) for anxiety (Baetz and Malcolm 1995). The patient recovered after both the drugs were discontinued and lorazepam was used to control agitation.

Tricyclic Antidepressants and Monoamine Oxidase Inhibitors. This combination is generally considered to be without risk of an interaction. However, serious side effects, including fatalities, have been reported with the combination of imipramine, a tricyclic antidepressant, and monoamine oxidase inhibitors (Brachfeld et al 1963). Clomipramine, a tricyclic antidepressant, is involved in several interactions with monoamine oxidase inhibitors.

Clomipramine, a tricyclic antidepressant, given together with moclobemide, a selective monoamine oxidase inhibitor, has been reported to produce serotonin syndrome fulfilling the criteria of Sternbach (Spigset et al 1993). Two fatal cases of serotonin syndrome due to simultaneous ingestion of an overdose of moclobemide and clomipramine have been reported (Neuvonen et al 1993).

Serotonin syndrome has also been reported as the result of an interaction between clomipramine and phenelzine, a monoamine oxidase inhibitor (Nierenberg and Semprebon 1993). A fatal serotonin syndrome occurred in a patient after taking moclobemide, amitriptyline, and clomipramine concomitantly (Kuisma 1995). The blood concentrations of all the drugs were within the normal range for each so that the syndrome was caused by drug interaction rather than an overdose.

Serotonin syndrome has been described in two patients as the result of an interaction between clomipramine and clorgyline when given 4 weeks after discontinuation of the monoamine oxidase inhibitor, clorgyline (Insel et al 1982).

Tricyclic Antidepressants and Serotonin Reuptake Inhibitors. Serotonin syndrome can result from a clomipramine (a serotonin reuptake inhibitor)-moclobemide (tricyclic antidepressant) interaction (Gillman 1997; Dardennes et al 1998).

Clomipramine and s-adenosylmethionine. S-adenosylmethionine stimulates serotonin and norepinephrine metabolism in the brain and is used in the treatment of depression. Serotonin syndrome has been reported in a patients with combined clomipramine and s-adenosylmethionine therapy and is attributed to the synergic action of these two drugs (Iruela et al 1993).

Clomipramine and Lithium. Serotonin syndrome has been reported after the addition of lithium to clomipramine therapy (Kojima et al 1993). Later, the patient was treated with lithium alone without recurrence of serotonin syndrome.

Monoamine Oxidase Inhibitor and Tricyclic Antidepressants. Selegeline, a selective monoamine oxidase inhibitor, is used in the treatment of Parkinson's disease. Selegiline's package insert was revised to reflect the potential risk of adverse effects when it is used in combination with selective serotonin reuptake inhibitors and tricyclic antidepressants.

Monoamine Oxidase Inhibitors and Serotonin Reuptake Inhibitors. Serotonin syndrome was reported in a patient receiving tranylcypromine after accidental ingestion of a single dose of venlafaxine, which inhibits neuronal uptake of serotonin, noradrenaline, and dopamine (Hodgman et al 1997). Accidental simultaneous ingestion of phenelzine and venlafaxine has been reported to cause serotonin syndrome (Weiner et al 1998). Several cases of serotonin syndrome have been reported following the start of venlafaxine therapy shortly after discontinuation of phenelzine therapy (Heisler et al 1996; Kolecki 1997; Diamond et al 1998).

These interactions are based on spontaneous reports. A clinical study of the interaction of fluoxetine (serotonin reuptake inhibitor) and moclobemide (monoamine oxidase inhibitor) failed to find a pharmacodynamic basis for this interaction (Dingemanse et al 1998). In an open-label study on 19 patients, moclobemide was used in combination with paroxetine or fluoxetine (selective serotonin reuptake inhibitors) for 6 weeks and only one patient was diagnosed to have developed a toxic serotonin syndrome (Hawley et al 1996).

Monoamine Oxidase Inhibitors and Tryptophan. The combination of monoamine oxidase inhibitors and tryptophan has been reported to cause behavioral or neurologic toxicity. Pope and colleagues presented eight cases of delirious syndromes in association with this combination of agents (Pope et al 1985). Two of these patients fit the description of serotonin syndrome. There are several case reports of serotonin syndrome after tryptophan administration in patients taking a monoamine oxidase inhibitor.

Monoamine Oxidase Inhibitors and Lithium. Serotonin syndrome has been reported following treatment with this combination (Mekler and Woggon 1997). It is possible that lithium may intensify the effect of serotonin although it is not involved in the metabolism of serotonin.

Monoamine Oxidase Inhibitors and Dextromethorphan. Serotonin syndrome has been reported to develop after taking an over-the-counter cold remedy containing dextromethorphan (Sovner and Wolfe 1988). A similar but fatal reaction was reported in a patient on phenelzine therapy who took a cough remedy containing dextromethorphan (Rivers and Harner 1970). Dextromethorphan has been shown to block the neural uptake of serotonin in rabbits (Sinclair 1973).

Monoamine Oxidase Inhibitors and Meperidine. Meperidine (pethidine) blocks the neuronal uptake of 5-hydroxytryptamine and its interaction with monoamine oxidase inhibitors can lead to serotonin syndrome (Stack et al 1988). The monoamine oxidase inhibitor/pethidine interaction has two distinct forms: an excitatory and a depressive form. Pethidine should not be used in the presence of monoamine oxidase inhibitors because of the risk of fatal excitatory interaction (serotonin syndrome). Morphine does not cause this excitatory reaction and is the drug of choice under these circumstances (Brown and Linter 1987).

Monoamine Oxidase Inhibitors and Ecstasy. One patient was reported to develop marked hypertension, diaphoresis, hypertonicity, and altered mental status after ingesting ecstasy and phenelzine (Smilkstein et al 1987). Sympathomimetic-monoamine oxidase inhibitor interaction can cause excessive release of endogenous bioactive amines leading to a reaction that resembles serotonin syndrome but does not fulfill the diagnostic criteria.

L-Dopa and Bromocriptine. L-dopa induced serotonin syndrome has been reported in a patient with Parkinson's disease on bromocriptine therapy (Sandyk 1986). Acute administration of levodopa-carbidopa could have produced a sudden displacement of endogenous serotonin into the synaptic cleft and on to serotonin receptor sites, thus increasing the availability of serotonin in the synapse. Since bromocriptine also enhances serotonin metabolism in the CNS, serotonin syndrome could have resulted from a synergistic effect of the two drugs.

Lithium and Clozapine. In one study, 4 of the 10 patients treated with a combination of lithium and clozapine developed reversible neurologic symptoms such as myoclonus and agitation (Blake et al 1992). Some of these neurologic symptoms appear to be early manifestations of serotonin syndrome and the pathomechanism of these symptoms may have been the interaction of the serotonergic effects of clozapine and lith-

ium. Lithium has also been shown to facilitate the onset of serotonin syndrome with L-tryptophan and monoamine oxidase inhibitor combination without rise of its serum levels.

Trazodone and Buspirone. Buspirone is a partial 5-hydroxytryptamine 1 agonist which can contribute to the development of serotonin syndrome in a patient who has been on trazodone therapy previously (Goldberg and Huk 1992). This patient was also on theophylline therapy which could increase the availability of tryptophan to the brain.

Trazodone with Isocarboxazid and Methylphenidate. A patient developed serotonin syndrome while taking trazodone (a nontricyclic, nontetracyclic antidepressant) and methylphenidate (Bodner et al 1995). Trazodone has a week 5-hydroxytryptamine reuptake inhibiting action and a metabolite, m-chlorophenylpiperazine, that has partial agonist activity at many 5-hydroxytryptamine subtypes.

Prognosis and Complications

Most patients recover from serotonin syndrome following drug withdrawal and minor supporting therapy as this is a self-limiting condition. There are, however, reports of severe complications such as seizures (Kline et al 1989; Beasley et al 1993; Neuvonen et al 1993), disseminated intravascular coagulation (Tackley and Tregaskis 1987; Miller et al 1991), respiratory failure (Graber et al 1994; Ruiz 1994), and severe hypothermia (Ooi 1991; Spigset et al 1993) with deaths in a few cases.

Prevention of Serotonin Syndrome

Substances that deplete 5-hydroxytryptamine or block 5-hydroxytryptamine receptors have been shown to prevent serotonin syndrome in experimental animals (Marley and Wozniak 1984). Blockade of 5-hydroxytryptamine 1 receptors rather than of 5-hydroxytryptamine 2 receptors is required (Luck et al 1984). Cyproheptadine, a nonspecific 5-hydroxytryptamine receptor antagonist, can block the serotonin syndrome in animal models (Gerson and Baldessarini 1980). β-blockers have been reported to block 5-hydroxytryptamine receptors and prevent serotonin syndrome (Weinstock et al 1977).

The combination of drugs known to produce serotonin syndrome should be avoided as a preventive measure. Caution should be exercised in prescribing serotomimetic agents after the discontinuation of a monoamine oxidase inhibitor or when commencing a monoamine oxidase inhibitor after discontinuation of a serotomimetic agent. Most of the monoamine oxidase inhibitors are irreversible enzyme inhibitors and following their cessation, enzyme replacement may take a few weeks. Serotonin syndrome has been reported in a patient prescribed clomipramine 4 weeks after terminating clorigiline (Insel et al 1982). Therefore, 4 to 6 weeks should elapse between the switchover of these two classes of medications. Long-term administration of high dose fluoxetine may require a 3-month washout period (Rosenstein et al 1991).

Management of Serotonin Syndrome

To reduce the occurrence, morbidity, and mortality of the serotonin syndrome, it must be both prevented by prudent pharmacotherapy and given prompt recognition when it is present. In clinical practice, serotonin syndrome is often transient and does not require discontinuation of the offending medication or any special treatment. If the clinical features are a cause for concern, the offending medication should be discontinued and supportive measures should be used.

There are no prospective studies of the evaluation of treatment of serotonin syndrome in man. Management strategies are based on studies in animal models and case reports on human patients. In most of the reported cases, symptoms resolved after discontinuation of the offending medications. Milder cases can be sent home after discontinuation of the contributing agents and followed up. Management of moderate to severe cases involves hospitalization with close monitoring and appropriate supporting measures. The following medications have been investigated for counteracting the serotonin syndrome.

- Lorazepam (Dursun et al 1993)
- Methysergide, a nonspecific 5-hydroxytryptamine antagonist for movement disorders (Sandyk 1986)
- Propranolol has a specific affinity for 5-hydroxytryptamine 1A receptor and suppresses the serotonin syndrome quite effectively (Guze and Baxter 1986; Yamada et al 1989).
- Cyproheptadine, a 5-HT_2 receptor antagonist, blunts the clinical manifestations of serotonin syndrome (Lappin and Auchincloss 1994; Graudins et al 1998). In a review of all published cases, Gillman (1999) found that the evidence for cyproheptadine less substantial, perhaps because the dose of cyproheptadine necessary to ensure blockade of brain 5-HT_2 receptors is 20–30 mg, which is higher than that used in the cases reported to date (4–16 mg).
- Nitroglycerin. This approach has been tried in a patient with severe vascular disease who developed hypertension during an episode of serotonin syndrome (Brown and Scop 1996). The rationale was based on the idea that enhancement of the endogenous counterregulatory mechanisms that normally restrain serotonergic activity might reduce the symptoms.
- Chlorpromazine (Graham 1997). An analysis of reported cases of serotonin syndrome treated with chlorpromazine showed that this drug was effective (Gillman 1999).

The following drugs have been used for alleviating rigidity and tremor but efficacy in alleviating serotonin syndrome has not been established:

- Clonazepam (Lejoyeux et al 1993)
- Benzatropine (Goldberg and Huk 1992)
- Diphenylhydramine (Hansen et al 1990)

For practical management of the patient, the following medications may be tried in the following order: (1) Lorazepam 1 mg to 2 mg by slow IV push until excessive sedation develops. If there is no improvement, use (2) propranolol 1 mg to 3 mg every 5 minutes up to 0.1 mg/kg. If the response is inadequate, try (3) cyproheptadine 4 mg orally every 4 hours up to 20 mg per 24 hours. If no response, try other experimental approaches, e. g., nitroglycerin.

In severe cases resembling monoamine oxidase inhibitor poisoning with hyperthermia, the treatment strategy recommended by the London National Poisons Information Service is to induce elective paralysis and ventilate them mechanically to increase the chances of survival (Henry 1994).

References

Ames D, Wirshing WC: Ectasy, the serotonin syndrome, and neuroleptic malignant syndrome—a possible link? (letter). JAMA 1993; 269: 869.

Apelland T, Gedde-Dahl T, Dietrichson T: Serotonin syndrome with fatal outcome caused by selective serotonin reuptake inhibitors. Tidsskr Nor Laegeforen 1999; 119(5): 647–650.

Baetz M, Malcolm D: Serotonin syndrome from fluvoxamine and buspirone. Canad J Psychiatry 1995; 40: 428–429.

Beasley CM, Masica DN, Heiligenstein JH, et al: Possible monoamine oxidase inhibitor-serotonin uptake inhibitor interaction: fluoxetine clinical data and preclinical findings. J Clin Psychopharmacol 1993; 13: 312–320.

Benazzi F: Serotonin syndrome with moclobemide-fluoxetine combination. Pharmacopsychiatry 1996; 29: 162.

Bhatara VS, Bandetti FC: Possible interaction between sertraline and tranlcypromine. Clin Pharm 1993; 12: 222–225.

Bhatara VS, Magnus RD, Paul KL, et al: Serotonin syndrome induced by venlafaxine and fluoxetine: a case study in polypharmacy and potential pharmacodynamic and pharmacokinetic mechanisms. Ann Pharmacother 1998; 32: 432–436.

Blake LM, Marks RC, Luchins DJ: Reversible neurologic symptoms with clozapine and lithium. J Clin Psychopharmacol 1992; 12: 297–299.

Bodner RA, Lynch T, Lewis L, et al: Serotonin syndrome. Neurology 1995; 45: 219–223.

Bogdanski DF, Weissbach H, Udenfriend S: Pharmacological studies with the serotonin precursor 5-hydroxytryptophan. J Pharmacol Exp Ther 1958; 122: 182–194.

Brachfeld J, Wirtshafter A, Wolfe S, et al: Imipramine-tranylcypromine incompatibility. JAMA 1963; 209: 1172–1173.

Brannan SK, Talley BJ, Bowden CH: Sertraline and isocarboxazid cause a serotonin syndrome. J Clin Psychopharmacol 1994; 14: 144–145.

Brodribb TR, Downey M, Gilbar PJ: Efficacy and adverse effects of moclobemide. Lancet 1994; 343: 475–476.

Brown B, Linter S: Monoamine oxidase inhibitors and narcotic analgesics. Br J Psychiatry 1987; 151: 210–212.

Brown TM, Scop BP, Mareth TR: Pathophysiology and management of the serotonin syndrome. Ann Pharmacother 1996; 30: 527–533.

Brown TM, Scop BP: Nitroglycerine in the treatment of serotonin syndrome (letter). Ann Pharmacother 1996; 30: 191.

Butzkueven H: A case of serotonin syndrome induced by moclobemide during an extreme heatwave. Austral N Z J Med 1997; 27: 603–604.

Coplan JD, Gorman JM: Detectable levels of fluoxetine metabolites after discontinuation: an unexpected serotonin syndrome (letter). Am J Psychiatry 1993; 150: 837.

Coppen A, Shaw DM, Farrell JP: Potentiation of antidepressant effect of monoamine oxidase inhibitor by tryptophan. Lancet 1963; 1: 79–81.

Dardennes RM, Even C, Ballon N, et al: Serotonin syndrome caused by a clomipramine-moclobemide interaction (letter). J Clin Psychiatry 1998; 59: 382–383.

Diamond S, Pepper BJ, Diamond ML, et al: Serotonin syndrome induced by transitioning from phenelzine to venlafaxine: four patient reports. Neurology 1998; 51: 274–276.

Dike GL: Triphasic waves in serotonin syndrome (letter). J Neurol Neurosurg Psychiatry 1997; 62: 200.

Dingemanse J, Wallnofer A, Gieschke R, et al: Pharmacokinetic and pharmacodynamic interactions between fluoxetine and moclobemide in the investigation of development of the "serotonin syndrome." Clin Pharmacol Ther 1998; 63: 403–413.

Dursun SM, Mathew VM, Reveley MA: Toxic serotonin syndrome after fluoxetine plus carbamazepine (letter). Lancet 1993; 342: 442–443.

Egberts AC, ter Borgh J, Brodie-Meijer CC: Serotonin syndrome attributed to tramadol addition to paroxetine therapy. Int Clin Psychopharmacol 1997; 12(3): 181–182.

Feigner JP, Boyer WF, Tyler DL, et al: Adverse effects of fluoxetine-MAOI combination therapy. J Clin Psychiatry 1990; 51: 222–225.

Fischer P: Serotonin syndrome in the elderly after antidepressive monotherapy. J Clin Psychopharmacol 1995; 15: 440–442.

Friedman R: Ectasy, the serotonin syndrome, and neuroleptic malignant syndrome—a possible link? (letter). JAMA 1993; 269: 869–870.

Gardner DM, Lynd LD: Sumatriptan complications and the serotonin syndrome. Ann Pharmacother 1998; 32: 33–38.

Gerson SC, Baldessarini RJ: Motor effects of serotonin in the central nervous system. Life Sci 1980; 27: 1435–1451.

Gill M, LoVecchio F, Selden B: Serotonin syndrome in a child after a single dose of fluvoxamine. Ann Emerg Med 1999; 33(4): 457–459.

Gillman PK: Serotonin syndrome—clomipramine too soon after moclobemide. International Clinical Psychopharmacology 1997; 12: 339–342.

Gillman PK: The serotonin syndrome and its treatment. J Psychopharmacol 1999; 13(1): 100–109.

Glasman AH, Platman SR: Potentiation of monoamine oxidase inhibitor by tryptophan. J Psychiatr Res 1969; 7: 83–88.

Goldberg RJ, Huk M: Serotonin syndrome from trazodone and buspirone. Psychosomatics 1992; 33: 235–236.

Graber MA, Hoehns TB, Perry PJ: Sertraline-phenelzine drug interaction: a serotonin syndrome reaction. Ann Pharmacother 1994; 28: 732–755.

Graham PM: Successful treatment of the toxic serotonin syndrome with chlorpromazine (letter). Med J Aust 1997; 166: 166–167.

Graudins A, Stearman A, Chan B: Treatment of the serotonin syndrome with cyproheptadine. J Emerg Med 1998; 16: 615–619.

Guze BH, Baxter LR: The serotonin syndrome: case responsive to propranolol (letter). J Clin Psychopharmacol 1986; 6: 119–120.

Hansen TE, Dieter K, Keepers GA: Interaction of fluoxetine and pentazocine (letter). Am J Psychiatry 1990; 147: 949–950.

Hawley CJ, McPhee S, Quick S, et al: Combining SSRIs and moclobemide. Pharm J 1996; 257: 506.

Hegerl U, Bottlender R, Gallinat J, et al: The serotonin syndrome scale: first results on validity. Eur Arch Psychiatry Clin Neurosci 1998; 248: 96–103.

Heisler MA, Guidry JR, Arnecke B: Serotonin syndrome induced by administration of venlafaxine and phenelzine (letter). Ann Pharmacother 1996; 30: 84.

Henry JA: Serotonin syndrome (letter). Lancet 1994; 343: 607.

Hess SM, Redfield BG, Udenfriend S: The effect of monoamine oxidase inhibitors and tryptophan on the tryptamine content of animal tissues and urine. J Pharmacol Exp Ther 1959; 127; 178–181.

Hodgman MJ, Martin TG, Krenzelok EP: Serotonin syndrome due to venlafaxine and maintenance tranylcypromine therapy. Hum Exp Toxicol 1997; 16: 14–17.

Hollander E, Fay M, Cohen R, et al: Serotonergic and noradrenergic sensitivity in obsessive-compulsive disorders: behavioral findings. Arch Gen Psychiatry 1988; 145: 1015–1023.

Humphrey PP, Fenuik W: Mode of action of the antimigraine drug sumatriptan. Trends Pharmacol Sci 1991; 12: 444–446.

Insel TR, Roy BF, Cohen RM, et al: Possible development of serotonin syndrome in man. Am J Psychiatry 1982; 139: 954–955.

Iruela LM, Minguez L, Merino J, et al: Toxic interaction of S-adenosylmethionine and clomipramine (letter). Am J Psychiatry 1993; 150: 522.

Jahn JS, Pisto JD, Gitlin MC, et al: The serotonin syndrome in a patient receiving sertraline after an ankle block. Anaesth Analg 1994; 79: 189–191.

Jain KK: High pressure neurological syndrome (HPNS). Acta Neurol Scand 1994; 90: 45–50.

John L, Perreault MM, Tao T, Blew PG: Serotonin syndrome associated with nefazodone and paroxitine. Ann Emerg Med 1997; 29: 287–289.

Kaminski CA, Robbins MS, Weibley RE: Sertraline intoxication in a child. Ann Emerg Med 1994; 23: 1371–1374.

Klaassen T, Ho Pian KL, Westenberg HG, et al: Serotonin syndrome after challenge with the 5-HT agonist metachlorophenylpiperazine. Psychiatry Res 1998; 79(3): 207–212.

Klawans HL, Goetz CG, Weiner WJ: 5-Hydroxytryptophan-induced myoclonus in guinea pigs and the possible role of serotonin in infantile myoclonus. Neurology 1973; 23: 1234–1240.

Kline SS, Mauro LS, Scala-Barnett DM, et al: Serotonin syndrome versus neuroleptic malignant syndrome as a cause of death. Clin Pharm 1989; 8: 510–514.

Kojima H, Terao T, Yoshimura R, et al: Serotonin syndrome during clomipramine and lithium treatment. Am J Psychiatry 1993: 150: 1897.

Kolecki P: Venlafaxine induced serotonin syndrome occurring after abstinence from phenelzine for more than two weeks. J Toxicol Clin Toxicol 1997; 35: 211–212.

Kudo K, Sasaki I, Tsuchiyama K, et al: Serotonin syndrome during clomipramine monotherapy: comparison of two diagnostic criteria. Psychiatry Clin Neurosci 1997; 51: 43–46.

Kuisma MJ: Fatal serotonin syndrome with trismus. Ann Emerg Med 1995; 26: 108.

Lane R, Baldwin D: Selective serotonin reuptake inhibitor-induced serotonin syndrome: review. J Clin Psychopharmacol 1997; 17(3): 208–221.

Lappin RI, Auchincloss EL: Treatment of serotonin syndrome with cyproheptadine. N Engl J Med 1994; 331: 1021–1022.

Lejoyeux M, Rouillon F, Ades J, et al: Prospective evaluation of the "serotonin syndrome" in depressed patients treated with clomipramine. Acta Psychiatr Scand 1993; 88: 369–371.

Lenzi A, Raffaelli S, Marazziti D: Serotonin syndrome like symptoms in a patient with obsessive compulsive disorder, following inappropriate increase in fluvoxamine dosage. Pharmacopsychiatry 1993; 26: 100–101.

Luck I, Noble MS, Frazer A: Differential action of serotonin antagonists on two behavior models of serotonin receptor activation in rat. J Pharmacol Exp Ther 1984; 1: 133–139.

Marley E, Wozniak KM: Interaction of non-selective monoamine oxidase inhibitors, tranylcypromine, and nialamide, with inhibitors of 5-hydroxytryptamine, dopamine, or noradrenaline uptake. J Psychiatr Res 1984; 18: 191–203.

Mathew NT, Tietjen GE, Lucker C: Serotonin syndrome complicating migraine pharmacotherapy. Cephalalgia 1996; 16: 323–327.

Mekler G, Woggon B: A case of serotonin syndrome caused by venlafaxine and lithium. Pharmacopsychiatry 1997; 30: 272–273.

Miller F, Friedman R, Tanenbaum J, et al: Disseminated intravascular coagulation and acute myoglobinuric renal failure: a consequence of serotonergic syndrome. J Clin Psychopharmacol 1991; 11: 277–279.

Neuvonen PJ, Pohjola-Sintonen S, Tacke U, et al: Five fatal cases of serotonin syndrome after moclobemide-citalopram or moclobemide-clomipramine overdoses. Lancet 1993; 342: 1419.

Nierenberg DW, Semprebon M: The central nervous system serotonin syndrome. Clin Pharmacol Ther 1993; 53: 84–88.

Nimmo SM, Kennedy BW, Tullett WM, et al: Drug-induced hyperthermia. Anesthesia 1993; 48: 892–895.

Oates JA, Sjoerdsma A: Neurologic effects of tryptophan in patients receiving a monoamine oxidase inhibitor. Neurology 1960; 10: 1076–1078.

Öhman R, Spigset O: Serotonin syndrome induced by fluvoxamine-lithium interaction. Pharmacopsychiatry 1993; 26: 263–264.

Ooi TK: The serotonin syndrome. Anesthesia 1991; 46: 597–608.

Pennings EJM, Verkes RJ, De Konig J, et al: Tranylcypromine intoxication with malignant hyperthermia, delirium, and thrombocytopenia. Journal of -clinical Psychopharmacology 1997; 17: 430–432.

Phillips SD, Ringo P: Phenelzine and venlafaxine interaction. Am J Psychiatry 1995; 152(9): 1400–1401.

Pope HG, Jonas JM, Hudson JI, et al: Toxic reactions to the combination of monoamine oxidase inhibitors and tryptophan. Am J Psychiatry 1985; 142: 491–492.

Power BM, Hackett LP, Dusci LJ, et al: Antidepressant toxicity and the need for identification and concentration monitoring in overdose. Clin Pharmacokinet 1995; 29: 154–171.

Rapport MM, Green AA, Page IH: Serum vasoconstrictor (serotonin) IV: isolation and characterization. J Biol Chem 1948; 176: 1243–1251.

Reeves RR, Bullen JA: Serotonin syndrome produced by paroxetine and low-dose trazodone. Psychosomatics 1995; 36(2): 159–160.

Rella JG, Hoffman RS: Possible serotonin syndrome for paroxetine and clonazepam. J Toxicol Clin Toxicol 1998; 36: 257–258.

Richard IH, Kurlan R, Tanner C, et al: Serotonin syndrome and the combined use of deprenyl and an antidepressant in Parkinson's disease. Neurology 1997; 48: 1070–1077.

Rivers N, Harner B: Possible lethal reaction between Nardil and dextromethorphan. Can Med Assoc J 1970; 103: 85.

Rosebush PI, Margetts P, Mazurek MF: Serotonin syndrome as a result of clomipramine monotherapy. J Clin Psychopharmacol 1999; 19(3): 285–287.

Rosenstein DL, Takeshita J, Nelson JC: Fluoxetine-induced elevation and prolongation of tricyclic levels in overdose. Am J Psychiatry 1991; 148: 807.

Ruiz E: Fluoxetine and serotonin syndrome. Ann Emerg Med 1994; 24: 983–985.

Sandyk R: L-dopa induced "serotonin syndrome" in a parkinsonian patient on bromocriptine (letter). J Clin Psychopharmacol 1986; 6: 194.

Schenck CH, Mahowald MW: Potential hazard of serotonin syndrome associated with dexfenfluramine hydrochloride (Redux) (letter). JAMA 1996; 276: 1220–1221.

Sinclair JG: Dextromethorphan-monoamine oxidase inhibitor interaction in rabbits. J Pharm Pharmacol 1973; 25: 803–808.

Skop BP, Finkelstein JA, Mareth TR, et al: The serotonin syndrome associated with paroxetine, an over-the-counter cold remedy, and vascular disease. Am J Emerg Med 1994; 12: 642–644.

Smilkstein MJ, Smolinske SC, Rumack BH: A case of MAO inhibitor/MDMA interaction: agony after ecstasy. Clin Toxicol 1987; 25: 149–159.

Smith B, Prockop DJ: Central nervous system effects of ingestion of L-tryptophan by normal subjects. N Engl J Med 1962; 267: 1338–1341.

Sobanski T, Bagli M, Laux G, et al: Serotonin syndrome after lithium add-on medication to paroxetine. Pharmacopsychiatry 1997; 30(3): 106–107.

Sovner R, Wolfe J: Interaction between dextromethorphan and monoamine oxidase inhibitor therapy with isocarboxazid (letter). N Engl J Med 1988; 319: 1671.

Spigset O, Mjörndahl T, Lövheim O: Serotonin syndrome caused by a moclobemide-clomipramine interaction (drug points). BMJ 1993; 306: 248.

Sporer KA: The serotonin syndrome. Drug Safety 1996; 13: 94–104.

Stack CG, Rogers P, Linter SPK: Monoamine oxidase inhibitors and anesthesia. Br J Anaesth 1988; 60: 222–227.

Steiner W, Fontaine R: Toxic reaction following combined administration of fluoxedtine and L-tryptophan: five case reports. Biol Psychiatry 1986; 21: 1067–1071.

Sternbach H: Danger of MAOI therapy after fluoxetine withdrawal (letter). Lancet 1988; 2: 850.

Sternbach H: The serotonin syndrome. Am J Psychiatry 1991; 148: 705–713.

Suchowersky O, deVries JD: Interaction of fluoxetine and selegiline. Can J Psychiatry 1990; 35: 571–572.

Tackley RM, Tregaskis B: Fatal disseminated intravascular coagulation following a monoamine oxidase inhibitor/tricyclic interaction. Anesthesia 1987; 42: 760–763.

Weiner LA, Smythe M, Cisek J: Serotonin syndrome secondary to phenelzine-venlafaxine interaction. Pharmacotherapy 1998; 18: 399–403.

Weinstock A, Weiss C, Gitter S: Blockade of 5-hydroxytryptamine receptors in the central nervous system by β adrenoceptor antagonists. Neuropharmacology 1977; 16: 273–276.

Yamada J, Sugimotot Y, Horisaka K: The evidence for the involvement of the 5-HT1A receptor in 5-HT syndrome induced in mice by 5-hydroxytryptamine. Jpn J Pharmacol 1989; 51: 421–424.

Yamawaki S, Yanagawak K, Hotta I, et al: Effect of long-term lithium treatment on serotonin syndrome in rats. Yakubutsu Seishin Kodo 1986; 6: 247–252.

Zohar J, Insel TR: Obsessive-compulsive disorders: psychobiological approaches to diagnosis, treatment and pathophysiology. Biol Psychiatry 1987; 22: 667–687.

Chapter 22
Drug-Induced Guillain-Barré Syndrome

Introduction

Guillain-Barré Syndrome (GBS) is an eponym derived from the description in 1916 by French neurologists Guillain and Barré combined with electrophysiological studies by Strohl (Ropper 1992). GBS is an acute inflammatory demyelinating polyradiculopathy (AIDP) causing progressive weakness of the limbs (Landry's ascending paralysis) and loss of tendon reflexes. The supporting clinical criteria are relatively symmetrical weakness, mild sensory signs, cranial nerve involvement (particularly facial), autonomic dysfunction, and absence of fever. The main supporting laboratory criterion is increase of protein concentration in CSF with normal cell count (albuminocytologic dissociation). Electrophysiological studies show slowing of nerve conduction suggesting demyelination. GBS is a significant cause of acute generalized paralysis with an annual incidence of 1–2 cases/100,000 population (Hughes 1990).

One of the important criteria for GBS is that the paralysis should not progress for longer than 4 weeks (Asbury 1978). If it does persist, the question rises whether the patient may be developing chronic polyradiculopathy, also referred to as chronic relapsing GBS. There is still controversy about the nomenclature and diagnostic criteria of GBS and Dyck (1993) has suggested that GBS or AIDP should be considered as a family of closely related disorders that might be divided by the following criteria:
- Class of axon involved: motor, sensory, autonomic, or mixtures
- Pathologic process: inflammatory, demyelinating, direct antibody attack, or others
- Preceding infection

- Associated antibody
- Underlying disease mechanisms
- Response to treatment

Pathophysiology

Approximately two-thirds of patients with GBS have presented after infections with organisms such as HIV, cytomegalovirus, Epstein-Barr virus and *Campylobacter jejuni*. Infections have been suggested as possible triggers of GBS and it is mediated, at least partially, by autoimmune mechanisms. The pathological concept of this syndrome as an inflammatory disorder is based on the classical studies showing lymphocytes and macrophages surrounding endoneural vessels and causing adjacent demyelination (Asbury et al 1969). Demyelination may be produced mainly by the T-lymphocytes in some cases whereas in others macrophages may be involved and the process may be antibody-mediated (Thomas 1992). Antibodies against gangliosides GM-1 and P-2, cerebroside, and peripheral myelin glycolipids, which are all components of myelin, have been identified in patients with GBS. These antibodies attack the myelin and remove it from intact axons.

Cytotoxins of *C. jejuni* are poorly understood and an immune mechanism remains the most likely explanation. The specific disease manifestations of post *C. jejuni* GBS may be determined by the location of the specific epitopes under attack in the peripheral nervous system – the myelin, the axolemma or both (Griffin and Ho 1993). Recent observations suggest that GBS may have more than one pathomechanisms.

Drug-Induced Guillain-Barré Syndrome

Various pharmaceutical preparations which have been reported to be associated with onset of GBS or Guillain-Barré-like syndromes are listed in Table 22.1.

Table 22.1. Drugs and other therapies that have been reported to be associated with onset of Guillain-Barré syndrome.

Drugs
Arsenicals (organic)
Cantharidin
Captopril
Corticosteroids
Fansidar
Gangliosides*
Gold salts
Ofloxacin
Oxytocin
Penicilla mine
Streptokinase*
Zimeldine (withdrawn from the market in 1983)

Vaccines
Hepatitis B vaccine
Influenza vaccines*
Measles mumps and rubella vaccine
Oral poliomyelitis vaccine
Rabies vaccine*
Tetanus toxoid
Typhoid vaccine

Therapeutic procedures
Bone marrow transplantation (Wen et al 1997)
Surgery with postoperative epidural morphine analgesia (Rosenberg and Stacey 1996)

*Well documented.

Arsenicals (Organic). These compounds are used for the treatment of human trypanosomiasis. Neurotoxicity of these compounds is known to manifest as encephalopathy (see Chapter 3). Gherardi et al (1990) have reported a Guillain-Barré-like syndrome in a patient treated with melarsoprol. Electrophysiological data in this case were misleading for GBS. Neuropathological findings included massive distal wallerian degeneration in peripheral nerves and abnormalities in the dorsal ganglia and spinal cord with vacuolation of anterior horn cells.

Cantharidin. Cantharides are herbal agents used as abortifacients and aphrodisiacs. Two cases of cantharidin toxicity with symptoms resembling GBS have been reported in South Africa (Harrisberg et al 1984). Cantharidin poisoning has not been reported in the United States where only the topical cantharides are available for application on benign epithelial lesions.

Captopril. This is an ACE inhibitor used for the treatment of hypertension. Peripheral neuropathy as an adverse reaction to the drug is described in Chapter 11. There are case reports of GBS as well during treatment with captopril (Chakraborty and Ruddell 1987; Atkinson et al 1980a and 1980b). Captopril is chemically similar to D-penicillamine (both have sulfhydryl groups) and causes similar side effects which appear to be due to an autoimmune reaction which may precipitate GBS.

Corticosteroids. Steiner et al (1986) reported three patients who developed GBS while on corticosteroid treatment. In each case the syndrome appeared while the dose of steroids was being tapered. The pathomechanism of GBS in these cases was postulated to be a selective effect of low dose steroids on a specific, perhaps suppressive lymphocytic subpopulation. One of the patients had a history of multiple sclerosis.

A case of GBS has been reported following danazol and corticosteroid therapy for hereditary angioedema (Hory et al 1985). Danazol is an androgenic anabolic agent and has been reported to exacerbate SLE. In this case either danazol or steroids or combination of both may have precipitated GBS.

Fansidar. This is an antimalarial drug and one case of GBS has been reported following its use as a prophylactic and it was considered to have been possibly precipitated by the drug (Lorentzon 1984).

Gangliosides. These have a role in promoting nerve repair by increasing collateral sprouting. They have not been proven to be effective as an adjuvant treatment for various neuropathies. The use of a parenteral bovine ganglioside (Cronassial) was suspended in Germany in 1989 because of the suspicion of their possible association with GBS. At least 20 of the approximately 14,000 patients treated with gangliosides are known to have suffered from neurological sequelae with characteristics of either amyotrophic lateral sclerosis or GBS. However, health authorities in Italy continued their surveillance on gangliosides, restricting its use to treatment of diabetic neuropathies and truncular lesions while banning its use in all autoimmune disorders (Raschetti et al 1992). Landi et al (1993) described 244 further cases of GBS after ganglioside treatment. The number exceeds the estimated number expected in the unexposed population and places the increased risk of GBS with ganglioside close to 200-fold. The Spanish national drug surveillance system has received 17 reports of acute motor polyneuropathies associated with the use of bovine glycosides of which 10 were diagnosed as GBS (Figueras et al 1992).

Antinuclear antibodies have been detected in sera of patients who developed GBS or motor neuron-like disorders following treatment with parenteral gangliosides (Latov et al 1991; Yuki et al 1991). Knorr-Held et al (1986) reported a patient with multiple sclerosis who developed acute polyradiculoneuritis 11 days after implantation of swine brain ganglioside. Sensitization against brain nucleotides could be demonstrated by lymphocyte transformation test. Schwerer et al (1994) reported the case of a 39-year old woman who developed progressive motor polyneuropathy following the use of IM gangliosides and recovered after discontinuation of the therapy and plasma exchanges. She had relapses and was found to have a high level of antiganglioside GM_1.

Gold Salts. Patients with rheumatoid arthritis treated with gold salts have been reported to develop GBS (Dick and Raman 1982; Schlumpf et al 1983; Vernay et al 1986). Miller-Fisher syndrome, a variant of GBS, has been reported to develop in patients with rheumatoid arthritis during treatment with gold salts (Roquer et al 1985).

Ofloxacin. This is one of the quinolone antibiotics which have been associated with adverse effects on the central as well as peripheral nervous systems. Schmidt et al (1993) reported GBS in a patient with urinary infection treated with ofloxacin with recovery after discontinuation and recurrence after resumption of therapy. They mentioned 10 similar cases which have

been reported to the manufacturer and in whom GBS coincided with ofloxacin treatment.

Oxytocin. One case of GBS is reported in a postpartum patient who used oxytocin spray to continue lactation during a period of separation from her infant and this followed the development of a syndrome of inappropriate secretion of antidiuretic hormone (SIADH) which led to hyponatremic encephalopathy (Seifer et al 1985). The patient did not have the characteristic EMG changes of GBS but gradually improved. Several other cases of GBS-like syndrome have been reported in association with SIADH. The causal relationship of oxytocin to GBS remains questionable.

Penicillamine. Two cases of GBS have been reported following use of D-penicillamine therapy but no satisfactory explanation was provided (Knezevic et al 1984; Pool et al 1981).

Streptokinase. Nine published case reports have implicated that streptokinase can precipitate GBS (Taylor et al 1995; Ancillo et al 1994; Barnes and Hughes 1992; Rocquer et al 1990; Cicale 1987; Arrowsmith et al 1985; Leaf et al 1984; Eden 1983). The pathomechanism is unclear but streptokinase is a foreign protein and may induce the immunological reaction that is presumed to be necessary for the development of GBS. GBS has also been reported to occur in 0.75–2/100,000 patients with myocardial infarction without treatment with streptokinase (McDonagh and Dawson 1987).

Zimeldine. This serotonin reuptake inhibitor antidepressant was reported to be associated with peripheral neuropathy (see Chapter 11). Fagius et al (1985) reviewed 13 cases of GBS in Sweden in association with introduction of zimeldine and found that risk of developing GBS was increased 25-fold in patients receiving zimeldine. An analysis of 9 of these cases by microcomputer-assisted Bayesian differential diagnosis revealed that these were probably causally related to zimeldine (Naranjo and Lanctot 1991). This drug was withdrawn from the market in 1983 because of its association with GBS as 10 cases in 200,000 prescriptions indicated that the population exposed to it was 25 times more liable to develop GBS than the unexposed population.

Vaccines

Evidence from published literature shows that GBS follows immunization in only a small percentage of cases. The following vaccines have been implicated.

Hepatitis B Vaccination. In post-marketing surveillance, GBS has been reported following hepatitis-B vaccination but this risk is unlikely to outweigh the prophylactic benefit of this vaccine (Shaw et al 1988; Tuohy 1989).

Influenza Vaccines. In the fall of 1976 there was a massive campaign in the United States for vaccination against an epidemic of influenza expected to affect the nation. The campaign was halted after 45 million immunizations with swine flue vaccine had been done and 1300 alleged cases of GBS had been reported to the Center for Disease Control. There was much confusion and controversy about the issue whether the cases fulfilled the criteria for the diagnosis of GBS (Kurland 1985). The explanation of the apparent epidemic of GBS following swine flue vaccine remains uncertain. A reassessment of this situation by Safranek et al (1991), using modified criteria for assessment of cases (Asbury et al 1978), showed that there was an increased risk of developing GBS only during the first 6 weeks following vaccination in the adults.

Hemophilus influenzae type B conjugate vaccine has also been associated with GBS (D'Cruz et al 1989). This vaccine contains the *H. influenzae* antigen and diphtheria toxoid. The syndrome resolved in all the patients and there has been no further reports of similar occurrences.

Measles Mumps and Rubella Vaccine (MMR). Morris and Rylance (1994) published the case of a child who developed GBS after MMR vaccine. The authors mentioned that 2 similar cases had been reported to the Medicines Control Agency in UK and a larger number (less than 20) were reported to the manufacturer. In view of the widespread use of this vaccine, this association is extremely rare.

Oral Poliomyelitis Vaccine (OPV). Increased incidence of GBS following oral poliomyelitis vaccination has been reported from Finland (Kinnunen et al 1989; Uhari et al 1989). However, there was no increase of such an incidence in the United States. One explanation of this is that immunization in the United States is exclusively with OPV whereas in Finland the routine immunization was with inactivated polio virus and OPV was given to individuals who may not have the same intestinal immunity as children given OPV (Salisbury 1998).

Rabies Vaccine. The neuroparalytic illness following rabies vaccination frequently resembles GBS (Griffin 1988). The incidence of neuroparalytic complications following the use of Semple vaccine in Thailand was in the order of 1:1000 to 1:4000 (Hemachuda et al 1987). Cases of GBS were also reported to follow a improved variety, the suckling mouse brain vaccine, which was used in Peru (Cabrera et al 1987). There is no theoretical reason why the human diploid cell culture derived rabies vaccine should produce GBS although two cases have been reported following this vaccine (Boe and Nyland 1980; Knittel et al 1989). The pathomechanism of rabies vaccine-induced GBS is not clear. It may be similar to experimental allergic neuritis but the identity of the antigen is not known. Sera of the patients with vaccine-induced GBS contain autoantibodies to myelin basic protein (MBP) but the distribution of MBP in the nervous system makes it an unlikely target for pathogenetically important autoimmune reactions in GBS (Hughes 1990).

Tetanus Toxoid. It may precipitate GBS when given alone (Newton and Janati 1987; Pollard and Selby 1978) or in combination with diphtheria toxoid. The evidence is not strong enough to forego tetanus toxoid in cases of potentially contaminated wounds but its use should be avoided in patients with a past history of GBS. A background rate of 0.3 cases of Guillain-Barré syndrome per million person-weeks has been estimated (Tuttle et al 1997). By chance, 2.2 persons with the syndrome would have received tetanus-toxoid-containing vaccine within the 6 weeks before onset, yet only 1 person had done so. If an association exists between tetanus toxoid and GBS, it must be extremely rare and not of public health significance.

Typhoid Vaccination. Cases of GBS following typhoid vaccination have been reported by Miller and Stanton (1954). It would be considered a rare occurrence.

A committee of the US National Academy of Sciences's Institute of Medicine has reviewed the evidence on this topic and accepted the causal relationship only of diphtheria and tetanus toxoids and oral polio vaccine to GBS (Stratton et al 1994).

Management of Guillain-Barré Syndrome

The prognosis of GBS is generally good with 80% of the patients making a good recovery. In case of suspected drug-induced GBS, the drug in question should be continued. The management is the same as GBS due to other non-drug-related causes. Supportive treatment includes respiratory intensive care management and monitoring of cardiorespiratory function. Complications associated with immobility should be prevented, particularly pneumonia and thromboembolism. Specific treatment includes plasma exchange and intravenous immune globulins. In a randomized trial, both of these therapies were found to be equally effective (Plasma Exchange/Sandoglobulin Guillain-Barré Syndrome Trial Group 1997).

References

Ancillo P, Duarte J, Cortina JJ: Guillain-Barré syndrome after acute myocardial infarction treated with anistreplase. Chest 1994; 105: 1301–1302.

Arrowsmith JB, Milstein JB, Kuritsky JB, et al: Streptikinase and Guillain-Barré syndrome. Ann Int Med 1985; 103: 302.

Asbury AK, Arnason BG, Adams RD: The inflammatory lesion in idiopathic polyneuritis: its role in pathogenesis. Medicine (Baltimore) 1969; 48: 173–215.

Asbury AK, Aronson BGW, Karp Hr, et al: Criteria for diagnosis of Guillain-Barré syndrome. Ann Neurol 1978; 3: 565–566.

Atkinson AB, Brown JJ, Lever AF, et al: Combined treatment of severe intractable hypertension with captopril and diuretic. Lancet 1980b; 2: 105–107.

Atkinson AB, Brown JJ, Lever AF, et al: Neurological dysfunction in two patients receiving captopril and cimetidine. Lancet 1980a; 2: 36–37.

Barnes D, Hughes RAC: Guillain-Barré syndrome after treatment with streptokinase. BMJ 1992; 304: 1225.

Boe E, Nyland H: Guillain-Barré syndrome after vaccination with human diploid cell rabies vaccine. Scand J Infect Dis 1980; 12: 231–232.

Cabrera J, Griffin DE, Johnson RT: Unusual features of GBS after rabies vaccine prepared in sucking mouse brain. J Neurol Sci 1987; 81: 239–246.

Chakraborty TK, Ruddell WSJ: Guillain-Barré neuropathy during treatment with captopril. Postgraduate Med J 1987; 63: 221–222.

Cicale MJ: Guillain-Barré syndrome after streptokinase therapy. South Med J 1987; 80: 1068.

D'Cruz OF, Shapiro ED, Spiegelman KN, et al: Acute inflammatory demyelinating polyradiculoneuropathy (Guillain-Barré syndrome) after immunization with Haemophilus influenzae type b conjugate vaccine. J Pediatr 1989; 115(5 Pt 1): 743–746.

Dick DJ, Raman D: The Guillain-Barré syndrome following gold therapy. Scand J Rheumatol 1982; 11: 119–120.

Dyck PJ: Is there an axonal variety of GBS? (editorial). Neurology 1993; 43: 1277–1280.

Eden KV: Possible association of Guillain-Barré syndrome with thrombolytilc therapy. JAMA 1983; 249: 2020–2021.

Fagius J, Osterman PO, Siden A, et al: Guillain-Barré syndrome following zimeldine treatment. JNNP 1985; 48: 65–69.

Figueras A, Morales-Olivas FJ, Capella D, et al: Bovine glycosides and acute motor polyneuropathy. BMJ 1992; 305: 1330–1331.

Gherardi RK, Chariot P, Vanderstigel M, et al: Organic arsenic-induced Guillain-Barré-like syndrome due to melaproprol: a clinical, electrophysiological, and pathological study. Muscle & Nerve 1990; 13: 637–645.

Griffin DE: Post-infectious and post-vaccinal disorders of the central nervous system. Immunol Allergy Clin North Am 1988; 8: 239–242.

Griffin JW, Ho TW: The Guillain-Barré syndrome at 75: The *Campylobacter* connection (editorial). Ann Neurol 1993; 34: 125–127.

Harrisberg J, Deseta J, Cohen L, et al: Cantharidine poisoning with neurological complications. S Afr Med J 1984; 65: 66–67.

Hemachuda T, Phanuphak P, Johnson RT, et al: Neurologic complications of Semple type rabies vaccine. Neurology 1987; 37: 550–557.

Holliday P, Bauer RB: Polyradiculoneuritis secondary to immunization with tetanus and diphtheria toxoids. Arch Neurol 1983; 40: 56–57.

Hory B, Blanc D, Boillot A, et al: Guillain-Barré syndrome following danazol and cortico steroid therapy for hereditary angioedema. Am J Med 1985; 79: 111–114.

Hughes RAC: Guillain-Barré syndrome, London, Springer-Verlag, 1990.

Kinnunen E, Farkkila M, Hovi T, et al: Incidence of Guillain-Barré syndrome during a nationwide oral poliomyelitis vaccine campaign. Neurology 1989; 39: 1034–1036.

Knezevic W, Quinter J, Mastaglia FL, et al: Guillain-Barré

syndrome and pemphigus foliatus associated with D-pencillamine therapy. Austr NZ J Med 1984; 14: 50–52.

Knittel T, Ramadori G, Meyer WJ, et al: Guillain-Barré syndrome and human diploid cell rabies vaccine. Lancet 1989; 1: 1334–1335.

Knorr-Held S, Brendel W, Kiefer H, et al: Sensitization against brain gangliosides after therapeutic swine brain implantation in a multiple sclerosis patient. J Neurol 1986; 233: 54–56.

Kurland LT, Wiederholt WC, Kirkpatrick JW, et al: Swine influenza vaccine and Guillain-Barré syndrome. Arch Neurol 1985; 42: 1089–1090.

Landi G, D'Alessandro R, Dossi BC, et al: Guillain-Barré syndrome after exogenous gangliosides in Italy. BMJ 1993; 307: 1463–1464.

Latov N, Koski CL, Walicke P: Guillain-Barré syndrome and parenteral gangliosides. Lancet 1991; 338: 757.

Leaf DA, McDonald I, Kliks B, et al: Streptokinase and Guillain-Barré syndrome. Ann Int Med 1984; 100: 617.

Lorentzon B: Guillain-Barré syndrome associated with fansidar intake. Lakartidningen 1984; 81: 2919.

McCarthy M: Adverse events and childhood vaccines. Lancet 1993; 342: 798.

McDonagh AJG, Dawson J: Guillain-Barré syndrome after myocardial infarction. BMJ 1987; 294: 213–214.

Miller HG, Stanton JB: Neurologic sequelae of prophylactic inoculation. Q J Med 1954; 23: 1–27.

Morris K, Rylance G: Guillain-Barré syndrome after measles, mumps, and rubella vaccine (letter). Lancet 1994; 343: 60.

Naranjo C, Lanctot KL: Microcomputer-assisted Bayesian differential diagnosis of severe adverse reactions to new drugs: a 4-year experience. Drug Information Journal 1991; 25: 243–250.

Newton LN, Janati A: Guillain-Barré syndrome after vaccination with purified tetanus toxoid. South Med J 1987; 80: 1053–1054.

Plasma Exchange / Sandoglobulin Guillain-Barré Syndrome Trial Group. Randomized trial of plasma exchange, intravenous immunoglobulin, and combined treatments in Guillain-Barré syndrome. Lancet 1997; 349: 225–230.

Pollard JD, Selby G: Relapsing neuropathy due to tetanus toxoid. J Neurol Sci 1978; 37: 113–125.

Pool KD, Feit H, Kirkpatrick J: Penicillamine-induced neuropathy in rheumatoid arthritis. Ann Int Med 1981; 95: 457–458.

Raschetti R, Maggini M, Popoli P: Guillain-Barré syndrome and ganglioside therapy in Italy. Lancet 1992; 340: 60.

Rocquer J, Herraiz J, Arnau d, et al: Guillain-Barré syndrome after treatment with streptokinase therapy. Acta Neurol Scand 1990; 82: 153.

Rocquer J, Herraiz J, Maymo J, et al: Miller-Fisher syndrome (Guillain-Barré syndrome with ophthalmoplegia) during treatment with gold salts in a patient with rheumatoid arthritis. Arthritis Rheum 1985; 28: 838–839.

Ropper AH: The Guillain-Barré Syndrome. NEJM 1992; 326: 1130–1136.

Rosenberg SK, Stacy BR: Postoperative Guillain-Barré syndrome, arachnoiditis, and epidural analgesia. Regional Anesthesia 1996; 21: 486–489.

Safranek TJ, Lawrence DN, Kurland LT, et al: Reassessment of the association between Guillain-Barré syndrome and receipt of swine influenza vaccine in 1976–1977: results of two state study. Am J Epidemiol 1991; 133: 940–951.

Salisbury DM: Association between oral poliovaccine and Guillain-Barré syndrome. Lancet 1998; 351: 79–80.

Schlumpf U, Meyer M, Ulrich J, et al: Neurologic complications induced by gold treatment. Arthritis Rheum 1983; 26: 825–831.

Schmidt A, Cordt-Schlegel A, Heitman R: Guillain-Barré syndrome during treatment with oflaxacin. J Neurol 1993; 240: 506–507.

Schwerer B, Pichler S, Bernheimer H, et al: Chronic progressive motor polyneuropathy after ganglioside treatment. JNNP 1994; 57: 238.

Seifer DB, Sandberg EC, Ueland K: Water intoxication and hyponatremic encephalopathy from the use of an oxytocin nasal spray. A case report. J Reprod Med 1985; 30(3): 225–228.

Shaw FE, Graham DJ, Guess HA, et al: Postmarketing surveillance for neurologic adverse events reported after hepatitis B vaccination. Am J Epidemiol 1988; 127: 337–352.

Steiner I, Wirguin I, Abramsky O: Appearance of Guillain-Barré syndrome in patients during corticosteroid treatment. J Neurol 1986; 233: 221–223.

Stratton KR, Howe KJ, Johnston RB: Adverse events associated with childhood vaccines other than pertussis and rubella. JAMA 1994; 271: 1602–1605.

Svennerholm L, Fredman P: Antibody detection in Guillain-Barré syndrome. Ann Neurol 1990; 27 (suppl): S36–S40.

Taylor BV, Mastaglia FL, Stell R: Guillain-Barré syndrome complicating treatment with streptokinase. Med J Aust 1995; 162(4): 214–5.

Thomas PK: The Guillain-Barré syndrome: no longer a simple concept. J Neurol 1992; 239: 361–362.

Tuohy PG: Guillain-Barré syndrome following immunization with synthetic hepatitis B vaccine. N Z Med J 1989; 102(863): 114–5.

Tuttle J, Chen RT, Rantala H, et al: The risk of Guillain-Barré syndrome after tetanus-toxoid-containing vaccines in adults and children in the United States. Am J Public Health 1997; 87(12): 2045–8.

Uhari M, Rantala H, Niemela M: Cluster of childhood Guillain-Barré cases after oral poliovaccine campaign. Lancet 1989; ii: 440–441.

Vernay D, Dubost JJ, Thevenet JP, et al: "Choree fibrillaire de Morvan" followed by Guillain-Barré syndrome in a patient receiving gold therapy. Arthritis Rheum 1986; 29(11): 1413–1414.

Wen PY, Alyea EP, Simon D, et al: Guillain-Barré syndrome following allogeneic bone marrow transplantation. Neurology 1997; 49(6): 1711–1714.

Yuki N, Sato S, Miyatake T, et al: Motor neuron disease-like disorder after ganglioside therapy. Lancet 1991; 337: 1109–1110.

Chapter 23
Neuroleptic Malignant Syndrome

Introduction

Neuroleptic malignant syndrome (NMS) is a rare but potentially fatal idiosyncratic reaction to neuroleptic medications characterized by muscular rigidity, fever, autonomic dysfunction, and altered consciousness. It was first noted during clinical trials of haloperidol and described in French literature as "syndrom malin" by Delay et al (1960). The first description in English was by Delay and Deniker (1968) in the *Handbook of Clinical Neurology*. Caroff (1980) presented the first detailed review of the clinical characteristics and differential diagnosis of NMS based on review of cases in the English literature. Several excellent reviews of this topic have appeared since then (Kornhuber and Weller 1994; Gratz and Simpson 1994; Caroff and Mann 1993; Kellam 1990; Tesar et al 1988; Addonizio et al 1987; Shalev and Munitz 1986; Mueller 1985; Levenson 1985; Kurlan et al 1984). There is a comprehensive book on this topic by Addonizio and Susman (1991).

Epidemiology

The prevalence of NMS among admissions to acute psychiatric wards has been estimated to vary from 0.2% to 2% (Keck et al 1991). In a 18-month prospective study of 679 hospitalized patients, NMS was diagnosed in six (0.9%) of cases (Keck et al 1987). In a study in China, 12 (0.012%) of 9792 inpatients exposed to neuroleptics developed NMS (Deng et al 1990). In a study in Japan, NMS occurred in 1.8% of patients who received antipsychotic therapy (Naganuma and Fujii 1994). The lack of consensus on diagnostic criteria of NMS makes comparison of incidence from various studies difficult.

Pathomechanism

Pathomechanism of NMS is not completely understood. It is generally agreed that alterations in dopaminergic transmission in the CNS associated with drug therapy is the most important factor in its etiology. This is caused either by treatment with dopamine receptor antagonists or by withdrawing dopamine receptor agonists. Acute dopamine transmission block in basal ganglia and the hypothalamus is considered to be the pathophysiological mechanism of NMS (Weller and Kornhuber 1992a, 1992b). In this respect NMS, "the malignant dopamine depletion syndrome" may be identical with akinetic parkinsonian crisis. Additionally an alteration of dopaminergic-serotonergic transmission in the body, an enhanced synthesis and action of prostaglandins E_1 and E_2, and a modification of calcium-mediated signal transduction in the body have been suggested (Ebadi et al 1990). Malfunction of the central N-methyl-D-aspartate-glutamate receptors has also been postulated as pathomechanism and forms the basis of recommendation of NMDA receptor antagonists as treatment for NMS. Based on the clinical effectiveness of benzodiazepines in reversing NMS, it has been suggested that GABA plays a role in the development of NMS. Many of the features of NMS suggest that sympathetic nervous system hyperactivity is involved in the pathophysiology of this disorder. Elevated urinary catecholamines and metabolites are a frequent but inconstant feature of NMS (Gurrera and Romero 1992). Schibuk and Schachter (1986) hypothesized that NMS is caused by a central imbalance between norepinephrine and dopamine and not by dopamine depletion. This view is supported by a case of NMS due to desipramine, a tricyclic antidepressant (Baca and Martinelli 1990). Desipramine inhibits the reuptake of norepinephrine with subsequent enhancement of central noradrenergic effects but does not significantly alter central dopaminergic levels.

Positron emission tomography studies using $C^{15}O_2$ and $^{15}O_2$ techniques show that cerebral oxygen metabolism and CBF are disturbed during NMS, indicating that not only dopaminergic but also the other neurotransmitter systems are involved (De Reuck et al 1991).

There is debate whether NMS is due to central or peripheral action of haloperidol. Downey et al (1992) described a patient with complete cervical cord transection who suffered a fatal hyperthermic episode after haloperidol administration which implies that NMS is this case was peripheral effect of haloperidol.

No definite pathological lesions have been identified in NMS. Necrosis in the anterior and lateral nuclei of hypothalamus, the regions concerned with temperature regulation, has been described in a case of NMS (Horn et al 1988). In other cases there are no abnormal findings in Parkinson's disease patients who suffer NMS, the brain pathology does not differ from that of Parkinson's disease patients without NMS.

Risk Factors

The following risk factors have been identified for NMS and these can be divided into risk factors involving the drugs and the patient risk factors.

Risk factors related to the drugs
- Patients on rapidly escalating doses of high potency neuroleptics given by intramuscular injections for long periods are more likely to develop NMS.
- Patients on neuroleptic therapy with concomitant use of lithium and antidepressants are at risk for developing NMS.

Risk factors related to the patient
- Young male patients are more likely to suffer.

Mean age of NMS patients has been estimated to be 40 years. The reasons for this are not clear. Perhaps younger patients receive higher doses of neuroleptics for longer periods than the elderly patients.
- Genetic factors may predispose to NMS as suggested by two case reports (Tu 1997).
- About of 40% of patients who develop NMS have an affective disorder (Pearlman 1986). These patients are more likely to develop NMS than those with schizophrenia.
- Patients with fluid and electrolyte disturbances such as dehydration, hyponatremia, and hypernatremia, which are common in psychiatric patients are at risk for development of NMS.
- Hypothyroidism (Moore et al 1990).
- Patients with existing brain damage may have marginal stores of dopamine in the hypothalamus and basal ganglia and are susceptible to dopamine blocking activity of even low doses of neuroleptics (Lazarus 1992). NMS has been reported in a patient with Alzheimer's disease after haloperidol administration (Serby 1986). Patients with Huntington's disease and alcohol-related organic brain disease are more susceptible to NMS. Patients with mental retardation, who often receive neuroleptics, are at risk for the development of NMS. Boyd (1993) has reviewed 29 such cases from medical literature.
- Levodopa withdrawal in patients with Parkinson's disease (Henderson and Wooten 1981).
- Patients with malignant disease (Woodruff et al 1991).
- Patients with medical disorders, and drug-related adverse effects which compromise thermoregulation, may be at risk for NMS.
- Stress and physical exhaustion predispose to onset of NMS.
- Premenstrual period. A case of a woman with Parkinson's disease who was on levodopa therapy developed a NMS-like condition during the premenstrual period without withdrawal of the drug (Mizuta et al 1993). This resolved during the menstruation and the authors postulated that the central dopaminergic system may have been affected by the menstrual cycle.

Clinical Features and Diagnosis of NMS

Although the classic features of NMS are well recognized, there is considerable controversy regarding the classification and diagnostic criteria of NMS. Reilly et al (1991) have presented a review of the various concepts as follows:

The Nihilistic View. There are those who do not believe that NMS is a valid entity. They suggest the term "neuroleptic induced extrapyramidal side-effects with fever" (Levinson and Simpson 1986).

The Traditional View. NMS has four features which must be present for diagnosis
– Muscular rigidity
– Hyperthermia (< 39°C)
– Altered consciousness (confusion, disorientation, mutism, stupor, or coma).
– Autonomic dysfunction. Two or more of the following (Adityanjee et al 1988):
  · rapid pulse (< 90/min)
  · rapid respiration (< 25/ min)
  · fluctuations of blood pressure (30 mmHg systolic or 15 mmHg diastolic)
  · excessive sweating
  · incontinence

The diagnostic criteria are based strictly on clinical findings and no laboratory data is taken into consideration for this.

The Operational View. This view, proposed by those who think that application of strict diagnostic criteria to a syndrome, the etiology and pathology of which is not well-understood, may hinder its further understanding. The criteria for guidance in the diagnosis of NMS should include the following manifestations:
– *Major.* Fever, rigidity, elevated CPK
– *Minor.* Tachycardia, abnormal blood pressure, tachypnea, altered consciousness, sweating, leucocytosis.

All the three major or two major and four minor manifestations indicate a high probability of the syndrome.

The Spectrum View. According to this view NMS is a spectrum of severe neuroleptic toxicity with varying combinations of extrapyramidal, cortical, and autonomic dysfunction. The spectrum approach proposed initially by Fogel and Goldstein (1985) and later by others is marked by a deliberate withdrawal of rigidly defined boundaries between NMS and extrapyramidal syndrome by combining them on a spectrum. This does not dismiss the core concept of NMS but places it at one extreme end of the spectrum of the neuroleptic-related toxicity. This concept has been criticized because its adoption removes guidelines for clinical decision making. The proponents of this view claim that it enables to identify prodromal forms of NMS prior to emergence of full blown NMS and the atypical cases of NMS are not missed (Nierenberg et al 1991).

DMS-IV Criteria of Diagnosis of NMS. These are shown in Table 23.1 and the most widely accepted guidelines for diagnosis of NMS.

Table 23.1. Criteria for the diagnosis of neuroleptic malignant syndrome according to DMS-IV (American Psychiatric Association 1994). Reproduced by permission.

A. The development of severe muscle rigidity and elevated temperature associated with the use of neuroleptic medication

B. Two (or more) of the following:
  1. diaphoresis
  2. dysphagia
  3. tremor
  4. incontinence
  5. changes in level of consciousness ranging from confusion to coma
  6. mutism
  7. tachycardia
  8. elevated or labile blood pressure
  9. leucocytosis
  10. laboratory evidence of muscle injury (e. g., elevated CPK levels)

C. The symptoms in criteria A and B are not caused by another substance (e. g., phencyclidine) or a neurological or other general medical condition (e. g., viral encephalitis)

D. The symptoms in criteria A and B are not better accounted for by a mental disorder (e. g., mood disorder with catatonic features)

CPK = creatine phosphokinase.

Laboratory Findings

Diagnosis of NMS is based on clinical and historical information. Laboratory data such as CPK and elevated WBC can be helpful in making the diagnosis but no laboratory finding is diagnostic of this disorder.

Creatine Phosphokinase (CPK). This is an enzyme found in significant concentrations in skeletal muscle, myocardium, and the brain. When tissue damage occurs in any of these areas, the level of serum CPK increases. The muscle isoenzyme can rise significantly in muscle trauma, exercise, intramuscular injection, seizures, etc. The cause of elevation of CPK is not known. Muscle biopsy shows acute fiber necrosis and absence of glycogen and lipid substrate stores in both types of muscle fibers suggesting depletion from metabolic consumption (Morris et al 1980). They suggested that these findings implied partial uncoupling of metabolic phosphorylation from muscle fiber contraction.

Leukocytosis. Elevated WBC counts or leucocytosis can be seen in various medical situations and may or may not be related to the disease process. NMS is often associated with mild leucocytosis (10,000 to 20,000/mm^3) which subsides as NMS resolves.

Other Investigations. Hypoferremia, proteinuria, and myoglobinuria are frequent findings in NMS. CT scan of the brain is usually normal in NMS. CSF is usually normal in cases where lumbar puncture is done. EEG is usually normal but may show non-specific slowing suggestive of metabolic encephalopathy.

Autopsy studies on patients who die are usually non-revealing. Laboratory tests may not be diagnostic of NMS but they help in ruling out other disorders.

Differential Diagnosis. Conditions which should be considered in the differential diagnosis of NMS are listed in Table 23.2.

Catatonia (see Chapter 5). Clinical picture of catatonia resembles that of NMS and distinction between the two may be difficult at times (Kontaxakis et al 1990; White 1992). Catatonia which progresses to agitation, mutism, hyperthermia

Table 23.2. Conditions to be considered in the differential diagnosis of neuroleptic malignant syndrome.

Akinetic mutism
Catatonia
Drug-induced extrapyramidal disorders with fever (Chapter 8)
Dystonia (neuroleptic-induced)
Encephalomyelitis
Heat stroke (complication of neuroleptic therapy)
Intercurrent febrile infections
Intermittent acute porphyria
Locked-in syndrome (brainstem stroke)
Malignant hyperthermia
NMS-like disorders with non-neuroleptic drugs
Polymyositis
Serotonin syndrome
Tetanus
Tetany

and dehydration may be lethal and shows a marked overlap with NMS (Arya 1992). NMS may be thought of as a variant of catatonia that has been triggered by a neuroleptic drug.

Important differences, however, exist between NMS and lethal catatonia. The latter existed before the introduction of neuroleptic therapy. Management approach to NMS is discontinuation of neuroleptics whereas these drugs are useful in the treatment of catatonia. According to Andersen (1991) electroconvulsive therapy gives better results than neuroleptics in catatonia.

Intercurrent Febrile Infections. Psychiatric patients also suffer from febrile illnesses unrelated to neuroleptic therapy. In a series of 34 suspected NMS patients, 10 were found to have intercurrent febrile infections (Sewell and Jeste 1992).

Malignant Hyperthermia (see Chapter 13). This is usually associated with administration of halogenated inhalational anesthetic agents. Symptoms include muscle rigidity, hyperthermia (up to 43°C), dramatic rise in CPK, and myoglobinuria. There is some suggestion of a potential association between malignant hypothermia and NMS because of similarities in clinical presentation and positive halothane muscle contracture test in some of NMS patients (Caroff et al 1987). Both syndromes exhibit rigidity and hyperthermia. Dantrolene has been found to useful for treating both these conditions. Malignant hypothermia is a genetic disorder and there is some suggestion that NMS may be genetically transmitted (Otani et al 1991). Caution should be exercised in giving anesthesia to a patient with history of NMS (Hard 1991).

Clinical Course of NMS

Typical cases of NMS develop early during treatment with neuroleptics and rapidly manifest over the course of a few days. Signs of NMS may persist for a few weeks but there is a wide range of variations. NMS may begin months after neuroleptic therapy (Caroff 1980) and it may occur in patients who had no complication during previous treatment with neuroleptics.

Rechallenge and Recurrences. Neuroleptic rechallenge was reported to result in recurrence in about one-third of patients and in some symptoms subsided despite continued neuroleptic therapy (Pearlman 1986). Rosebush (1989) reported that 87% of patients who suffered an episode of NMS were able to take neuroleptics again. The choice of a neuroleptic lower in potency and dosage than that which precipitated the original episode of NMS was not related to successful regime. However, close monitoring for NMS is mandatory and a minimum period of five days before rechallenge may reduce the recurrence of NMS (Wells et al 1988). Neuroleptics should not be reintroduced before the initial episode of NMS has completely resolved (Susman and Addonizio 1988). Successful rechallenge has been performed with clozapine in a patient with prior NMS as a reaction (Cohen 1994).

Drugs Associated with NMS

Although classically only neuroleptics were considered to induce NMS, several other drugs have been associated with NMS (Table 23.3).

Antidepressants. A MEDLINE analysis has revealed 23 cases of antidepressant-induced NMS reported in the literature with different pathophysiological hypotheses for the precipitation of

Table 23.3. Drugs associated with neuroleptic malignant syndrome.

Antipsychotics
- Bromperidol
- Chlorpromazine
- Flupenthixol (Singh and Al-Baranzanchi 1995)
- Fluphenazine
- Haloperidol
- Levomepromazine
- Loxapine (Chong and Abbott 1991; Ewert et al 1983)
- Molindone hydrochloride (Gordon 1991)
- Perphenazine
- Promazine
- Thioridazine
- Trifluoperazine
- Zuclopenthixol (Kemperman and van den Hoofdakker 1990)

Atypical antipsychotics (see comments in text)

Other Drugs (isolated case reports)
- Amphetamine
- Antidepressants
  - Desipramine (Baca and Martinelli 1990;Sumiyoshi et al 1982)
  - Amitriptyline (Heyland and Sauve 1991)
  - Fluoxetine (Halman and Goldbloom)
- Antiparkinsonian drugs withdrawal
- Amantadine (Toru et al 1981; Simpson and Davis 1984)
- Antidepressants (see comments in text)
- Levodopa (see comments in text)
- Carbamazepine (see comments in text)
- Cocaine
- Cyclobenzaprine (Theoharides et al 1995)
- Fenfluramine
- Lithium (Susman and Addonizio 1987)
- Methylphenidate (Ehara et al 1998)
- Metoclopramide (Bakri et al 1992; Donnet et al 1991; Le Couteur and Kay 1995; Henderson and Longdon 1991; Nonino and Campomori 1999)
- Phencyclidine (PCP)
- Sulpride (Yokoyama et al 1995)
- Tetrabenazine (Mateo et al 1992; Burke et al 1981; Ossemann et al 1996)
- Tiapride (Sanchez-Trenado and Rodriguez-Vidigal 1995; Bobolakis 1995)

Anticholinergic drug withdrawal (Spivak et al 1996)

Neuroleptics cited without source are quoted from Addonizio and Susman (1991).

NMS (Assion et al 1998). The results show no hard evidence of an antidepressant-induced NMS. There have been a few reports of NMS associated with tricyclic antidepressants and selective serotonin reuptake inhibitors. One case of paroxetine-associated NMS has been reported (Heinemann et al 1997). Serotonergic system may have a possible role in the pathophysiology of NMS. NMS is a very rare complication due to pretreatment with neuroleptics causing chronic dopamine blockade and elevation of plasma levels of neuroleptics with the introduction of antidepressants.

Carbamazepine. The first case of NMS in a patient with combined carbamazepine and clozapine therapy was reported by Müller et al (1988). This was a poorly documented report where NMS was likely due to a combination of lithium and clozapine. However, this case is frequently quoted as carbamazepine-induced NMS. The second case (Goldwasser et al 1989) had a previous episode of NMS with thioridazine and carbamazepine was started six days after discontinuation of thioridazine with recurrence of NMS. The role of carbamazepine in the precipitation of NMS which was atypical (no fever) was speculative. The third case was that of a women who developed forme fruste of NMS (absence of fever) after taking an overdose of trifluoperazine and carbamazepine (Dalkin and Lee 1990). In the fourth case NMS developed after withdrawal of carbamazepine and start of loxapine therapy (Keepers 1990). A fifth case of NMS was attributed to carbamazepine (O'Griofa and Voris 1991). A critical review of these cases reveals no hard evidence that carbamazepine has any role in the pathogenesis of NMS. This comment is important because carbamazepine is an important alternative to neuroleptics in the management of psychiatric illnesses and has been used without complications in patients with previous history of NMS.

Atypical Antipsychotics. Initially it was expected that the atypical antipsychotics would be less likely to cause NMS. However, case reports have been published, first about clozapine and later about risperidone which was the next atypical antipsychotic to be introduced. Some of these case reports are cited here. Reports have also started to appear about olanzapine (Burkhard et al 1999; Johnson and Bruxner 1998) and remoxipride (Koponen et al 1993).

Several cases of neuroleptic malignant-like syndrome have been reported with the use of clozapine, an atypical neuroleptic (Goates and Escobar 1992; Pope et al 1986; Thornberg and Ereshefsky 1993; Redding et al 1993; Sachdev et al 1995; Ganelin et al 1996). Clozapine seems to be more selective for the mesolimbic and mesocortical than the striatonigral dopamine pathways and would not be expected to be associated with NMS or extrapyramidal effects. There were several confounding factors in the cases reported. Clozapine can cause self-limiting fever and elevation of CPK as well as muscle stiffness. One hypothesis is that some patients may be hypersensitive to dopamine blockade. In these patients even a weak blockade of D_1 and D_2 receptors such as that produced by clozapine may produce NMS-like clinical picture (Das Gupta and Young 1991).

Similar cases of NMS have been reported following introduction of risperidone (Webster and Wijeratne 1994; Raitasuo et al 1994; Murray and Haller 1995; Dave 1995; Singer et al 1995; Najara and Enikeev 1995; Sharma et al 1996; Tarsy 1996; Bajjoka et al 1997; Newman et al 1997).

Hasan and Buckley (1998) carried out a MEDLINE literature search and identified 19 cases of NMS associated with clozapine and 13 cases associated with risperidone. These cases were analyzed against 3 sets of criteria for the diagnosis of NMS. Results showed that 9/19 clozapine cases and 8/13 risperidone cases had a high probability of being NMS and the remaining cases had a low probability of being NMS. These authors pointed out that diagnosis of NMS is complicated when a patient is under treatment with an atypical antipsychotic. The adverse events are likely to be attributed to NMS because of resemblance. At present, there is no firm evidence to link atypical antipsychotics to NMS.

Neuroleptic Malignant-Like Syndrome after Levodopa Withdrawal

Neuroleptic malignant-like syndrome has been reported in patients with idiopathic parkinsonism following withdrawal of levodopa (Sechi et al 1984; Friedman et al 1985; Keyser and Rodnitzky 1991). The akinetic crisis in an "off" stage of levodopa in a patient with Parkinson's disease with clinical signs resembling NMS (Bachli and Albani 1994). While NMS is due to dopaminergic receptor blockade or dopamine depletion, akinetic crisis can occur despite adequate dopaminergic therapy as a symptom of severe basal ganglia dysfunction related to the advanced stage of Parkinson's disease.

Levodopa withdrawal is more likely to precipitate NMS when the patient is receiving concomitant neuroleptic therapy for psychiatric problems. Reutens et al (1991) described a case which they described as NMS after withdrawal of low-dose levodopa for mild Parkinson's disease. This patient did not fulfil the traditional criteria of NMS and should be described as neuroleptic malignant-like syndrome. Temperature elevation was only 38.5° C and it subsided after reintroduction of levodopa but rigidity was slow to resolve and required additional treatment with dantrolene. Granner and Wooten (1991) have suggested the term "parkinsonian hyperpyrexia" for such a condition because of the overlap in the clinical features of NMS and parkinsonism. There are one case reports where NMS was diagnosed during treatment of Parkinson's disease with controlled release delivery of levodopa (Cunningham et al 1991). In this case there might have been fluctuations in the levels of levodopa or withdrawal effect of amantadine (Weller and Kornhuber 1993). In another case NMS with disseminated intravascular coagulation developed while the patient was receiving levodopa, bromocriptine, and amantadine (Yamawaki and Ogawa 1992). The patient was treated successfully with dantrolene sodium while the antiparkinsonian medications were continued.

Another situation where levodopa withdrawal may produce a NMS-like syndrome is in the postoperative period. One case of NMS was reported in a patient where levodopa was temporarily discontinued according to the experimental protocol while the patient underwent an adrenal medulla-caudate transplant for Parkinson's disease (Young and Kaufman 1995). The patient recovered after restoration of the levodopa dose.

Evaluation of NMS due to any drug in a patient with Parkinson's disease (PD) patient is problematic because the disease itself predisposes to NMS. Central dopaminergic and possible noradrenergic activity contributes to NMS development in an elderly population of PD patients. Measuring CSF levels of monoamine metabolites may provide a means for identifying NMS susceptibility in PD patients (Ueda et al 1999).

Medical Complications of NMS. These are as follows:
- *Pulmonary.* Delaney and Deniker (1968) believed that "signs in the lungs" were among the cardinal features of NMS. Now it is known that they are secondary phenomena or complications. Aspiration pneumonia, pulmonary edema, and pulmonary embolism may occur.
- *Cardiovascular.* Arrhythmias, myocardial infarction, cardiac arrest, and disseminated intravascular coagulation.
- *Renal.* Renal failure may occur secondary to rhabdomyolysis.
- *Death.* Pearlman (1986) calculated two separate mortality rates; 22% for cases prior to 1980, and 4% for cases thereafter. This decrease of mortality is attributed to better awareness of NMS, early detection and improved management.
- *Late neurological sequelae.* Some of the long-term neurological and psychological sequelae of NMS are listed in Table 23.4.

Table 23.4. Long-term neurological and psychological sequelae of neuroleptic malignant syndrome.

Amnesic disorder (van Harten and Kemperman 1991)
Cerebellar degeneration due to hyperpyrexia (Lal et al 1997)
Cerebral hypoxic encephalopathies
Dementia (Welch 1993)
Depression(Koponen et al 1991)
Parkinsonism (Koponen et al 1991)
Progression of dementia
Tardive dyskinesias

Management

Discontinuation of the neuroleptics and basic supportive care of the patient are the most important steps. These involve correction of fluid and electrolyte imbalance, cooling the patient, and treatment of pulmonary, renal, and cardiac complications.

Pharmacotherapy. Several drugs have been tried for the treatment of NMS and include the following:

- Dantrolene
- Bromocriptine
- Benzodiazepines (Lew and Tollefson 1983; Kumar 1987)
- Lisuride (de Mar et al 1991)
- N-methyl-D-aspartate (NMDA) receptor agonists

Dantrolene has been successfully used by several investigators. It has been shown to restore the level of CSF homovanillic acid which is lowered during NMS (Nisijima and Ishiguro 1993).

Bromocriptine, a dopamine agonist has been used successfully for treatment of NMS (Mueller et al 1983; Thomas et al 1993). Bromocriptine has been used concomitantly with thioridazine to counteract its effect and keep the patient under cover of neuroleptic (Goldwasser et al 1989).

Roberts et al (1991) are sceptical and their prospective studies do not show a useful role for either dantrolene or bromocriptine in the treatment of NMS. In spite of this, Sakas et al (1991) found that these agents lower the mortality in case-controlled studies.

NMDA receptor agonists: amantadine and memantine have been advocated by Kornhuber et al (1993) for the management of akinetic hyperthermic episodes and NMS-like states in patients with Parkinson's disease which are resistant to anticholinergic therapy.

Carbamazepine may also be used as an alternative to neuroleptics. A case is reported of NMS during treatment with sulpride which was discontinued and replaced by carbamazepine which has psychotropic action and the patient recovered (Peet and Collier 1990).

High dose vitamin E and B_6. This was used successfully as an adjunct to supportive care in a patient with NMS induced by risperidine (Dursun et al 1998).

Another alternative is to replace neuroleptic treatment in NMS by electroconvulsive therapy in cases who do not respond to medical treatment (Nisijima and Ishiguro 1999).

Concluding Remarks

NMS is probably should not as called "malignant," a word which suggests progressive deterioration with death. The mortality of this condition has declined considerably during the past decade due to early recognition and improved management. NMS is not seen exclusively with neuroleptics as other drugs produce similar syndromes and in two-third of patients, neuroleptics have been resumed without recurrence of the syndrome. The syndrome needs to be redefined and criteria for discontinuation of neuroleptics need to be formulated.

References

Addonizio G, Susman VL, Roth SD: Neuroleptic malignant syndrome: review and analysis of 115 cases. Biol Psychiatry 1987; 22: 1004–1020.

Addonizio G, Susman VL: Neuroleptic malignant syndrome, St. Louis, Mosby-Year Book, 1991.

Adityanjee, Singh S, Sing G, et al: Spectrum concept of neuroleptic malignant syndrome. Br J Psychiatry 1988; 153: 107–111.

American Psychiatric Association: DSM-IV. Washington, DC, American Psychiatric Association, 1994.

Andersen WH: Lethal catatonia and the neuroleptic malignant syndrome. Crit Care Med 1991; 19: 1333–1334.

Arya DK: Neuroleptic malignant syndrome and catatonia—other diagnostic considerations. J Roy Soc Med 1992; 85: 60.

Assion HJ, Heinemann F, Laux G: Neuroleptic malignant syndrome under treatment with antidepressants? A critical review. Eur Arch Psychiatry Clin Neurosci 1998; 248(5): 231–239

Baca L, Martinelli L: Neuroleptic malignant syndrome: a unique association with a tricyclic antidepressant. Neurology 1990; 40: 1797–1798.

Bachli E, Albani C: Dia akinetische Krise beim Morbus Parkinson. Schweiz Med Wochenschr 1994; 124: 1017–1023.

Bajjoka I, Patel T, O'Sullivan T: Risperidone-induced neuroleptic malignant syndrome. Ann Emerg Med 1997; 30: 698–700.

Bakri YN, Khan R, Subhi J, et al: Neuroleptic malignant syndrome associated with metoclopramide antiemetic therapy. Gynecologic Oncology 1992; 44: 189–190.

Bobolakis I: Neuroleptic malignant syndrome following tiapride treatment of clonazepam withdrawal. Eur Psychiatry 1995; 10: 110–111.

Boyd RD: Neuroleptic malignant syndrome and mental retardation: review and analysis of 29 cases. Am J Ment Retard 1993; 98: 143–155.

Burke RE, Fahn R, Mayeux R, et al: Neuroleptic malignant syndrome caused by dopamine depleting drugs in a patient with Huntington's disease. Neurology 1981; 31: 1022–1026.

Burkhard PR, Vingerhoets FJ, Alberque C, et al: Olanzapine-induced neuroleptic malignant syndrome. Arch Gen Psychiatry 1999; 56(1): 101–102.

Caroff SN, Mann SC: Neuroleptic malignant syndrome. Med Clin North Am 1993; 77: 185–202.

Caroff SN, Rosenberg H, Fletcher JE, et al: Malignant hyperthermia susceptibility in neuroleptic malignant syndrome. Anesthesiology 1987; 67: 20–25.

Caroff SN: The neuroleptic malignant syndrome. J Clin Psychiatry 1980; 41: 79–83.

Chong LS, Abbott PM: Neuroleptic malignant syndrome secondary to loxapine. Br J Psychiatry 1991; 159: 572–573.

Cohen SA: Successful clozapine rechallenge following prior intolerance to clozapine (letter). J Clin Psychiatry 1994; 55: 498–499.

Cunningham MA, Darby DG, Donan GA: Controlled release delivery of L-dopa associated with non-fatal hyperthermia, rigidity, and autonomic dysfunction. Neurology 1991; 41: 942–943.

Dalkin T, Lee AS: Carbamazepine and forme fruste neuroleptic malignant syndrome. Br J Psychiatry 1990; 157: 437–438.

Das Gupta K, Young A: Clozapine-induced neuroleptic malignant syndrome. J Clin Psychiatry 1991; 52: 105–107.

Dave M: Two cases of risperidone-induced neuroleptic malignant syndrome. Am J Psychiatr 1995; 152: 1233–1234.

de Mari M, Lamberti P, Simone F, et al: Intravenous administration of lisuride in the treatment of neuroleptic malignant syndrome. Funct Neurol 1991; 6: 285–288.

De Reuck J, Van Aken J, Van Landegem W, et al: Positron emission tomographic studies of changes in cerebral blood flow and oxygen metabolism in neuroleptic malignant syndrome. Eur Neurol 1991; 31: 1–6.

Delay J, Deniker P: Drug-induced pyramidal syndromes. In Vibken PJ, Bruyn GW (Eds.): Handbook of clinical neurology, vol 6, New York, Elsevier-North Holland Inc, 1968, pp 248–266.

Delay J, Pichot P, Lemperiere T, et al: Un neuroleptique majeur non-phenothiazine et non-reserpine, l'haloperidol, dans la traitment des psychoses. Ann Med Psychol 1960; 118: 145–152.

Deng MZ, Chen GQ, Phillips MR: Neuroleptic malignant syndrome in 12 of 9,792 chinese inpatients exposed to neuroleptics: a prospective study. Am J Psychiatry 1990; 147: 1149–1155.

Donnet A, Harle JR, Dumont JC, et al: Neuroleptic malignant syndrome induced by metoclopramide. Biomed & Pharmacother 1991; 45: 461–462.

Downey RJ, Downey JA, Newhouse E, et al: Fatal hyperthermia in a quadriplegic man. Chest 1992; 101: 1728–1730.

Dursun SM, Oluboka OJ, Devarajan S, et al: High-dose vitamin E plus vitamin B6 treatment of risperidone-related neuroleptic malignant syndrome. J Psychopharmacol 1998; 12(2): 220–221.

Ebadi M, Pfeiffer RF, Murrin LC: Pathogenesis and treatment of neuroleptic malignant syndrome. Gen Pharmacol 1990; 21: 367–386.

Ehara H, Maegaki Y, Takeshita K: Neuroleptic malignant syndrome and methylphenidate. Pediatr Neurol 1998; 19(4): 299–301.

Ewert AL, Kloek J, Wells B, et al: Neuroleptic malignant syndrome associated with loxapine. J Clin Psychiatry 1983; 44: 37–38.

Fogel BS, Goldberg RJ: Neuroleptic malignant syndrome (letter). NEJM 1985; 313: 1292.

Friedman JH, Feinberg SS, Feldman RG: A neuroleptic malignant-like syndrome due to levodopa therapy. JAMA 1985; 254: 2792–2795.

Ganelin L, Lichtenberg PS, Marcus EL, et al: Suspected neuroleptic malignant syndrome in a patient receiving clozapine. Ann Pharmacother 1996; 30: 248–250.

Goates MG, Escobar JI: An apparent neuroleptic malignant syndrome without extrapyramidal symptoms upon initiation of clozapine therapy: report of a case and results of clozapine rechallenge. J Clin Psychopharmacol 1992; 12: 139–140.

Goldwasser HD, Hooper JF, Spears NM: Concomitant treatment of neuroleptic malignant syndrome and psychosis. Br J Psychiatry 1989; 154: 102–104.

Gradon JD: Neuroleptic malignant syndrome possibly caused by molindone hydrochloride. DICP Ann Pharmacother 1991; 25: 1071–1072.

Granner MA, Wooten GF: Neuroleptic malignant syndrome or parkinsonism hyperpyrexia syndrome. Sem Neurol 1991; 11: 228–235.

Gratz SS, Simpson GM: Neuroleptic malignant syndrome. CNS Drugs 1994; 2: 429–439.

Gurrera RJ, Romero JA: Sympathomedullary activity in the neuroleptic malignant syndrome. Biol Psychiatry 1992; 32: 334–343.

Halman M, Goldbloom DS: Fluoxetine and neuroleptic malignant syndrome. Biol Psychiatry 1990; 28: 518–521.

Hard C: Neuroleptic malignant syndrome versus malignant hyperthermia. Am J Med 1991; 91: 322–323.

Hasan S, Buckley P: Novel antipsychotics and the neuroleptic malignant syndrome;: a review and critique. Am J Psychiatr 1998; 155: 1113–1116.

Heinemann F, Assion HJ, Hermes G, et al: Paroxetine-induced neuroleptic malignant syndrome. Nervenarzt 1997; 68(8): 664–666.

Henderson A: Fulminant metoclopramide induced neuroleptic malignant syndrome rapidly responsive to intravenous dantrolene. Austr NZ J Med 1991; 21: 742–743.

Henderson VW, Wooten GF: Neuroleptic malignant syndrome—a pathological role for dopamine receptor blockade? Neurology 1981; 31: 132–137.

Heyland D, Sauve M: Neuroleptic malignant syndrome without the use of neuroleptics. Can med Assoc J 1991; 145: 817–819.

Horn E, Lach B, Lapierre Y, et al: Hypothalmic pathology in neuroleptic malignant syndrome. Am J Psychiatry 1988; 145: 617–620.

Johnson V, Bruxner G: Neuroleptic malignant syndrome

associated with olanzapine. Aust N Z J Psychiatry 1998; 32(6): 884–886.

Keck PE, McElroy SL, Popee HG: Neuroleptic malignant syndrome. Current Opinion in Psychiatry 1991; 4: 34–37.

Keck PE, Pope HG, McElroy SL: Frequency and presentation of neuroleptic malignant syndrome: a prospective study. Am J Psychiatry 1987; 144: 1344–1346.

Keepers GA: Neuroleptic syndrome associated with withdrawal from carbamazepine. Am J Psychiatry 1990; 147: 1687.

Kellam AMP: The (frequently) neuroleptic (potentially) malignant syndrome. Br J Psychiatry 1990; 157: 169–173.

Kemperman CJF, van den Hoofdakker RH: Neuroleptic malignant syndrome (NMS): challenge with zuclopenthixol and follow-up—a case report. Europ Neuropharmacol 1990; 1: 67–69.

Keyser DL, Rodnitzky RL: Neuroleptic malignant syndrome in Parkinson's disease after withdrawal or alteration of dopaminergic therapy. Arch Int Med 1991; 151: 794–796.

Kontaxakis VP, Vaikadis NM, Christodoulou GN, et al: Neuroleptic-induced catatonia or a mild form of neuroleptic syndrome. Neuropsychobiology 1990; 23: 38–40.

Koponen H, Lepola UM, Leinonen EVJ: Neuroleptic malignant syndrome during remoxipride treatment. A case report. Eur Neuropharmacol 1993; 3: 517–519.

Koponen H, Repo E, Lepola U: Long-term outcome after neuroleptic malignant syndrome. Acta Neurol Scand 1991; 84: 550–551.

Kornhuber J, Weller M: Neuroleptic malignant syndrome. Curr Opin Neurol 1994; 7: 353–357.

Kornhuber J, Weller M, Reifer P: Glutamate receptor agonists for neuroleptic malignant syndrome and akinetic hyperthermic parkinsonian crisis. J Neural Transm (P-D Sect) 1993; 6: 63–72.

Kumar V: A case of neuroleptic malignant syndrome treated with diazepam. Canad J Psychiatry 1987; 32: 815–816.

Kurlan R, Hamill R, Shoulson I: Neuroleptic malignant syndrome. Clin Neuropharmacol 1984; 7: 109–120.

Lal V, Sardana V, Thussu A, et al: Cerebellar degeneration following neuroleptic malignant syndrome. Postgrad Med J 1997; 73(865): 735–6.

Latz SR, McCracken JT: Neuroleptic malignant syndrome in children and adolescents: two case reports and a warning. J Child Adolesc Psychopharmacol 1992; 2: 123–129.

Lazarus A: Neuroleptic malignant syndrome and preexisting brain damage. J Neuropsychiat Clin Neurosci 1992; 4: 185–187.

Le Couteur DG, Kay T: Delayed neuroleptic malignant syndrome following cessation of prolonged therapy with metoclopramide. Aust N Z J Med 1995; 25(3): 261.

Levenson JL: Neuroleptic malignant syndrome. Am J Psychiatry 1985; 142: 1137–1145.

Levinson DF, Simpson GM: Neuroleptic-induced extrapyramidal symptoms with fever. Arch Gen Psychiatry 1986; 43: 839–848.

Lew TY, Tollefson G: Chlorpromazine-induced neuroleptic malignant syndrome and its response to diazepam. Biol Psychiatry 1983; 18: 1441–1446.

Mateo D, Munoz-Blanco L, Gimenez-Roldan S: Neuroleptic malignant syndrome related to tetrabenazine introduction and haloperidol discontinuation. Clin Neuropharmacol 1992; 15: 63–68.

Mizuta E, Shunzou N, Kuno S: Neuroleptic malignant syndrome in parkinsonian woman during the premenstrual period. Neurology 1993; 43: 1048–1049.

Moore AP, Macfarlane IA, Blumhardt LD: Neuroleptic malignant syndrome and hypothyroidism. J Neurol Neurosurg Psychiatry 1990; 53: 517–8.

Morris HH, McCormick WF, Reinarz JA: Neuroleptic malignant syndrome. Arch Neurol 1980; 37: 462–463.

Mueller PS, Vester JW, Fermaglich J: Neuroleptic malignant syndrome. JAMA 1983; 249: 386–387.

Mueller PS: Neuroleptic malignant syndrome. Psychosomatics 1985; 26: 654–662.

Müller T, Becker T, Fritze J: Neuroleptic malignant syndrome after clozapine plus carbamazepine (letter). Lancet 1988; ii: 1500.

Murray S, Haller E: Risperidone and NMS? Psychiatric Services 1995; 46: 951.

Naganuma H, Fujii I: Incidence and risk factors in neuroleptic malignant syndrome. Acta Psychiatrica Scandinavica 1994; 90: 424–426.

Najara JE, Enikeev ID: Risperidone and neuroleptic malignant syndrome: a case report. J Clin Psychiatr 1995; 56: 534–535.

Newman M, Adityanjee, Jampala C, et al: Atypical neuroleptic malignant syndrome associate with risperidone treatment. Am J Psychiatr 1997; 154: 1475.

Nierenberg D, Disch M, Manheimer E, et al: Facilitating prompt diagnosis and treatment of the neuroleptic malignant syndrome. Clin Pharmacol Ther 1991; 50: 580–586.

Nisijima K, Ishiguro T: Electroconvulsive therapy for the treatment of neuroleptic malignant syndrome with psychotic symptoms: a report of five cases. J ECT 1999; 15(2): 158–63

Nisijima K, Ishiguru T: does dantrolene influence central dopamine and serotonin metabolism in the neuroleptic malignant syndrome? A retrospective study. Biol Psychiatry 1993; 33: 45–48.

Nonino F, Campomori A: Neuroleptic malignant syndrome associated with metoclopramide. Ann Pharmacother 1999; 33(5): 644–645.

O'Griofa FM, Voris JC: Neuroleptic malignant syndrome associated with carbamazepine. Southern Med J 1991; 84: 1378–1380.

Ossemann M, Sindic CJM, Laterre C: Terbenazine as a cause of neuroleptic malignant syndrome. Mov Dis 1996; 11: 95.

Otani K, Horiuchi M, Kondo T, et al: Is the predisposition to neuroleptic malignant syndrome genetically transmitted? Br J Psychiatry 1991; 158: 850–853.

Pearlman CA: Neuroleptic malignant syndrome: a review of the literature. J Clin Psychopharmacol 1986; 6(5): 257–273.

Peet M, Collier J: Use of carbamazepine in psychosis after neuroleptic malignant syndrome. Br J Psychiatry 1990; 156: 579–581.

Pope HG, Aizley HG, Keck PE, et al: Neuroleptic malignant syndrome: long-term follow-up of 20 cases. J Clin Psychiatry 1991; 52: 208–212.

Pope HG, Cole JO, Choras PT, et al: Apparent neuroleptic malignant syndrome with clozapine and lithium. J Nerv Ment Dis 1986; 174: 493–495.

Raitasuo V, Vataja R, Elomaa E: Risperidone-induced neuroleptic malignant syndrome in young patient (letter). Lancet 1994; 344: 1705.

Redding S, Minnema AM, Tandon R: Neuroleptic malignant syndrome and clozapine. Ann Clin Psychiatry 1993; 5: 25–27.

Reilly JR, Crowe SF, Lloyd JH: Neuroleptic toxicity syndromes: a clinical spectrum. Austr NZ J Psychiatry 1991; 25: 499–505.

Reutens DC, Harrison WB, Goldswain PRT: Neuroleptic malignant syndrome complicating levodopa withdrawal. Med J Aust 1991; 155: 53–54.

Rosebush PI, Stewart T, Mazrek MF: The treatment of neuroleptic malignant syndrome. Are dantrolene and bromocriptine useful adjuncts to supportive care? Br J Psychiatry 1991; 159: 709–712.

Rosebush PI, Stewart TD, Gelenberg AJ: Twenty neuroleptic rechallenges after neuroleptic malignant syndrome in 15 patients. J Clin Psychiatry 1989; 50: 295–298.

Sachdev P, Kruk J, Kneebone M, et al: Clzapine-induced neuroleptic malignant syndrome: review and report of new cases. J Clin Psychopharmacol 1995; 15: 365–371.

Sakas P, Davies JM, Janicak PG, et al: Drug treatment of neuroleptic malignant syndrome. Psychopharmacology Bull 1991; 27: 381–384.

Sanchez-Trenado JM, Rodriguez-Vidigal FF: Malignant neuroleptic syndrome during tiapride treatment. Farmacia Clinica 1995; 12: 614–615.

Schibuk M, Schachter D: A role for catecholamines in the pathogenesis of neuroleptic malignant syndrome. Canad J Psychiatry 1986; 31: 66–69.

Sechi GP, Tanda F, Mutani R: Fatal hyperpyrexia after withdrawal of levodopa. Neurology 1984; 34: 249–251.

Serby M: Neuroleptic malignant syndrome in Alzheimer's disease. JAGS 1986; 34: 895–896.

Sewell DD, Jeste DV: Distinguishing NMS from NMS-like medical illness. A study of 34 cases. J Neuropsychiatry 1992; 4: 265–269.

Shalev A, Munitz H: The neuroleptic malignant syndrome: agent and host interaction. Acta Psychiatr Scand 1986; 73: 337–347.

Sharma R, Trappler B, Ng YK, et al: Risperidone-induced neuroleptic malignant syndrome. Ann Pharmacother 1996; 30: 775–778.

Simpson DM, Davis GC: Case report of neuroleptic malignant syndrome associated with withdrawal from amantadine. Am J Psychiatry 1984; 141: 796–797.

Singer S, Richards C, Boland RJ: Two cases of risperidone-induced neuroleptic malignant syndrome. Am J Psychiatry 1995; 152(8): 1234.

Singh AN, Al-Baranzanchi AJ: Neuroleptic rechallenge

after neuroleptic malignant syndrome in a 73-year old woman with schizophrenia—four year's follow-up. J Drug Develop Clin Practice 1995; 7: 63–65.

Spivak B, Gonen N, Mester R, et al: Neuroleptic malignant syndrome associated with abrupt withdrawal of anticholinergic agents. Int Clin Psychopharmacol 1996; 11(3): 207–209.

Sumiyoshi A, Oguchi T, Takahyshi A: Two cases of syndrome malin induced by tricyclic antidepressants. Folia Psychiatr Neurol Jpn 1982; 36: 461–463.

Susman VL, Addonizio G: Recurrence of neuroleptic malignant syndrome. J Nerv Ment Dis 1988; 176: 234–241.

Susman VL, Addonizio G: Reintroduction of neuroleptic malignant syndrome by lithium. J Clin Psychopharmacol 1987; 7: 339–341.

Tarsy D: Risperidone and neuroleptic malignant syndrome. JAMA 1996; 275: 446.

Tesar GE: Neuroleptic malignant syndrome. Prob Crit Care 1988; 2: 149–158.

Theoharides TC, Harris RS, Weckstein D: Neuroleptic malignant-like syndrome due to cyclobenzaprine? J Clin Psychopharmacol 1995; 15: 79–81.

Thomas K, Rajeev KK, Abraham OC, et al: Management of neuroleptic malignant syndrome—a series of eight cases. J Assoc Physicians of India 1993; 41: 91–93.

Thornberg SA, Ereshefsky L: Neuroleptic malignant syndrome associated with clozapine monotherapy. Pharmacotherapy 1993; 13: 510–514.

Toru M, Matsuda O, Makiguchi K, et al: Neuroleptic malignant syndrome-like state following withdrawal of antiparkinsonian drugs. J Nerv Ment Dis 1981; 169: 324–327.

Tu JB: Psychopharmacogenetic basis of medication-induced movement disorders. International Clinical Psychopharmacology 1997; 12: 1–12.

Ueda M, Hamamoto M, Nagayama H, et al: Susceptibility to neuroleptic malignant syndrome in Parkinson's disease. Neurology 1999; 52(4): 777–81.

van Harten PN, Kemperman CJF: Organic amnestic disorder: a long-term sequel after neuroleptic malignant syndrome. Biol Psychiatry 1991; 29: 407–410.

Webster P, Wijeratne C: Risperidone-induced neuroleptic malignant syndrome. Lancet 1994; 344: 1228–1229.

Welch JB: Dementia as a consequence of neuroleptic syndrome (letter). Am J Psychiatry 1993; 150: 1561–1562.

Weller M, Kornhuber J: A rationale for NMDA receptor antagonist therapy for neurologic malignant syndrome. Med Hypotheses 1992b; 38: 329–333.

Weller M, Kornhuber J: Amantadine withdrawal and neuroleptic malignant syndrome (letter). Neurology 1993; 43: 2155.

Weller M, Kornhuber J: Pathophysiologie und Therapie des maligen neuroleptischen Syndroms. Nervenarzt 1992a; 63: 645–655.

Wells AJ, Sommi RW, Crismon ML: Neuroleptic rechallenge after neuroleptic malignant syndrome: case report and literature review. Drug Intell Clin Pharm 1988; 22: 475–480.

White DA: Catatonia and NMS—a single entity? Br J Psychiatry 1992; 161: 558–560.

Woodruff PWR, Palazidou E, Cranson I, et al: Neoplasia and neuroleptic malignant syndrome. Human Psychopharmacology 1991; 6: 257–260.

Yamawaki Y, Ogawa N: Successful treatment of levodopa-induced neuroleptic malignant syndrome (NMS) and disseminate intravascular coagulation in a patient with Parkinson's disease. Int Med 1992; 31: 1298–1302.

Yokoyama N, Takeuchi I, Uehara T: A case of elderly patient with neuroleptic malignant syndrome induced by sulpride of total amount of 200 mg. Seishin Igaku 1995; 37: 668–669.

Young CC, Kaufman BS: Neuroleptic malignant syndrome: postoperative onset due to levodopa withdrawal. J Clin Anesth 1995; 7: 652–656.

Chapter 24
Subacute Myelo-Optico-Neuropathy (SMON)

Introduction

A myelitis-like illness with peripheral neuropathy and visual loss, preceded by abdominal disorders was reported sporadically in Japan from 1955 to 1960. It reached an epidemic proportion in the following decade with several thousand cases. Subacutemyelo-opticoneuropathy (SMON) was recognized as a distinct syndrome by Tsubaki et al (1965). It was suspected to be linked to use of clioquinol for gastrointestinal disorders. A SMON Commission was organized in Japan in 1969 to investigate this problem. Based on the opinion of the Commission that SMON is caused by clioquinol, the Japanese government banned the sale of clioquinol in 1970 and this was followed by dramatic disappearance of new cases. The work of the SMON Commission was concluded in 1972 and the following statement was issued:

"On the basis of epidemiological facts and of experimentation, it can be concluded that in the majority of patients diagnosed as having SMON the neurological symptoms have arisen as a result of oral use of chinoform preparations. Nevertheless, as has been stated in reports by the various committees, there are many obscure points in regard to the mechanism of occurrence of SMON and such problems remain as that of SMON patients who have not used chinoform preparations. Research must continue on these points in the future."

A historical account of SMON has been given by Takasaki and Kanamaru 1974). The results of the work of SMON Commission were published in a special issue of the *Japanese Journal of Medical Sciences* (1975: vol 28). Important documents related to SMON/clioquinol are shown in Table 24.1.

Clioquinol

Clioquinol or iodochlorhydroxyquinoline is a dihalogenated derivative of 8-hydroxyquinoline. The drug was first introduced in Japan in 1929 and initially considered to be non-absorbable after oral ingestion, but now it is known that 25% of it is absorbed and 70% of circulating clioquinol is bound to the serum albumin, the maximum concentration being present four hours after ingestion (Jack and Riess 1973).

Table 24.1. Important documents (monographs/symposia/book chapters) on SMON/Clioquinol (modified from Gelzer 1991).

Year	Editor(s)/Author(s)	No. of pages	Principle message
1974	Takasaki & Kanamaru	213	More research needed to determine the cause
1976	Gent & Shigematsu	337	Clioquinol is a hazard and should be discontinued
1977/1978	WHO	12	Clioquinol benefit insufficiently documented
1979	Soda	514	Clioquinol is a major harmful drug
1979	Hansson	168	Pharmaceutical giants and the SMON scandal
1980	Izumi	54	Clioquinol responsible for harm
1983	Carlsson et al	89	Clioquinol: etiology of SMON not entirely solved
1986	Mann	8	Paradoxes of SMON; clioquinol should go

Epidemiology

The epidemiology of SMON has been reviewed by Yamamoto et al (1975). The number of cases reported in Japan had reached 8500 by the end of 1972. Male to female ratio was 1:2.5 and middle-aged women were affected most frequently. Point prevalence at the end of 1968 was 4.5/100 000 population (4355 cases). The following points were left for future investigation:
- Study of SMON patients who did not take clioquinol.
- Dose response relationship in patients who has SMON at a lower dose of clioquinol.
- Explanation of sex, age, and geographical differences.

Only 238 non-Japanese cases of hydroquinolone neurotoxicity were reported worldwide between 1935 and 1980 and these have been analyzed by Baumgartner et al (1979) and Thomas (1984). Of these cases, 27% had a probable relationship to hydroxyquinolones, 39% a possible relationship, and 34% were unlikely or not related to the drug. Peripheral neuropathy was not found to be a prominent part of the neurotoxicity.

Clinical Aspects

Clinical features of SMON have been reviewed by Sobue (1979). The illness is described to be preceded by abdominal disorders. The onset was acute in 60% and subacute in 40% of the cases. Complete manifestations usually took several days and sometimes progressed over 1–2 months.

Neurological Manifestations. The initial manifestations were paresthesias of the lower extremities in 80% of the cases and these developed in an ascending progression. Motor weakness was seen in 50% of the cases and predominantly involved the legs. About 75% of the patients were ataxic and bladder disorders were encountered in 15–20% of the patients. Bilateral decrease of visual acuity was seen in 27.6% of the cases and optic discs were atrophic in patients with severe loss of vision. Encephalopathy with seizures, loss of consciousness and cognitive impairment was reported rarely.

Laboratory Diagnosis. Diagnosis of SMON was made clinically but the following laboratory tests were used in some of the cases:
- Blood counts. There were no characteristic changes.
- Blood chemistry. There were no specific findings related to SMON.
- CSF. Slight rise of protein content was found in 10.5% of cases.
- EMG. In 100 cases studied electrophysiologically, EMG of tibialis anterior and gastrocnemius muscles revealed reduction of interference pattern in 37% to 52% of cases, of fibrillation potentials in 16% to 21%, and of high amplitude potentials in 3% to 9% (Iida et al 1971). Motor conduction velocity was reduced in 28% to 31% and evoked potentials in 56% to 59% of cases.
- EEG. There were no significant changes.
- Immunologic tests. Immunoglobulins, examined by single diffusion method, showed high values in 48.2% of 112 cases examined (Sobue et al 1971). IgG abnormalities were higher than those of IgA and IgM and were of longer duration. There was no fixed pattern of these abnormalities on long-term follow-up.
- Sural nerve biopsy. Characteristic findings of this examination were:

Table 24.2. Diagnostic guidelines of the SMON Commission (Kono 1975).

Cardinal symptoms
- Abdominal symptoms preceding neurological symptoms
- Neurological symptoms
- Acute or subacute onset
- Sensory disturbances in the lower extremities

Other frequent symptoms
- Motor disturbances
- Bilateral decrease of vision leading to blindness
- Psychological disturbances
- Bladder paralysis
- Greenish fur on the tongue

Other features
- Prolonged clinical course. Relapses not rare.
- Rare in infants and children
- No abnormality found in blood or CSF by ordinary examination

- Axonal swelling and degeneration was recognized 10 to 14 days after onset of illness.
- Demyelination of nerve fibers.
- Fibrous proliferation of the interstitial tissue and Schwann cells.

An abbreviated version of the diagnostic guidelines suggested by the SMON Commission is shown in Table 24.2.

Differential Diagnosis. There are several neurological illnesses which may resemble SMON but those that were emphasized in the differential diagnosis of SMON by Japanese neurologists are summarized in Table 24.3.

Table 24.3. Conditions to be considered in the differential diagnosis of SMON with characteristic features of each which differ from SMON.

Anterior poliomyelitis
- Sensory disturbances are not usual in poliomyelitis
- CSF cells and proteins are increased
- Diagnosis confirmed by isolation of virus and immunology

Devic's disease (optico-myelitic type of multiple sclerosis)
- No prodromal abdominal symptoms
- Disseminated neurological signs
- Abnormal CSF findings
- No axon degeneration in sural nerve biopsy

Coeliac disease
- Steatorrhea in childhood
- Glove and stocking type of anesthesia in extremities
- Disturbances of eye movements
- Mental deterioration

Guillain-Barré syndrome
- Ascending paralysis with cranial nerve involvement
- No optic atrophy
- CSF shows albumino-cytologic dissociation
- Course is fluctuating with recovery

Course and Prognosis. Analysis of 981 cases by the SMON Commission revealed the following points (Sobue et al 1975).

- There was no prognostic difference between males and females but the elderly over 60 had a poor outcome.
- The cumulative death rate of SMON was twice the generally expected rate.
- Approximately 80% of the patients showed some sort of improvement 7 to 12 months after onset.
- Complete recovery from sensory disturbances was rare. Recovery of motor deficits was more

favorable. Approximately 40% of those with visual disturbances recovered or showed considerable improvement, whereas 9% of them detriorated.

- The rate of relapse was 16.7% and 68% of the relapses occurred within the first 18 months.
- About 10% of the patients were unable to walk or needed assistance.

Pathophysiology. Initially an infectious agent (virus) was considered to be the causative agent but this was excluded because no virus could be isolated and no virus particles could be seen on electron microscopic examination of tissues from SMON patients or experimentally inoculated animals. Pesticides were also considered possible culprits because of their widespread use in Japan at that time. This combined with excessive use of drugs by the Japanese led to the toxic hypothesis of SMON which was soon abandoned as clioquinol was pinned down as the cause for the following reasons:

- The number of SMON cases increased with the increase in import and production of clioquinol.
- Extraction of chinoform (chelated form of clioquinol) from the green pigment of the tongue and urine of SMON patients.
- Neuropathologic studies showing the relation between the dose and severity of pathologic changes in the nervous system and induction of SMON in experimental animals by administration of clioquinol.
- Animal experimental studies with radionuclide labelled clioquinol as tracer in vivo (Toyokura et al 1975). High levels of accumulation of the tracer were found in the peripheral nerves, the dorsal columns of the spinal cord, and the retina which are the sites of lesions in SMON.

The criticism of this concept is based on rarity of SMON outside of Japan and also the fact that 5% of SMON patients in Japan were not exposed to clioquinol. A hypothesis to explain some of these consistencies has been put forward by Tsälve et al (1984). Clioquinol can increase the penetration of metallic ions through the cellular membranes by forming lipophilic metal chelates. It is suggested that pathogenesis of SMON may involve an accumulation of toxic metals in the tissues of the nervous system. The Japanese have been more heavily exposed to metals by environmental pollution than inhabitants of most other countries. Okada et al (1984) investigated the role of concomitant medications containing metals consumed by SMON patients by a retrospective cohort study. Their conclusion was that aluminum and bismuth containing drugs demonstrated the strongest association with clinical features of SMON whereas those containing copper had little association.

Neuropathology and Clinicopathological Correlation of SMON

This subject has been reviewed by Shiraki (1979).

Experimental Neuropathology. Experiments were carried on different species by a large number of investigators. Dogs and cats were the most sensitive animals and most pronounced changes were in the spinal cord and the optic nerves. The human SMON pathology could be nearly reproduced.

Neuropathological Examination in SMON Cases. All of 113 SMON cases which were autopsied showed significant degeneration of the cervical and lumbar regions of the spinal cord. Most of the cases showed damage to the posterior columns but only slight to moderate lesions in the corticospinal tracts. This corresponds to the higher incidence of sensory disturbances as compared to the motor deficits. There was effective regeneration of the axon collaterals in the anterior spinal nerve roots even in the subacute stage corresponding to the motor recovery seen in SMON patients. The regeneration of sensory nerve fibers was unsuccessful with degeneration of dorsal root ganglia corresponding to incomplete recovery from sensory disturbances. Visual impairment due to disintegration of the inner ganglia cells of the retina and not associated with optic nerve lesions explains the improvement in 40% of the cases.

Clioquinol-induced SMON was considered to be an excellent model of a systemic, non-progressive combined degeneration of the long tracts of the spinal cord associated with polyneuropathy, which involves the peripheral nervous system, the sympathetic system, and the optic nerves. The myelo-optic neuropathy is suggestive of a "dying back process" (see Chapter 11).

SMON-like Syndromes due to Drugs other than Clioquinol

Several drugs can produce a combination of optic neuropathy with myelopathy and/or peripheral neuropathy (see Chapter 10, 11, and 14). Some of these drugs are listed in Table 24.4.

None of these drugs have been linked to SMON with the exception of antitubercular

Table 24.4. Drugs that produce SMON-like syndromes.

Amiodarone
Antineoplastics
Chloramphenicol
Disulfiram
Ethambutol
Isoniazid
Oral contraceptives
Vaccines

Table 24.5. Guidelines for the management of SMON (Sobue 1979).

I.   General measures
         1. Rest
         2. Nutrition
         3. Prevention of infection
II.   Management of abdominal symptoms
III. Treatment of neurological symptoms
         A. Medicinal treatment
            1. Steroids
            2. Vitamins and nerve metabolism activators
            3. Drugs to regulate autonomic disturbances
            4. Vasodilators
            5. Muscle relaxants
         B. Control of paresthesias
            1. Epidural infusion of lidocaine
            2. Acupuncture
         C. Hyperbaric oxygen treatment
IV.   Ophthamologic management of visual disorders
V.   Daily life guidance
VI.   Psychological guidance
VII. Rehabilitation

drugs. There are two case reports of SMON-like syndromes associated with ethambutol (Donati et al 1990; Lappert and Waespe 1988).

Management of SMON

Guidelines for management of SMON, summarized from those that were recommended by the SMON Commission (Sobue 1979), are shown in Table 24.5.

Not all the patients affected by SMON received the recommended treatment. Most of the medical treatments were empirical. It is difficult to evaluate the role of treatment in the recovery of patients.

A Critical Re-Evaluation of SMON

Rose and Gawel (1984) reviewed the SMON episode and made the following points:
- Abdominal symptoms were considered to be cardinal features of SMON. It is difficult to distinguish the abdominal symptoms for which the drug is given from the symptoms resulting from the drug.
- Guidelines for the diagnosis of SMON recommended by the Commission were not adhered to and it is difficult to determine the number of cases which fulfilled the criteria.
- Clinical presentation of SMON outside Japan was very different. Peripheral neuropathy was reported in 38% (less than in Japan). Non-Japanese cases involved children with neurotoxicity presenting as optic atrophy in 38% (children were affected rarely in Japan).
- Oral preparations of clioquinol were available in Japan since 1929 but the first case of SMON was not reported till 1955.
- Banning of fungicides in 1965 and chlorinated hydrocarbons in 1968–69 in Japan may be relevant to disappearance of SMON.

Pallis (1984) has put forward the suggestion that the adequate number of neurologists in Japan as compared to the few neurologists available in India might explain the disparity in number of cases reported in these countries where the use of clioquinol was widespread. Only nine cases of SMON were diagnosed in India during 1967 to 1976 (Wadia 1984). Myelopathy with more distal dysthesias was seen more often than the full-blown picture of SMON and peripheral neuropathy was not a constant or an important part. No explanation was given for this regional difference. Paradoxes and open questions about SMON are listed in Table 24.6.

Table 24.6. Paradoxes and open questions about SMON (from Mann 1986).

Incidence before 1970 not known. Clioquinol in use since 1929
SMON was considered to be an overdose effect of clioquinol but cases have occurred where drug was used within therapeutic limits
No SMON epidemic in Indonesia with greater per capita consumption of clioquinol than in Japan since 1970
SMON is rare in children
Genetic factors which predispose the Japanese to SMON
Dietary factors peculiar to Japan
Drug interaction, e. g., with belladona
Clioquinol plus a viral infection
Clioquinol facilitates the passage of toxic metals into CNS
Species differences in susceptibility to SMON: Mongrel dogs versus beagles

Recent epidemic of optic neuritis in Cuba has drawn attention to a similar problem where no therapeutic drug has been implicated. Over 50,000 cases have been reported and various nutritional toxic and metabolic causes have been considered (MMWR 1994).

Clioquinol is no longer recommended for the traveller's diarrhoea and it has been removed from the WHO list of essential drugs. Restrictions on the use of clioquinol in various countries vary according to the importance of diarrheal illness in each country. In India the need for a cheap effective drug for amoebic dysentary is important and clioquinol has been retained as a prescription only drug and a warning on its potential neurotoxicity has been included in the package insert.

In conclusion, there is no doubt that clioquinol is neurotoxic in long-term use but the mystery of epidemic of SMON in Japan and its relation to clioquinol has not been cleared up as yet.

References

Baumgartner G, Gawel MJ, Kaeser HE, et al: Neurotoxicity of halogenated hydroxyquinolines: clinical analysis of cases reported outside of Japan. JNNP 1979; 42: 1073–1083.

Donati E, Bargnani C, Besana R, et al: Subacute myelo-optic neuropathy (SMON) induced by antituberculous treatment in uremia. Functional Neurology 1990; 5: 151–154.

Gelzer J: Discovery of adverse drug reactions: debate on the paradox of clioquinol and SMON. In Report on the Meeting on Methods for the Detection and Study of Unwanted Drug Effects, Kiel, Germany, Institut für Gesundheits-System-Forschung, 1991: 128–142.

Gent M, Shigematsu I (Eds.): Epidemiological issues in reported drug-induced illnesses—SMON and other examples. Hamilton, Canada, McMaster University Library Press, 1978.

Hansson O: Arzneimittel-Multis und der SMON-Skandal. Basel, Z-Verlag, 1979.

Iida M, Hirose K, Sobue I: Electrophysiological studies on the pathophysiology of SMON (Japanese). Clin Enceph 1971; 13: 235–245.

Izumi H: Organizing Committee of the Geneva Press Conference on SMON—Proceedings, Geneva, Simul International Inc., 1980.

Jack DB, Riess W: Pharmacokinetics of iodochlorhydroxyquine in man. Br J Pharm Sci 1973; 62: 1929–1932.

Kono R: Introductory view of subacute myelo-opticoneuropathy (SMON) and its studies done by the SMON research Commission. Jpn J Med Sci & Biol 1975; 28 (suppl): 1–21.

Lappert D, Waespe W: Neurotoxicity of antituberculous drugs in a patient with active tuberculosis. Ital J Neurosci 1988; 9: 31–34.

Mann RD: Drug-induced disorders of the central nervous function—section on SMON. In D'ArcyPF, Griffin JP (Eds.): Iatrogenic Diseases. Oxford, Oxford University Press, 3rd ed, 1986: 604–612.

MMWR: Epidemic Neuropathy—Cuba, 1991–1994. MMWR 1994; 43: 183, 189–192.

Okada H, Aoki K, Ohno Y, et al: Effects of metal-containing drugs taken simultaneously with clioquinol upon clinical features of ISMON. J Toxicol Sci 1984; 9: 327–341.

Pallis C: Some thoughts on SMON. Acta Neurol Scand 1984; 70 (suppl 100): 147–153.

Rose FC, Gawel M: Clioquinol neurotoxicity: an overview. Acta Neurol Scand 1984; 70(suppl 100): 137–145.

Shiraki H: Neuropathological aspects of etiopathogenesis of SMON. In Vinken PJ: Handbook of Clinical Neurology. Amsterdam, North Holland Publishing Co, 1979: 141–198.

Sobue I, Aoki K, Ohtani M: Prognosis of SMON patients. Jpn J Med Sci & Biol 1975; 28 (suppl): 89–103.

Sobue I: Clinical aspects of subacute-myelo-opticoneuropathy. In Vinken PJ: Handbook of Clinical Neurology, Amsterdam, North Holland Publishing Co, 1979: 115–139.

Soda T (Ed.): Drug-induced Sufferings. Medical, Pharmaceutical, and Legal Aspects. Amsterdam, Excerpta Medica, 1980.

Takasaki H, Kanamaru M: Subacute Myelo-optico Neuropathy. Tokyo, Igaku Shoin Ltd, 1974 (English translation in 1976 distributed at "Honolulu Symposium").

Thomas PK: Neurotoxicity of halogenated hydroxyquinolines: non-Japanese cases. Acta Neurol Scand 1984; 70(suppl 100): 155–158.

Tjälve H: The aetiology of SMON may involve an interaction between clioquinol and environmental metals. Medical hypotheses 1984; 15: 293–299.

Toyokura Y, Takasu T, Mitsuoka O: Experimental studies utilizing radio-nuclides of clioquinol as tracer in vivo. Jpn J Med Sci & Biol 1975; 28 (suppl): 001–008.

Tsubaki T, Honma Y, Hoshi M: Subacute myelo-opticneuropathy following abdominal symptoms. Jpn J Med 1965; 4: 181.

Wadia NH: SMON as seen from Bombay. Acta Neurol Scand 1984; 70 (suppl 100): 159–164.

World Health Organization (WHO): Clioquinol and SMON. Drug Information Bulletin 1977; 113: 9–15.

World Health Organization (WHO): Clioquinol and amoebiasis. Drug Information Bulletin 1978; 115: 9–13.

Yanagawa H, Yamamoto S, Nakae N: Epidemiological approach to SMON. Jpn J Med Sci & Biol 1975; 28(suppl): 23–33.

Chapter 25
Drug-Induced Pituitary Disorders

Introduction

Several drugs affect the pituitary gland but there is a paucity of studies on this organ of the effect of xenobiotics (pharmacologically, endocrinologically and toxicologically active substances which are not produced endogenously). According to Walker and Cooper (1992), reasons for the relative shortage of studies of the toxic effects of xenobiotics on the pituitary are as follows:

- Relatively low exposure of the pituitary cells to xenobiotics as the vascular supply and concentrating ability of the gland are less than the major organs of excretion and metabolism such as the liver and the kidneys.
- Low frequency of published reports describing histopathologic lesions in the pituitary as compared with other endocrine glands.
- Manifestations of pituitary toxicity are usually expressed as functional and structural changes in target endocrine glands under its control, thus shifting attention away from it.

Toxic substances affect the pituitary gland function or structure in following ways:
- Disturbance of pituitary function by direct effect on cells within the gland.
- Producing complications in preexisting lesions within the pituitary gland such as tumors.
- Vascular disturbances in the pituitary gland.
- Disturbances of other endocrines and peripheral hormones which disturb the pituitary function.
- Alteration of neurogenic signals (neuropeptides/neurotransmitters) that regulate the activity of the adenohypophyseal cells.
- A combination of more than one of the above.

Direct Effects on the Pituitary

This has been studied mostly in animal toxicology studies. An unidentified "novel anticancer drug" produced vacuolation and apopstosis in monkey anterior pituitary cells without predilection for any particular cell type (Gopinath et al 1987). Hypertrophy and hyperplasia of lactotrophs has been observed in experimental animals administered natural or synthetic estrogens (Lloyd 1983). This is similar to the pituitary enlargement that occurs during pregnancy when endogenous estrogens are produced in large quantities and the effect is considered to be directly on estrogen receptors in the pituitary. In animals hypertrophy may proceed to neoplasm formation but estrogen treatment does not induce tumor formation de novo in humans (Reichlin 1980).

Complications Related to Preexisting Lesions in the Pituitary

This is a significant factor because of the following reasons:
- Some drugs are used to treat pituitary tumors
- Silent pituitary tumors discovered at autopsy are present in as high as 20% of the general population.

Various lesions that have been encountered are:
- Pituitary apoplexy (infarction or hemorrhage)
- Enlargement of a pituitary tumor
- Cerebrospinal fluid leakage due to shrinking of the pituitary tumor.

Pituitary Apoplexy

Various causes of pituitary apoplexy are shown in Table 25.1. Postpartum ischemic necrosis of the anterior pituitary was described as occurring due to spasm of the infundibular arteries (Sheehan 1937). However, since the original description of Sheehan's syndrome the disorder is seen most frequently from severe hemorrhage of the capillary network during parturition, but may also result from anesthesia or poisoning (Doniach and Walker 1946; Smith and Howard 1959; Murdoch 1962; Harlin and Givens 1968).

Table 25.1. Causes of pituitary apoplexy.

Post-partum pituitary necrosis (Sheehan's syndrome)
Spontaneous hemorrhages in adenomas
Idiopathic pituitary hemorrhages
Iatrogenic pituitary infarction due to surgery in sellar
    or parasellar region
Drugs
    – Anesthesia
    – Anticoagulants
    – Bromocriptine
    – Chlorpromazine
    – Clomiphene
    – Estrogens
    – Hormones for testing pituitary function: insulin
    – Hormones for diagnosis of pituitary adenomas:
       TRH and GnRH
    – Luteinizing-hormone releasing hormone
       LHRH) used therapeutically: leuprorelin

Precipitating Factors for Pituitary Apoplexy. Presence of pituitary tumors predisposes to pituitary apoplexy which occurs frequently in glands in which adenomas are present (Lock and Tyler 1961; Taylor 1968; Dawson and Kothandaram 1972) and is seen more commonly with somatotroph, lactotroph or corticotroph adenomas. Softening or degenerative changes within the adenoma may predispose to hemorrhage. Pituitary apoplexy may be precipitated by the administration of estrogens or anticoagulants (Veldhuis and Hammond 1980). Heparin therapy for myocardial infarction trigger pituitary apoplexy in one case (Oo et al 1997).

Pituitary Apoplexy after Pituitary Function Tests. Apoplexy may occur in a pituitary with little or no evidence of previous disease. Pituitary apoplexy can follow pituitary stimulation tests (Vassallo et al 1994). Harvey et al (1989) presented a case of in which pituitary infarction was precipitated by hypoglycemia induced by insulin stress testing for suspected hypothyroidism. Preoperative assessment of pituitary adenomas includes a combined testing of growth hormone (GH) and ACTH release stimulated by hypoglycemia, thyroid stimulating hormone (TSH) release by thyroid releasing hormone (TRH), and gonadotropin release by gonadotropin-releasing hormone (GnRH). Complications with these tests are rare but several cases have been reported of pituitary apoplexy with combined dynamic testing of pituitary hormones (Bernstein et al 1984; Chapman et al 1985). A single intravenous administration of GnRH led to infarction of the pituitary in a patient with prolactinoma (Arafah et al 1989). Repeat injection after removal of the hemorrhage and adenoma did not produce any adverse effects. Pituitary apoplexy has also occurred in a patient with glycoprotein secreting adenoma after GnRH administration (Masson et al 1993).

Pituitary infarction occurred in another case of follicle stimulating hormone (FSH) secreting pituitary adenoma two hours after therapeutic injection of luteinizing hormone releasing hormone (LHRH) which normalized FSH level (Korsic et al 1984). Pituitary apoplexy has been reported after injection of goserelin (LHRH analog) in a patient with advanced prostatic carcinoma (Ando et al 1995). Masago et al (1995) reported two cases of pituitary apoplexy following a dynamic combined test of pituitary function involving intravenous injection of TRH, GnRH and regular insulin. These authors also reviewed the literature on this topic and found 22 cases that had precipitation of pituitary apoplexy following pituitary function tests.

Pathomechanism. The pathomechanism of apoplexy is not understood but mechanisms related to functional tests are:

– TRH has vasoactive properties and also elevates serum levels of norepinephrine. TRH-induced vasospasm or pressor effect may precipitate pituitary infarction. TRH also directly activates tumor cells. The subsequent increase in blood flow, blood volume and tumor size may lead to stretch and occlusion of many vessels resulting in their rupture.

- GnRH may increase the cell metabolism underlying the excessive Gonadotropin production to such an extent that a vascular accident can occur.
- Insulin induces hypoglycemia which reduces CBF. Catecholamine release in response to hypoglycemia may affect the cerebrovascular circulation.

Pituitary Apoplexy as an Adverse Effect of Drugs. There are only a few drugs involved and a limited number of case reports in the literature. Some of these are:

Bromocriptine. Bromocriptine which is used for treatment of prolactinomas has been found to be associated with intratumoral hemorrhage (Wakai et al 1981; Cardoso and Peterson 1984; Onesti et al 1990; Endoh et al 1994; Lazaro et al 1994). Bromocriptine is said to lead to rapid shrinkage of the prolactin-secreting tumor cells and this may lead to disruption of the tissue texture and hemorrhage (Landolt et al 1987; Shirataki et al 1988).

Chlorpromazine. One case of pituitary apoplexy in a prolactinoma was reported following chlorpromazine injection (Silverman et al 1978). Postural hypotension induced by chlorpromazine was considered to be the precipitating factor.

Clomiphene. This is used for the treatment of infertility. One case of clomiphene-induced pituitary apoplexy occurred in a young women with acromegaly (Walker et al 1996). This was treated surgically.

Leuprorelin. This is used for the treatment of prostate cancer based on the inhibition of pituitary gonadal function and suppression of gonadal steroid hormone. The aim of therapy is inhibition of sex hormone-dependent tumors. One patient developed pituitary apoplexy after the first injection of leuprorelin depot (Reznik et al 1997). MRI scan showed hemorrhage in a previously undiagnosed pituitary adenoma which was removed surgically.

Clinical Manifestations of Pituitary Apoplexy. These include deterioration of vision, ophthalmoplegia, and headache. Hemiparesis and coma may occur in severe cases.

Diagnosis. This is established by CT scan and MRI.

Treatment. Surgical treatment of pituitary apoplexy is transsphenoidal removal of the necrotic mass. The results of surgery are usually good with recovery of vision but in some cases the visual deficits do not recover. Some cases have been managed conservatively and followed up by MRI examinations.

Cerebrospinal Fluid Rhinorrhea (CSF) due to Shrinking of Prolactinoma

CSF rhinorrhea has been reported in ten cases as a sequel of shrinking of macroprolactinomas as an effect of bromocriptine therapy (Clayton et al 1985; Bronstein et al 1989; Eljamel et al 1992; Coculescu and Finer 1994; Barlas et al 1994; Pascal-Vigneron et al 1994). Some of these tumors invade the sella floor and plug it. Shrinking of the tumor mass unplugs this leading to CSF leakage. In some cases discontinuation of bromocriptine led to cessation of CSF leak. The risk of meningitis requires closure of the CSF fistula. The treatment is surgical repair of the CSF leak or as an alternative a CSF shunting procedure is done to promote healing of the CSF fistula.

Pituitary Insufficiency

Hypopituitarism is the partial or complete insufficiency (panhypopituitrism) of anterior-pituitary hormone secretion and results from pituitary or hypothalamic disease. The manifestations may be due to deficiency of corticotrophin, Gonadotropins, androgen or growth hormone (Lamberts et al 1998). Drugs may induce hypopituitarism and some examples are.

- Antineoplastic drugs
- Interferon-α-2b (Sakane et al 1995)
- Corticosteroids (Kobayashi et al 1997; Kamoda et al 1998)

Effect of drugs on various pituitary hormones will be discussed in the following sections.

Drug-Induced Disorders of the Pituitary due to Disturbances of Other Endocrines

Pituitary is the master gland of the endocrine orchestra and is affected by the brain as well as feedback influences from the target glands and their effects on the peripheral tissues. The relationships of the pituitary are shown schematically in Figure 25.1.

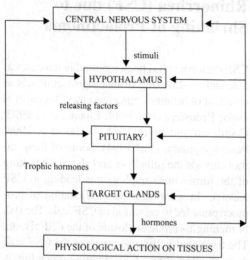

Figure 25.1. Relationships of the pituitary.

Several drugs have a secondary effect on the pituitary via induction of changes in the other endocrine function. The scope of this work does not allow any discussion of the complex endocrine interrelationships and adverse effects of drugs on other endocrines. Drug may also influence the pituitary via their effects on the central nervous systems and neurotransmitter changes. Some adverse reactions involving various hypothalamo-pituitary-target endocrine axes will be mentioned briefly.

Hypothalamo-Pituitary-Thyroid Axis

Therapeutic doses of thyroid hormone can suppress TSH secretion. In addition to this several glucocorticoids and dopaminergic drugs can inhibit thyroid stimulating hormone (TSH) secre-

tion and reduce the TSH response to thyroid releasing hormone (TRH). Neuroleptics such as chlorpromazine and haloperidol can raise basal TSH levels and enhance the TSH response to goitrogenic medications that produce hypothyroidism. This leads to a compensatory increase in TSH levels. Drugs which alter thyrotropin secretion are listed in Table 25.2.

Table 25.2. Drugs that alter thyrotropin secretion.

Increase	Decrease
Domperidone	Androgens
Estrogens	Antiepileptics: carbamazepine,
Lithium	phenytoin
Metachlopramide	Dopamine agonists: bromo-
Glucocorticoids	criptine, levodopa
Sulpiride	Verapamil

Hypothalmo-Pituitary-Adrenal (HPA) Axis

Arginine vasopressin is the most important of various hormones that influence adrenocorticotrophin (ACTH) secretion by the pituitary. ACTH secretion is impaired by the feedback effect on the hypothalamus and the pituitary of prolonged high dose glucocorticosteroid therapy. Drugs which alter ACTH secretion are shown in Table 25.3.

Iatrogenic Cushing's syndrome can occur with pharmacological doses of glucocorticoids or ACTH. Cytokines activate the HPA axis and cause release of ACTH and glucocorticoids (Rivier and Rivest 1993). Interleukin (IL)-1 is one of the most potent activators of HPA axis,

Table 25.3. Drugs that alter ACTH secretion.

Increase	Decrease
Alcohol	Glucocorticoids
CNS stimulants: amphetamine,	Opiates
methylphenidate	
Cytokines: IL-2, IL-6, TNF-α	
Nicotine	
Opiate antagonists	
Physostigmine	
Tricyclic antidepressants:	
imipramine, desipramine	

but other cytokines such as IL-2, IL-6, and tumor necrosis factor (TNF)-α can act synergistically with it. Peripheral or central administration of IL-1 or IL-6 causes release of corticotrophin releasing hormone (CRH), which subsequently, stimulates the release of ACTH and glucocorticoids, although cytokines can act directly at the level of the pituitary.

Hypothalamo-Gonadal Axis

The secretion of Gonadotropin-releasing hormone (GnRH), follicle stimulating hormone (FSH), and luteinizing hormone (LH) are under the negative feedback control of testosterone and estradiol. Drugs that alter Gonadotropin secretion are listed in Table 25.4.

Glucocorticoid excess can inhibit pituitary

Table 25.4. Drugs that alter gonadotropin secretion.

Increase	Decrease
Alcohol	Androgen
Antineoplastic agents	Cytokines: IL-1
Ketoconazole	Digitoxin
Opiate antagonists	Dopamine agonists: bromocriptine
	Estrogens
	Glucocorticoids
	Opiates
	Verapamil

Gonadotropin secretion. Chronic administration of IL-1β into the CNS disrupts the estrous cycle by inhibiting the synthesis and release of luteinizing hormone releasing hormone (LHRH) and inhibits luteolysis via increased production of prolactin (Rivest and Rivier 1993).

Hypothalamo-Pituitary-Prolactin Secretion

Prolactin is a polypeptide trophic hormone secreted by the anterior pituitary. Its secretion is primarily under the inhibitory control of hypothalamic dopamine and stimulatory influence of serotonergic system. TRH is also a stimulant of prolactin.

Hyperprolactinemia

Various physiological stimuli such as sleep, stress, exercise, sexual intercourse, menstrual cycle, and pregnancy also stimulate prolactin secretion. Hyperprolactinemia frequently produces galactorrhea. Occasionally galactorrhea can occur without hyperprolactinemia. About 20% of the women with galactorrhea have prolactinomas of the pituitary demonstrated radiologically. This frequency increases to 34% in women with galactorrhea and amenorrhea. Causes of hyperprolactinemia are shown in Table 25.5 and drugs which can induce hyperprolactinemia are shown in Table 25.6.

Table 25.5. Causes of hyperprolactinemia.

Hypothalamic lesions
 – Infiltrative diseases: sarcoidosis
 – Ischemia
 – Neuraxis radiation
 – Trauma
 – Tumors
Pituitary lesions
 – Acromegaly
 – Cushing's Disease
 – Empty sella syndrome
 – Pituitary stalk section
 – Prolactinomas
Neurogenic
 – Breast stimulation
 – Chest wall lesions
 – Spinal cord lesions
Other conditions
 – Chronic renal failure
 – Cirrhosis of liver
 – Hypothyroidism
Drugs (see Table 25.3)
Idiopathic

Pathomechanism. Many of these drugs act on the hypothalamus via neurotransmitter systems and some of the examples are:
 – *Depletion of catecholamine stores.* For example, reserpine and methyldopa.
 – *Blockage of dopamine receptors*: Antipsychotic (neuroleptic) phenothiazines and butyrophenones block dopamine receptors (Tolis et al 1974). Proliferative adenohypophyseal lesions involving lactophs occur in animals treated with neuroleptics which are dopamine antagonists (Horowski and Graf 1979).

Table 25.6. Drugs that cause hyperprolactinemia.

Alcohol
Anesthetics
Antidepressants
  – tricyclic
    • amitriptyline
    • clomipramine
    • imipramine
  – monoamine oxidase inhibitors
Antiemetics
  – metoclopramide
  – sulpride
Antihypertensives
  – methyldopa
  – reserpine
Antipsychotics
  – phenothiazines
    • chloropromazine
    • fluphenazine
    • perphenazine
    • prochlorperazine
    • promazine
    • thioridazine
    • trifluoperazine
  – haloperidol
Benzodiazepines: chlordiazepoxide
Cocaine
Dexamphetamine and phenfluramine
H_2-receptor blockers
  – cimetidine
  – ranitidine
Hormones
  – estrogens
  – oral contraceptives
  – thyrotropin-releasing hormone
Nicotine
Opioids
Physostigmine
Serotonin precursors: tryptophan
Verapamil

Clozapine is a an antipsychotic agent that displays atypical pharmacological and clinical properties as compared to classic antipsychotics. It has a relatively weak central dopaminergic activity (Fitton and Heel 1990) and affects serum prolactin levels in a manner different from other antipsychotics. In rats, clozapine produces rapid elevations in serum prolactin levels similar in magnitude to those produced by haloperidol but they are of much shorter duration than those elicited by haloperidol (Gudelsky et al 1987). In humans treated with clozapine under a single-dose schedule, prolactin levels are normal most of the time. Clozapine's weak D_2-receptor blocking effects, combined with increased activity of tuberoinfundibular neurons, may explain its weak effect on prolactin secretion (Kane et al 1981). Secondary effects of hyperprolactinemia such as amenorrhea, galactorrhea, and gynecomastia are seldom seen in patients on clozapine therapy.

– *Disturbances of serotonin.* Antidepressants probably stimulate prolactin release by blocking the reuptake of serotonin or enhancing the sensitivity of postsynaptic serotonin receptors (Gadd et al 1987). Monoamine oxidase inhibitors may shift the balance between dopaminergic inhibition and serotonergic stimulation of prolactin release (Slater et al 1977).

– *Increased responsiveness to prolactin releasing stimuli.* Estrogens may increase mean serum prolactin levels by this mechanism (Frantz 1978).

– *Histamine.* Brain histamine may play a role in prolactin release. Antihistaminic cimetidine may rarely increase prolactin secretion and produce galactorrhoea (Ehrinpreis et al 1989).

Management of Hyperprolactinemia

Hyperprolactinemia is a frequent cause of amenorrhea, infertility, and galactorrhea in women and decreased libido and impotence in men. Investigations of patients with raised serum prolactin levels includes search for pituitary prolactinomas, drugs, and other causes listed in Table 25.2. If no cause can be demonstrated, it is labeled as idiopathic hypoprolactinemia and is treated with drugs. Prolactinomas can be treated with drugs, surgery, or radiation therapy.

Bromocriptine has been the standard therapy for hyperprolactinemia for the over 20 years. It is a dopamine agonist that not only inhibits the synthesis and secretion of prolactin but also reduces cellular DNA synthesis and tumor growth. Approximately 80% of the patients with prolactinomas respond to bromocriptine with shrinkage of the tumor and substantial reduction of the serum prolactin levels (Serri 1994). New dopamine agonists drugs including quinagolide, pergolide, and cabergoline have been developed as alternatives for patients who do not tolerate bromocriptine.

In drug-induced hyperprolactinemia consideration is given to the withdrawal of the offending drug if possible. Treatment cannot be always discontinued in psychiatric patients with neuroleptic-induced hyperprolactinemia. Smith (1992) used concomitant bromocriptine with neuroleptics in six psychiatric outpatients with neuroleptic-induced hyperprolactinemia with amenorrhea/oligomenorrhea. Three of the patients had the menstrual irregularity corrected successfully with bromocriptine. Controlled clinical studies are required to evaluate this combination. As an alternative classical neuroleptics can be switched over to clozapine which is unlikely to induce hyperprolactinemia.

Hypothalamic-Pituitary-Growth Hormone Axis

Various organs and hormones involved in this axis are:
- *Hypothalamus:* Growth hormone releasing hormone stimulates growth hormone (GH) gene transcription and GH secretion whereas somatostatin inhibits GH secretion.
- *Pituitary:* GH stimulates insulin-like growth factor (IGF)-1 production and antagonizes insulin action.

Drugs may affect growth through their effect on GH secretion at hypothalamic or pituitary level through effect on IGF-1 which can be produced in the liver and extrahepatic tissues and stimulates bone growth and cell replication. Prolonged use of steroids in children may affect growth but it is not certain if the effect is due to alteration of growth hormone secretion or direct effect on the target tissues. Drugs which affect growth hormone secretion are shown in Table 25.7.

Posterior Pituitary

This will be considered because of its connection with the syndrome of inappropriate antidi-

Table 25.7. Drugs that influence growth hormone (GH) secretion.

Increase of GH secretion
α-agonists: clonidine, apomorphine
β-blockers: propranolol
Androgens
CNS stimulants: amphetamine, methylphenidate, nicotine
Dopamine agonists: levodopa, bromocriptine
Estrogens
Fentanyl
GABAergic drugs: baclofen, diazepam
Opioids: methadone, nalorphine
Physostigmine
Pyridostigmine
Serotonin precursors: tryptophan
Tricyclic antidepressants: imipramine, desipramine

Decrease of GH secretion
α-blockers: phentolamine, phenoxybenzamine
Atropine
Cimetidine
Dopamine receptor blockers: chlorpromazine, haloperidol
Glucocorticoids
Serotonin receptor blockers: cyproheptadine
Somatostatin

uretic hormone secretion which has been described as an adverse reaction to several drugs. The antidiuretic hormone (ADH) is synthesized in the supraoptic and paraventricular nuclei of the hypothalamus and transported down to axon terminals in the posterior pituitary where it is stored until release into peripheral circulation. A large number of stimuli such as vomiting and hypoglycemia can cause release of ADH. Under normal condition, the major regular of water homeostasis is plasma osmotic pressure which exerts its influence through specific osmoreceptor neurons located in the anterior hypothalamus. In the kidneys, the antidiuretic effect of ADH is mediated mainly by vasopressin-2 receptors located on the cells of the collecting ducts. These cells are relatively impermeable to water in the absence of ADH and the receptors initiate the series of steps that increase the permeability of the cells lining the lumen of collecting ducts so that reabsorption of water is facilitated along a concentration gradient.

Syndrome of Inappropriate Secretion of Antidiuretic Hormone (SIADH)

This syndrome was first described by Bartter and Schwartz (1967). It is characterized by sustained release of ADH in the absence of either osmotic or non-osmotic stimuli or by an enhanced renal action of ADH. The patients are unable to excrete a diluted urine and ingested water is retained leading to hyponatremia. Symptoms of hyponatremia usually do not appear until serum sodium level falls below 130 mmol/L. Common early symptoms are weakness, confusion, lethargy, headache, and weight gain. Persistent severe hyponatremia may lead to convulsions and coma.

Causes. Various causes of SIADH are shown in Table 25.8.

Table 25.8. Causes of the syndrome of inappropriate secretion of antidiuretic hormone (SIADH).

Malignant tumors producing ADH
- small cell lung carcinoma, cancer of the pancreas, prostate, and duodenum
- carcinomas of the reticuloendothelial system
- malignant thymomas
Pulmonary diseases
- acute respiratory failure
- chronic obstructive pulmonary disease
- empyema
- pneumonia
- tuberculosis
Disorders of the central nervous system
- cerebrovascular accidents; subarachnoid hemorrhage
- cerebral atrophy
- encephalitis
- head injuries: skull fracture, subdural hematoma
- hydrocephalus
- infections: meningitis, brain abscess
- postoperative: neurosurgical procedures in the pituitary area
Drugs (see Table 25.6)

Investigations. The investigation of a patient with SIADH includes a careful history taking with the various causes in mind and a list of medications that the patient may be taking. In addition to the basic laboratory investigations, the following special tests should be done:
- serum electrolytes and osmolality
- urine electrolytes and osmolality, specific gravity

- endocrine function screening tests
- EEG in patients with hyponatremic encephalopathy
- Diagnostic tests according to the cause suspected

Drug-Induced SIADH

Various drugs which have been reported to cause SIADH are listed in Table 25.9. Causes diagnosis and management of SIADH have been reviewed by Chan (1997).

Pathomechanism. Some of the basic mechanisms of ADH increase are not well understood but some of the mechanisms which are applicable to drug-induced SIADH are as follows:
- *Increased ADH production.* Noradrenaline induces release of ADH via α_1-adrenergic receptors. Stimulation of serotonergic systems also increase ADH. Antidepressants, antipsychotics and dopaminergic drugs may induce SIADH by these mechanisms.
- *Increased responsiveness of distal renal tubules to ADH.* Carbamazepine is an example.
- *Role of dopamine.* This has both a stimulatory as well as an inhibitory effect on ADH release. Under certain circumstances such as schizophrenic patients with low plasma osmolality, dopamine-antagonist neuroleptics may have an increase in ADH secretion. Dopamine agonists such as bromocriptine are known to stimulate both central and peripheral dopaminergic receptors predominantly in the kidney. They can modify diuresis and sodium excretion. Damase-Michel et al (1993) have described a patient with Parkinson's disease who developed hyponatremia following treatment with bromocriptine.
- *Hypotension.* Drug induced hypotension may cause SIADH (Zabik et al 1993).

Drugs Involved in SIADH. Although a large number of drugs are reported to produce SIADH, most of the published reports concern vasopressin and its analogues, thiazide diuretics, antipsychotics, antidepressants and carbamazepine.
- *Vasopressin.* This drug as well as its analogues are used in the treatment of cranial diabetes

Table 25.9. Drugs reported to induce syndrome of inappropriate secretion of ADH.

ACE inhibitors
Amiloride
Anesthesia
Antiepileptic drugs
  – carbamazepine*
  – oxcarbazepine*
Antineoplastics
  – cyclophosphamide
  – etoposide
  – vinca alkaloids
Antipsychotics*
  – clozapine
  – chlorpromazine
  – fluphenazine
  – flufenthioxol
  – haloperidol
  – trifluoperazine
  – thioridazine
  – thiothixene
Antidepressants
  – Tricyclic antidepressants*
    • amoxapine
    • clomipramine
    • desipramine
    • dothiepin
    • doxepin
    • imipramine
  – Selective serotonin reuptake inhibitors
    • citalopram
    • fluoxetine
    • fluvoxamine
    • paroxetine
    • sertraline
    • venlafaxine
  – Trazodone
  – MAO inhibitors: tranylcypromine
Benzodiazepines
Bromocriptine
Clofibrate
Chloropropamide*
Non-steroidal anti-inflammatory drugs
Omeprazole
Posterior pituitary hormones*
  – vasopressin
  – desmopressin
  – oxytocin
Thiazide diuretics*

*Well documented. Other drugs are linked with SIADH in isolated case reports.

inspidus. Desmopressin has a longer duration of action than vasopressin. Water intoxication, hyponatremia and seizures are well recognized complications of treatment with vasopressin and its analogues, particularly by the use of intranasal desmopressin for nocturnal enuresis in children (Kallio et al 1993).

– *Thiazide diuretics.* These often cause a syndrome resembling SIADH except that the hyponatremia is accompanied by hypokalemia and alkalosis. Strictly speaking, it cannot be called SIADH because ADH secretion is physiologically appropriate in this case.

– *Carbamazepine.* Hyponatremia is a well known adverse effect of carbamazepine in patients with epilepsy and trigeminal neuralgia with an incidence as high as 22% (Lahr 1985). Including psychiatric disorders as indications for treatment, CBZ-induced hyponatremia has been reported to range from 4.8 to 40% (Van Amelsvoort et al 1994) and 33 to 50% (Gandelman 1994). It is postulated to be due to antidiuretic effect by stimulation of ADH release as a consequence of altered sensitivity of hypothalamic osmoreceptors to serum osmolality. Carbamazepine, in doses of 600 to 2000 mg per day, produces statistically significant hyponatremia in patients with affective disorders but clinical manifestations are rare (Joffe et al 1986). Oxcarbazepine, which is structurally similar to carbamazepine, has similar effect in producing hyponatremia and has been reported in a 25% of epileptic patients treated with this medication (Friis et al 1993).

– *Antidepressants and antipsychotics.* Hyponatremia associated with administration of antipsychotics and antidepressants has been reviewed by Spigset and Hedenmalm (1995). In evaluating the development of hyponatremia in psychiatric patients, the following factors should be taken into consideration:

· An important risk factor for the development of SIADH is psychiatric disorders with polydipsia
· There is a transient increase in the release of ADH during exacerbation of psychosis
· Anticholinergic effects of tricyclic antidepressants may lead to dry mouth and increased thirst
· Drug interactions

Management. Patients with serum sodium values around 125 mmol/L and no clinical manifestations can be managed conservatively by water restriction and change of therapy. The dose of the suspected drug may be reduced or switched over to a drug not associated with this adverse reaction. Patients with serum sodium values below 125 mmol/L and clinical manifestations, who do not respond to withdrawal of the offending drug and water restriction, should receive infusion of hypertonic sodium chloride. Rapid sodium correction should be avoided because of danger of central pontine myelinolysis (Sterns et al 1986). In patients with chronic an infusion of 0.9% saline has been recommended (Höjer 1994). Furosemide, which enhances the excretion of hypotonic urine, may be used as an adjunct (Riggs et al 1991).

After the initial hyponatremia has improved, rechallenge with the suspected drug may be considered for determination of the causal role. If the use of the drug inducing hyponatremia is essential for the patient, water restriction and sodium supplementation may be tried. Demeclocycline (a tetracycline derivative) inhibits the renal effects of ADH and has been used successfully in patients who do not respond to water restriction. Brewerton and Jackson (1994) have used demeclocycline successfully in prevention of hyponatremia in six psychiatric patients on carbamazepine therapy. Lithium also inhibits the renal action of ADH and has been used with some success in the management of chronic SIADH.

Diabetes Insipidus

This is a condition that is characterized by excretion of large amounts of dilute urine.Thirst and polydipsia are prominent features. There are relatively few physical signs. Routine laboratory rests are usually normal. Plasma osmolality and sodium concentration are not significantly elevated. Any abnormalities seen are usually due to underlying disease. There are two main types of diabetes insipidus which should be differentiated from primary polydipsia (excessive water intake) which may be psychogenic or due to medical disorders.

Neurogenic or central diabetes insipidus. This is due to vasopressin deficiency which may be due to increased metabolism such as in pregnancy or due to decreased secretion which may occur in the following conditions:
- Trauma: accidental or surgery
- Malignant tumors in the sellar region
- Infections
- Vascular lesions: aneurysm, ischemia
- Anorexia nervosa
- Exposure to environmental toxins: carbon monoxide
- Congenital malformations
- Adverse effects of drugs

Vasopressin resistant or nephrogenic diabetes insipidus. This may be due to several underlying diseases or drugs. Drugs leading to nephrogenic diabetes insipidus are shown in Table 25.10. Of these, lithium is the most commonly involved.

Table 25.10. Drugs that have been reported to induce nephrogenic diabetes insipidus.

Demeclocycline
Ifosfamide
Lithium toxicity (long-term administration)
Methicillin
Methoxyflurane

References

Ando S, Hoshino T, Mihara S: Pituitary apoplexy after goserelin (letter). Lancet 1995; 345: 458.

Arafah BM, Taylor HC, Salazar R, et al: Apoplexy of a pituitary adenoma after dynamic testing with Gonadotropin-releasing hormone. Am J Med 1989; 87: 103– 105.

Barlas O, Bayindir C, Hepgul K, et al: Bromocriptine-induced cerebrospinal fistula in patients with macroprolactinomas: report of three cases and a review of the literature. Surg Neurol 1994; 41: 486–489.

Bartter FC, Schwartz WB: The syndrome of inappropriate secretion of antidiuretic hormone. Am J Med 1967; 42: 790–806.

Bernstein M, Hegele RA, Gentili F, et al: Pituitary apoplexy associated with a triple bolus test. Case report. J Neurosurg 1984; 61: 586–590.

Brewerton TD, Jackson CW: Prophylaxis of carbamazepine-induced hyponatremia by demeclocycline in six patients. J Clin Psychiatry 1994; 55: 249–251.

Bronstein MD, Musolino NR, Benabou S, et al: Cerebrospinal fluid rhinorrhea occurring in long-term bromocriptine treatment for macroprolactinomas. Surg Neurol 1989; 32: 346–349.

Cardoso ER, Peterson EW: Pituitary apoplexy: a review. Neurosurgery 1984; 14: 363–373.

Chan TYK: Drug-induced syndrome of inappropriate antidiuretic hormone secretion. Drugs & Aging 1997; 11: 27–44.

Chapman AJ, Williams G, Hockley AD, et al: Pituitary apoplexy after combined tests of anterior pituitary function. BMJ 1985; 291: 26–27.

Clayton RN, Webb J, Heath DA, et al: Dramatic and rapid shrinkage of a massive invasive prolactinoma with bromocriptine, a case report. Clin Endocrinol 1985; 22: 573–581.

Coculescu R, Finer N: Cerebrospinal fluid rhinorrhea and meningitis after bromocriptine therapy for an invasive macroprolactinoma. J Endocrinol 1994; 140(suppl): 57.

Damase-Michel C, Sarrail E, Lans J, et al: Hyponatremia in a patient treated with bromocriptine. Drug Investigation 1993; 5: 285–287.

Dawson BH, Kothandaram P: Acute massive infarction of pituitary adenomas. J Neurosurg 1972; 37: 275.

Doniach I, Walker AHC: Combined anterior pituitary necrosis and bilateral cortical necrosis of kidneys following concealed accidental hemorrhage. J Obstetr Gynecol Br Emp 1946; 53: 140.

Ehrinpreis MN, Dhar R, Narula A: Cimetidine-induced galactorrhoea. Am J Gastroenterol 1989; 84: 563.

Eljamel MS, Foy PM, Swift AC, et al: Cerebrospinal fluid rhinorrhea occurring in long-term bromocriptine treatment for macroprolactinomas (letter). Surg Neurol 1992; 38: 321.

Endoh M, Wakai S, Iouh S, et al: Massive intraventricular hemorrhage from prolactinoma during bromocriptine therapy: case report. No Shinkei Geka 1994; 22(7): 661–664.

Fitton A, Heel RC: Clozapine: a review of its pharmacological properties, and therapeutic use in schizophrenia. Drugs 1990; 40: 723–747.

Frantz AG: Prolactin. NEJM 1978; 298: 201.

Friis ML, Kristensen O, Boas J, et al: Therapeutic experiences with 947 epileptic out-patients in oxcarbazepine treatment. Acta Neurol Scand 1993; 87: 224–227.

Gadd EM, Norris CM, Beeley L: Antidepressants and galactorrhoea. Int Clin Psychopharmacol 1987; 2: 361.

Gandelman MS: Review of carbamazepine-induced hyponatremia. Prog Neuropsychopharmacol Biol Psychiatry 1994; 18: 211–233.

Gopinath C, Prentice DE, Lewis DJ: Atlas of experimental toxicological pathology, vol 13, Boston, MTP Press, 1987, pp 104–121.

Gudelsky GA, Koening JI, Simonovic M, et al: Differential effects of heloperidol, clozapine and fluperlapine on tubuloinfundibular dopamine neurons and prolactin secretion in the rat. J Neural Transm 1987; 68: 227–240.

Harlin RS, Givens JR: Sheehan's syndrome associated with eclampsia and small sella turcica. Southern Med J 1968; 61: 900.

Harvey R, Michelagnoli M, McHenry P, et al: Pituitary apoplexy (letter). BMJ 1989; 298: 258.

Höjer J: Management of symptomatic hyponatremia: dependence on the duration of treatment. J Intern Med 1994; 235: 497–501.

Horowski R, Graf JK: Neuroendocrine effects of neuro-

psychotropic drugs and their possible influence on toxic reactions in animals and man—the role of dopamine-prolactin system. Arch Toxicol 1999; suppl 2: 93–104.

Joffe RT, Post RM, Uhde TW: Effects of carbamazepine on serum electrolytes in affectively ill patients. Psychol Med 1986; 16: 331–335.

Kallio J, Rautava P, Huupponen R, et al: Severe hyponatremia caused by intranasal desmopressin for nocturnal enuresis. Acta Paediatr 1993; 82: 881–2.

Kamoda T, Nakahara C, Matsui A: A case of empty sella after steroid pulse therapy for nephrotic syndrome. J Rheumatology 1998; 25: 822–823.

Kane JM, Cooper TB, Sacher EJ, et al: Clozapine: plasma levels and prolactin response. Psychopharmacology 1981; 73: 184–187.

Kobayashi S, Warabi H, Hashimoto H, et al: Hypopituitarism with empty sella syndrome after steroid pulse therapy. J Rheumatology 1997; 24: 236–238.

Korsic M, Lelas-Bahun N, Surdonja P, et al: Infarction of FSH-secreting pituitary adenoma. Acta Endocrinologica 1984; 107: 149–154.

Lahr MB: Hyponatremia during carbamazepine therapy. Clin Pharmacol Ther 1985; 37: 693–6.

Lamberts SWJ, de Herder WW, van der Lely AJ: Pituitary insufficiency. Lancet 1998; 352: 127–134.

Landolt AM, Osterwalder V, Landolt T: Storage and release of secretary granules in prolactinomas: modification by bromocriptine. J Endocrinol 1987; 113: 495–499.

Lazaro CM, Guo WY, Sami M, et al: Hemorrhagic pituitary tumors. Neuroradiology 1994; 36: 111–114.

Lloyd RV: Estrogen-induced hyperplasia and neoplasia in the rat anterior pituitary gland. Am J Pathology 1983; 113: 198–206.

Locke S, Tyler HR: Pituitary apoplexy. Am J Med 1961; 30: 643.

Masago A, Ueda Y, Kanai H, et al: Pituitary apoplexy after pituitary function test: a report of two cases and review of the literature. Surgical Neurology 1995; 43: 158–165.

Masson EA, Atkin SL, Diver M, et al: Pituitary apoplexy and sudden blindness following the administration of Gonadotropin releasing hormone. Clin Endocrinol 1993; 38: 109–110.

Murdoch R: Sheehan's syndrome. Survey of 57 cases since 1950. lancet 1962; i: 1327.

Onesti ST, Wisnewski T, Post KD: Clinical versus subclinical pituitary apoplexy: presentation, surgical management, and outcome in 21 patients. neurosurgery 1990; 26: 980–986.

Oo MM, Krishna AY, Bonavita GJ, et al: Heparin therapy for myocardial infarction: an unusual trigger for pituitary apoplexy. Am J Med Sci 1997; 314(5): 351–353

Pascal-Vigneron V, Werya G, Braun M, et al: La rhinorrhee et l'otorrhea: des complication rares du traitment medical des prolactinomes invasifs. Ann Endocrinol (Paris) 1994; 54: 347–351.

Reichlin S: Etiology of pituitary adenomas. In Post KD (Ed.) The pituitary adenoma, New York, Plenum Press, 1980, pp 29–45.

Reznik Y, Chapon F, Lahlou N, et al: Pituitary apoplexy

of a gonadotroph adenoma following Gonadotropin releasing hormone agonist therapy for prostatic cancer. J Endocrinol Invest 1997; 20(9): 566–8.

Riggs AT, Dysken MW, Kim SW, et al: A review of the disorders of water homeostasis in psychiatric patients. Psychosomatics 1991; 32: 133–148.

Rivest S, Rivier C: Centrally injected interleukin 1-β inhibits the hypothalamic LHRH secretion and circulating LH levels via prostaglandin. J Neuroendocrinology 1993; 5: 445–450.

Rivier C, Rivest S: Corticotrophin Releasing Factor. In Vale WW (Ed.), Ciba Foundation Symposium, No. 172, Chichester, Wiley, 1993, pp 204–225.

Sakane N, Yoshida T, Yashioka K: Reversible hypopituitarism after interferon α therapy. Lancet 1995; 345: 1305.

Serri O: Progress in the management of hyperprolactinemia (editorial). NEJM 1994; 331: 942–944.

Sheehan HL: Post-partum necrosis of the anterior pituitary. J Pathol Bacteriol 1937; 45: 189–214.

Shirataki K, Chihara K, Shibata Y, et al: Pituitary apoplexy manifested during a bromocriptine test in a patient with growth hormone- and prolactin-producing pituitary adenoma. Neurosurgery 1988; 23: 395–398.

Silverman VE, Boyd AE, McCrary JA, et al: Pituitary apoplexy following chlorpromazine stimulation. Arch Int Med 1978; 138: 1738–1739.

Slater SL, Lipper S, Shilling DJ, et al: Elevation of plasma prolactin by monoamine oxidase inhibitors. Lancet 1977; ii: 275.

Smith CW, Howard RP: Variations in endocrine gland function in postpartum pituitary necrosis. J Clin Endocrinol 1959; 19: 1420.

Smith S: Neuroleptic associated hyperprolactinemia. Can

it be treated with bromocriptine? J Reproductive Medicine 1992; 37: 737–740.

Spigset O, Hedenmalm K: Hyponatremia and the syndrome of inappropriate antidiuretic hormone secretion (SIADH) induced by psychotropic drugs. Drug Safety 1995; 12: 209–225.

Sterns RH, Riggs JE, Schochet SS: osmotic demyelination syndrome following correction of hypernatremia. NEJM 1986; 314: 1535–1542.

Taylor AL: Pituitary apoplexy in acromegaly. J Clin Endocrinol 1968; 28: 1784.

Tolis G, Somma M, Campenhout JV, et al: Prolactin secretion in 65 patients with galactorrhoea. Am J Obstet Gynecol 1974; 118: 91.

Van Amelsvoort T, Bakshi R, Devaux CB, et al: Hyponatremia associated with carbamazepine and oxcarbazepine therapy: a review. Epilepsia 1994; 35: 181–188.

Vassallo M, Rana Z, Allen S: Pituitary apoplexy after stimulation tests. Postgrad Med J 1994; 70: 444–445.

Veldhuis JD, Hammond JM: Endocrine functions after spontaneous infarction of the human pituitary. Report, review and reappraisal. Endocrin Rev 1980; 1: 100.

Wakai S, Fukushima T, Teramoto A, et al: Pituitary apoplexy: its incidence and clinical significance. Neurosurgery 1981; 55: 187–193.

Walker AB, Eldridge PR, MacFarlane IA: Clomiphene-induced pituitary apoplexy in a patient with acromegaly. Postgrad Med J 1996; 72(845): 172–173.

Walker RF, Cooper RL: Toxic effects of xenobiotics on the pituitary gland. In Atterwill CK, Flack JD (Eds.) Endocrine toxicology, Cambridge, Cambridge University Press, 1992, pp 51–82.

Zabik JE, Sprague JE, Odio M: Interactive dopaminergic and noradrenergic systems in the regulation of thirst in the rat. Physiol Behav 1993; 54: 29–33.

Index of Drugs

Symptom Index

A symptom index has been added to lead the reader to the appropriate table in the text which lists the drugs associated with that symptom or disease. A description of the role of individual drugs can be found in the following text in the same chapter. The letter t following the page number indicates that the information is in a table.